Patient Care Skills

Patient Care Skills

SEVENTH EDITION

Mary Alice Duesterhaus Minor, PT, MS
Clinical Assistant Professor, Retired
Department of Physical Therapy
Clarkson University, Potsdam, New York

Scott Duesterhaus Minor, PT, PhD
Associate Professor
Department of Physical Therapy
Clarkson University, Potsdam, New York

PHOTOGRAPHY
Sarah Ruth Minor, MA, MS
Minor Manor Enterprises, Incorporated, Potsdam, New York, and Chicago, Illinois

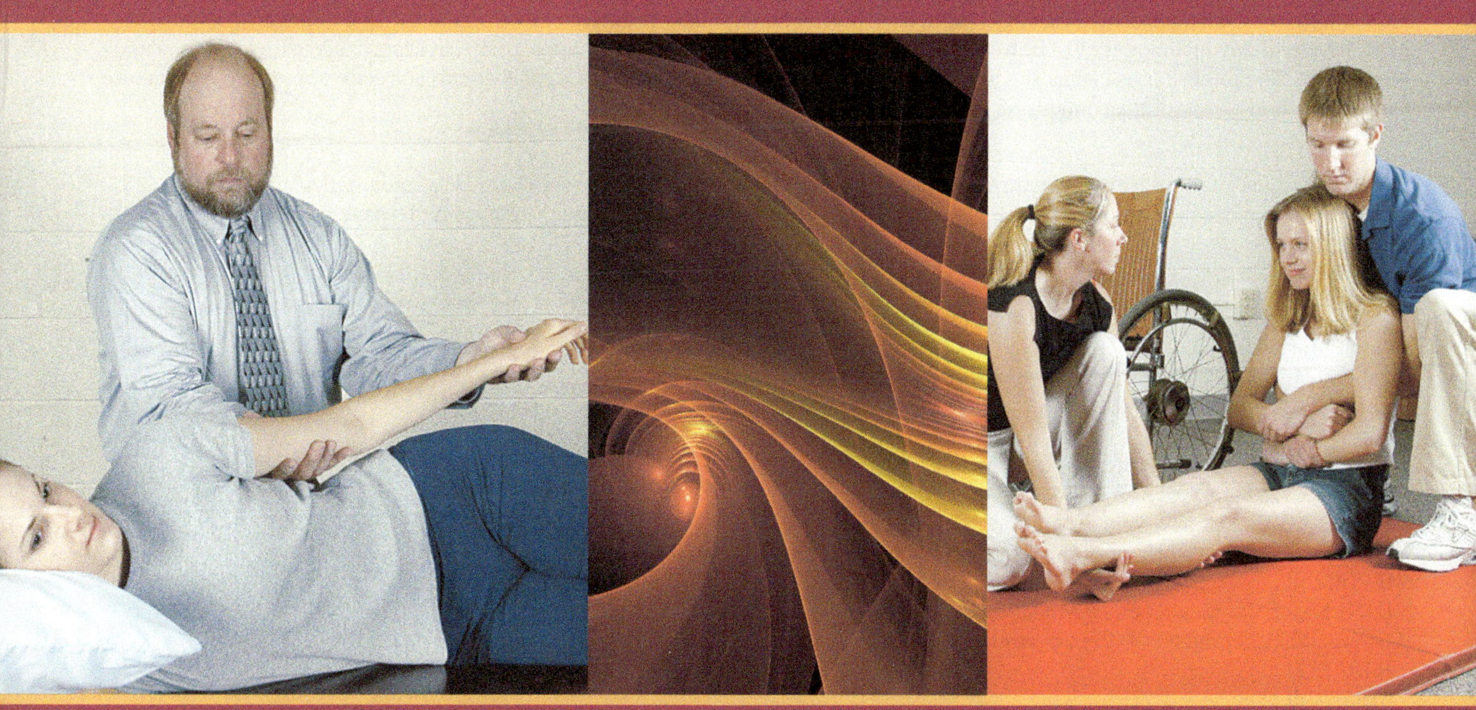

PEARSON

Boston Columbus Indianapolis New York San Francisco Upper Saddle River
Amsterdam Cape Town Dubai London Madrid Milan Munich Paris Montreal Toronto
Delhi Mexico City Sao Paulo Sydney Hong Kong Seoul Singapore Taipei Tokyo

Publisher: Julie Levin Alexander
Publisher's Assistant: Regina Bruno
Editor in Chief: Marlene McHugh Pratt
Executive Editor: John Goucher
Editorial Program Manager: Monica Moosang
Editorial Assistant: Ericia Vivani
Development Editor: Andrea M. Klingler
Director of Marketing: David Gesell
Marketing Manager: Katrin Beacom
Marketing Specialist: Michael Sirinides
Project Management Team Lead: Cindy Zonneveld
Project Manager: Patricia Gutierrez
Senior Operations Specialist: Nancy Maneri-Miller
Art Director: Mary Siener
Cover/Text Designer: Mary Siener
Cover/Chapter Opener Art: Fotolia, © DrHitch
Media Producer: Amy Peltier
Lead Media Project Manager: Lorena Cerisano
Full-Service Project Management: Rebecca Lazure
Composition: Laserwords, Inc.
Printer/Binder: LSC Communications
Cover Printer: LSC Communications
Text Font: 10/12, TimesTenLTStd

Credits and acknowledgments for content borrowed from other sources and reproduced, with permission, in this textbook appear on appropriate page within text.

Library of Congress Cataloging-in-Publication Data

Minor, Mary Alice D.
Patient care skills / Mary Alice Duesterhaus Minor, Scott Duesterhaus Minor ; photography, Sarah Ruth Minor.—Seventh edition.
p. cm.
Includes bibliographical references and index.
ISBN-13: 978-0-13-305587-0
ISBN-10: 0-13-305587-6
I. Minor, Scott Duesterhaus, author. II. Minor, Sarah Ruth, photographer. III. Title.
[DNLM: 1. Physical Therapy Modalities. 2. Asepsis—methods. 3. Orthopedic Equipment. 4. Transportation of Patients—methods. WB 460]
RT87.T72
610.73—dc23

2013024527

6 17

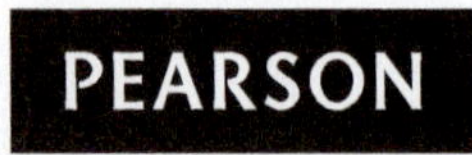

ISBN 10: 0-13-305587-6
ISBN 13: 978-0-13-305587-0

Dedication

This book is dedicated to better care for all patients.

Preface

As the authors of the first text in physical therapy on these topics, first published in 1982, it is exciting to see a seventh edition come to fruition 32 years later. This effort continues to be truly a family project. Our daughter, Sarah, born during the first year of publication, has been a photographic subject in earlier editions and has become the photographer for the last three editions of this text.

We feel extremely fortunate for the continued acceptance of this text by physical therapists, physical therapy providers, and other healthcare providers. We appreciate the faith our colleagues have demonstrated by allowing us to assist them in teaching new generations of physical therapists and physical therapist assistants over the past three decades. We have been fortunate to have received, and we continue to seek, critical commentary and counsel from students and colleagues who have used earlier editions of this text. We extend our appreciation and thanks to those who have provided information and critical commentary that assisted us as we have moved forward through seven editions.

As in previous editions, a large number of procedures and variations are included in this text, although it is not all inclusive. There are numerous choices to make in all patient interventions. When choosing among alternative methods or procedures, the most important consideration is to use the safest and most beneficial method for patients and physical therapists/assistants. In some cases, this will require modification of previously learned procedures. In all cases, practice will develop safe and efficient performance.

We find that when teaching these procedures, instructors can help students learn both the specifics of the procedures as well as general rules of good body mechanics, patient handling, and safety for patients and physical therapists/assistants. Students may require assistance in problem solving when applying procedures in a variety of patient-care situations. To assist student learning and problem solving, Suggested Activities and Case Studies continue to be included in the text. Instructors may also visit the Instructor Resource Center at www.pearsonhighered.com to find videos for students on topics such as body mechanics, passive range of motion, transfers and ambulation with ambulatory assistive devices.

For this seventh edition we revised Chapters 1 and 2 extensively. Included in Chapter 1 is an introduction to legislation that has driven rehabilitation over the past five decades. Chapter 2 includes increased emphasis on communication and documentation skills.

Each chapter and major section is introduced by a general explanation of the basis for performing the procedures to be described and by a presentation of general rules or guidelines that are generic to a series of procedures. Wording of instructions in the text are repeated in a similar format to enhance generic application when appropriate. For each procedure presented, step-by-step illustrations are accompanied by brief written explanations. Following the sequence of illustrations for a specific procedure decreases the need for extensive explanations in the text and provides students with a visual reference to determine whether the sequence of steps they are performing matches the sequence of steps presented. We recognize that there may be a need to adapt procedures to meet the abilities and needs of patients and physical therapists/assistants. Each chapter concludes with Review Questions that provide students an opportunity to test newly acquired knowledge. Review Questions can also be used as a study guide by reviewing the questions *before* beginning study of a chapter's content.

Finally, we wish to comment on the terms *patient* and *physical therapist/assistant.* We have used *patient* throughout the text to designate the individual receiving care. This term has been used for its general sense of meaning for consistency throughout the text. We have used *physical therapist/assistant* throughout the text to designate the potential individuals providing care. In cases where decision making is to be performed (from our perspective) by a physical therapist before delegating care to a physical therapist assistant, we have used only the term *physical therapist.*

We expect that in addition to physical therapists and physical therapist assistants, many healthcare providers, including home health aides, medical assistants, nurses, nurses' aides, nursing home attendants, occupational therapists, occupational therapy assistants, and orderlies will perform these procedures. Therefore, we hope this text will be useful to the practitioners providing, and the many individuals receiving, care.

Mary Alice Duesterhaus Minor
Scott Duesterhaus Minor
Potsdam, NY

Acknowledgments

No authors can create a text and then perform by themselves all the additional tasks required to transform the text into a book and place it before the public. Having created six previous editions, we are very aware that this is not possible.

The six previous editions acknowledged significant numbers of people who contributed to each of those editions, and the numbers increase as we acknowledge those who have contributed significantly to this seventh edition.

First, we thank our daughter, Sarah Minor, photographer, for the photographs on which this book depends. We are grateful to Sarah for her critical eye, suggestions, attention to detail, and diligent work in creating the photographic illustrations, as well as for her willingly putting her education and training as a professional photographer at our disposal.

Second, we thank our colleague, Vicki L. LaFay, PT, DPT, Director of Clinical Education, Clarkson University, for her outstanding contributions to Chapters 1 and 2. Her enthusiasm and professionalism are exemplary and much appreciated.

We must acknowledge our appreciation to the Pearson Education personnel who have provided patience, support, and assistance as we have prepared this seventh edition. We are grateful to Mark Cohen, Editor-in-Chief, John Goucher, Executive Editor, and Melissa Kerian and Monica Moosang, Program Managers, for guiding this project from inception to completion and for their perseverance in continuing the existence of this text. We are most grateful to Andrea Klingler, Development Editor, Silverwood Editorial & Communications, for her support and assistance while providing the prodding any author will agree is necessary for a successful text. We are fortunate that her prodding has been low key and friendly. Her work has been indispensible to this seventh edition.

For their participation and contributions to this seventh edition, we thank Paige Baritot-Finnerty, Jerome Castillo, Megan McClure, and Cindy Zhang for their participation as participants in photography sessions.

Finally, to acknowledge that this is the seventh edition of a successful text, we wish to remember those who contributed to the first six editions. This list is long, as we are fortunate to have created so many editions. For their participation and contributions to the first two editions, we thank Jim York, photographer, Gary Bergner, Freda Bowden, Mary Edna Harrell, Marvin Levand, Julie Leidecker, and Jennifer McFarland. We thank Cheryl L. Mehalik, Editor, and Sondra Greenfield, Production Editor, for their contributions to the third edition. For their participation and contributions to the fourth edition, we thank Lin Marshall, Editor, Robert Morrison, photographer, Arnie Berger, Deborah Bosse, Jeffrey Bosse, Bettina Brown, Suzanne Cornbleet, Kathleen Dixon, Mustafa Koluman, Janice Loudon, and Sarah Minor. For their participation and contributions to the fifth edition we thank Ruth Ann Bosse, Christin Cavoretto, Michelle Deslauriers, Jason Garner, Pradip Grosh, Chuck Gulas, Buddy Heimburger, Nick Heimburger, Kristen Hobgood, Bonnie Hogenkamp, MaryClare Krusing, Chrysta Lloyd, Lewis Mueller, Patty Navarro, Jason Rubel, Abby Schilly, Debbie Schilly, Kathryn Schopmeyer, Joe Shapiro, Tina Shapiro, Sarah Stawizynski, and Michelle Unterberg for their participation in photography sessions. For their participation and contributions to the sixth edition we thank Anne Gilbert, Kelly McGuire, and Michael Richards as participants in photography sessions.

We thank Gerald Bunker, Heather Caswell, George Fulk, Natalie Gilbert, Justin Hetu, Ellie O'Neill, and King Wilcox for their participation in videography sessions for the companion website that accompanies the sixth edition. We thank Rebecca Lazure of Laserwords Maine for her work as Production Editor and Patricia Gutierrez, for her assistance as Project Manager.

For arranging the loan and use of patient care equipment we thank Joe Neels of Provider Plus Inc. (St. Louis, MO), Philip Lyons of Orthotic Mobility Systems, Inc. (Kensington, MD), and Marra's Home Care Equipment and Supply (Potsdam, NY).

For their contributions of facilities and equipment for our work for all editions we acknowledge and express our appreciation to Wichita State University, Maryville University–St. Louis, Washington University–St. Louis, and Clarkson University.

Reviewers

James Bellew, EdD, PT
University of Indianapolis
Indianapolis, IN

Kathleen Cook, PT, DPT
Washtenaw Community College
Axnn Arbor, MI

Lisa R. Dehner, PT, PhD
College of Mount St. Joseph
Cincinnati, OH

Wing Fu, PT, PhD(c), OCS, PCS
Long Island University
Brooklyn, NY

Carla Gleaton, B.S., M.Ed., PT
Kilgore College
Kilgore, TX

Lois Harrison, PT, DPT, MS
Concordia University Wisconsin
Mequon, WI

Cindy Lavine, PTA, MPH
Kilgore College
Kilgore, TX

Twala H. Maresh, PT, DPT
University of Central Arkansas
Conway, AR

Julianne Martin, B.S., PT, M.S.
Broome Community College
Binghamton, NY

Nelson Marquez, PT, EdD
Polk Community College
Winter Haven, FL

Jennifer McDonald, PT, DPT, MS
SUNY Canton
Canton, NY

Deirdra Murphy, PT, DPT, MS, MHA
University Massachusetts Lowell
Lowell, MA

Jeffrey Rothman, PT, EdD
College of Staten Island
Staten Island, NY

Shannon Tripod, PTA
Arkansas State University
Jonesboro, AR

Contents

Procedures

Introduction to Patient Care

LEARNING OUTCOMES

Upon completion of this chapter, you will be able to:

1. State the purposes of patient care.
2. Discuss models of the healthcare practitioner and patient/client relationship.
3. Describe the Nagi, International Classification of Function (ICF), and National Center for Medical Rehabilitation Research Classification (NCMRR) models of the continuum from health to disability.
4. Describe major federal legislation enacted since 1968 related to healthcare and enhancing the quality of life of persons with disabilities, and resources to locate updated information.
5. Describe the purposes of the Health Insurance Portability and Accountability Act of 1996 (HIPAA).
6. List the 18 identifiers used in medical records specific to the HIPAA.
7. Describe why these patient identifiers are protected by the HIPAA.
8. List the rights and responsibilities outlined in the Patient's Bill of Rights.
9. Describe specific requirements for selected architectural environments as presented in the Americans with Disabilities Act of 1990 (ADA).

KEY TERMS

Active pathology
Americans with Disabilities Act of 1990 (ADA)
Disability
Education for All Handicapped Children Act of 1975 (EHA)
Functional limitation
Health and disease models
Health Insurance Portability and Accountability Act of 1996 (HIPAA)
Impairment
Individually identifiable health information (18 HIPAA identifiers that are "protected information")
Individuals with Disabilities Education Act of 1990 (IDEA)
International Classification of Function (ICF) model
Nagi model
National Center for Medical Rehabilitation Research (NCMRR) classification model
Patient Protection and Affordable Care Act of 2010 (ACA)
Patient's Bill of Rights
Rehabilitation Act of 1973 (504 Act)
Riser height
Tread depth

Introduction

Patient care is intended to enhance function, participation in society (work/school and leisure), and the quality of life for patients. Although patients are the obvious focus of care, services provided to patients to relieve their impairments and limitations will also affect family members and caregivers. The term *patient* refers to patients or clients (patients/clients) with temporary or long-term disabilities. The term *family* is meant in a broad sense to include related and unrelated significant others—basically all relevant people in patients' lives.

The provision of healthcare to patients and their families is influenced by many factors. These influences range from federal legislation, to the technical and thinking skills of the individual healthcare practitioner, as well as the specific characteristics of patients themselves. This text provides some of the information healthcare professionals, especially physical therapists and physical therapist assistants, need to improve function, participation, and quality of life for patients.

Models of Healthcare Professional and Patient Relationships

Healthcare in the past was a "top-down," provider-centered model, with patients relying almost exclusively on the judgment of healthcare professionals. Decisions were made about patient care with little or no input or regard as to patients' desires or concerns regarding care. Healthcare transitioned to a more patient-centered model that placed emphasis on patients being active participants in their healthcare, thereby aligning their care with their needs and preferences. Recognizing that patients do not exist in isolation, a family-centered model acknowledges the importance of the context in which a patient's care is provided. This context includes, but is not limited to, the patient's family members, culture, roles in family and society, and home/work/school/leisure environments. In this model, healthcare professionals function as team members whose roles and importance change in response to the needs of patients and their families.

■ Take Note

Patients are considered in context.

Models of Health and Function

Healthcare professionals use models of health and disability to assist in identifying the causes of impairments and limitations that affect a patient's function, participation in society, and, quality of life. Recognizing specific causes and effects, and knowing a patient's priorities, healthcare professionals are best able to recommend effective and efficacious interventions. A number of models exist to describe a person's state of health.

Nagi[1–3] described a model with four sequential phases: (a) active pathology, (b) impairment, (c) functional limitation, and (d) disability (Figure 1–1 ■). The first phase, **active pathology**, is the interruption of normal body function at the cellular level. The second phase, **impairment**, results when the body cannot compensate or heal itself, with the result that the individual sustains loss of normal function of a system. The third phase, **functional limitation**, occurs when the loss of a system is sufficient to prevent the performance of routine tasks by an individual, such as performing activities of daily living (ADLs) independently and in a timely manner. The fourth phase, **disability**, occurs when functional limitations prevent an individual from fulfilling life roles. *The Guide to Physical Therapist Practice*[4] is based conceptually on the Nagi disablement model. The following models emerged to define further relationships and factors that have an impact on patient function and quality of life.

■ Take Note

An example of the Nagi Model: Active pathology—osteoarthritis of hip; Impairment—decreased hip extension; Functional limitation—decreased ambulation distance; Disability—Unable to do grocery shopping.

Pathology → Impairment → Functional Limitation → Disability

FIGURE 1–1 ■ Nagi Model of Disability.

The World Health Organization (WHO) presents the **International Classification of Function (ICF)**[5] **model** (Figures 1–2 ■ and 1–3 ■), which considers that a person's health influences, and is influenced by, any disease or disorder that affects body functions and structures. Changes in body functions and structures may cause limitations in activities and social participation. Contextual factors include a patient's personal factors and the environment in which the patient lives, works/attends school, and plays. All phases of the ICF model combine to affect a person's quality of life.

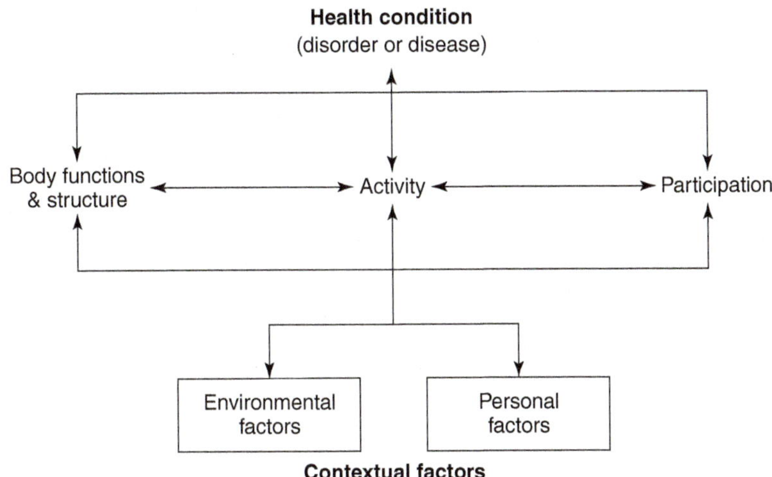

FIGURE 1–2 ■ International Classification of Function, Disability, and Healthcare (ICF) Model.

	Part 1: Functioning and Disability		Part 2: Contextual Factors	
Components	Body functions and structures	Activities and participation	Environmental factors	Personal factors
Domains	Body functions and structures	Life areas (tasks, actions)	External influences on functioning and disability	Internal influences on functioning and disability
Constructs	Change in body functions (physiological) Change in body structures (anatomical)	Capacity executing tasks in a standard environment Performance executing tasks in the current environment	Facilitating or hindering impact of features of the physical, social, and attitudinal world	Impact of attributes of the person
Positive aspect	Functional and structural integrity	Activities and participation	Facilitators	Not applicable
	Functioning			
Negative aspect	Impairment	Activity limitation and participation restriction	Barriers/hindrances	Not applicable
	Disability			

FIGURE 1–3 ■ Overview of ICF Model.

Table 1–1 ■ An example of delineating the aspects of the ICF Model for a patient referred to physical therapy with a medical diagnosis of low back pain*

Body function and structure impairments	Activity limitations	Social participation restrictions	Personal factors	Environmental factors
1. Low back pain on lumbar flexion. 2. Strain of left lumbar erector spinae. 3. Limited trunk flexion and rotation range of motion.	Unable to: 1. Lift 2. Sit for extended periods 3. Sit-to-stand and reverse 4. Stand for extended periods 5. Perform activities of daily living easily	Unable to: 1. Perform lifting task for job 2. Lift child 3. Carry groceries 4. Bowl	To consider: 1. Gender 2. Age 3. Height 4. Weight 5. General health 6. Health habits 7. Nutrition 8. Family and other life roles 9. Family support	To consider: 1. Job environments and requirements (e.g., tools, air quality) 2. Home environment (e.g., stairs, furniture) 3. Postures and positions 4. Family responsibilities

*Patient long-term goals are usually related to activity and participation limitations. Patient short-term goals focus on correction of problems related to body functions and structures. Note that the items within each column are not exhaustive and may be unique to each patient.

As the ICF model is complex, an example may assist with understanding (Table 1–1 ■). A patient referred to physical therapy with a medical diagnosis of back pain is examined by a physical therapist to determine the body functions and structures involved, what activities can or cannot be performed, and the effect the back pain has on the ability of the patient to fulfill life roles, such as supporting his or her family by working.

The **National Center for Medical Rehabilitation and Research (NCMRR)**[6] presents a disablement model derived from both the Nagi and the WHO models. The NCMRR model uses the term *societal limitations,* replacing the term *handicap,* which has potential negative connotations. A classification for *functional limitation,* defined as the "restriction or lack of ability to perform an action in the manner or range consistent with the purpose of an organ or organ system,"[7] was also added. As an example, for a patient with low back pain, a *functional limitation* might be the inability to bend forward from the waist, with the resulting *disability* being unable to lift his/her child from the floor.

A schematic comparison of the three models is presented in Table 1–2 ■

Legislation

Patient Confidentiality and Rights

Federal legislation was enacted to ensure that patients are knowledgeable about their rights as healthcare consumers and are empowered to make educated decisions on how personal health information will be used. The Health Insurance Portability and Accountability Act, Patient Protection and Affordable Care Act, and Patient's Bill of Rights define and provide for these patient protections and establish regulatory expectations for healthcare providers and organizations.

HEALTH INSURANCE PORTABILITY AND ACCOUNTABILITY ACT OF 1996 (PL 104–191) The **Health Insurance Portability and Accountability Act (HIPAA)**[8] established national standards for the privacy and security of health information. These standards are known as the HIPAA Security Rule. The Department of Health and Human Services published a final Security Rule, which delineates standards for protecting the confidentiality,

Table 1–2 ▪ Comparison of terminology between the three models of health and disability

Model	Terminology	Description
Nagi Scheme	Active pathology*	Impedes normal processes and efforts to regain nonpathological state
	Impairment†	Pathological condition or loss of anatomical, physiological, mental, emotional functions
	Functional limitation‡	Whole person or whole organism limitation in performance
	Disability§	Performance limitation of socially defined roles and tasks within sociocultural and physical environments
WHO International Classification of Impairments, Disabilities, and Handicaps (1980)	Disease*	Intrinsic pathology or disorder
	Impairment†	Psychological, physiological, or anatomical structure or function abnormality or loss
	Disability‡	Performance of activity in non-pathological manner restricted
	Handicap§	Disadvantage resulting from impairment or disability limiting or preventing fulfillment of a normal role-based on age, gender, sociocultural factors
National Center for Medical Rehabilitation Research Classification (1992)	Pathophysiology*	Normal physiological developmental processes or structures interrupted
	Impairment†	Cognitive, emotional, physiological, anatomical structure, or function abnormality or loss
	Functional limitation‡	Performance of actions in the manner or range consistent with purpose of an organ or organ system restricted
	Disability§	Performance of tasks, activities, and roles at expected levels within physical and social contexts limited or not possible
	Social limitation	Restriction attributable to social policy or barriers that limit fulfillment of all roles

Items with the same symbols indicate equivalent categories within each of the three models. There is no equivalent category in the Nagi or WHO models with respect to social limitation in the NCMRRC mode. Adapted from material presented in the *Guide to Physical Therapist Practice.*

integrity, and availability of protected health information (PHI). The HIPAA Privacy Rule defines the privacy regulations governing **individually identifiable health information** with compliance required for all "covered entities." A "covered entity" is defined as health plans, healthcare clearinghouses, and any healthcare provider that conducts electronic transmission of patient health information.

The primary purpose of HIPAA is to standardize the exchange of financial and administrative data, while ensuring each patient's health information is properly protected and to avoid confidential patient information being revealed or used inappropriately.

Although **protected information** is usually considered to be health information and is called protected health information, protected information also covers any personal information. HIPAA established requirements for the storage and dissemination (electronic, written, or oral) of patient information between healthcare providers and between healthcare providers and insurers. Examples of revealing patient information inappropriately are when healthcare providers discuss a patient or his/her care in public venues, such as hallways, elevators, or cafeterias, or when medical records are left accessible to persons who do not have the right to view such information. Inappropriate use of information might occur by either lack of understanding or intentional disregard of HIPAA mandates; thus all healthcare providers have the responsibility to be aware of, and follow, HIPAA requirements and the processes and procedures instituted by their organization/employer for compliance.

■ Take Note

Permission to release or share patient information is required and must be in writing.

Within HIPAA, 18 individual pieces of information are designated identifiers that could allow intentional or unintentional identification of an individual and their health information. Although a direct connection may not be able to be made between health information and a specific person without additional effort, knowledge of any one of the 18 identifiers could provide an opportunity for others to connect a person with their personal or medical information. The identifiers are

- Names/initials
- All geographic identifiers smaller than a state, including county, city, street address, precinct, zip code, and their equivalent geocodes
- All elements of dates (except year) directly related to an individual; all ages 90 years and above; and all elements of dates (including year) indicative of such age (except for aggregate categorization of ages 90 and above)
- Telephone numbers
- Fax numbers
- Electronic mail addresses
- Social Security numbers
- Medical record numbers
- Health-plan beneficiary numbers
- Account numbers
- Certificate and license numbers
- Vehicle identifiers and serial numbers, including license plate numbers
- Medical device identifiers and serial numbers
- Internet universal resource locators (URLs)
- Internet protocol (IP) addresses
- Biometric identifier including fingerprints and voice prints
- Full-face photographic images and any comparable images
- Any other unique identifying number, characteristic, or code, except that covered identities may, under certain circumstances, assign a code or other means of record identification that allows de-identified information to be reidentified

To provide full confidentiality, none of the 18 identifiers can be released without a patient's written permission. Permission must be requested by each facility with which a patient has a relationship. Facilities are required to provide each patient with written notification of policies and procedures relating to patient confidentiality under HIPAA regulations, and each patient must sign a statement indicating that he or she has been informed of such policies. Institutions are required to inform patients/clients how medical information will be shared. Often this is in the form of a brochure that provides a short synopsis of the institution's confidentialty policies. A second form, which may be called a *Patient Authorization Form, Informed Consent Form,* or *Release Form,* is then provided to patients for signature. The original signed form is retained as part of the patient's medical record.

PATIENT PROTECTION AND AFFORDABLE CARE ACT OF 2010 (PL 111–148)[9] The **Patient Protection and Affordable Care Act** (commonly called the Affordable Care Act, or ACA) requires hospitals provide patients with a copy of the **Patient's Bill of Rights**, a list of guarantees for those receiving medical care. Many facilities voluntarily adopted versions of a Patient's Bill of Rights as healthcare became more patient and family focused. A legislative version of a Patient's Bill of Rights was originally developed as a portion of a Senate bill (The Bipartisan Patient Protection Act) in 2001, which was never voted into law. A Patient's Bill of Rights did become law with passage of the ACA. Healthcare facilities and providers are required to follow the legislated Patient's Bill of Rights and may be required to follow a facility's individually adopted additional rights. All healthcare providers have the responsibility to be aware of, and follow, the requirements of the Patient's Bill of Rights and the processes and procedures instituted by their organization/employer for compliance. The ACA Patient's Bill of Rights:

- Provides coverage to Americans with preexisting conditions
- Protects a patient's choice of doctors
- Young adults under 26 may be eligible for coverage under their parents' health plan
- Ends lifetime limits on coverage for all new health insurance plans
- Ends pre-existing condition limitations/exclusions for children under 19
- Ends arbitrary withdrawals of insurance coverage
- Requires insurance companies to justify publicly unreasonable rate hikes
- Requires insurance premium dollars to be spent primarily on health care, and not administrative costs
- Restricts annual dollar limits on coverage by 2014
- Removes insurance company barriers to emergency services so patients can seek emergency care at a hospital outside their health plan's network.

The American Physical Therapy Association (APTA) has a growing compliance section[10] that can help clinicians learn more about Medicare, HIPAA, ACA, and other regulatory requirements as they pertain to the practice of physical therapy. The site provides direct links to the respective organizations for more detailed information (www.apta.org/compliance).

■ Take Note
Professional organizations offer information and assistance to members on being in compliance with laws.

Accessibility

Management of patient impairments and limitations does not ensure a patient's ability to participate in society. A person's quality of life is reduced without the availability of an accessible environment. In the United States, federal legislation is instrumental in promoting quality of life by influencing funding, rights, and opportunities for all. Some federal legislation specifically addresses integration of individuals with disabilities into society. Enacting federal legislation requires considerable effort on the part of concerned citizens, but the effects on a person's quality of life, and society in general, can be profound.

REHABILITATION ACT OF 1973 (PL93–112)[11] The **Rehabilitation Act** (often referred to as the 504 Act) addresses civil rights of individuals with disabilities. Section 504 of the act created and extended civil rights to people with disabilities. The act itself addresses two major issues: (1) the provision of reasonable accommodations, and (2) a specification that no federal funding may be received by any entity that excludes the participation of qualified individuals solely on the basis of disability.

EDUCATION FOR ALL HANDICAPPED CHILDREN ACT OF 1975 (PL 94–142)[12] The **Education for All Handicapped Children Act** (EHA) focuses on ensuring all children, including those with disabilities, have access to free and appropriate public education (FAPE). A major requirement of this act mandates children receive education in the least restrictive environment, resulting in children with disabilities being educated alongside children without disabilities to the greatest extent possible. Schools are required to provide necessary services, such as occupational, physical, and speech therapy services to provide the assistance disabled children need to be successful. Parent rights are addressed by requiring parent participation in development of individualized education programs (IEPs) for each child.

INDIVIDUALS WITH DISABILITIES EDUCATION ACT OF 1990 (PL 101–476)[13]/2004 (PL 108–446)[14] The EHA was replaced with the **Individuals with Disabilities Education Act (IDEA)**, which extends services to infants and toddlers. Early intervention (EI) services are recognized as providing the most significant opportunity to improve outcomes. Services for infants and toddlers are provided in a natural, patient- and family-focused environment. The Individuals with Disabilities Education Improvement Act (IDEA) of 2004 (PL 108-446) amended the IDEA of 1990.

The Rehabilitation Act of 1973, in conjunction with the EHA and IDEA provides individuals with disabilities opportunities to have a better quality of life and to participate in society. These laws improved the public's perception of disability and accessibility, providing opportunities for people with disabilities to be accepted and to participate more fully in society.

ARCHITECTURAL BARRIERS ACT OF 1968 (PL 90–480)[15] The first federal effort addressing architectural barriers was the Architectural Barriers Act of 1960 (ABA). The ABA focused on accessibility to, and within, federal buildings.

AMERICANS WITH DISABILITIES ACT OF 1990 (PL 101–336)[16] The second federal effort addressing architectural, transportation, and work site barriers was the **Americans with Disabilities Act (ADA)**. The quality of life for person with disabilities is often less then optimal because of accessibility issues. The ADA contains five titles:

- Title I—Employment
- Title II—Public Services and Transportation
- Title III—Public Accommodations
- Title IV—Telecommunications
- Title V—Other Provisions

The purpose of the ADA is to provide "a clear and comprehensive national mandate for the elimination of discrimination against individuals with disabilities."[14] Titles II and III address physical accessibility. Title II provides for accessible transportation, which permits individuals with disabilities "to gain employment"[14] and "allows individuals with disabilities to enjoy cultural, recreational, commercial and other benefits that society has to offer."[14] Title III provides individuals with disabilities the "full and equal enjoyment of the goods, services, facilities, privileges, advantages, or accommodations of any place of public accommodation."[16]

Requirements for accessibility must take into account a variety of disabilities resulting from a range of impairments. For example, requirements for ground- and floor-surface guidelines must take into account their effect on patients in wheelchairs and those who are visually impaired. Curb cuts may be advantageous for people in wheelchairs but may present a hazard to patients who are visually impaired. Accessibility designs must accommodate a broad spectrum of disabilities, rather than identifying each barrier to accessibility with a single impairment.

Limitations for many individuals arise because they use wheelchairs and ambulatory assistive devices such as crutches or walkers. The ADA provides standardized space requirements for accessibility in a variety of environments such as hallways, elevators, bathrooms, and work/leisure spaces. These standards provide for people using wheelchairs or ambulatory/assistive devices to maneuver safely in a variety of environments. Although the ADA has certain specific requirements, matching the environment to the patient is of utmost importance in decreasing functional limitations. This may mean that designing accessible spaces necessitates going beyond the minimal requirements of the ADA.

Eventually the standards required by the ABA and ADA were conjoined under the aegis of the U.S. Access Board (USAB), which publishes the ADA-ABA Accessibility Guidelines.[15] Practitioner knowledgeable of basic ADA/ABA Accessibility Guidelines, and the knowledge of how to access these guidelines, can assist in the design and implementation of physically accessible spaces.

RULES, REGULATIONS, AND ENFORCEMENT The language of laws cannot possibly or appropriately contain provisions for every potential situation that arises. Therefore, rules, regulations, and guidelines for implementation of laws are issued following passage of a new law. More specific interpretation of the law and its rules, regulations, and guidelines occurs as the result of administrative rulings and legal opinions in response to complaints and lawsuits filed by those who believe they have been subjected to discrimination. Definitive interpretations of specific requirements of federal law become known as the result of such administrative rulings or legal opinions.

In the case of the ADA, the government agencies primarily responsible for developing rules and regulations and enforcing the law are the Equal Employment Opportunity Commission (EEOC) and the Department of Justice (DOJ). Laws pertaining to EHA, IDEA, 504, and HIPAA are within the jurisdiction of the Department of Health and Human Services.

Resources

Resources for accessibility criteria and ADA compliance are available from public and private entities. Accessibility criteria, including *A Guide to the New ADA–ABA Accessibility Guidelines* and the full text and diagrams of the *Guidelines,* are available from the USAB. The text and diagrams can be downloaded directly from the Internet:

United States Access Board
1331 F Street, N.W., Suite 1000
Washington, DC 20004–1111
(800) 872–2253 (voice)
(800) 993–2822 (TTY)
www.access-board.gov

■ **Take Note**
Resources for accessibility guidelines.

Several private reporting services provide monthly updates regarding changes and recent legal opinions. The listing of one such service follows. This is a proprietary service with which the authors are most familiar. The listing of this service does not imply an endorsement of this service by the authors. The cost of a service such as this is higher than the cost for government or quasi-government publications. The benefits of such services are more timely and in-depth research and information.

Thompson Publishing Group, Inc.
Americans with Disabilities Act—ADA Compliance Guide
805 15th Street N.W., 3rd floor
Washington, D.C. 20005
(800) 677–3789
www.thompson.com

Selected ADA Requirements for Accessibility

Several architectural barriers are commonly encountered in the home and workplace. A clinician should be readily aware of architectural requirements for these selected barriers to make home and work environments accessible and functional. Information related to other requirements can be obtained from the sources cited earlier in this Resources section.

In addition to the specific architectural requirements listed here, diagrams of an expanded selection of ADA architectural requirements for accessibility are presented at the end of this Resources section.

RESTROOMS AND BATHROOMS Restrooms or bathrooms that are designed with dimensions and fixtures appropriate for accessible restrooms or bathrooms, but that are not on an accessible route, cannot be considered accessible. A significant number of dimensions and configurations conform to the requirements of an accessible restroom or bathroom. Diagrams for many of these are presented in this Resources section.

RAMPS AND LANDINGS Any portion of an accessible route with a grade greater than 1:20 (5%) must be considered a ramp. Transitions of greater than 0.5 inch between two connected surfaces require a ramp. Ramps must use the least grade possible, and the grade may not be greater than 1:12 (8.3%) for new construction. A landing is required when a ramp has a continuous vertical rise exceeding 30 inches in height. For existing construction, two criteria apply when a grade of 8.3% cannot be achieved. First, a ramp with a grade of 1:10 (10%) is allowable as long as vertical rise is limited to 6 inches or less before a landing is provided. Second, a ramp with a grade of 1:8 (12.5%) is allowable as long as the vertical rise is limited to 3 inches or less before a landing is provided. Ramps must have a cross grade no greater than 1:50 (2%). Ramp width must not be less than 36 inches.

■ **Take Note**
Useful information for patients and families.

Landings must be provided for any vertical rise greater than 30 inches in height (limited to 6 inches in height for a 10% grade, and 3 inches in height for a 12.5% grade). Landings must be provided at the top and bottom of each run of a ramp. They must be not less than 60 inches in length and at least as wide as the ramp. When a change in ramp direction or doorway occurs at a landing, the landing must meet the required landing clear space of 60 inches by 60 inches.

Handrails are required for a ramp with a vertical rise of 6 inches in height or more, or for a horizontal run of 72 inches or more. They must be provided along both sides of the ramp and must meet the general requirements listed under *Handrails.*

HANDRAILS Handrails are required for ramps as indicated above, and for stairs. Circular handrails must have a diameter not less than 1.5 inches and not more than 2 inches. Noncircular handrail dimensions, both cross-section and perimeter, are presented in **Figure 1–4** ■. The horizontal distance between handrails and wall and vertical distance between handrails and horizontal projections below handrails must be 1.5 inches. The top gripping surface of handrails must not be less than 34 inches or greater than 38 inches in the vertical dimension from the floor or stair tread.

Handrails along stairs must have an extension not less than 12 inches at the top of the stairs, and an extension not less than one tread depth at the bottom of the stairs. Handrail extensions must be parallel to the level floor surface at the ends of ramps, and at the tops of stairs, but must be parallel to the slope of the stair flight (not parallel to the floor) at the bottom of the stairs, as presented in **Figures 1–5** ■ through **1–7** ■. The ends of handrails must be rounded, or returned smoothly to the floor, a wall, or a post. All handrails must be secured and must not rotate within fittings.

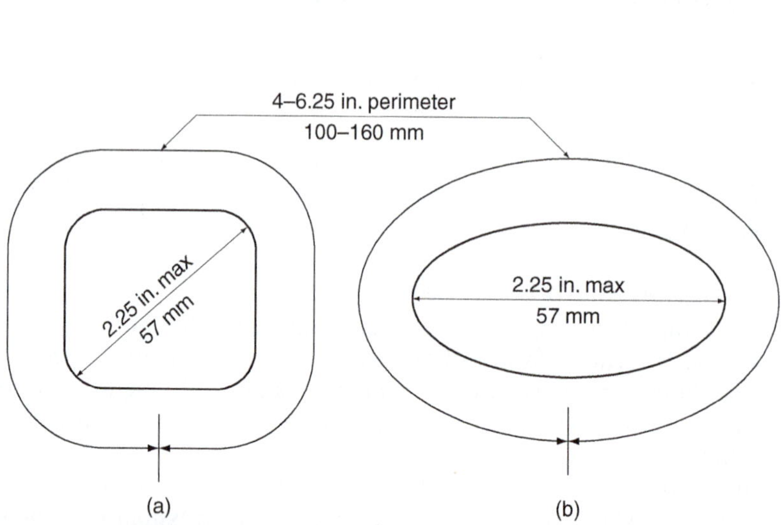

FIGURE 1–4 ■ Noncircular handrail dimensions.

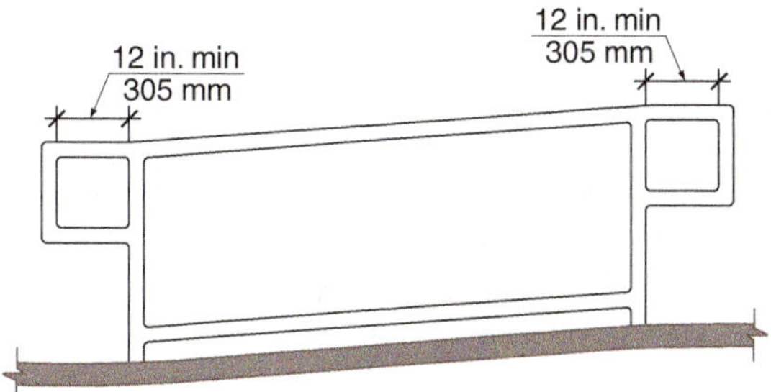

FIGURE 1-5 ■ Handrail extensions for ramps.

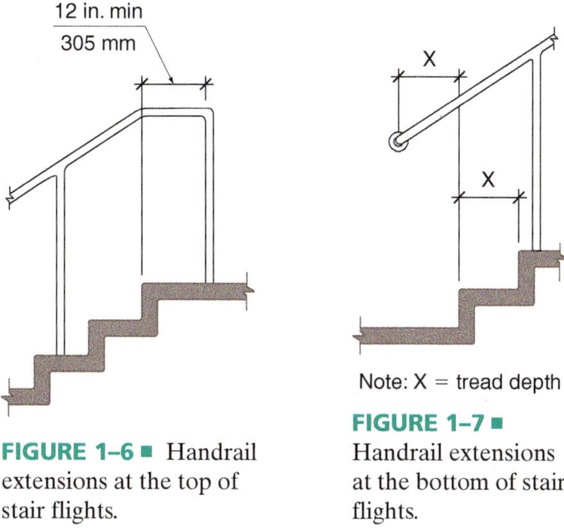

FIGURE 1-6 ■ Handrail extensions at the top of stair flights.

FIGURE 1-7 ■ Handrail extensions at the bottom of stair flights.

STAIRS **Riser height**, the vertical dimension that separates one stair tread from the next stair tread, must be not less than 4 inches or greater than 7 inches in height. Angulation of risers (lowest point to highest point for each stair) must not exceed 30 degrees. Open risers, a lack of the vertical board at the back of each stair, are not permitted. **Tread depth**, the horizontal dimension of a step, must be not less than 11 inches. Tread nosing, the front edge of a tread, must not project greater than 1.5 inches beyond the riser below it, with a radius of curvature for the nosing of not greater than 0.5 inch. For any given set of stairs, dimensions and configuration must be consistent for all stairs. Outdoor stairs and paths must be designed to avoid accumulation of moisture. Handrails must be provided along both sides of the stairway, except in assembly areas, and must conform to the guidelines presented previously under *Handrails.*

GROUND AND FLOOR SURFACES Ground and floor surfaces must be stable, firm, and slip resistant. Carpet must be securely attached, with exposed edges fastened to the floor, and have trim along the full length of exposed edges. Pile thickness must not be greater than 0.5 inch.

Grating spaces must be no greater than 0.5 inch in any dimension. If elongated openings are used, the long dimension of the opening must be oriented perpendicular to the dominant direction of travel.

TRANSITIONS Transitions between connected surfaces up to 0.25 inch may be left untreated. Transitions between 0.25 and 0.5 inch must have a beveled edge with a grade no greater than 1:2 (50%). Ramp guidelines must be used to accommodate transitions greater than 0.5 inch.

CLEAR SPACES Clear spaces are the areas in which patients maneuver when using wheelchairs or other ambulation devices. A significant number of dimensions and configurations conform to the requirements of clear spaces. Diagrams for many of these are presented at the end of this Resources section.

Consideration of uncluttered clear spaces is important not only as part of accessibility regulations, but also for safe patient care in facilities. As examples, consider carefully the amount of clear space required for persons (a) moving through doorways, and the direction in which the doors open, and (b) maneuvering along hallways and ramps and up and down stairs.

Additional ADA Requirements

Figures 1–8 ▪ through 1–49 ▪ illustrate additional ADA requirements.

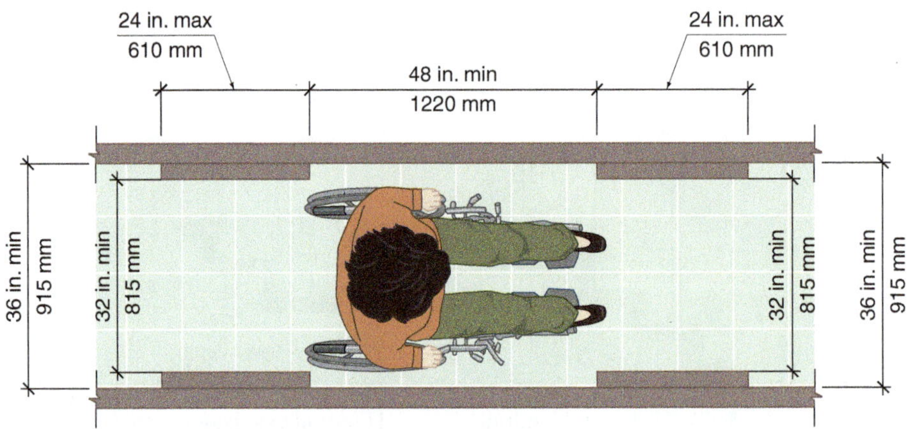

FIGURE 1–8 ▪ Clear width of an accessible route.

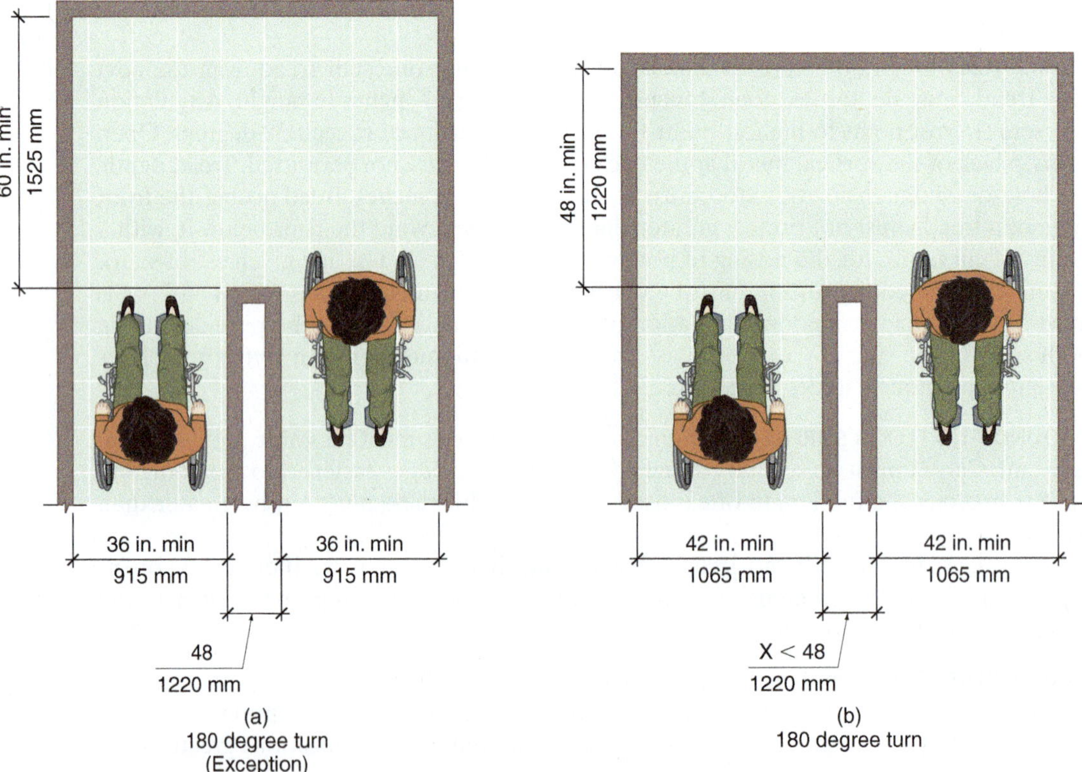

FIGURE 1–9 ▪ Clear width for turning 180 degrees on an accessible route.

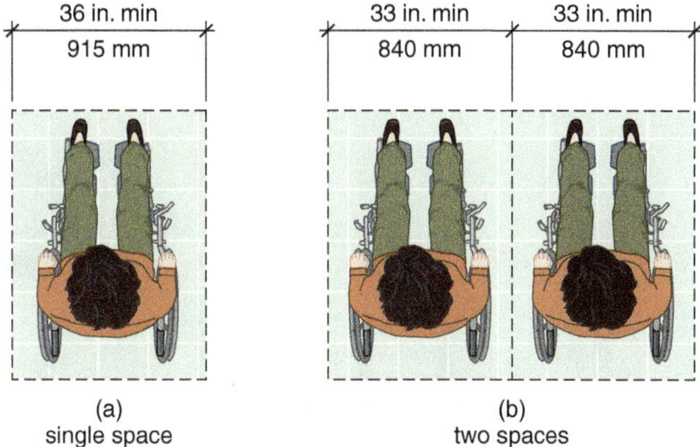

FIGURE 1–10 ■ Width of wheelchair spaces in assembly and auditorium areas.

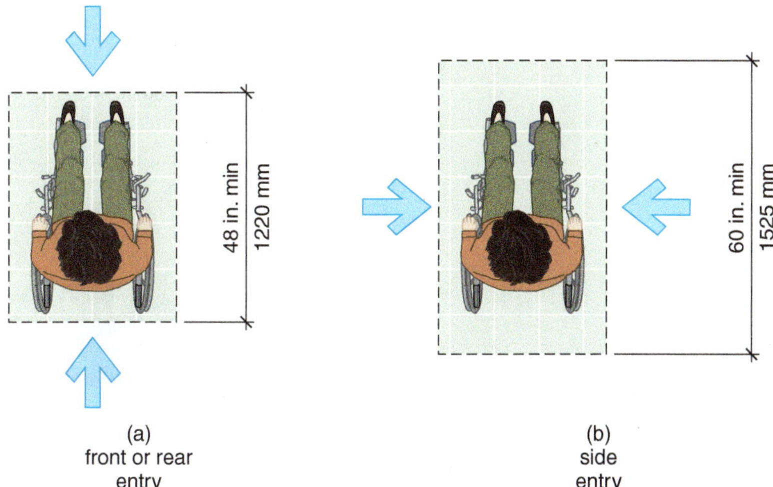

FIGURE 1–11 ■ Depth of wheelchair spaces in assembly and auditorium areas.

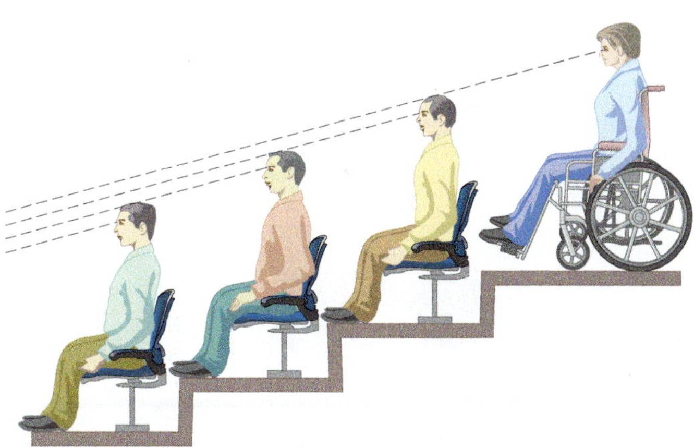

FIGURE 1–12 ■ Sight-line elevation over the heads of seated patrons.

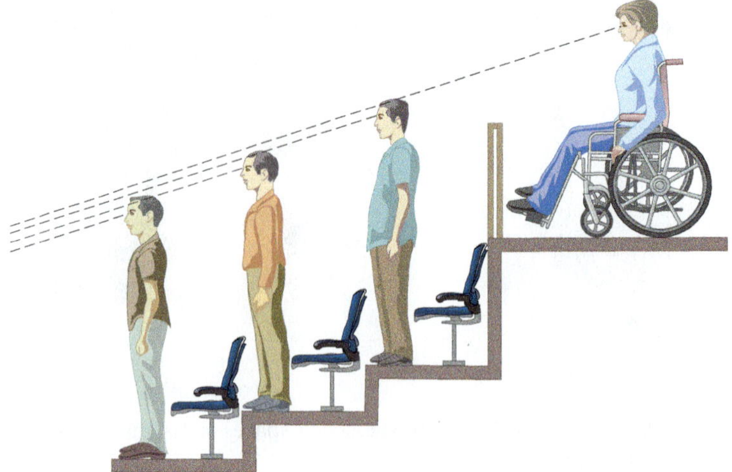

FIGURE 1–13 ■ Sight-line elevation over the heads of standing patrons.

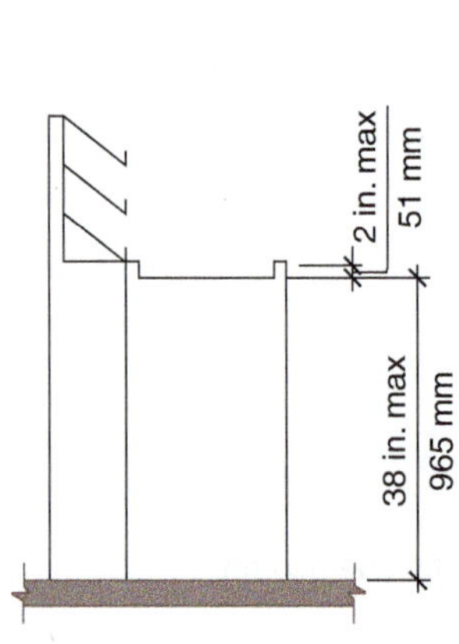

FIGURE 1–14 ■ Check-out aisle counters.

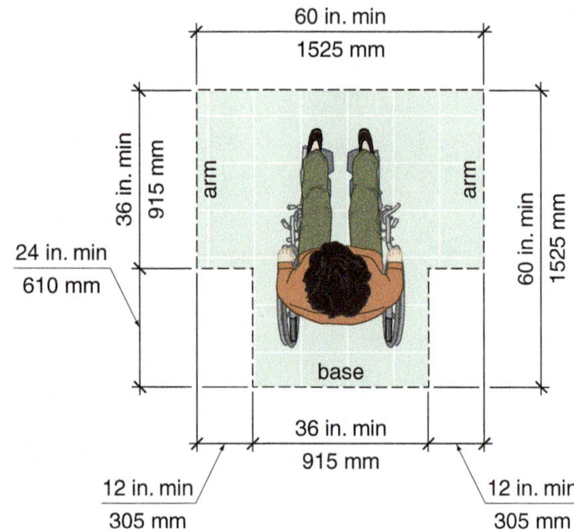

FIGURE 1–15 ■ T-shaped turning spaces.

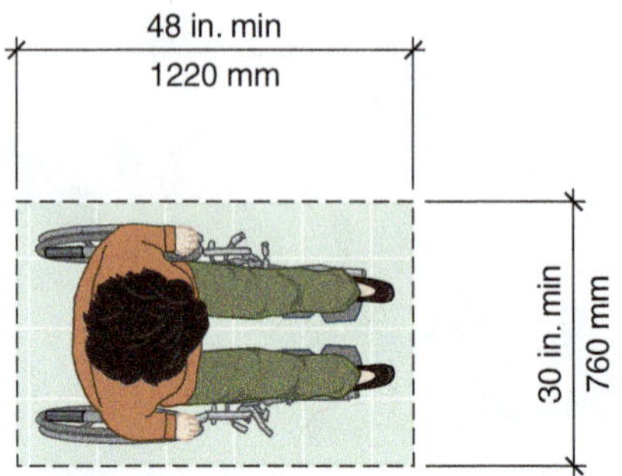

FIGURE 1–16 ■ Clear-area requirements for wheelchairs.

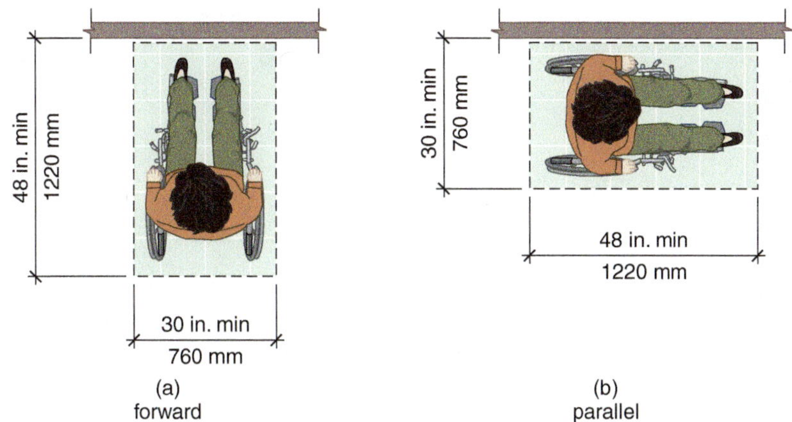

FIGURE 1–17 ■ Orientation of clear area for wheelchairs.

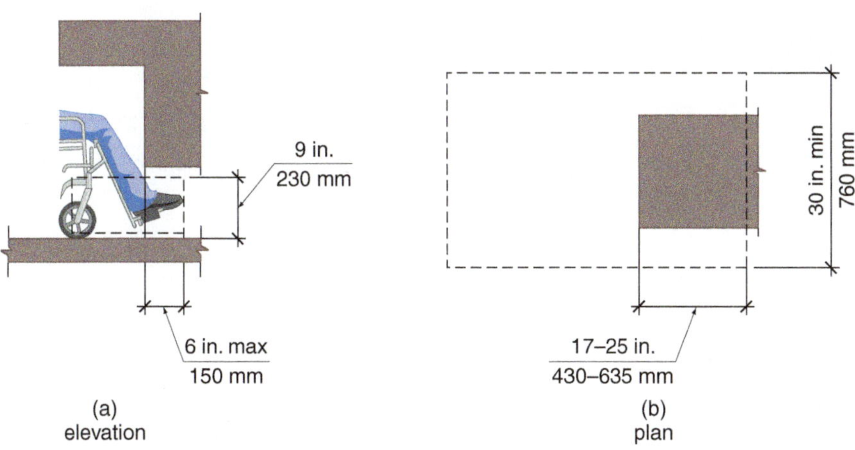

FIGURE 1–18 ■ Toe clearance requirements.

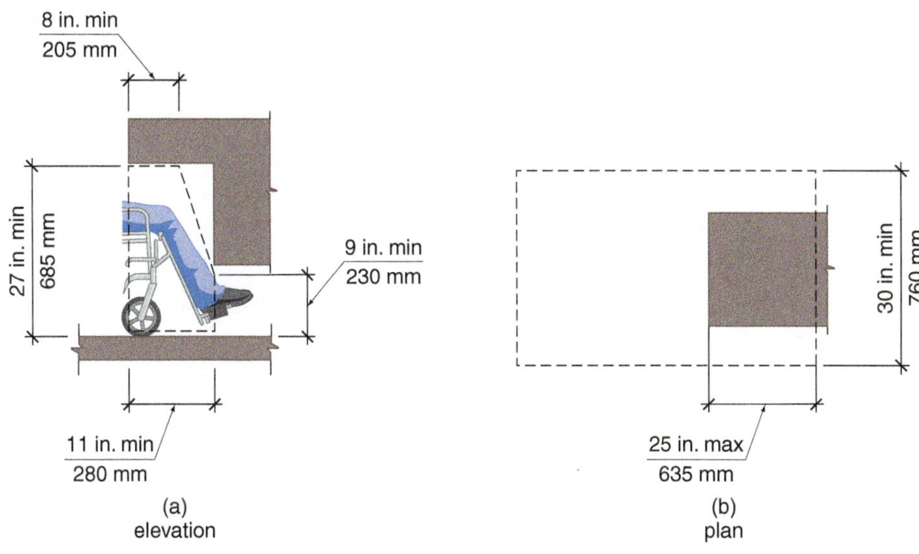

FIGURE 1–19 ■ Knee clearance requirements.

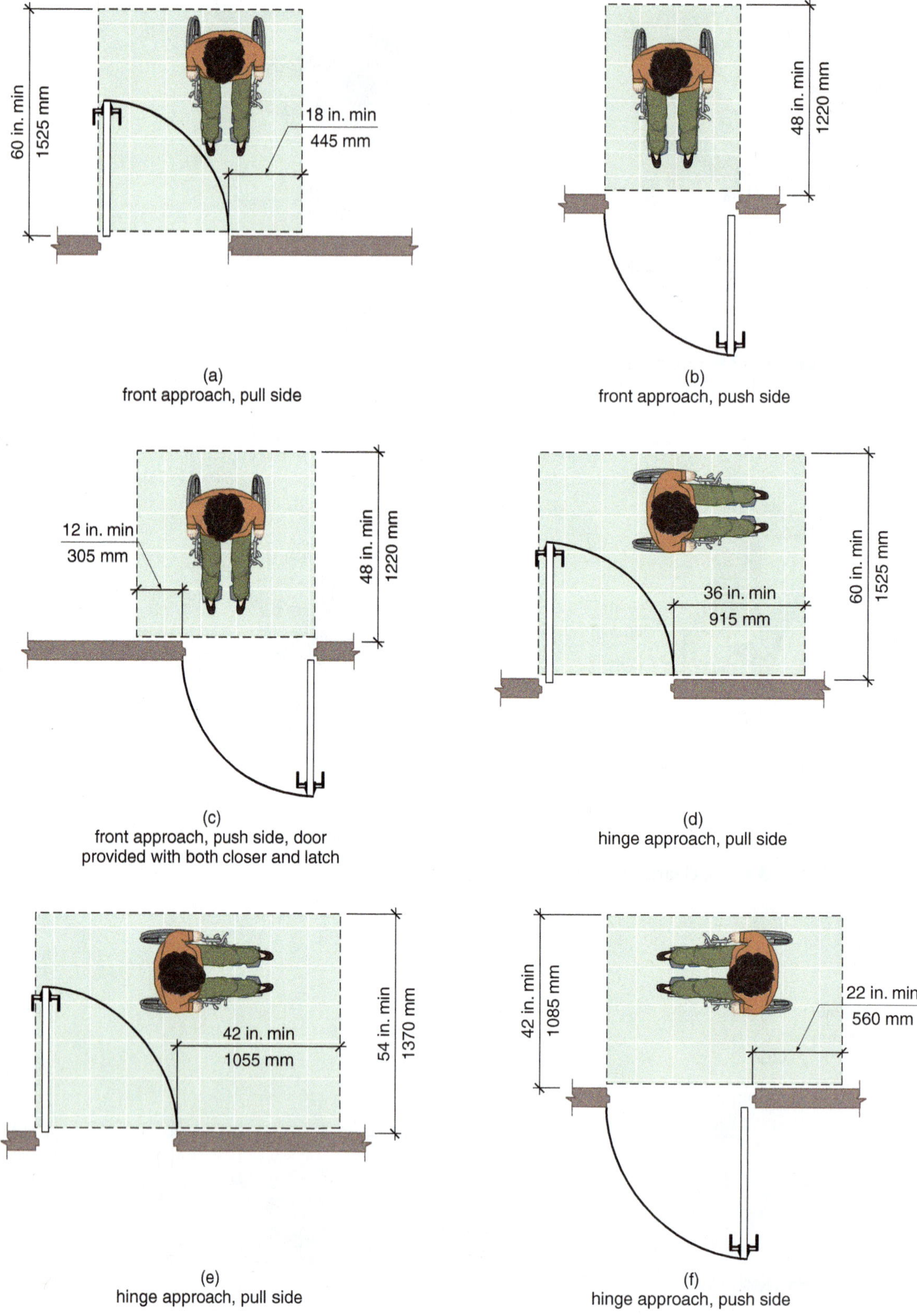

FIGURE 1–20 ■ Clear-space configurations for manual swinging doors.

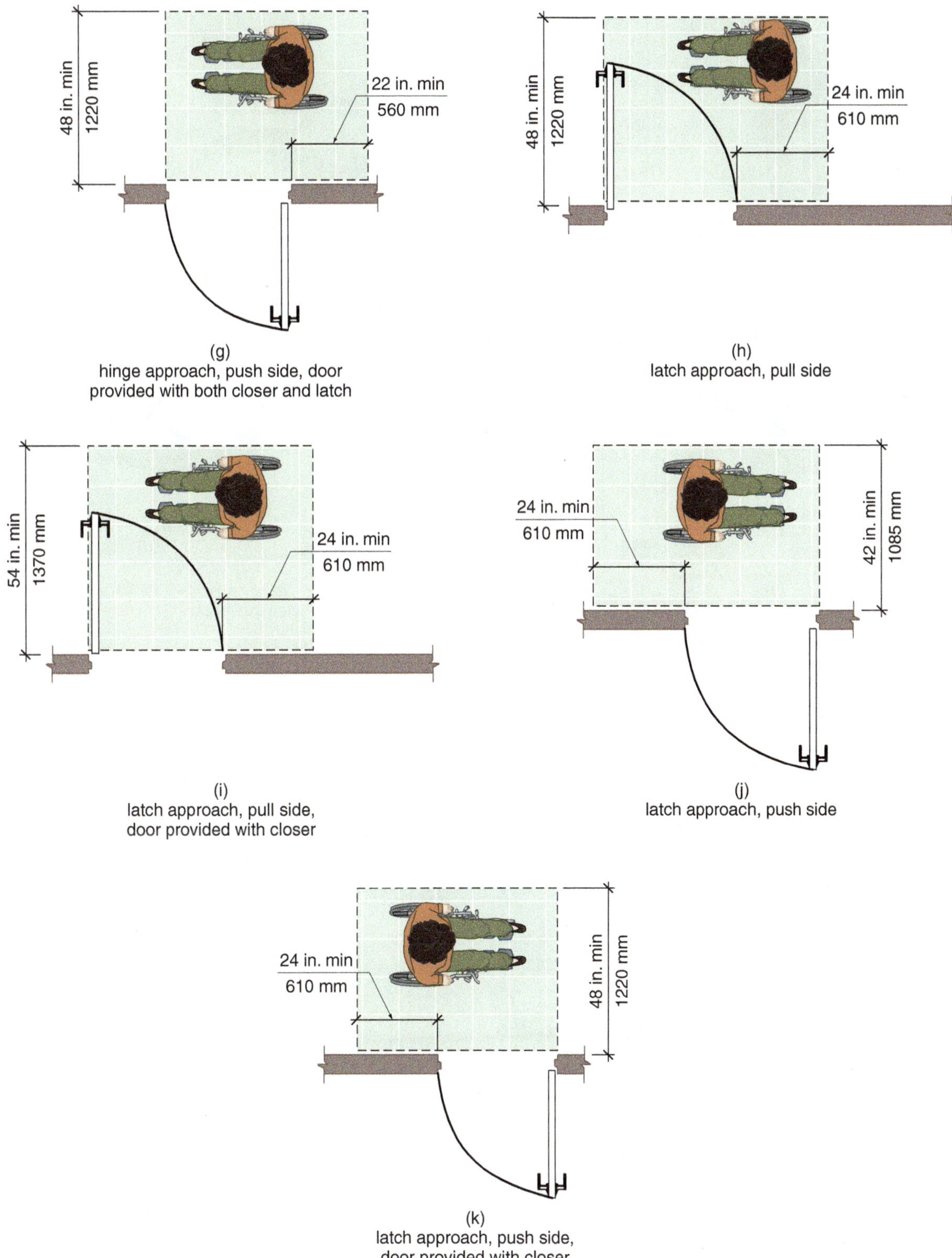

FIGURE 1–20 ■ Clear-space configurations for manual swinging doors (*continued*).

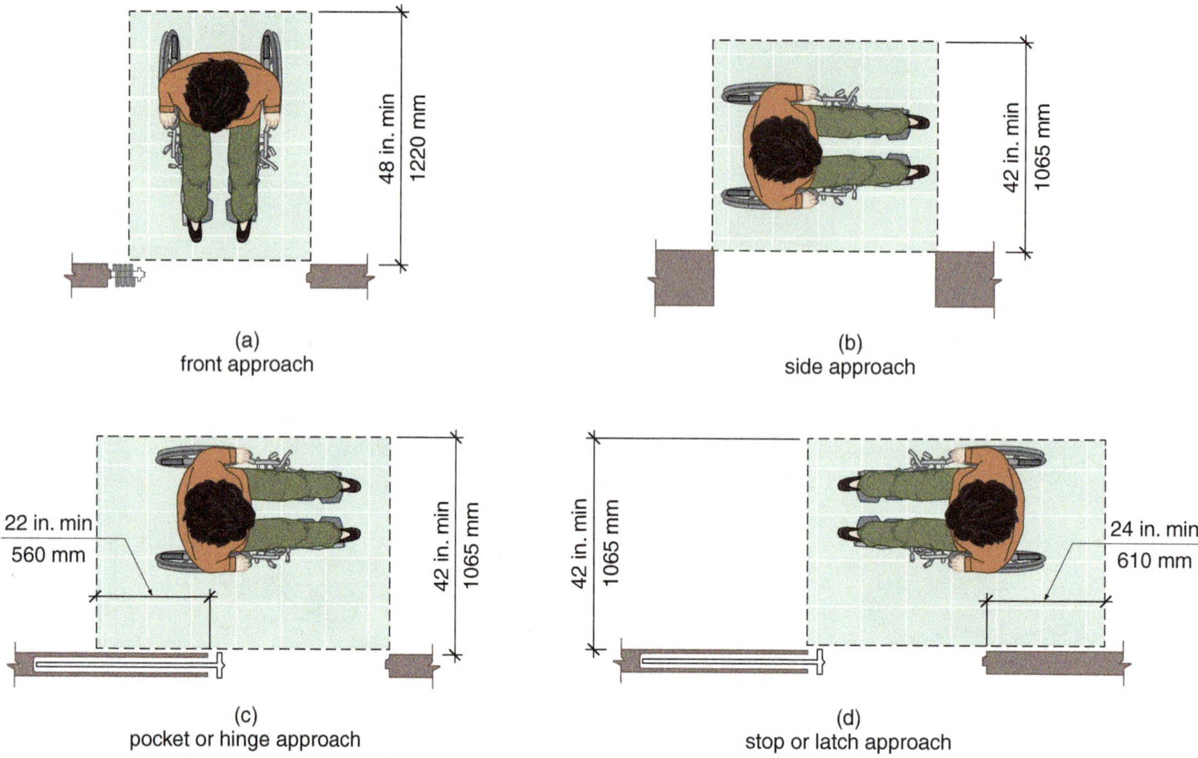

FIGURE 1–21 ■ Clear-space configurations for sliding and folding doors.

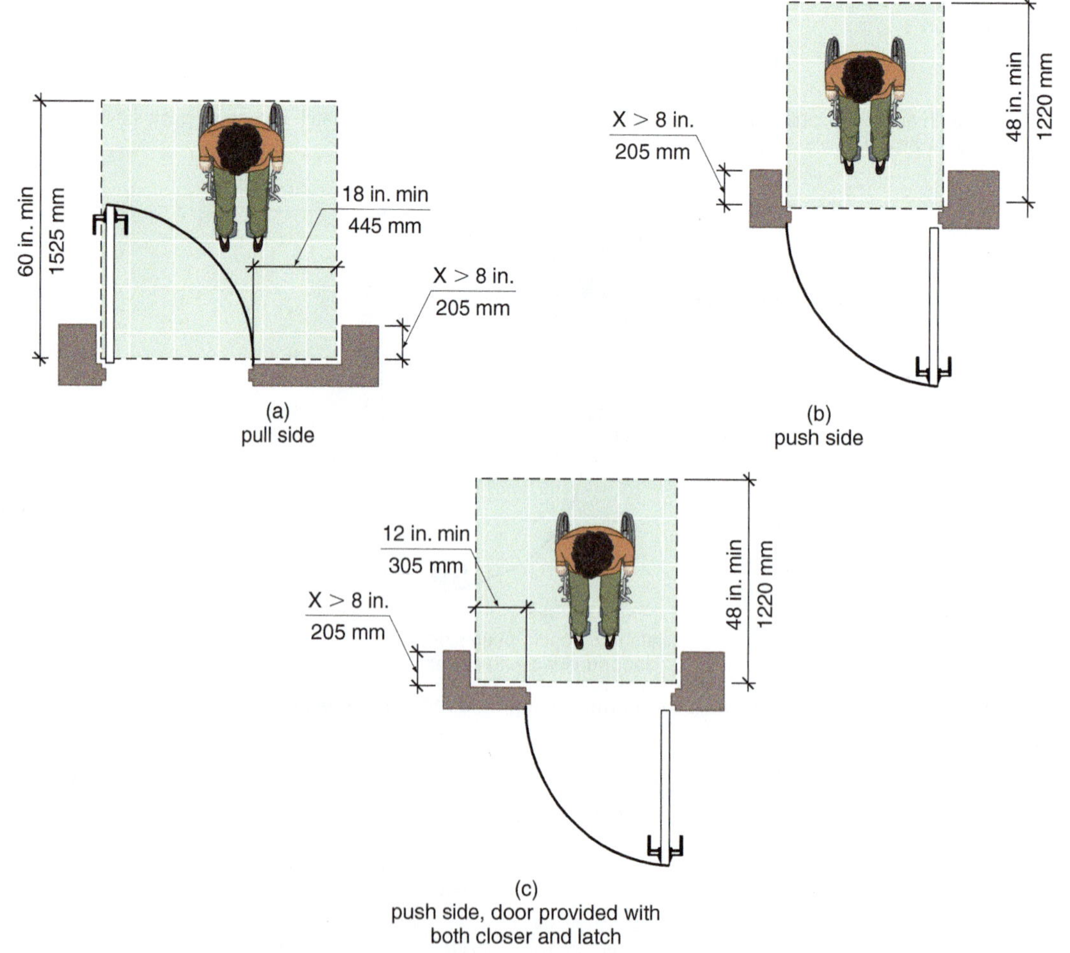

FIGURE 1–22 ■ Clear-space configurations for recessed doors.

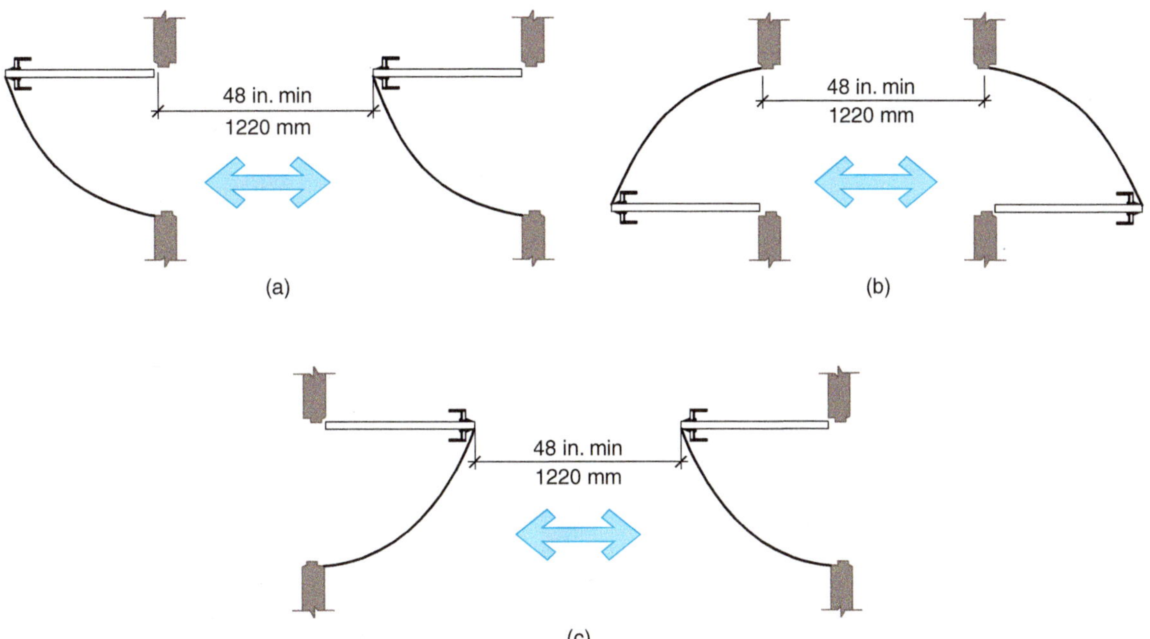

FIGURE 1–23 ■ Clear-space configurations for doors in series.

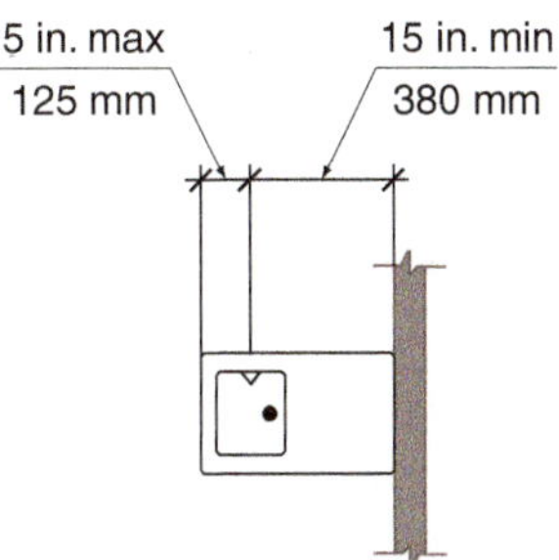

FIGURE 1–24 ■ Positioning requirements for drinking fountains.

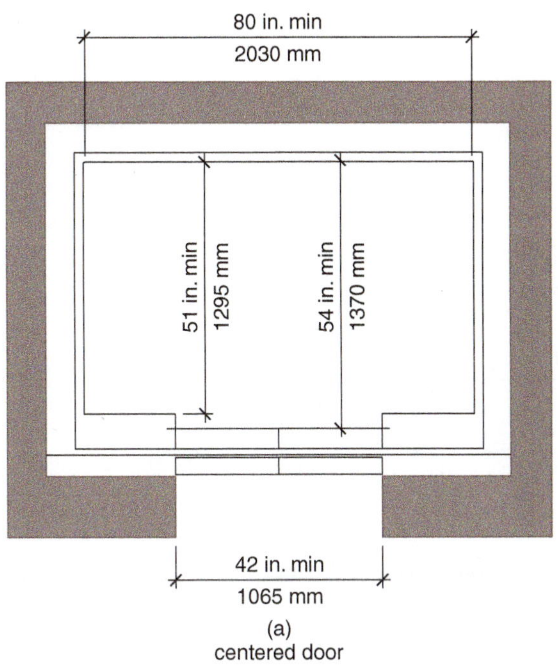

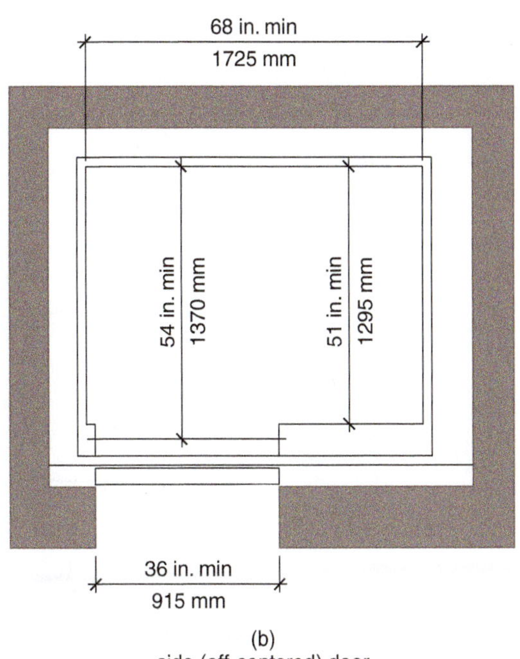

FIGURE 1–25 ■ Elevator car configurations.

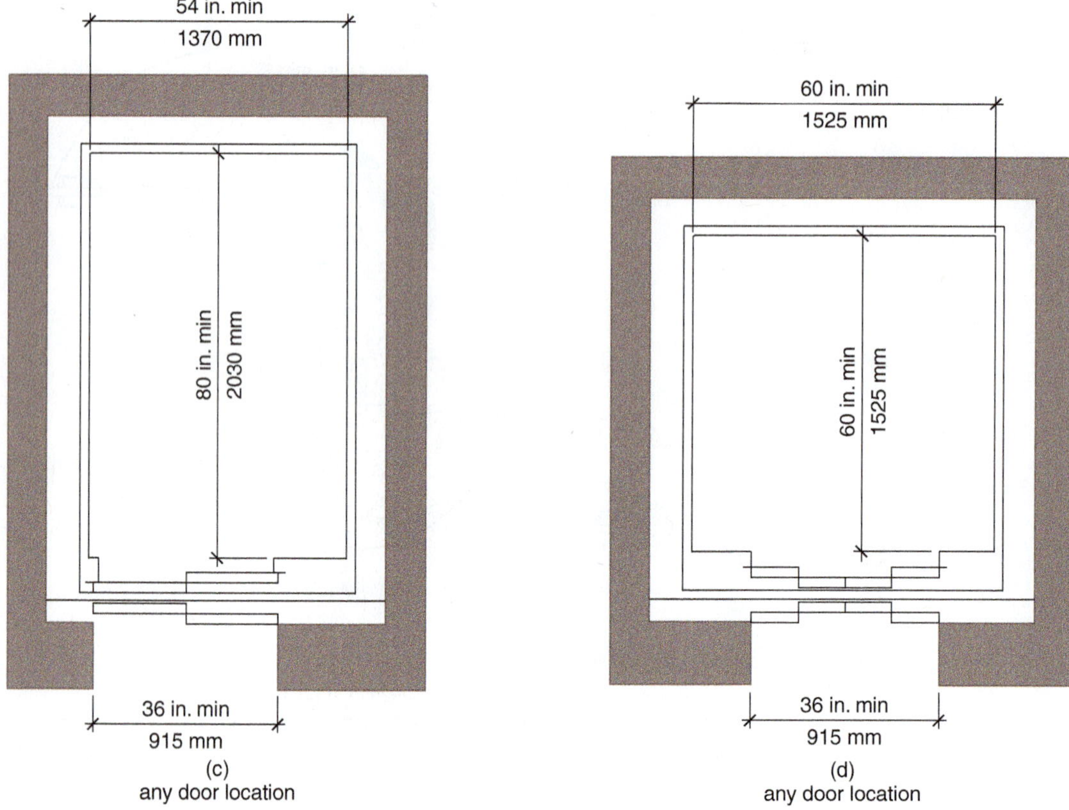

FIGURE 1–25 ■ Elevator car configurations (*continued*).

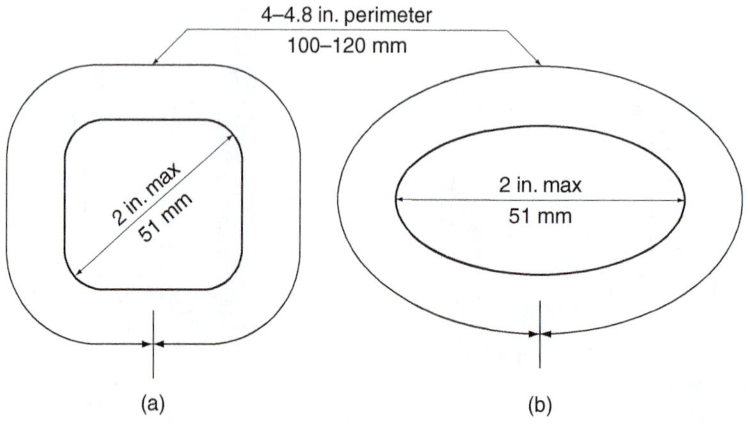

FIGURE 1–26 ■ Noncircular grab bar dimensions.

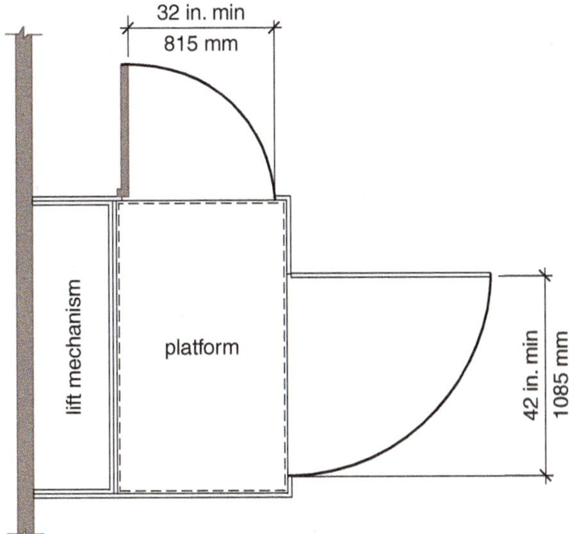

FIGURE 1–27 ■ Dimensions and configuration of platform lifts.

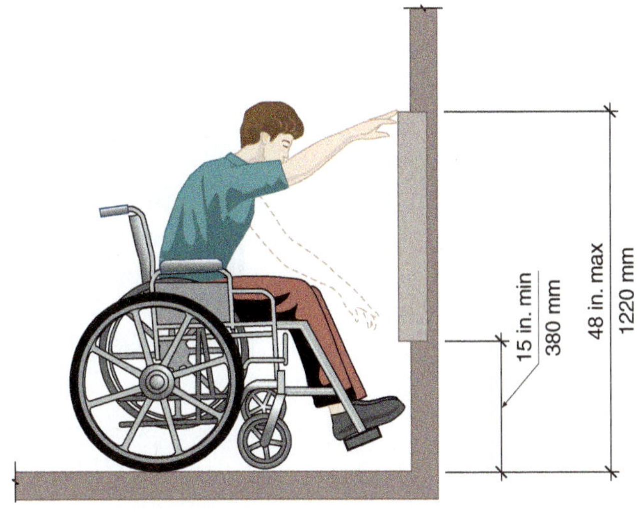

FIGURE 1–28 ■ Reach range—unobstructed forward reach.

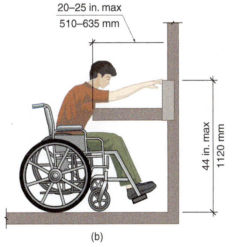

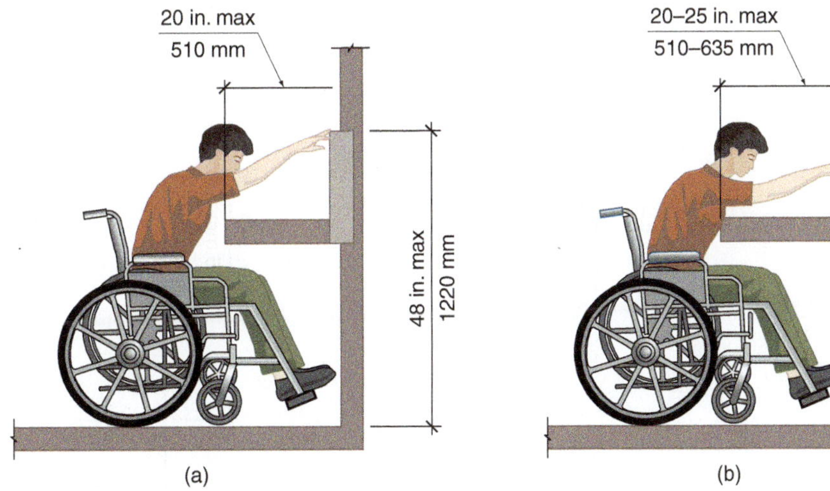

FIGURE 1–29 ■ Reach range—obstructed high forward reach.

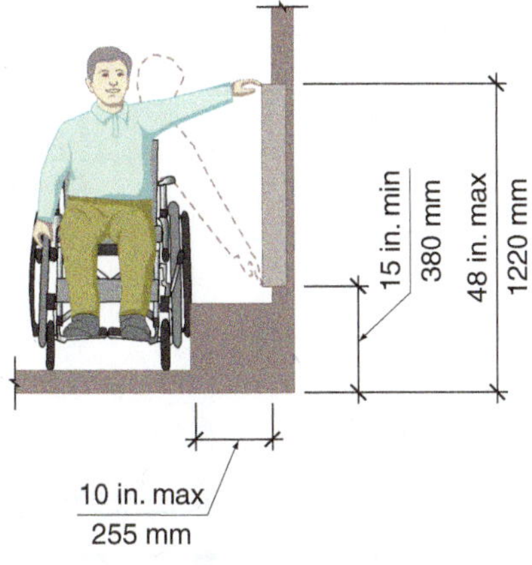

FIGURE 1–30 ■ Reach range—unobstructed side reach.

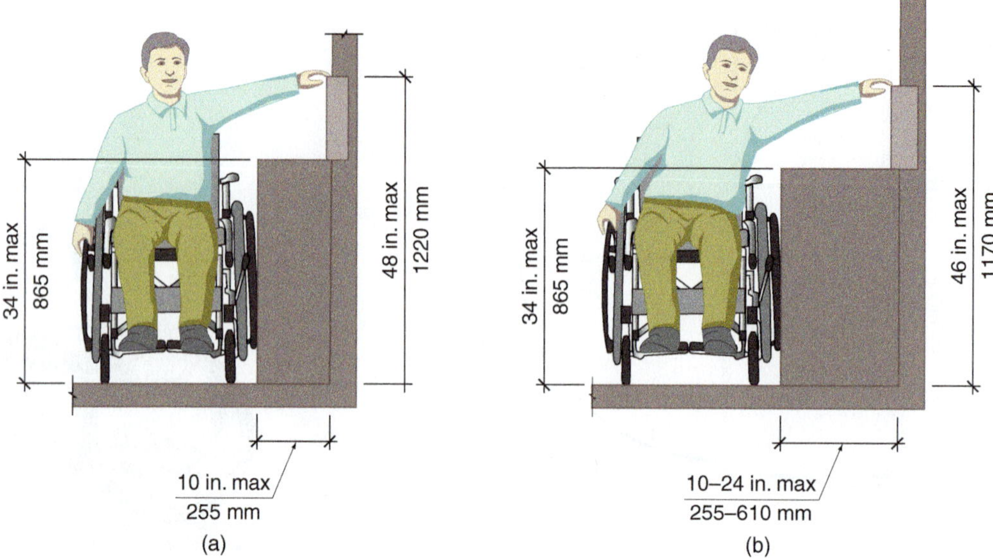

FIGURE 1–31 ■ Reach range—obstructed high side reach.

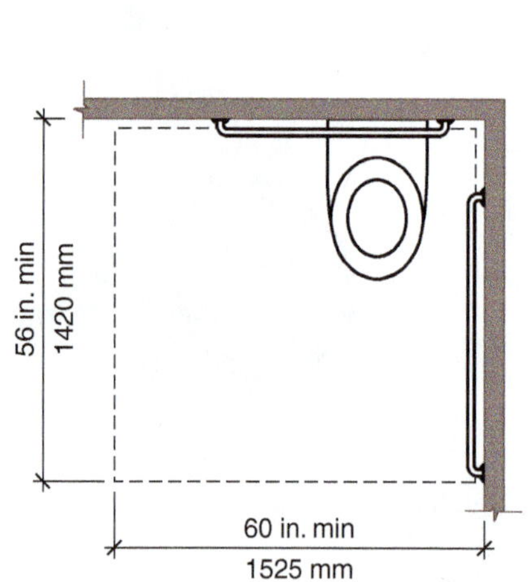

FIGURE 1–32 ■ Clearance for water closets.

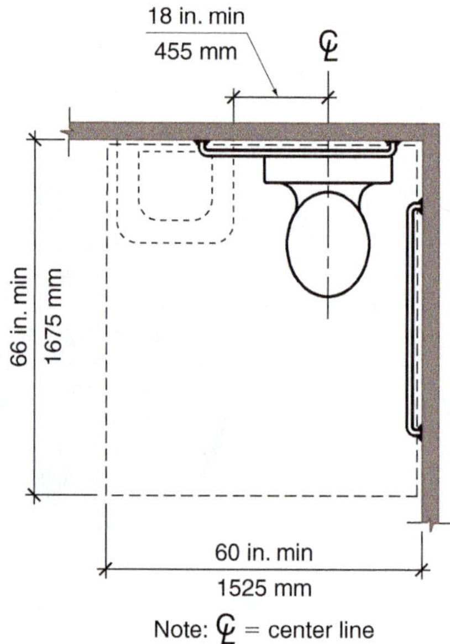

FIGURE 1–33 ■ Overlap of water closet clearance in residential bathrooms.

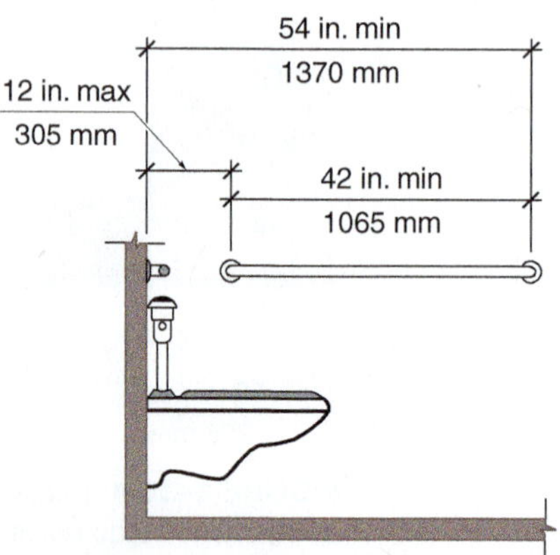

FIGURE 1–34 ■ Sidewall placement of grab bars in water closets.

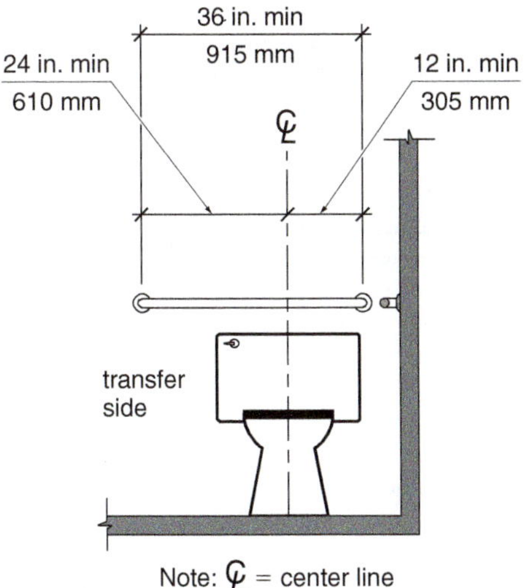

FIGURE 1–35 ■ Rear wall placement of grab bars in water closets.

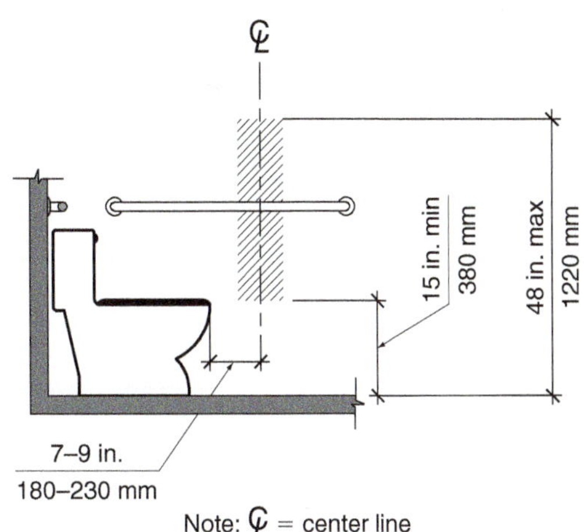

FIGURE 1–36 ■ Placement of toilet paper dispenser in water closets.

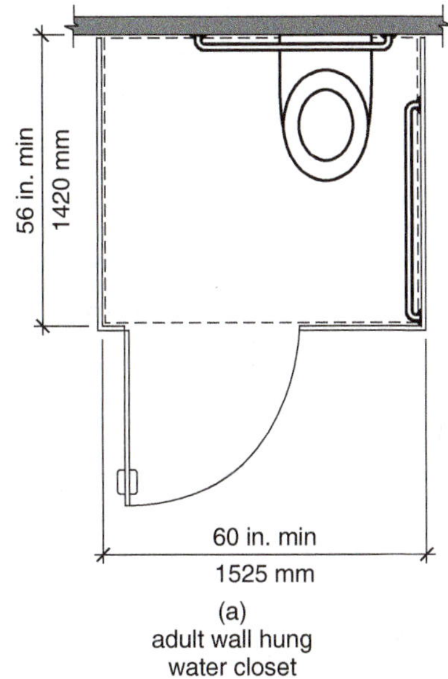

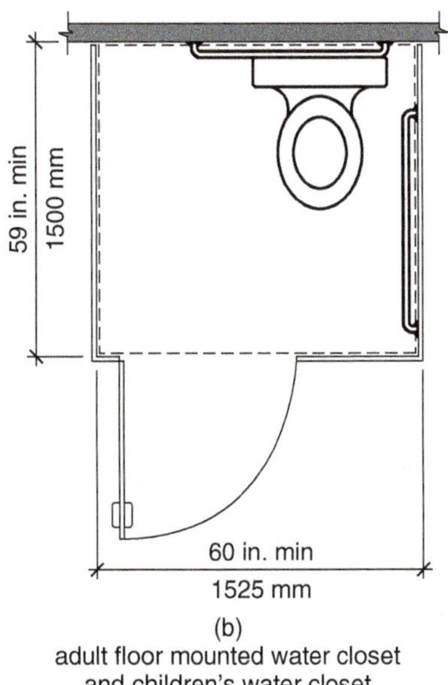

FIGURE 1–37 ■ Dimensions of wheelchair-accessible water closets.

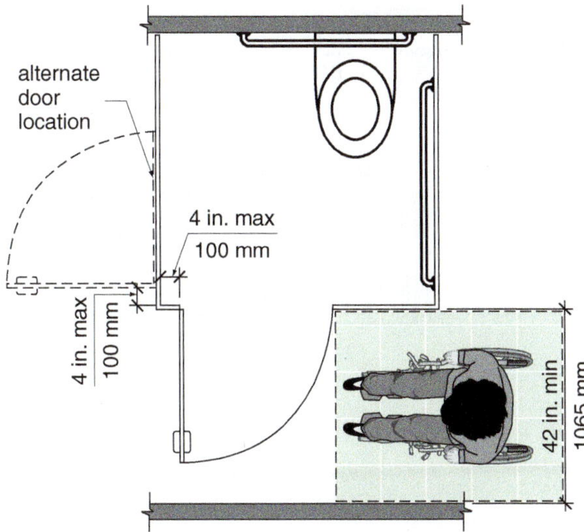

FIGURE 1–38 ■ Door dimensions of wheelchair-accessible water closets.

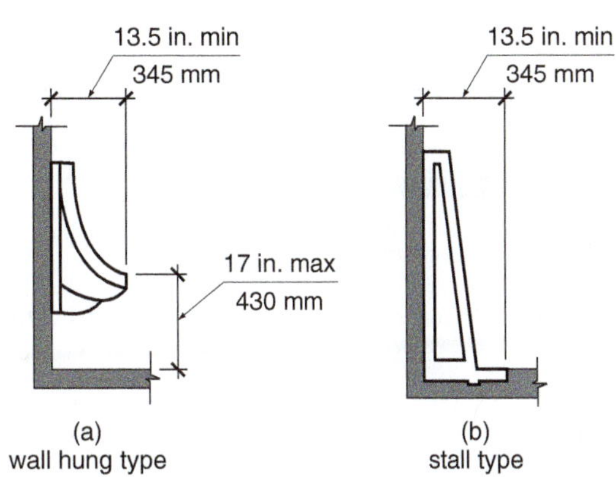

FIGURE 1–39 ■ Placement dimensions for urinals.

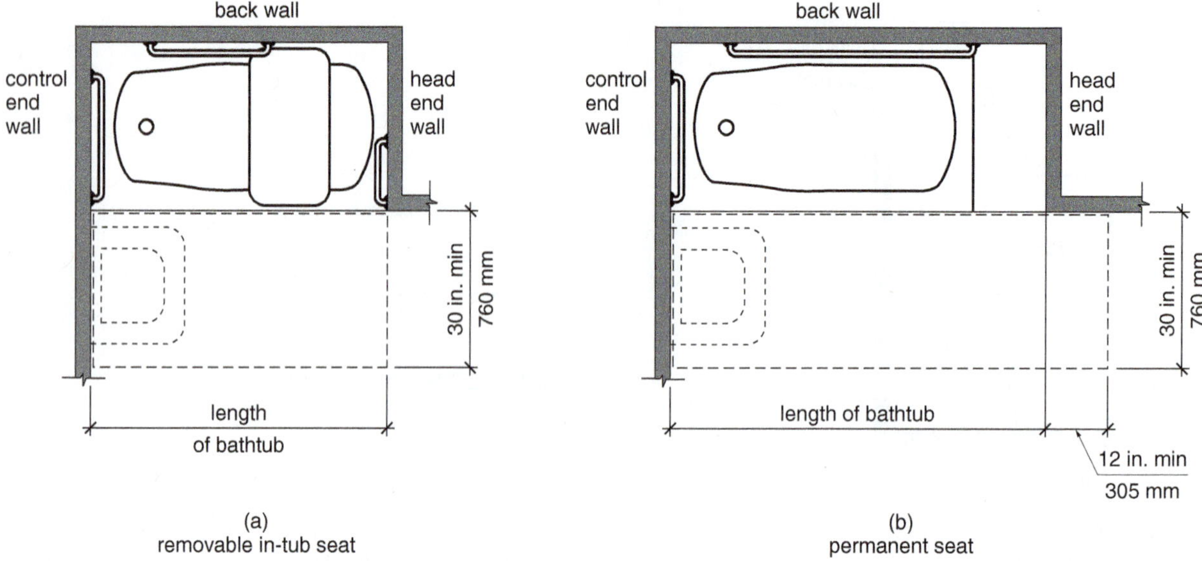

FIGURE 1–40 ■ Clearance dimensions for bathtubs.

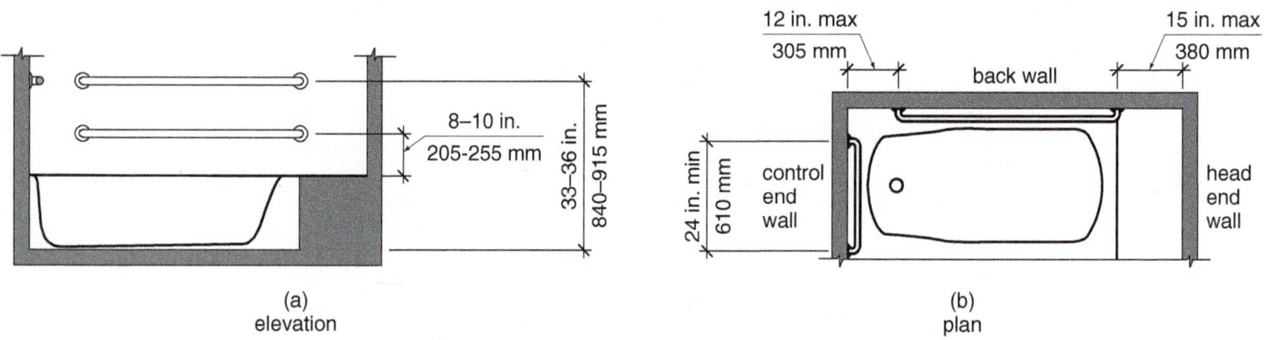

FIGURE 1–41 ■ Placement of grab bars for bathtubs with permanent seats.

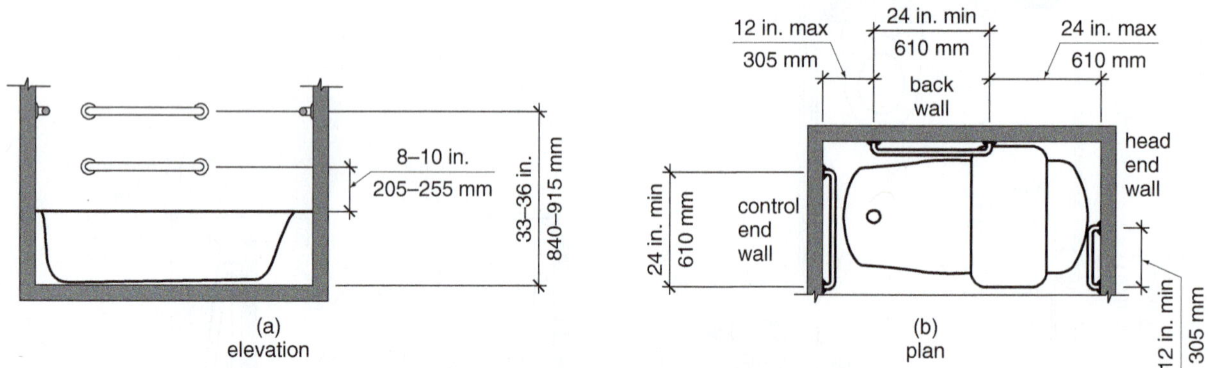

FIGURE 1–42 ■ Placement of grab bars for bathtubs with removable seats.

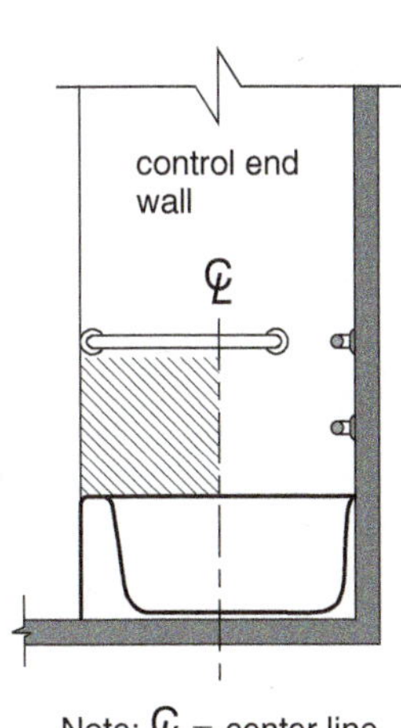

FIGURE 1–43 ■ Placement of water controls in bathtubs.

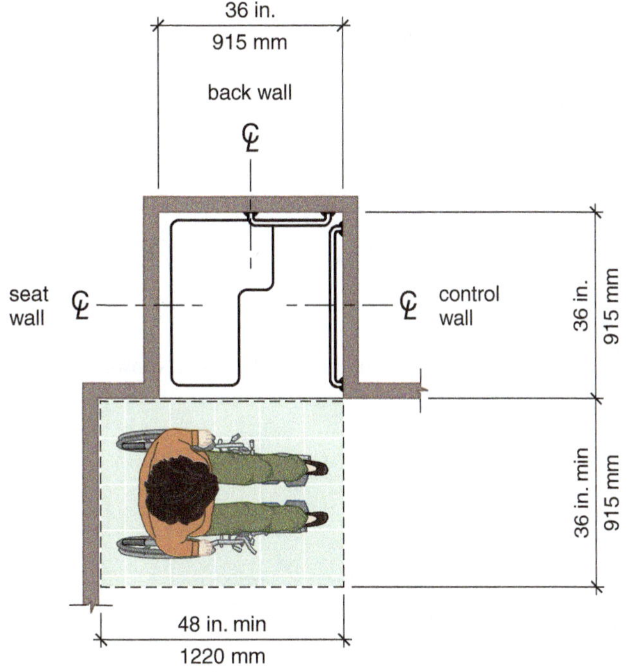

FIGURE 1–44 ■ Dimensions for transfer-type shower compartments.

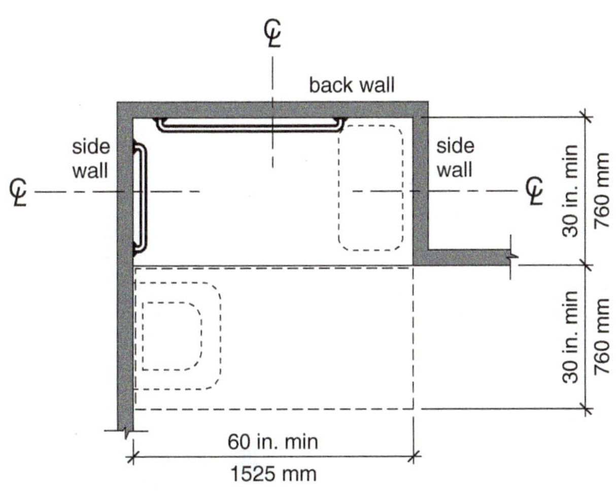

FIGURE 1–45 ■ Dimensions for standard roll-in-type shower compartments.

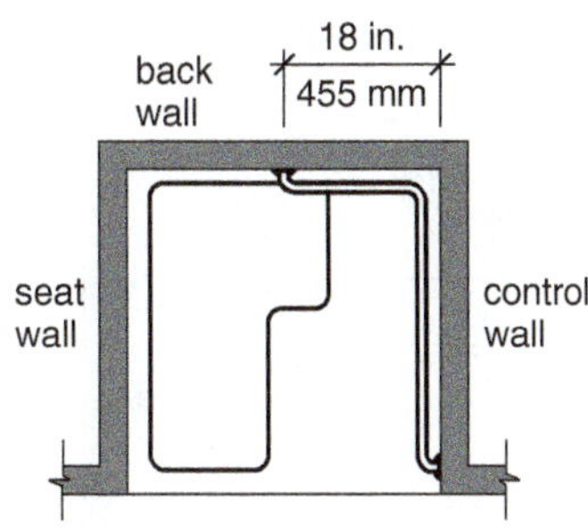

FIGURE 1–46 ■ Placement of grab bars in transfer-type shower compartments.

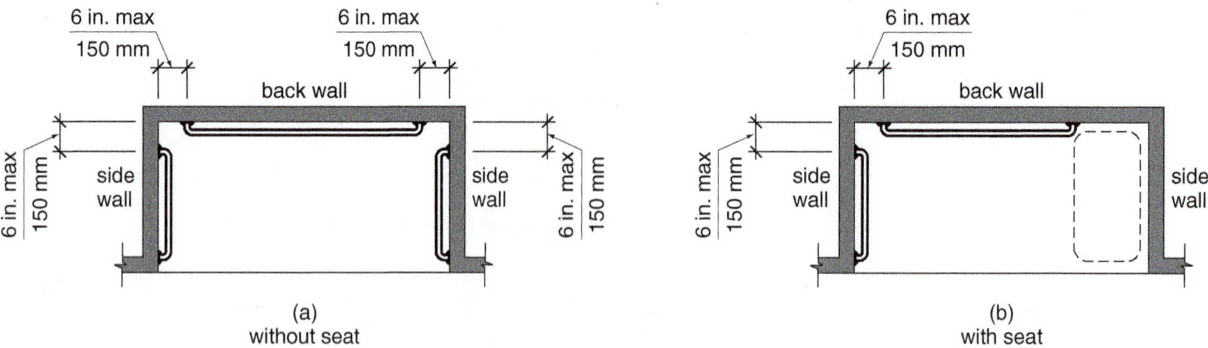

FIGURE 1–47 ■ Placement of grab bars in standard roll-in-type shower compartments.

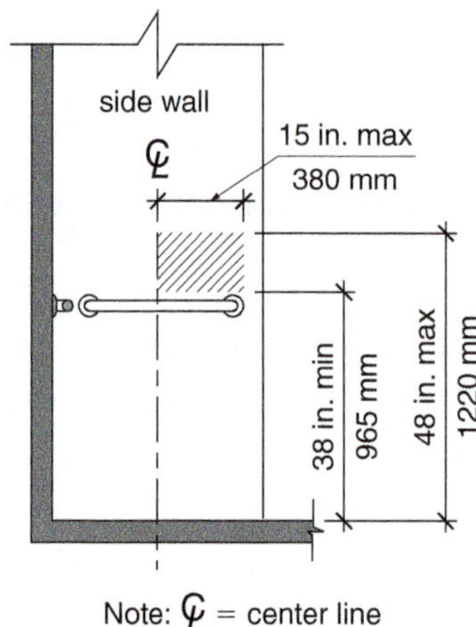

FIGURE 1–48 ■ Placement of water controls in transfer-type shower compartments.

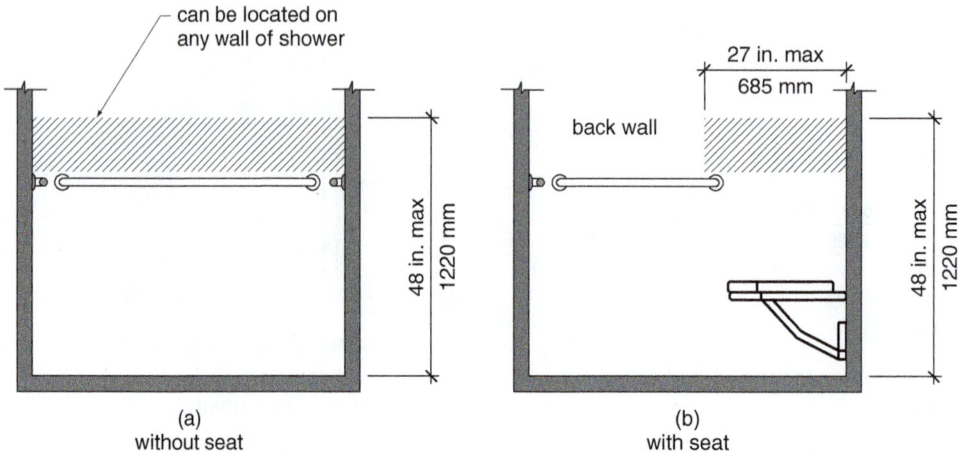

FIGURE 1–49 ■ Placement of water controls in standard roll-in-type shower compartments.

Table 1–3 ■ Clear-space requirements for manual swinging doors

Type of Use		Minimum Maneuvering Clearance	
Direction of Approach	Door or Gate Side	Perpendicular to Doorway	Parallel to Doorway*
From front	Pull	60 inches (1525 mm)	18 inches (455 mm)
From front	Push	48 inches (1220 mm)	0 inches (0 mm)[1]
From hinge side	Pull	60 inches (1525 mm)	36 inches (915 mm)
From hinge side	Push	54 inches (1370 mm)	42 inches (1065 mm)
From hinge side	Push	42 inches (1065 mm)[2]	22 inches (560 mm)
From latch side	Pull	48 inches (1220 mm)[3]	24 inches (610 mm)
From latch side	Push	42 inches (1065 mm)[4]	24 inches (610 mm)

*Beyond latch side, unless noted.
[1]Add 12 inches (305 mm) if closer and latch are provided.
[2]Add 6 inches (150 mm) if closer and latch are provided.
[3]Beyond hinge side.
[4]Add 6 inches (150 mm) if closer and latch are provided.

Review Questions

1. What are some examples of the purposes of patient care?
2. What is the family-centered model of the healthcare practitioner and patient/client relationship?
3. What are the components of the International Classification of Function (ICF) model?
4. What are examples of each component of the ICF model for an elderly man after total hip replacement?
5. What are some of the benefits gained through acts to permit free and appropriate education of children with disabilities?
6. What are the purposes of the Health Insurance Portability and Accountability Act of 1996 (HIPAA)?
7. What are the 18 identifiers used in medical records specific to the HIPAA?
8. Why are these patient identifiers protected by the HIPAA?
9. What are the rights and responsibilities outlined in the *Patients' Bill of Rights*?
10. What are the specific requirements for ramps as presented in the Americans with Disabilities Act of 1990 (ADA)?

Suggested Activities

1. Explore the websites provided in this chapter related to IDEA, HIPAA, and ADA and determine what information is available.
2. Examine specific areas of your campus for accessibility. Suggested areas include classrooms, restrooms, computer labs, building entryways, cafeteria, dormitory rooms, and access to rooms other than those on the ground floor. Use information on the ABA/ADA website to determine whether accessibility requirements are being met.

3. Determine appropriate recommendations to modify one area you found that lacked full accessibility.
4. Obtain a copy of a HIPAA form used by a local healthcare facility to determine if it meets requirements of the law.
5. Develop a Patients' Bill of Rights applicable for a pediatric physical therapy practice.
6. Research resources in your community for professional foreign language interpreters able to provide translation services in medical environments.

Case Studies

1. A patient requiring a wheelchair for ambulation lives in a home with a 6 inch step to enter. The clear space for the ramp is 18 feet along the front of the home to the driveway with 20 feet between the front of the building and the sidewalk. Design an appropriate ramp including location, length, width, and landings if needed.
2. Design a form that meets the requirements for HIPAA to be used in a physical therapy out-patient practice.

References

1. Nagi, S. (1965). Some conceptual issues in disability and rehabilitation. In M. Sussman (Ed.), *Sociology and rehabilitation* (pp. 100–113). Washington, DC: American Sociological Association.
2. Nagi, S. (1969). *Disability and rehabilitation.* Columbus: Ohio State University Press.
3. Nagi, S. (1991). Disability concepts revisted: Implications for prevention. In A. Pope & A. Tarlov (Eds.), *Disability in America: Toward a national agenda for prevention* (pp. 307–327). Washington, DC: Institute of Medicine, National Academy Press.
4. American Physical Therapy Association. (2003). *Guide to physical therapist practice* (2nd ed.). Alexandria, VA: Author. http://guidetoptpractice.apta.org/ (On-line edition. Must be APTA member to log-on) Accessed January 26, 2013.
5. http://www.who.int/classifications/icf/site/beginners/bg.pdf. Accessed January 26, 2013.
6. National Institutes of Health. (1992). *National Advisory Board on Medical Rehabilitation Research, Draft V: Report and plan for medical rehabilitation research.* Bethesda, MD: Author.
7. Jette, A. M. (1994). Physical disablement concepts for physical therapy research and practice. *Physical Therapy, 74,* 381.
8. http://www.gpo.gov/fdsys/pkg/PLAW-104publ191/pdf. Accessed January 26, 2013.
9. http://www.gpo.gov/fdsys/pkg/PLAW-111publ148/pdf/PLAW-111publ148.pdf. Accessed January 26, 2013.
10. http://www.apta.org/Compliance/. Accessed January 26, 2013.
11. https://www.civilrights.dot.gov/page/rehabilitation-act-1973. Accessed January 26, 2013.
12. http://www.venturacountyselpa.com/Portals/45/Users/Public%20Law%2094.pdf. Accessed January 26, 2013.
13. http://www.unc.edu/~ahowell/exceplaw.html#educationlaw. Accessed January 26, 2013.
14. http://idea.ed.gov/download/statute.html. Accessed January 26, 2013
15. http://www.usbr.gov/cro/pdfsplus/arcbarr.pdf. Accessed January 26, 2013.
16. http://scholarship.law.georgetown.edu/cgi/viewcontent.cgi?article=1069&context=cong. Accessed June 10, 2013.
17. http://www.nhlbi.nih.gov/guidelines/obesity/bmi_tbl.pdf. Accessed January 26, 2013.

2

Communication and Patient/Client Management Process

LEARNING OUTCOMES

Upon completion of this chapter, you will be able to:

1. Describe the elements of the Patient/Client Management process presented in the *Guide to Physical Therapist Practice* (Guide).
2. Describe the purposes of an initial interview with the patient.
3. Describe the two styles of questions, and when they are used, in an interview.
4. List and provide examples of the content included in an initial patient interview.
5. List the purposes of documentation in the healthcare system.
6. Discuss the requirements of adequate documentation.
7. Describe two formats of medical records: discipline-specific medical record and problem-oriented medical record.
8. Describe two formats of documentation within the medical record: SOAP note format and guide note format.
9. Discuss resources related to Medicare requirements for documentation.
10. Write examples of patient goals, using appropriate criteria for content and format.
11. Describe the purposes of medical records audits.
12. List the information necessary to perform an appropriate medical records audit.
13. List the information provided by an appropriate medical records audit.
14. Describe the purposes and characteristics of instructions and verbal cues.

KEY TERMS

Active listening
Audits
Chart review
Closed-ended questions
Diagnosis
Discharge plan
Documentation
ECHOWS
Effective communication
Episode of physical therapy
Evaluation
Examination
Explanatory Model
Feedback
Goals (long term and short term)
Instructions
Intake form
Interventions
Open-ended questions
Outcomes
Patient/client management
Plan of care
Preferred practice patterns
Prognosis
Red flag
Signs
SOAP notes
- Subjective
- Objective
- Assessment
- Plan

Symptoms
Systems review
Tests and measures
Verbal cues
Yellow flag

Introduction

Effective communication is essential to quality patient care and effective patient/client management. Physical therapists/assistants must be able to communicate effectively with each other, patients and their families/caregivers, and other healthcare providers. Communication methods include oral, written, and physical. Physical communication includes body language and touch. Effective communication is characterized by being timely, accurate, appropriate, clear, precise, concise, and organized. Trust and respect between patients and healthcare providers, and among healthcare providers, is fostered by effective communication. Several important aspects of communication and ways to communicate will be considered in this chapter.

Throughout this chapter, we will use a mock patient, Mr. John Doe, to illustrate points or provide examples. To follow this thread throughout the chapter, examples and interactions with Mr. Doe will be set in italic.

Aspects of Effective Communication

Effective communication, both oral and written, promotes understanding of what is being communicated. Although presentation may be effective, consideration must be given to reception and interpretation of the information. Correct terminology and appropriate levels of terminology enhance communication.

The environment in which oral communication occurs can also affect understanding. Noisy or distracting environments make concentration difficult, both for the provider and recipient of information. Attention to the person(s) involved in communication is important. Body language and touch can either enhance or degrade the quality of communication. Effective communication is sensitive to personal factors, such as gender, age, educational level, culture, religion, and language.

■ **Take Note**

Step one is establishing effective communication.

Effective communication includes factors of **active listening**:

- Be "present" when communicating with patients/families and other healthcare practitioners: Give the person with whom you are communicating your full attention.
- Show interest by making eye contact and addressing the person by his/her preferred name. *As an example, addressing a patient as "Mr. Doe" unless given permission to call him "John" is preferable.*
- Be aware of the message your body language is conveying. For example, crossed arms or turning your body away from the patient can be interpreted as defensive or uninterested.
- Staying focused on the topic. When more than one topic needs to be addressed, complete each topic before moving to the next one.
- Summarize your discussion. To check your understanding of information provided by the patient, present a brief summary of the discussion, asking the patient if your recitation of information is accurate. *As an example: "Mr. Doe, I want to make sure I understand what you have told me today. After I summarize our discussion, let me know if my understanding is accurate."*
- After information is clarified, patient/client management tasks will be discussed. Then it is important to ascertain that patients understand what you have told them. To check for understanding of information provided by you, ask the person to summarize, or restate, elements of the discussion in their own words. Do not just ask, "Do you understand?" *As an example: "Mr. Doe, could you please tell me in your own words what I have told you?"*

To participate effectively during examinations and interventions, patients must know what they are to do, how to perform it, and when they are to do it. Patients must be able to hear and understand instructions, cues, and feedback when presented. When patients cannot hear or do not understand spoken words, gestures and demonstrations may convey necessary meanings. For a patient who uses hearing aids, it is important to check that the hearing aid is being worn, is turned on, and is working properly. Professional interpreters are to be used when you are not fluent in a patient's primary language and the patient does not understand English. When interpreters are used, speak directly to the patient, and wait for the interpreter to translate. A patient's family and friends may offer to interpret; however, they may not be able to accurately translate to or from patients.

Communication with patients occurs when providing instruction prior to performance of activities, verbal cueing during performance of activities, and feedback after the performance of activities. **Instructions** inform patients what is to be performed and provide information as part of the teaching process. Instructions may include oral description, visual demonstration, and written description. **Verbal cues** are auditory cues to patients and are provided during activity performance. Prior to activity performance, patients should be instructed about the verbal cues that will be provided during activity performance.

■ **Take Note**

Instructions are given before and cues are given during activity performance.

Instructions must be simple, informative, and in a language and terms patients can understand. Lay language should be used unless patients readily understand medical terminology. Starting each session by describing to patients and families the general sequence of events that will occur and what they will be expected to do during that session enhances safety and learning.

Before proceeding with an activity, determine that patients understand instructions of what they are expected to do. Asking a patient, "Do you understand the instruction?" does not ensure understanding. Having patients repeat instructions in proper sequence indicates an appropriate level of understanding and provides an opportunity for mental rehearsal of the task. Verbal cues focus patients' attention on specifically desired actions. Verbal cues must be clear, brief, specific, properly timed, and spoken in appropriate tone and volume. Tone and volume vary as a situation requires. Generally, cues spoken in a sharp or loud manner receive quick responses, and cues spoken in a soft or low manner elicit slower responses.

Patients may become confused when provided a long series of actions to perform but only one cue. In many situations, each specific action may require a specific verbal cue. Verbal cues must be specific to the action desired. For example, counting to three does not direct a patient to perform a specific action. When a patient is to look up, the instruction may be "I will count to three and then say 'look up.' When I say 'look up,' you should look up." The verbal cue is "look up," which is a specific cue and does not require translating the word *three* into "look up." In this example, a patient has been provided an instruction that includes the verbal cue to be used and the expected response. Cues must be timed for each action to occur in the proper sequence and at the appropriate time so an entire activity is completed safely and effectively.

Feedback is provided after performance of an activity. In the early learning of an activity, feedback is given about how well the skill was performed, followed by instruction on ways to improve performance. Feedback should not be too lengthy or cover too many aspects of performance. As patients practice, feedback is given less frequently. Pausing to let patients assess their own performance and give self-assessments prior to your feedback is important to fostering learning.

■ **Take Note**

Feedback—important for learning.

Physical Therapist Patient/Client Management

The American Physical Therapy Association's *Guide to Physical Therapist Practice*[6] (*Guide*) describes physical therapy practice and presents the Physical Therapist Patient/Client Management Process. The *Guide*[6] presents the concepts of the sequential manner in which physical therapists approach patient care and categorize movement system disorders. These aspects are The Physical Therapist Patient/Client Management Process[6] and Preferred Physical Therapist Practice Patterns.[6]

The **Physical Therapist Patient/Client Management Process** is the process by which physical therapists generate and implement a plan of care for a specific patient. Physical therapist patient/client management must be within the scope of physical therapy practice. Physical therapist patient/client management is individualized through implementation of six elements: (1) examination, (2) evaluation, (3) diagnosis, (4) prognosis (including plan of care), (5) intervention, and (6) outcomes (Figure 2–1 ■).

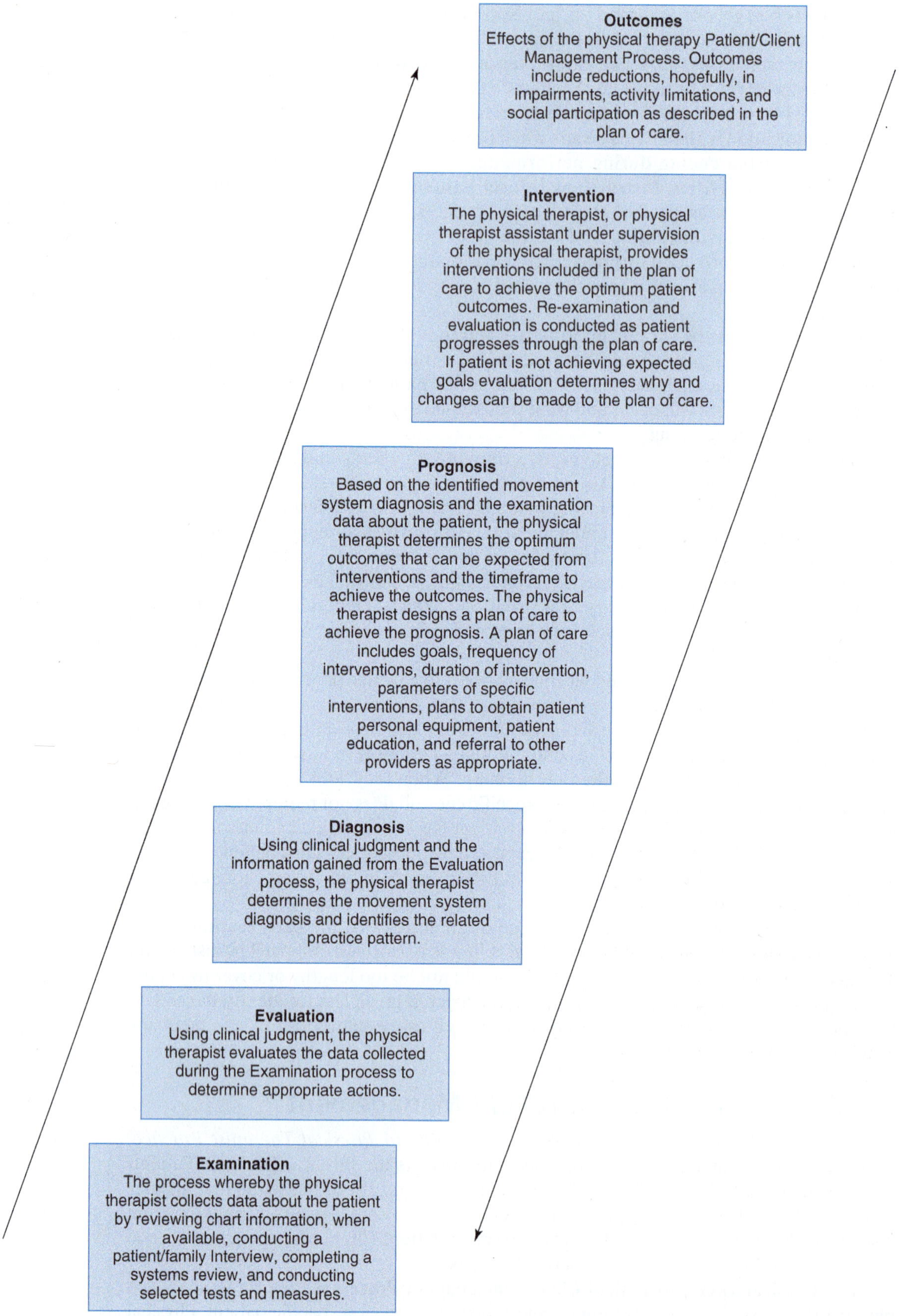

Outcomes
Effects of the physical therapy Patient/Client Management Process. Outcomes include reductions, hopefully, in impairments, activity limitations, and social participation as described in the plan of care.

Intervention
The physical therapist, or physical therapist assistant under supervision of the physical therapist, provides interventions included in the plan of care to achieve the optimum patient outcomes. Re-examination and evaluation is conducted as patient progresses through the plan of care. If patient is not achieving expected goals evaluation determines why and changes can be made to the plan of care.

Prognosis
Based on the identified movement system diagnosis and the examination data about the patient, the physical therapist determines the optimum outcomes that can be expected from interventions and the timeframe to achieve the outcomes. The physical therapist designs a plan of care to achieve the prognosis. A plan of care includes goals, frequency of interventions, duration of intervention, parameters of specific interventions, plans to obtain patient personal equipment, patient education, and referral to other providers as appropriate.

Diagnosis
Using clinical judgment and the information gained from the Evaluation process, the physical therapist determines the movement system diagnosis and identifies the related practice pattern.

Evaluation
Using clinical judgment, the physical therapist evaluates the data collected during the Examination process to determine appropriate actions.

Examination
The process whereby the physical therapist collects data about the patient by reviewing chart information, when available, conducting a patient/family Interview, completing a systems review, and conducting selected tests and measures.

FIGURE 2–1 ■ Elements of the Physical Therapist Patient/Client Management Process. The steps (elements) are used in ascending order to achieve appropriate outcomes. When desired outcomes are not attained, the steps are reviewed in descending order to determine appropriate modifications. (Adapted from content generated by the American Physical Therapy Association and presented in the *Guide to Physical Therapist Practice, 2nd ed.*[6])

Preferred practice patterns describe elements of evidence-based patient/client management for specific diagnoses. Preferred practice patterns guide management of patients/clients, but do not prescribe specifics of patient/client management. The *Guide*[6] describes four preferred practice patterns within the scope of physical therapy practice: (1) musculoskeletal, (2) neuromuscular, (3) cardiovascular/pulmonary, and (4) integumentary. A physical therapist preferred practice pattern is a categorization of movement system disorders. Each practice pattern details the elements of the Physical Therapist Patient/Client Management Process appropriate for the specific movement system disorder (Figure 2–2 ■).

■ **Take Note**

Patient/Client Management process is used to ensure patients/clients receive the most appropriate care.

Physical Therapist Practice Patterns

Musculoskeletal

- ☐ Pattern A: Primary prevention/risk reduction for skeletal demineralization.
- ☐ Pattern B: Impaired posture.
- ☐ Pattern C: Impaired muscle performance.
- ☐ Pattern D: Impaired joint mobility, motor function, muscle performance, and range of motion associated with connective tissue dysfunction.
- ☐ Pattern E: Impaired joint mobility, motor function, muscle performance, and range of motion associated with localized inflammation.
- ☐ Pattern F: Impaired joint mobility, motor function, muscle performance, range of motion, and reflex integrity associated with spinal disorders.
- ☐ Pattern G: Impaired joint mobility, muscle performance, and range of motion associated with fracture.
- ☐ Pattern H: Impaired joint mobility, motor function, muscle performance, and range of motion associated with joint arthroplasty.
- ☐ Pattern I: Impaired joint mobility, motor function, muscle performance, and range of motion associated with bony or soft tissue surgery.
- ☐ Pattern J: Impaired motor function, muscle performance, range of motion, gait, locomotion, and balance associated with amputation.

Neuromuscular

- ☐ Pattern A: Primary prevention/risk reduction for loss of balance and falling.
- ☐ Pattern B: Impaired neuromotor development.
- ☐ Pattern C: Impaired motor function and sensory integrity associated with non-progressive disorders of the central nervous system-congenital origin or acquired in infancy or childhood.
- ☐ Pattern D: Impaired motor function and sensory integrity associated with non-progressive disorders of the central nervous system-acquired in adolescence or adulthood.
- ☐ Pattern E: Impaired motor function and sensory integrity associated with progressive disorders of the central nervous system.
- ☐ Pattern F: Impaired peripheral nerve integrity and muscle performance associated with peripheral nerve injury.
- ☐ Pattern G: Impaired motor function and sensory integrity associated with acute or chronic polyneuropathies.
- ☐ Pattern H: Impaired motor function, peripheral nerve integrity, and sensory integrity associated with non-progressive disorders of the spinal cord.
- ☐ Pattern I: Impaired arousal, range of motion, and motor control associated with coma, near coma, or vegetative state.

Cardiovascular/Pulmonary

- ☐ Pattern A: Primary prevention/risk reduction for cardiovascular/pulmonary disorders.
- ☐ Pattern B: Impaired aerobic capacity/endurance associated with deconditioning.
- ☐ Pattern C: Impaired ventilation, respiration/gas exchange, and aerobic capacity/endurance associated with airway clearance dysfunction.
- ☐ Pattern D: Impaired aerobic capacity/endurance associated with cardiovascular pump dysfunction or failure.
- ☐ Pattern E: Impaired ventilation and respiration/gas exchange associated with ventilator pump dysfunction or failure.
- ☐ Pattern F: Impaired ventilation and respiration/gas exchange associated with respiratory failure.
- ☐ Pattern G: Impaired ventilation, respiration/gas exchange and aerobic capacity/endurance associated with respiratory failure in the neonate.
- ☐ Pattern H: Impaired circulation and anthropometric dimensions associated with lymphatic system disorders.

Integumentary

- ☐ Pattern A: Primary prevention/risk reduction for integumentary disorders.
- ☐ Pattern B: Impaired integumentary integrity associated with superficial skin involvement.
- ☐ Pattern C: Impaired integumentary integrity associated with partial-thickness skin involvement and scar formation.
- ☐ Pattern D: Impaired integumentary integrity associated with full-thickness skin involvement and scar formation.
- ☐ Pattern E: Impaired integumentary integrity associated with skin involvement extending into fascia, muscle, or bone and scar formation.

FIGURE 2–2 ■ Physical therapist preferred practice patterns. (Adapted from content generated by the American Physical Therapy Association and presented in the *Guide to Physical Therapist Practice, 2nd ed.*[6])

Physical Therapist Patient/Client Management Process

The six aspects of the Physical Therapist Patient/Client Management Process are presented in the order in which they are performed (see Figure 2–1).

Examination

Examination is the process of generating a patient/client history, reviewing all physiologic systems, and applying tests and measures. Examination is about collecting data about the patient. This includes chart review, review of intake forms, interview, systems review, tests, and measures. Each of these aspects is presented separately within this section. Patient interviewing requires specific skills, which are presented in the interview subsection. There are several types of data that must be obtained through a chart review and interview (Figure 2–3 ■).

When available, information about a patient is reviewed prior to the physical therapy interview. This review assists in focusing the interview and examination and provides a check on the accuracy of a patient's reports, both to the physical therapist and in the chart. A patient's medical information may be available in either paper or electronic form. Access to medical information in either format is subject to HIPAA regulations. Complete charts are typically available for inpatient care in hospitals and residential environments. Outpatient charts often contain information specific to the current episode of care only. Initial reviews of patient charts are performed by physical therapists prior to the first patient contact. **Chart reviews** before each treatment are necessary to determine any relevant changes in patient status or orders. When chart reviews are conducted by physical therapist assistants and changes in patient status or orders are noted, physical therapists must be informed immediately to determine if modification of the plan of care or patient reassessment is required. When physical therapist assistants provide most of the direct patient care, physical therapists must periodically review charts and consult with the

■ **Take Note**
Chart review

Demographics
Age
Sex
Race/ethnicity
Language
Education

Social History
Cultural background
Family/caregiver resources
Interactions/activities
Support systems

Employment/Work/School/Play
Current employment
Past employment
Job requirements
Level of schooling
Leisure activities

Growth/Development
Infants/young children

Living Environment
Home/work/community
Physical barriers
Adaptive equipment
Discharge environment

General Health Status
Self/family perception
Limitations or restrictions

Social/Health Habits/Risks
Smoking
Alcohol use
Recreational drugs
General exercise level
Non-traditional/alternative health practices

Clinical Tests
Diagnostic tests
Laboratory
Imaging
Functional

Family Medical History
Family diseases
Relatives

Medical/Surgical History
Prior problems-any system
Physical, mental, surgical
Current problems-any system
Physical, mental, surgical

Current Condition Chief Complaint
Signs and symptoms
Pattern of signs and symptoms
Previous occurrences
Interventions previously received (PT)
Mechanism of injury (when known)
Date of onset
Course of events
Expectations or goals (PT)
Prior experience (PT)
Emotional reactions

Functional Status
Activity limitations
Social restrictions
Current level of function
Level prior to current condition

Medications
Current medication list
Prescription/over-the-counter
Prescriber
Dosage
Current condition
Other conditions

FIGURE 2–3 ■ Data that should be determined during a chart review and interview. (Adapted from content generated by the American Physical Therapy Association and presented in the *Guide to Physical Therapist Practice, 2nd ed.*[6])

physical therapist assistant to ensure patients are receiving best care through appropriate clinical decision making, communication, and continuity of care.

Intake history in medical charts usually contains information about (1) general patient demographics, (2) current condition or chief complaint, (3) medical/surgical history, (4) general health status, (5) social history, (6) family history, (7) social health habits, (8) previous and present functional status, (9) medications, and (10) clinical tests ordered and their results. When patients are children, a review of developmental milestones may be included. Initial information related to a patient's status is in the intake history, but continually updated information concerning the patient's status, medications, and other orders will be recorded in appropriate sections of the chart.

In outpatient settings, patients may complete an **intake form** on arrival for their first appointment. The intake form helps guide the patient interview. These forms may allow patients to list current and prior medical conditions, note pertinent family history, and provide basic information about their current complaint before being seen by a physical therapist. During an interview, information supplied by patients is reviewed, and additional information is elicited to complete any missing or incomplete, but necessary, information. Clinics may have a generic form or a form for specific referrals. A sample form for chart review and intake, Documentation: Chart Review/Intake, with suggested information to be gathered, is available in the Resources section of this chapter.

▪ **Take Note**

Chart Review/Intake Form—Resources section

Patient interviews are a key component of the Patient/Client Management Process. One of the first components of each session is an interview of the patient. Family members and caregivers may be interviewed when patients are not able to be interviewed or may supplement information patients provide. Physical therapists/assistants should request of and receive permission from the patient, family, or caregiver to conduct an interview prior to proceeding. When English is a second language, inquire if the patient would like an interpreter. A plan and structure for interviews permits physical therapists/assistants to elicit information efficiently and effectively. Initial patient interviews are conducted by physical therapists and lay the framework for an open atmosphere for communication throughout a patient's episode of care.

▪ **Take Note**

Patient interviews

Physical therapists/assistants should introduce themselves by stating their full name and professional title. Physical therapists/assistants should use the patient's full name initially and may then ask the patient how they wish to be addressed. Only when a patient indicates that less formality is acceptable or desired should a patient be addressed by his/her first name. Physical therapists/assistants are responsible for ensuring that patients know the professional level of whoever is providing their care.

> *As examples: "Good morning, Mr. Doe, my name is ____ ____. I am a doctor of physical therapy and will be working with you today. Please feel free to call me ____. How do you prefer to be addressed?"*
>
> *"Good afternoon, Mr. Doe, my name is ____ ____ and I am a physical therapist assistant and will be working with you today. Please feel free to call me _____. How do you prefer to be addressed?"*

▪ **Take Note**

Include your professional title as you introduce yourself.

When patient comfort and safety are established, the interview can proceed.

Physical therapists initiate collection of information about patients as soon as a patient is observed. As an example, physical therapists can learn a great deal about a patient by how they get up out of a chair and walk into a treatment room. Patients also begin judging physical therapists/assistants when they are first seen and introduced. Professional clothing/attire, grooming and hygiene, body language, and general demeanor convey a message that may be more powerful than words. Healthcare professionals are responsible for establishing an appropriate environment and interactions with patients/clients based on mutual trust and initial first impressions.

During an initial physical therapy session, an interview is usually extensive. In subsequent sessions, interviews address changes since the previous session and compliance with the established plan of care. These subsequent brief interviews should be conducted by physical therapists whenever possible, but may be conducted by physical therapist assistants. As with chart reviews, when follow-up interviews by physical therapist assistants reveal significant changes in patient status, the physical therapist must be informed as soon as possible.

During an interview, information about the patient's general health is sought, as well as information about the specific reason for the current referral. Information gathered during chart and intake reviews should be discussed with the patient to determine accuracy and completeness. Specifics of the chief complaint(s) should be explored in a structured and systematic way, allowing for the development of hypotheses to guide the physical examination process. Physical therapists should summarize patient responses periodically and use additional questions to clarify details. Two main types of questions are used during interviews, open-ended and close-ended questions. The desired flow of an interview determines the types of questions to be asked. **Open-ended questions** allow patients to tell their story in their own words and cannot be answered with a simple "yes" or "no." This type of question allows physical therapists to direct the interview in a number of ways: (1) to explore, "Can you tell me more about it?" or "What problems are you having?"; (2) to encourage the patient, "And then what happened?"; (3) to focus an aspect of the interview, "I would like to clarify this aspect ... ?"; and (4) to paraphrase for clarity, "Am I correct in saying that you feel ... ?" Open-ended questions allow physical therapists to probe deeper when a patient's answer to a question is unclear or incomplete, but can make it difficult to elicit or clarify specific information.

■ **Take Note**
Types of questions

Closed-ended questions are used to focus the discussion and to obtain or confirm specific information. Closed-ended questions: (1) allow for "funneling" of information from very general to very specific responses; (2) are often used most effectively as follow-up on responses from open-ended questions; (3) can be answered with a single word or a brief phrase, such as "Yes," "No," or "Yes, once or twice before"; and (4) elicit specific information patients may not have thought to include. An example of a closed-ended question is: "Have you ever had this pain before?"

Interviews are concluded by asking the patient if there is any additional information they believe to be relevant to their care.

By chart review and interview, key information about Mr. Doe is obtained. His chief complaint is mild to moderate left knee pain of six months' duration. He reports becoming increasingly fearful of falling when on uneven ground, and having increased pain with "time on his feet" since the pain began 6 months ago. He experienced a significant exacerbation of pain 3 weeks prior to this initial physical therapy session when he "twisted" his left knee walking on his lawn. He did not report falling. X-rays taken during an appointment with an orthopedist indicated moderate osteoarthritis of his left knee. He does not wish to pursue surgery (i.e., total knee replacement) at this time and is managing his pain with over-the-counter (OTC) nonsteroidal anti-inflammatory drugs (NSAIDs). Since twisting his knee three weeks ago, he uses a cane or walker to ambulate in the home and curtailed all his usual leisure activities (i.e., golfing and attending his grandchildrens' sporting events). He reports frustration with loss of independence in activities of daily living, such as gait and transfers. He is retired and lives with his wife in a two-story home with children close by in the community. He has hypertension and heart disease, managed with medication, of note in his medical history.

Arthur Kleinman[7] proposed the **Explanatory Model** to assist in developing an understanding of the patients' perspective or explanation of their condition. Use of this model will often elicit cultural related information. Near the end of the interview, asking the patient a series of questions similar to the following provides patients an opportunity to share their perspective. Introduce the questions with a statement such as, "As different people view illness in different ways, it will be helpful to me to know your understanding of your condition."

"What do you call the problem?
What do you think the illness does?
What do you think the natural course of the illness is?
What do you fear?
Why do you think this illness or problem has occurred?
How do you think the sickness should be treated?
Who should be involved in the decision making?"[8]

Patient interviewing is a skill that can be honed with practice. Physical therapy students and new clinicians often struggle to refine the collection of patient data during an interview. **ECHOWS**,[9] a physical therapy patient-interview assessment tool, is useful in identifying aspects of the interview process that may be improved. The ECHOWS tool assesses how a student or clinician: **E**stablishes rapport, elicits information about the **C**hief complaint, collects the **H**ealth history, **O**btains psychosocial perspective, and performs an interview **W**rap-up. An overall **S**ummary of performance provides a comparison of characteristics between a skilled and novice interviewer. Scoring is based on whether the interviewer completed the ECHOW elements during the patient interview. The **S**ummary section allows for scoring the interview based on minimum competencies for a new physical therapy graduate, from "needs improvement" to "satisfactory" to "superior." Using this tool may assist students to reflect upon, and improve, interview skills.

After the patient interview, a survey and examination of all physiologic systems is performed. A **systems review** is a "brief or limited examination of (1) the anatomical and physiological status of the cardiovascular/pulmonary, integumentary, musculoskeletal, and neuromuscular systems and (2) the communication ability, affect, cognition, language, and learning style of the patient."[6] The purpose of a systems review is to obtain information related to the general health of a patient prior to a detailed examination regarding the chief complaint(s), and it begins the hands-on part of the examination. A sample form for systems review, Documentation: Systems Review, is available in the Resources section at the end of this chapter.

■ **Take Note**
Systems review

The Systems Review for Mr. Doe indicated the following.

Cardiovascular/Pulmonary System
Heart Rate (bpm): 87
Respiratory Rate (bpm): 12
Blood Pressure (mm Hg): 128/90
Further examination not indicated
Integumentary System
No disruption of skin
No unusual coloration or texture of skin
Further examination not indicated
Neuromuscular System
No loss of peripheral or central function
Further examination not indicated
Musculoskeletal System
No loss of function of upper extremity, head, neck, or trunk
Pain in left knee
Further examination is indicated

Physical therapists perform **tests and measures** to rule in or rule out causes of impairment and functional limitations. Appropriate tests and measures are selected by a physical therapist based on information obtained during chart review/intake form, interview data, and systems review. Before conducting tests and measures, patients should be informed by physical therapists about the tests and measures to be performed. Tests and measures are performed after the patient has consented.

■ **Take Note**
Tests and measures

Examples of tests and measures categories for each of the four preferred physical therapist practice patterns include, but are not limited to, aerobic endurance, integumentary integrity, joint mobility and integrity, and sensory integrity. Tests and measures vary in their validity and reliability to confirm or refute a potential diagnosis. Physical therapists select these tests and measures based on the individual or combined utility of tests to establish a diagnosis, prognosis, and plan of care. Interventions are determined by goals set within the plan of care. A sample form for examination, Documentation: Examination, is available in the Resources section of this chapter.

Tests and measures for Mr. Doe include:

Anthropometric characteristics
Height
Weight
Circumferential girth measurements

Circulation
Pulses
Environmental, home, work barriers
Home stairs, doors, floors
Gait, locomotion, and balance
Gait analysis
Balance testing
Joint integrity and mobility
Special tests
Muscle performance
Manual muscle testing
Muscle endurance
Muscle power
Orthotics, protective, and supportive devices
Ambulatory assistive devices
Pain
Intensity
Location
Duration
Frequency
Posture
Standing
Range of motion
Joint range of motion
Muscle length
Reflex integrity
Deep tendon reflexes
Self-care and home management
Activities of daily living (ADLs)
Instrumental ADLs (IADLs)
Sensory integrity
Peripheral (light touch, deep pressure)

Evaluation

Evaluation is the process whereby physical therapists use clinical judgement based on professional knowledge when using interview, systems review, and examination data to identify body structure and function impairments, activity limitations, and social restrictions. This then leads to the generation of a diagnosis, prognosis, and a plan of care. Evaluation is the synthesis and analysis of data collected during chart/intake form review, interview, systems review, and implementation of tests and measures. Physical therapists, and only physical therapists, make clinical judgements from these data with regard to diagnosis, prognosis, and plan of care for physical therapy. Physical therapists must discriminate between data that indicates a need for physical therapy services and factors related to conditions beyond the scope of physical therapy practice. Risk factors raise cautionary **yellow** - and warning - **red** - flags. These flags may be raised because of data in a patient's history or from their current signs and symptoms. Discrimination of this type should be an ongoing process during patient care.

■ **Take Note**
Clinical judgement by a physical therapist

A sample form for evaluation, Documentation: Evaluation, is available in the Resources section of this chapter.

An example of such decision making occurs if Mr. Doe presents with bilateral sensory loss in his feet, determined by sensory testing. The bilateral nature of this finding indicates a pattern of sensory loss not related to left knee pain, thus indicating a referral to a physician is warranted.

Results of Mr. Doe's evaluation are

Problem List: Impairments
Impaired joint mobility
Impaired gait

Pain
Impaired balance
Impaired muscle strength
Impaired coordination
Edema
Activity Limitation
Impaired gait
Limitations in self-care
Social Restrictions
Limitations in leisure activities
Limitations in home management
Contextual Factors (Environmental Factors)
Home barriers
Environmental barriers
Clinical Impression

Mr. John Doe is a 72-year-old male with significant limitations in left knee ROM, strength, and weight-bearing tolerance. He has significant pain and edema in his left leg. As a result, patient is limited in transfers, ambulation, and activities of daily living (ADLs). Patient requires assistance for ADLs and the use of an assistive device for transfers and gait. Patient was independent in all activities and moderately active 6 months ago. He is otherwise in good health with good family support. Mr. Doe requires physical therapy to resume his normal independent activity level. Because of a history of heart disease and hypertension, his cardiovascular status will need to be closely monitored.

Diagnosis

Diagnosis is assignment of a concise label that states the categorization or classification of problems identified through examination and evaluation. The diagnosis is selected from the practice pattern or diagnostic category (see Figure 2–2 ■) that most closely describes a patient's/client's impairments and functional limitations. A diagnosis by a physical therapist is related to the impact of a condition on function at a system level. This diagnosis directs the development of a prognosis and plan of care. There may be times when a physical therapist cannot place a patient in a diagnostic category, or the evaluation raises concerns about presentation of signs or symptoms that are not in one of the four practice patterns. A patient's impairment may be outside the scope of physical therapy practice, or additional assessment is required to address concerns in addition to those within the scope of physical therapy practice. In these cases, as part of a plan of care, physical therapists refer patients to other appropriate healthcare practitioners.

The term *differential diagnosis* is used in two ways. First, differential diagnosis is the process (an active process) in which data are interpreted to determine the most probable cause of a patient's impairments of body structure and function, functional activity limitations, and social participation restrictions. Second, a differential diagnosis is the most probable cause (a specific label) of a patient's impairments of body structure and function, functional activity limitations, and social participation restrictions. Physical therapists using the active process of differential diagnosis first determine if patients' complaints result from movement system impairments. When a medical condition is suspected, physical therapists make a referral to the appropriate healthcare provider. Patients often have both medical conditions and movement system disorders. Determining the exact movement system disorder, a differential diagnosis, is the result of evaluation of the data collected during the history, systems review, and physical therapy examination. Goodman and Synder[10] is one example of a source of information on common medical conditions that may be comorbidities, minic neuromusculoskeltal impairments, or cause movement system impairments. Physical therapists must be able to distinguish when a patient's medical conditions warrant referral.

■ **Take Note**
Diagnostic process and identification

Physical therapists classify patient conditions within specific practice patterns and assign movement systems disorder diagnostic labels that provide a basis for prognosis and directing plan of care. Patients often have conditions related to more than one practice pattern. Appropriate identification of all involved practice patterns is part of a differential diagnosis. The standard method of classifying diagnoses is called the International Statistical Classification of Diseases and Related Health Problems (ICD codes).

Our patient, John Doe, may be classified into the Guide[6] patient/client diagnostic classification of impaired joint mobility, motor function, muscle performance, and range of motion associated with localized inflammation (Pattern E within the musculoskeletal practice pattern). This diagnosis by the physical therapist is consistent with his diagnosis from his referring physician, left knee osteoarthritis.

Medical Diagnosis
715.36—osteoarthritis of knee, localized
Treatment Diagnosis
781.2—abnormality of gait

Prognosis

Prognosis[6] is the determination of an optimal level of improvement and the time necessary to achieve the projected outcomes. Physical therapists predict optimal levels of improvement in function and a time frame in which that will be achieved, which is a prognosis. The optimal level of function, or goal, may be based on a patient's prior level of function, or a higher level deemed attainable through therapy. A prognosis may also include predictions of intermediate levels of improvement and the time anticipated to attain these intermediate outcomes during the course of physical therapy.

Mr. Doe's prognosis might be:

Prognosis is good to excellent. He is predicted to achieve anticipated goals in 8 weeks. This will be demonstrated through optimal joint mobility, motor function, muscle performance, and range of motion and the highest level of functioning in the home, community and leisure environments. "During this episode of care, Mr. Doe will achieve the anticipated goals and expected outcomes of the interventions described in the plan of care and the global outcomes for patients classified in this pattern."

■ **Take Note**
Plan of care

Plan of care[6] is an outline of physical therapy management that specifies physical therapy goals, interventions, outcomes, and an anticipated timeline. A plan of care also includes, but is not limited to, referrals to other healthcare practitioners, ordering equipment for the patient, and discharge planning. Referrals to other healthcare practitioners may also include referrals to other physical therapists with specialized knowledge and skills.

A plan of care specifies the goals, outcomes, interventions, education, informed consent, and discharge planning necessary for a patient's care. Designing this plan of care is the responsibility of physical therapists. Physical therapists may delegate implementation of appropriate interventions within the plan of care to physical therapist assistants. A plan of care also includes necessary coordination, communication, and documentation for effective and efficient patient care.

■ **Take Note**
Goals

Goals are written with respect to the length of stay in a particular environment. They are not goals to be achieved over the total time of patient treatment unless the patient receives the full duration of all treatment in one environment.

Physical therapists, patients, and their families contribute to setting goals. Physical therapists establish diagnosis(es) and prognosis(es). **Goals**,[6] the clarification and description of expected patient outcomes, describe specific, objective, and measurable patient behaviors related to function. Descriptions of what a physical therapist will do, or listing an intervention, are not goal statements. **Long-term goals** (LTGs) are statements describing functional capabilities a patient will attain to be discharged from physical therapy. **Short-term goals** (STGs) are specific milestones a patient will attain building toward the expectations stated in long-term goals. A clear progression of short-term goals provides the basis for successful attainment of long-term goals. "Writing goals in functional terms is important because they support both the medical necessity of the physical therapy services and the need for the skilled intervention of the physical therapists or physical therapist assistants. The functional goals are a physical therapist's means of conveying to external stakeholders why this patient/client requires physical therapy services, rather than simply a checklist of what needs to be accomplished."[11]

Kettenbach[12] proposed the use of ABCD as a mnemonic to ensure the inclusion of components of a well-written goal. The mnemonic ABCDFT based on Kettenbach's work ensures that the behavior of the short-term goals' relation to function, the long-term goal, and the time to achieve the goal are included.

▪ **Take Note**
Goal components and format

The components of the ABCDFT mnemonic are

- **A**udience
  The audience is the person(s) to whom the goal applies. This may be the patient, patient's family, or caregivers.
- **B**ehavior
  Behavior is what the patient is expected to perform, described in observable and measurable terms. Long-term goals are typically defined as activities and social participation, such as transfers, ambulation, and work tasks. Short-term goals are related to remediating body functions and structures, impairments, and activity limitations necessary to achieve long-term goals. Examples of short-term goal behaviors are level of strength, range of motion, gait speed, and distance of ambulation.
- **C**onditions
  Conditions are variables that describe how behaviors are performed. Examples of conditions include the type of assistive device used, speed of performance, and type or amount of assistance required.
- **D**egree
  Degree is a statement of how often the patient is expected to perform the behavior under the conditions described. An example of a degree is "walking to the bathroom five times each day." When no specific degree is stated, patients are expected to perform the behavior to the condition described every time the behavior is required.
- **F**unction
  Behaviors must be related to specific functional abilities. As an example, a behavior in a short-term goal may be to increase strength as a requirement for the long-term goal's behavior of ambulation, a functional ability. Connecting behaviors of short-term goals to functional abilities identified in long-term goals assists patients, physicians, and third-party payers, among others, in understanding patient management progression.
- **T**ime
  Time is how long it will take a patient to achieve a short- or long-term goal. Time may be quantified by number of treatment sessions or number of weeks. Time necessary for attainment of goals is related to the environment in which physical therapy services are provided. An example is that acute care stays are often a few days or a week, whereas rehabilitation stays may be weeks or months.

A sample form for plan of care, Documentation: Plan of Care, is available in the Resources section at the end of this chapter.

Goals related to pain for Mr. Doe, might be stated as follows.

Long-term goal

Patient (audience) will ambulate (behavior) independently in the home and community (function) without pain (degree) and without an assistive device (condition) after 4 weeks (time).

Short-term goal

Patient (audience) will report (behavior) left knee pain less than 2/10 (degree) on visual analog scale during ambulation in home and community (function) with a single straight cane (condition) in 2 weeks (time).

Interventions

"**Intervention** is the purposeful interaction of physical therapists with the patient/client and, when appropriate, other individuals involved in patient care."[6] Diagnosis, prognosis, and patient goals direct the selection of specific physical therapy interventions designed to meet the established goals. Physical therapist interventions include procedural interventions

Mr. Doe instructed in use of cryotherapy at home for L knee. Instructed to place wet towel around L knee. Place bag of ice over towel for up to 10 minutes.

Cryotherapy to be used immediately after exercise/walking. May be repeated every two (2) hours when experiencing pain or swelling L knee.

Mr. Doe repeated instructions correctly, indicating level of understanding. Written instruction on cryotherapy provided.

FIGURE 2–4 ■ Documentation of an intervention for Mr. Doe.

such as therapeutic exercise, modalities, selection of, and training in, the use of patient care equipment, patient education, and instruction. Interventions are linked directly to the established goals.

As an example, one of the interventions to address Mr. Doe's left knee pain and edema might be cryotherapy. This intervention might be documented in the form of a treatment session note as seen in **Figure 2–4 ■**.

After physical therapists have determined the movement system disorder diagnosis, worked with the patient and family to develop goals, and outlined interventions to achieve the goals, patients are asked to consent to the plan of care. Physical therapists make sure patients are aware that they can refuse any interventions. At each treatment session, consent to the interventions being provided is to be obtained by the treating physical therapist/assistant.

■ **Take Note**
Discharge plan

A **discharge plan** is a plan indicating duration of care, referrals and follow-ups, and equipment requirements and a plan to obtain necessary equipment for a patient to achieve goals. It should be established for each episode of physical therapy care. An **episode of physical therapy** is defined as all physical therapy services provided without a break in care for a given condition or problem. A patient is discharged from care when the anticipated goals and expected outcomes have been met or there is a defined reason for discontinuation of services. Discharge plans, with a documented summary of the episode of care, is submitted to the referring physician and payor(s), when applicable or required.

As an example, Mr. Doe's discharge plan will be to discharge him to his home without need for an ambulatory assistive device and instructions for a home exercise program. No follow-up in physical therapy is required. He is to follow up with his family physician and his orthopedist as needed.

As an example of a discharge summary: Mr. Doe was discharged from physical therapy on this date, having successfully met the goals established for him. He was discharged with a home exercise program and education on self-management of pain and edema.

Outcomes

Outcomes[6] are the end result, the functional level, the patient will attain through physical therapy. Outcome measures are measures of function and quality of life that are used to assess achievement of long-term goals.

Documentation

Documentation[11, 12, 16] is a recording of data about patients, care provided, the provider of care, and results of care, entered into the patient's medical record immediately following such actions. Documentation is a medicolegal aspect of patient care. Events and actions must be documented and are deemed not to have occurred if not documented. There are many aspects of patient care and many individuals involved in the care of each patient. Coordination of patient care requires a high level of communication among all concerned. A patient's medical record serves as a repository of pertinent information concerning the patient's history, condition(s), and treatment and is a legal document. Appropriate documentation is paramount to ensure payment for the services provided to patients. Documentation must coincide with, and support, billing for services provided. With proper documentation, those involved with providing care for the patient, and support for the patient's family, will have sufficient information available regarding the physical therapy plan of care. Medical records and related documentation may be maintained as either physical or electronic files.

■ **Take Note**

Appropriate documentation is as essential as any other part of the patient management process.

Physical therapists/assistants, as well as other healthcare professionals, are held to increasingly stringent standards to communicate clearly, coordinate care, and provide best practices evidence-based care. Documentation, a form of communication, is critical and must be complete, accurate, precise, concise, and timely. "Medicare and third-party payers determine the physical therapy benefit or continuation of physical therapy services based on evidence of a significant functional change in a reasonable amount of time."[13] Documentation must demonstrate correlation among all aspects of the physical therapy patient/client management process. As an example, interventions implemented must be for a documented condition. Interventions for a diagnosis that is not documented are not eligible for reimbursement. Documentation must demonstrate that skilled physical therapy services are required to attain established goals. An example of documented skilled physical therapy service is "patient ambulation for 40 feet requiring frequent verbal cues to advance an ambulatory assistive device, and contact guarding to prevent falling."

REQUIREMENTS FOR ADEQUATE DOCUMENTATION The role of documentation is to enhance communication for medical and legal purposes. The rules of proper grammar are followed. An important aspect of medical documentation is the presentation of information in a manner that can be read and interpreted quickly and efficiently. Outline format may be significantly more concise than prose. Flowcharts and tables can be used to report individual and serial test results, enabling communication of large amounts of information in formats that can be read quickly and interpreted easily. Abbreviations (see Glossary of Abbreviations) may be used only if they are generally accepted abbreviations.

Documentation must be timely, accurate, appropriate, clear, precise, concise, organized, complete, and legible. Accurate documentation requires that recorded information be correct. Precise documentation requires that recorded information be provided in terms that state exactly what is intended to be conveyed. Concise documentation requires that information be organized effectively, conveying important information in a brief, clear, and unfettered fashion. Only relevant information is to be included. Complete documentation requires that all necessary information be included. Legible documentation requires that written, printed, or electronic media chart entries can be read easily. Timely documentation requires that notes be entered into the medical record as required by rule or regulation.

■ **Take Note**

Timely, accurate, appropriate, clear, precise, concise, organized, complete, and legible

Notes must contain the date of services provided and be signed by the physical therapist/assistant providing the services. The professional designation (PT or PTA) is part of the signature. Some institutions and states require that the practitioner's license number accompany the signature. Written notes should be entered using nonerasable ink. Corrections are made by drawing one line through the error, and the initials of the practitioner and date of correction are entered above the correction. When additions are made within existing notes, an inverted "V" (∧) is used to indicate where the addition is made, and the initials of the practitioner and date of addition are entered above the existing text and before the addition.

Regardless of the medical record or note format used, all documentation must meet basic documentation requirements. The Centers for Medicare and Medicaid Services (CMS) developed the Comprehensive Error Rate Testing program (CERT)[14] and the Hospital Payment Monitoring Program (HPMP)[15] to review claims submitted to Medicare. The 2007 CERT Report[14] found a high error rate for certain physical therapy services and that it was primarily due to errors in documentation. Insufficient documentation led to almost $34 million in projected improper payments for the service of therapeutic exercise alone. Findings such as these have led to increasingly stringent documentation and billing standards.

The APTA has numerous resources[16] that provide valuable information about patient care documentation. Some of these resources relate to documentation guidelines that span practice settings and patient populations. Other resources provide additional guidelines for unique practice settings (i.e., hospitals, skilled nursing facilities, outpatient clinics), that apply specifically to student physical therapists/assistants or to meet additional requirements set forth by states, payers, and accrediting organizations. Some of the documentation resources available to APTA members through the APTA (at http://www.apta.org/Documentation/DefensibleDocumentation/) are

- Introduction to Defensible Documentation
- General Documentation Guidelines
- Setting Specific Considerations in Documentation
- Components of Documentation in the Patient/Client Management Model
- General Guidelines
- Improving your Documentation: Reflecting Best Practice
- Defensible Documentation: Case Examples

Documentation may be deemed insufficient for a number of reasons. According to the APTA's Defensible Documentation[16] resources, the top ten payer complaints about documentation, leading to denials, are "(1) poor legibility, (2) incomplete documentation, (3) no documentation for date of service, (4) abbreviations—too many or cannot understand, (5) documentation does not support billing, (6) does not demonstrate skilled care, (7) does not support medical necessity, (8) does not demonstrate progress, (9) repetitious daily notes showing no change in patient status, and (10) interventions with no clarification of time, frequency, duration."[16]

FORMATS OF MEDICAL RECORDS There are several formats of medical records. The source-oriented method and the problem-oriented medical record (POMR) are two popular formats. Ideally all departments within a facility will use the same method of documentation. Documentation formats must provide appropriate information in a "user-friendly" manner, both for the person providing the documentation and for those reviewing it.

In the source-oriented method, charts are divided into sections for each healthcare profession providing service for a patient (e.g., clinical lab results, physical therapy notes, physician notes, dietary or nursing notes). The source-oriented system segregates patient information by discipline, necessitating that all healthcare providers review all discipline-specific sections of the record. A narrative format is usually used for writing notes in source-oriented charts.

The Problem-Oriented Medical Record (POMR) system, introduced by Lawrence Weed,[17] was designed to facilitate care provided to patients by organizing each medical record in a format based on identified patient problems, rather than by professional discipline. The POMR is composed of (1) database, (2) problem list, and (3) notes. In the POMR system, the **S**ubjective–**O**bjective–**A**ssessment–**P**lan (**SOAP**) format is used for note writing.

FORMATS OF NOTES

Narrative Notes Narrative notes can be unstructured, so headings and subheadings may or may not be used to organize information. The complexity and detail required in initial, evaluation, progress, and discharge notes may be difficult to achieve when using the narrative format.

SOAP Notes The **SOAP** acronym denotes section headings in the note: (1) **S**ubjective, (2) **O**bjective, (3) **A**ssessment, and (4) **P**lan. Each section of the SOAP note need not be included in every note. Initial notes, however, should include all sections. Progress notes should include only those sections necessary for indicating changes in patient status or plan of care.

In a SOAP note, a section identifying the patient often precedes the first section (**S**). This section contains information such as name, gender, age and date of birth, primary and secondary diagnoses, and physicians. Others, however, may place this information in the "Subjective" section even though this information is not truly subjective. "**S**" denotes **subjective** data. A patient's report of his/her history and symptoms, such as functional problems, pain, and the date of onset, are considered subjective data. **Symptoms** are a patient's subjective perceptions. A patient's goals of treatment are included in the subjective section.

"**O**" denotes **objective** data, which are verifiable data. These data include examination results, observations by healthcare providers, interventions, and patient response to interventions. **Signs** are objective evidence perceptible by healthcare providers. Subheadings are helpful in organizing the content of this section.

"**A**" denotes **assessment** of data gleaned through the Patient/Client Management Process. Included in this section is list of patient impairments/limitations/restrictions, diagnosis, and prognosis, with justification.

"**P**" denotes a **plan of care** for a patient. Each plan has a number of components for the care of a specific patient, such as interventions, coordination, and discharge planning. In some facilities, goals of treatment are included in the plan section, whereas other facilities include goals in the analysis section of the note.

An example of documentation in a SOAP note for Mr. Doe is available in the Resources section at the end of this chapter.

Patient/Client Management Notes The Patient/Client Management Note Format (Figure 2–5 ■) is based on the elements of the Patient/Client Management Process.[6] Examination, evaluation, and plan of care, elements of the Patient/Client Management Process, provide the major headings for a note in this format. Subheadings within each heading are included as deemed necessary to convey patient information in an accurate, precise, and concise manner. As an example, subheadings under Examination are History, Systems Review, and Tests and Measures. Other subheadings may be added as necessary for complete patient presentation. Each subheading may be divided further by using sub-subheadings. As an example, Social History might be a sub-subheading within the subheading History, within the heading Examination. Use of this outline format makes it easy to organize notes, ensure all necessary information is included, and retrieve information in notes.

Although the ICF Model for the provision of health care has become widely accepted conceptually, a documentation framework to integrate ICF into clinical documentation is not yet well established.[10,18,19]

A Sample Patient/Client Management Note Format for Mr. Doe is available in the Resources section at the end of this chapter.

MEDICARE GUIDELINES Medicare guidelines are issued by the Center for Medicare and Medicaid Services (CMS).[13] These guidelines must be followed if reimbursement for services rendered under Medicare is expected. CMS guidelines change relatively frequently, requiring updates, which can be obtained online from the federal government website (http://www.cms.hhs.gov/manuals). Of specific interest may be section 220, Coverage of Outpatient Rehabilitation Therapy Services (Physical Therapy, Occupational Therapy, and Speech-Language Pathology) Under Medical Insurance. This section appears in Chapter 15, Covered Medical and Other Health Services, within the Medicare Benefit Policy Manual. In a significant number of cases, Medicare guidelines are adopted by nonfederal government agencies and third-party payers, necessitating an understanding of CMS rules and regulations for more than just services rendered under Medicare.

■ **Take Note**

Professional organizations and government agencies offer information to ensure documentation meets requirements.

Highlights of Medicare documentation guidelines include a variety of topics:

- Conditions of coverage for patients requiring physical therapy services
    - Patient is under the care of a physician/NPP who is certified to approve plans of care.
    - Services are required because of medical necessity.
    - Plans for services developed by physical therapists must be certified by a physician.
    - Physician recertification of plans of care for therapy services must occur every 30 days.

PATIENT/CLIENT MANAGEMENT NOTE FORMAT

EXAMINATION		
History		
General Demographics	Social History	Employment/Work (Job/School/Play)
Growth and Development	Living Environment	General Health Status
Social/Health Habits	Family History	Medical/Surgical History
Current Conditions	Functional Status and Activity Level	Medications
Other Clinical Tests		
Systems Review		
Cardiovascular/Pulmonary	Integumentary	Musculoskeletal
Neuromuscular	Communication	Affect
Cognition	Language	Learning Style
Tests and Measures		
Aerobic Capacity/Endurance	Anthropometric Characteristics	Arousal, Attention/Cognition
Assistive and Adaptive Devices	Circulation	Cranial/Peripheral Nerve Integrity
Environmental/Home/Work Barriers	Ergonomics and Body Mechanics	Gait/Locomotion and Balance
Integumentary Integrity	Joint Integrity	Motor Function
Muscle Performance	Neuromotor Development and Sensory Integration	Orthotic/Protective Devices
Pain	Posture	Prosthetics
ROM/Muscle Length	Reflex Integrity	Self-Care/Home Management
Sensory Integrity	Ventilation/Respiration	Work/Community, Leisure Integration
EVALUATION		
Diagnosis	Prognosis (Timeframe and Outcomes/Goals)	Preferred Practice Pattern (Cardiovascular/pulmonary, integumentary, musculoskeletal, and neuromuscular)
PLAN OF CARE		
Interventions and Parameters (Specifics of interventions)	Frequency (Number of times/week)	Duration (Number of weeks or treatment sessions for plan of care)
Equipment and Devices (Assistive/Adaptive)	Coordination of Services	Re-examination Timeline

FIGURE 2–5 ■ Physical Therapist Patient/Client Management note format: headings and subheadings.

- Physical therapy services must be of a complexity that requires the clinical decision-making skills of a physical therapist and the intervention skills of either physical therapists or physical therapist assistants.
- Physical therapy services may only be rendered by physical therapists or physical therapist assistants under the supervision of a physical therapist.

- Contents of Physical Therapy Plans of Care
  - Each patient's Plan of Care must be consistent with evaluation results.
  - Diagnosis.
  - Long-term treatment goals.
  - Services are of appropriate type, frequency, intensity, and duration for the individual needs of the patient.
- Documentation requirements
  - Consistently and accurately reported.
  - Legible, relevant, and sufficient to justify services.
  - Evaluation and Plan of Care.
  - Certification.
  - Indication of active participation by a physical therapist during each progress report period.
  - Progress reports shall be at least once every 10 treatment days, or within one certification cycle.
  - Complete progress reports shall be written by physical therapists.
  - Physical therapist assistants may write certain elements of progress reports.
  - Treatment/daily notes for each treatment day.
  - Treatment/daily notes may be written by either a physical therapist or physical therapist assistant.

AUDIT OF PATIENT CARE Periodic and consistent evaluation of patient care activities is necessary to measure, analyze, and ensure the quality of patient care. **Audits** are systematic reviews of documentation that examine the efficacy and efficiency of patient care outcomes with respect to interventions used. Proper content and procedures for documentation are to be included in department policy and procedure manuals, and all personnel are responsible to follow these policies and procedures. Proper content and consistent implementation of policies and procedures in documentation facilitate productive audits.

A partial list of information a physical therapy departmental audit may yield is whether:

- Individual physical therapists are following departmental policies and procedures relating to documentation.
- Interventions being implemented are appropriate to diagnosis and goals for the patient.
- Patients achieve expected outcomes.
- Changes in departmental policy or procedures are necessary.
- Changes in treatment protocols are necessary.
- Continuing education is necessary to improve patient care skills.

An internal audit checklist is frequently used to determine if a patient's medical record and related documentation meet general documentation standards and additional compliance standards set forth by payers, state law, or accreditation agencies.

Internal audits to measure and analyze the quality of patient care assist in preparing for external compliance audits. External audits are performed by healthcare accreditation agencies such, as The Joint Commission (TJC) and DNV Healthcare, by Federal (Centers for Medicaid and Medicare Services, or CMS) or state agencies (State Department of Health, State Board for Workers' Compensation), or by private insurance companies that reimburse for physical therapy services. Each of these organizations has detailed requirements for acceptable documentation and billing.

▪ Take Note

Audits are an important part of ensuring best practice is being followed and patients receive the best care.

Resources

Patient Name ____________ ____________ ____________ **Date** ____________
Last First
Patient ID

Admission Date ____________ **Date of Birth** ____________
Race ____________
Ethnicity ____________
Language ____________

Education
Highest grade achieved ______
Some college/technical school ______
College graduate ______
Graduate school/advanced degree ______

Advance Directive
Completed by patient? ☐ Yes ☐ No

Referred by ____________
Medical diagnosis ____________
Reasons for referral
____
____

Cultural/Religious
Beliefs/customs/practices/wishes to be respected
____
____

Living arrangement	Upon Admission	Expected at Discharge
Alone	☐	☐
Spouse	☐	☐
Spouse and other(s)	☐	☐
Child	☐	☐
Other relatives	☐	☐
Group setting	☐	☐
Personal Care Attendant	☐	☐
Other ____________		
Unknown		

Support
Emotional ☐ Yes ☐ No
Intermittent support with ADL/IADLs ☐ Yes ☐ No
Daily support with ADL/IADLs ☐ Yes ☐ No
Transportation ☐ Yes ☐ No

Employment/Job/School/Play
Retired ☐ Yes ☐ No
Unemployed ☐ Yes ☐ No
Occupation ____________
Time ☐ Full time ☐ Part time
Student ☐ Yes ☐ No

Gender ____Male ____Female

Adaptive equipment (Describe)
____
____

Type of residence	Upon Admission	Expected at Discharge
Private home	☐	☐
Private apartment	☐	☐
Rented room	☐	☐
Assisted living/group home	☐	☐
Homeless	☐	☐
Long-term care facility	☐	☐
Hospice	☐	☐
Other ____________		
Unknown	☐	☐

Environmental barriers
Stairs to enter no railing ☐ Yes ☐ No
Stairs to enter railing ☐ Yes ☐ No
Interior stars with railing ☐ Yes ☐ No
Ramps ☐ Yes ☐ No
Elevator ☐ Yes ☐ No
Types of floor coverings ____________
Location of bedroom ____________
Location of bathroom ____________

Social/Health Habits
Alcohol ☐ Yes ☐ No
_______Frequency _______Amount
Smoking ☐ Yes ☐ No
_______Frequency _______Amount
Recreational Drugs ☐ Yes ☐ No
_______Frequency _______Amount
____

Exercise
Type ____________
Frequency ____________
Duration ____________

Family health history	Condition	Relative
Heart disease	______	______
Hypertension	______	______
Renal disease	______	______
Respiratory disease	______	______
Diabetes	______	______
Cancer	______	______
Other ____________	______	______

Documentation: Chart Review/Intake. (Adapted from content generated by the American Physical Therapy Association and presented in the *Guide to Physical Therapist Practice, 2nd ed.*[6])

Patient Medical/Surgical History

____
____
____
____

Patient General Health Status (include co-morbidities)

____
____
____
____

Medications (include dose)

____
____
____
____
____

Lab/Imaging Reports

____
____
____

Current Chief Complaint (by patient report)

____
____
____

Major Activity Limitations (by patient report)

____
____
____

Major Social Restrictions (by patient report)

____
____
____

Current Level of Function

____
____
____
____
____

Level of Function Prior to Current Condition

____
____
____
____
____

Anthropometrics

Height__________ Weight__________

Vital Signs	At rest	After activity
BP	______	______
HR	______	______
RR	______	______
Pain	______(0–10)	______(0–10)

Areas needing physical therapy assessment (to be completed by physical therapist)

- Aerobic capacity/endurance ☐
- Arousal, Attention, Cognition ☐
- Circulation ☐
- Cranial and peripheral nerve integrity ☐
- Ergonomics and body mechanics ☐
- Balance ☐
- Locomotion-all surfaces ☐
- Gait ☐
- Integumentary integrity ☐
- Joint integrity ☐
- Joint ROM/muscle length ☐
- Motor function (motor control and learning) ☐
- Muscle strength ☐
- Muscle endurance ☐
- Neuromotor development ☐
- Sensory integration ☐
- Orthotic, protective, and supportive devices ☐
- Pain ☐
- Posture
  - Sitting ☐
  - Standing ☐
- Prosthetic requirements ☐
- Reflex integrity ☐
- Self-care-ADLs and IADLs ☐
- Sensory integrity ☐
- Ventilation and respiration/O2 saturation ☐

Patient Name: ______________________ ______________________ ______________________
Last First Date

COMMUNICATION

Arousal	☐ Impaired	☐ Not impaired	
Cognition	☐ Impaired	☐ Not impaired	
Communication	☐ Appropriate	☐ Not appropriate	
Hearing	☐ Impaired	☐ Not impaired	☐ Uses hearing aid
Learning style	☐ Seeing	☐ Hearing ☐ Reading	☐ Able to read English
Orientation	☐ Impaired	☐ Not impaired	

Preferred language ______________________

Further examination needed ☐ Yes ☐ No

Comments

____

____

ANTHROPOMETRICS

Height _______ Weight_________ BMI ________

Hand Dominance ___R ___L

Comments

____

____

CARDIOVASCULAR/PULMONARY SYSTEMS

Vital Signs	HR_______ RR_______	BP ________
Edema	☐ Yes	☐ No
Location of edema	______Bilateral LE	______Unilateral LE___R___L
	______Bilateral UE	______Unilateral UE___R___L
Complaint SOB with activity	☐ Yes	☐ No
Persistent cough	☐ Yes	☐ No
Further examination needed	☐ Yes	☐ No

Comments

____

____

NEUROMUSCULAR SYSTEM

Transition between sitting and standing	☐ Impaired	☐ Not impaired
Gait	☐ Impaired	☐ Not impaired
Balance	☐ Impaired	☐ Not impaired
Mobility	☐ Impaired	☐ Not impaired

Describe Type of Mobility

____

Further examination needed ☐ Yes ☐ No

Comments

____

____

Documentation: Systems Review. (Adapted from content generated by the American Physical Therapy Association and presented in the *Guide to Physical Therapist Practice, 2nd ed.*[6])

INTEGUMENTARY SYSTEM

Color	☐ Uniform/Normal	☐ Not Uniform/Normal
Bruising	☐ Present	☐ Not present
Location ____________		
Texture	☐ Impaired	☐ Not impaired
Wounds	☐ Present	☐ Not present
Location ____________		
Scars	☐ Present	☐ Not present
Type ____________		
Location ____________		
Further examination needed	☐ Yes	☐ No

Comments

____

____

MUSCULOSKELETAL SYSTEM

Gross range of motion	☐ Impaired	☐ Not impaired
Gross muscle strength	☐ Impaired	☐ Not impaired
Gross posture	☐ Impaired	☐ Not impaired
Pain	☐ Present	☐ Not present

At rest _______(0–10) Pain with activity: ________(0–10)

Description

☐ Burning	☐ Itching	☐ Sting	☐ Throbbing
☐ Aching	☐ Numbing	☐ Pulling	☐ Pins/Needles
☐ Constant	☐ Brief	☐ Sharp	☐ Jabbing
☐ Shooting	☐ Electric		

_____Other (describe)

____

Further examination needed	☐ Yes	☐ No

Comments

____

____

Patient Name: ______________________ ______________________ ______________________
Last First Date

TESTS AND MEASURES

Based on the results of the chart review, patient/family interview, and systems review, indicate the appropriate tests and measures to be conducted. Indicate all that apply

☐ Aerobic capacity/endurance
☐ Assistive and adaptive equipment
☐ Circulation
☐ Cranial and peripheral nerve integrity
☐ Locomotion-all surfaces
☐ Integumentary integrity
☐ Joint ROM/muscle length
☐ Motor function (motor control and learning)
☐ Muscle endurance
☐ Sensory integration
☐ Orthotic, protective, and supportive devices
☐ Posture ☐sitting ☐standing
☐ Reflex integrity
☐ Sensory integrity
☐ Ventilation and respiration/O_2 saturation
☐ Arousal, Attention, Cognition
☐ Balance
☐ Circumference
☐ Ergonomics and body mechanics
☐ Gait
☐ Joint integrity
☐ Muscle strength
☐ Neuromotor development
☐ Pain
☐ Prosthetic requirements
☐ Self-care ADLs and IADLs
☐ Sensory integration
☐ Work/School/Play Integration

TESTS/OUTCOME MEASURES CONDUCTED AND RESULTS

Documentation: Examination. (Adapted from content generated by the American Physical Therapy Association and presented in the *Guide to Physical Therapist Practice, 2nd ed.*[6])

Patient Name: ______________________ ______________________ ______________________
Last First Date

DIAGNOSIS

Based on results of the chart review, patient/family interview, systems review, and examination, select the appropriate Physical Therapy Practice Pattern. Select all that apply.

Musculoskeletal

☐ Pattern A: Primary prevention/risk reduction for skeletal demineralization
☐ Pattern B: Impaired posture
☐ Pattern C: Impaired muscle performance
☐ Pattern D: Impaired joint mobility, motor function, muscle performance, and range of motion associated with connective tissue dysfunction.
☐ Pattern E: Impaired joint mobility, motor function, muscle performance, and range of motion associated with localized inflammation.
☐ Pattern F: Impaired joint mobility, motor function, muscle performance, range of motion, and reflex integrity associated with spinal disorders.
☐ Pattern G: Impaired joint mobility, muscle performance, and range of motion associated with fracture.
☐ Pattern H: Impaired joint mobility, motor function, muscle performance, and range of motion associated with joint arthroplasty.
☐ Pattern I: Impaired joint mobility, motor function, muscle performance, and range of motion associated with bony or soft tissue surgery.
☐ Pattern J: Impaired motor function, muscle performance, range of motion, gait, locomotion, and balance associated with amputation.

Neuromuscular

☐ Pattern A: Primary prevention/risk reduction for loss of balance and falling.
☐ Pattern B: Impaired neuromotor development.
☐ Pattern C: Impaired motor function and sensory integrity associated with non-progressive disorders of the central nervous system-congenital origin or acquired in infancy or childhood.
☐ Pattern D: Impaired motor function and sensory integrity associated with non-progressive disorders of the central nervous system-acquired in adolescence or adulthood.
☐ Pattern E: Impaired motor function and sensory integrity associated with progressive disorders of the central nervous system.
☐ Pattern F: Impaired peripheral nerve integrity and muscle performance associated with peripheral nerve injury.
☐ Pattern G: Impaired motor function and sensory integrity associated with acute or chronic polyneuropathies.
☐ Pattern H: Impaired motor function, peripheral nerve integrity, and sensory integrity associated with non-progressive disorders of the spinal cord.
☐ Pattern I: Impaired arousal, range of motion, and motor control associated with coma, near coma, or vegetative state.

Cardiovascular/Pulmonary

☐ Pattern A: Primary prevention/risk reduction for cardiovascular/pulmonary disorders.
☐ Pattern B: Impaired aerobic capacity/endurance associated with deconditioning.
☐ Pattern C: Impaired ventilation, respiration/gas exchange, and aerobic capacity/endurance associated with airway clearance dysfunction.
☐ Pattern D: Impaired aerobic capacity/endurance associated with cardiovascular pump dysfunction or failure.
☐ Pattern E: Impaired ventilation and respiration/gas exchange associated with ventilator pump dysfunction or failure.
☐ Pattern F: Impaired ventilation and respiration/gas exchange associated with respiratory failure.
☐ Pattern G: Impaired ventilation, respiration/gas exchange and aerobic capacity/endurance associated with respiratory failure in the neonate.
☐ Pattern H: Impaired circulation and anthropometric dimensions associated with lymphatic system disorders.

Integumentary

☐ Pattern A: Primary prevention/risk reduction for integumentary disorders.
☐ Pattern B: Impaired integumentary integrity associated with superficial skin involvement.
☐ Pattern C: Impaired integumentary integrity associated with partial-thickness skin involvement and scar formation.
☐ Pattern D: Impaired integumentary integrity associated with full-thickness skin involvement and scar formation.
☐ Pattern E: Impaired integumentary integrity associated with skin involvement extending into fascia, muscle, or bone and scar formation.

PROGNOSIS STATEMENT

____
____
____

Documentation: Evaluation. (Adapted from content generated by the American Physical Therapy Association and presented in the *Guide to Physical Therapist Practice, 2nd ed.*[6])

Patient Name: ______________ ______________ ______________
Last First Date

PLAN OF CARE
Duration of PT Services: ______________
Frequency of PT Services: ______________
Anticipated Date of Discharge: ______________

LONG-TERM GOALS
A. ______________
B. ______________
C. ______________

SHORT-TERM GOALS
A. ______________
B. ______________
C. ______________
D. ______________
E. ______________

INTERVENTIONS AND PARAMETERS

Intervention	Parameters	Person to Perform	Expected Changes	Flags: Red/Yellow

EDUCATION SERVICES REQUIRED

Topic	Methods	To Whom Given	By

RE-EVALUATION DATE ______________

DISCHARGE PLAN
____
____
____
____
____
____

PATIENT/FAMILY CONSENT TO PLAN OF CARE

______________ ______________
Print Name Date

____
Signature

____
Patient/Relationship to Patient

______________ ______________
Physical Therapist Signature Date

____
Physical Therapist License Number

Documentation: Plan of Care. (Adapted from content generated by the American Physical Therapy Association and presented in the *Guide to Physical Therapist Practice, 2nd ed.*[6])

John Doe DOB: 07/23/1941

S. *Mr. John Doe's chief complaint is mild to moderate left knee pain of six months' duration. He reports becoming increasingly fearful of falling when on uneven ground, and having increased pain with "time on his feet" since the pain began 6 months ago. He experienced a significant exacerbation of pain 3 weeks prior to this initial physical therapy session when he "twisted" his left knee walking on his lawn. He did not report falling. He reports X-rays taken during an appointment with an orthopedist indicated moderate osteoarthritis of his left knee. He does not wish to pursue surgery (i.e., total knee replacement) at this time and is managing his pain with over-the-counter (OTC) nonsteroidal anti-inflammatory drugs (NSAIDs). Since twisting his knee three weeks ago, he uses a cane or walker to ambulate in the home and curtailed all his usual leisure activities (i.e., golfing and attending his grandchildren's sporting events). He reports frustration with loss of independence in activities of daily living, such as gait and transfers. He is retired and lives with his wife in a two-story home with children close by in the community. He has hypertension and heart disease, managed with medication, of note in his medical history.*

O. *The Systems Review for Mr. Doe indicated the following.*

Cardiovascular/Pulmonary System:Heart Rate (bpm): 87; Respiratory Rate (bpm): 12; Blood Pressure (mm Hg): 128/90; Further examination not indicated

Integumentary System: No disruption of skin. No unusual coloration or texture of skin. Further examination not indicated.

Neuromuscular System: No loss of central function. Loss of sensation in feet. Further examination indicated.

Musculoskeletal System: No loss of function of upper extremity, head, neck, or trunk. Pain and decreased ROM in left knee. Further examination is indicated.

Tests and measures:

Anthropometric characteristics: Height-5' 10" Weight-150 lbs.

Circulation: Pulses regular, reduced in bilateral LE present at femoral triangle.

Environmental: Home 4 stairs at entrance, full flight to second floor, carpet throughout

Gait, locomotion, and balance: Decreased stance time on left, short step with right. Two-minute walk test 125 meters. Timed-up-and-go test 14 seconds.

Muscle performance: UE, R LE, L hip, and trunk strength good. L knee strength not tested due to pain

Orthotics, protective, and supportive devices: Uses a cane or walker

Pain: left knee 4/10 in morning and 8/10 by end of day. Pain is constant.

Posture: Stands with weight shifted to right LE

Range of motion: ROM of left knee: 10 to 100; other ROM adequate for function.

Circumference: Left knee circumference $\frac{3}{4}$ inch larger than right at joint space, non-pitting edema

Reflex integrity: DTRs normal except bilateral ankle which are reduced

Self-care and home management: Able to do most ADLs but slower due to pain. No longer participating in golf and attending sport events of grandchildren.

Sensory integrity: Bilateral sensory loss in feet.

Note for Mr. Doe in SOAP Note Format.

A. *Results of Mr. Doe's evaluation are*

Problem List: Impairments

Impaired left knee joint mobility

Impaired gait

Pain

Impaired balance

Impaired muscle strength

Edema

Activity Limitations

Able to walk short distances only

Self-care taking extra time

Social Restrictions

Limitations in leisure activities: golf and attending grandchildren's sport events

Limitations in home management: unable to do usual tasks such as lawn mowing and snow removal.

Contextual Factors—Environmental Factors: Home barriers-stairs and carpets

Mr. Doe presents with bilateral sensory loss in his feet, determined by sensory testing. The bilateral nature of this finding indicates a pattern of sensory loss not related to left knee pain.

Mr. Doe's left knee pain and edema are reducing his left knee ROM, gait, function, and quality of life.

Medical diagnosis: Osteoarthritis; left knee trauma

Movement systems diagnosis: Musculoskeletal pattern E—Impaired joint mobility, motor function, muscle performance, and range of motion associated with localized inflammation.

P. *Recommend Mr. Doe see his primary care physician for evaluation of bilateral loss of sensation in feet and decreased bilateral ankle DTRs.*

Physical therapy is recommended to reduce left knee edema and pain to improve his gait and quality of life.

LTG: Mr. Doe will resume playing golf and attending sport events of grandchildren within three weeks.

STG: Mr. Doe will report left knee pain of no more than 4/10 at end of day to improve his ability to attend sport events of grandchildren within 10 days.

STG: Mr. Doe's left knee circumference will be no more than $\frac{1}{2}$ inch larger than the right knee within 2 treatments to improve his gait.

STG: Mr. Doe will increase walking speed to 200 meters in two minutes as measured by the two-minute walk test in two weeks to increase community participation.

STG: Mr. Doe will decrease TUG to 10 seconds in two weeks to reduce risk of falls.

Interventions: Mr. Doe will receive physical therapy to include cryotherapy, massage, exercise, and ADL training three times a week for two weeks.

M. Major, DPT/27-12345

05/05/2013

Note for Mr. Doe in SOAP Note Format (*continued*)

John Doe DOB: 07/23/1941

HISTORY

Social, employment/leisure, living environment: Mr. John Doe is retired and lives with his wife in a two-story home, bed and bath on first floor. Until recent injury he was independent in ADLs, and IADLs, golfed and attended sport events of his grandchildren.

General health issues: hypertension and heart disease managed with medications.

Functional status and activity level: Before present injury independent in all ADLs and IADLs. Played golf twice a week.

Current Condition: Mr. John Doe's chief complaint is mild to moderate left knee pain of 6 months' duration. He reports becoming increasingly fearful of falling when on uneven ground, and having increased pain with "time on his feet" since the pain began 6 months ago. He experienced a significant exacerbation of pain 3 weeks prior to this initial physical therapy session when he "twisted" his left knee walking on his lawn. He did not report falling. He reports radiographs taken during an appointment with an orthopedist indicated moderate osteoarthritis of his left knee. He does not wish to pursue surgery (i.e., total knee replacement) at this time and is managing his pain with over-the-counter (OTC) nonsteroidal anti-inflammatory drugs (NSAIDs). Since twisting his knee three weeks ago, he uses a cane or walker to ambulate in the home and curtailed all his usual leisure activities.

SYSTEMS REVIEW

Cardiovascular/Pulmonary System: Heart Rate (bpm): 87; Respiratory Rate (bpm): 12; Blood Pressure (mm Hg): 128/90; Further examination not indicated.

Integumentary System: No disruption of skin. No unusual coloration or texture of skin. Further examination not indicated.

Neuromuscular System: No loss of central function. Loss of sensation in feet. Further examination indicated.

Musculoskeletal System: No loss of function of upper extremity, head, neck, or trunk. Pain and decreased ROM in left knee. Further examination is indicated.

Communication: Speaks and understands English. Effectively communicated current conditions.

Affect: He reports frustration with loss of independence in activities of daily living, such as gait and transfers.

Cognition: Intact.

Learning Style: Prefers demonstrations.

TESTS AND MEASURES

Anthropometric characteristics: Height-5' 10" Weight-150 lbs.

Circulation: Pulses regular, reduced in bilateral LE present at femoral triangle.

Environmental: Home 4 stairs at entrance, full flight to second floor, carpet throughout.

Gait, locomotion, and balance: Decreased stance time on left, short step with right. Two-minute walk test 125 meters. Timed-up-and-go test 14 seconds.

Muscle performance: UE, R LE, L hip, and trunk strength good. L knee strength not tested due to pain.

Orthotics, protective, and supportive devices: Uses a cane or walker.

Pain: left knee 4/10 in morning and 8/10 by end of day. Pain is constant.

Posture: Stands with weight shifted to right LE.

Range of motion: ROM of left knee: 10 to 100; other ROM adequate for function.

Circumference: Left knee circumference $\frac{3}{4}$ inch larger than right at joint space, non-pitting edema.

Reflex integrity: DTRs normal except bilateral ankle, which are reduced.

Note for Mr. Doe in Patient/Client Management Note Format.

Self-care and home management: Able to do most ADLs but slower due to pain. No longer participating in golf and attending sport events of grandchildren.

Sensory integrity: Bilateral sensory loss in feet.

EVALUATION

Problem List: Impairments

Impaired left knee joint mobility

Impaired gait

Pain

Impaired balance

Impaired muscle strength

Edema

Activity Limitations

Able to walk short distances only

Self-care taking extra time

Social Restrictions

Limitations in leisure activities: golf and attending grandchildren's sport events

Limitations in home management: unable to do usual tasks such as lawn mowing and snow removal.

Contextual Factors—Environmental Factors: Home barriers-stairs and carpets

Mr. Doe presents with bilateral sensory loss in his feet, determined by sensory testing. The bilateral nature of this finding indicates a pattern of sensory loss not related to left knee pain.

Mr. Doe's left knee pain and edema are reducing his left knee ROM, gait, function, and quality of life.

Medical Diagnosis: Osteoarthritis; acute trauma left knee.

Preferred Practice Pattern: Musculoskeletal pattern E—Impaired joint mobility, motor function, muscle performance, and range of motion associated with localized inflammation.

Prognosis: Prognosis for recovery of function is good given Mr. Doe's general good health, short duration of systems, and his motivation.

PLAN OF CARE

Physical therapy is recommended to reduce left knee edema and pain to improve his gait and quality of life.

Equipment: Mr. Doe should continue use of cane during ambulation.

LTG: Mr. Doe will resume playing golf and attending sport events of grandchildren within three weeks.

STG: Mr. Doe will report left knee pain of no more than 4/10 at end of day to improve his ability to attend sport events of grandchildren within 10 days.

STG: Mr. Doe's left knee circumference will be no more than $\frac{1}{2}$ *inch larger than the right knee within 2 treatments to improve his gait.*

STG: Mr. Doe will increase walking speed to 200 meters in two minutes as measured by the two-minute walk test in two weeks to increase community participation.

STG: Mr. Doe will decrease TUG to 10 seconds in two weeks to reduce risk of falls.

Interventions: Cryotherapy instructions, massage, graded exercise, and ADL training.

Frequency/duration: three times a week for two weeks.

Coordination of Services: Recommend Mr. Doe see his primary care physician for evaluation of bilateral loss of sensation in feet and decreased bilateral ankle DTRs.

Reexamination: Reevaluation after two treatment sessions.

M. Major, DPT/27-12345

05/05/2013

Note for Mr. Doe in Patient/Client Management Note Format (*continued*)

Review Questions

1. What are the elements of the Patient/Client Management Process presented in the *Guide to Physical Therapist Practice* (Guide)? Describe each.
2. What types of information are obtained during initial patient interviews?
3. What are open-ended and close-ended questions? Provide examples for use during patient interviews.
4. What are the purposes for open-ended and close-ended questions used in patient interviews?
5. What are the purposes of documentation in the healthcare system?
6. What are the requirements of adequate documentation of healthcare provider–patient interactions?
7. What are the similarities and differences between the two formats of medical records: discipline-specific medical record and problem-oriented medical record?
8. What are the similarities and differences between the two formats of documentation within the medical record: SOAP note format and Guide note format?
9. What resources are available to assist with meeting Medicare requirements for documentation?
10. How do medical records audits contribute to quality patient care?
11. What are the purposes and characteristics of instructions, verbal cues, and feedback?

Suggested Activities

1. Write examples of patient goals, using appropriate format (ABCDFT) and criteria.
2. Create lists of the information that should be collected during a medical record audit of physical therapists' patient notes.
3. In groups of three, practice interviewing using the ECHOWS tool; rotate roles so each person is interviewer, interviewee, and observer completing the ECHOWS tool and noting questions used.
   a. Review with the interviewer the questions used, noting appropriate use of open-ended and close-ended questions.
   b. Review the ECHOWS tool and discuss results.
   c. Develop an action plan to improve interview skills.
4. Using the information about Mr. Doe, write two notes one in SOAP format and one in Patient/Client Management format. Create new goals using the ABCDFT format.
5. In the following table, indicate the appropriate section of SOAP notes and Patient/Client Notes for each of the statements in the table.

SOAP Note	Patient/Client Note	Patient information
		ROM: R shoulder flexion 0–85
		The family reports that the patient fell during the night.
		Patient is to receive treatment 2×/week for 3 weeks.
		The patient can ambulate with a small base quad cane on all surfaces for 150 ft without fatigue in 4 weeks.
		Pain was 5/10 following intervention with TENS.
		Patient's pain level decreased following interventions.
		Patient ↑↓ 12 stairs step over stop using the hand rail 4 times.
		The patient's ability to assume standing from sitting is impaired because of weakness of bilateral quadriceps muscles.

Case Studies

1. Mr. Jimenez, a 67-year-old man, is 2 days post left total knee replacement. He is to be discharged to the hospital's skilled nursing facility in 2 days for additional physical therapy. Mr. Jimenez's goal is to be a community ambulator without any ambulatory assistive device. The physician has indicated that when Mr. Jimenez has 90 degrees of left knee flexion, good strength of left knee flexors and extensors, and can ambulate independently 200 ft × 4, he can be discharged to his home. Mr. Jimenez reports pain of 4/10 about the incision. The approximately 5-inch incision is anterior over the left knee in a proximal distal direction. Some clear discharge is noted at the end of the incision. The incision is closed with staples. The circumference of the left knee at 2 inches above the tibial tuberosity is ¾ inch greater than on the right knee.

Eduardo Jiminez	SSN: 123-45-6789
415 Main St.	DOB: 05/08/45
Any City, USA	Record: 444-3-45-897
Phone: (555) 212-2222	

   a. Using this information, identify and list information that is covered by HIPAA regulations.
   b. Organize the narrative note into a SOAP note format and a Patient/Client Management note format.
   c. Write two short-term goals based on Mr. Jimenez's long-term goal.

2. All physical therapists/assistants in the department are contributing to the development of a documentation checklist to ensure quality documentation of patient care. As a member of the department, develop a list of items to be included on the documentation checklist with justification for inclusion of each item.

References

1. Nagi, S. (1965). Some conceptual issues in disability and rehabilitation. In M. Sussman (Ed.), *Sociology and rehabilitation* (pp. 100–113). Washington, DC: American Sociological Association.
2. Nagi, S. (1969). *Disability and rehabilitation.* Columbus: Ohio State University Press.
3. Nagi, S. (1991). Disability concepts revisited: Implications for prevention. In A. Pope & A. Tarlow (Eds.). *Disability in America: Toward a national agenda for prevention.* Washington, DC: Institute of Medicine, National Academy Press.
4. World Health Organization. (2001). *ICIDH-2: International classification of function, disability and healthcare.* Geneva, Switzerland. Retrieved January 26, 2013, from http://www.who.int/classifications/icf/site/beginners/bg.pdf
5. *National Advisory Board on Medical Rehabilitation Research, Draft V: Report and Plan for Medical Rehabilitation Research.* (1992). Bethesda, MD: National Institute of Health.
6. The American Physical Therapy Association. (2003). *The guide to physical therapist practice* (2nd ed.). Alexandria, VA: Author. Retrieved January 26, 2013, from http://guidetoptpractice.apta.org
7. Kleinman, A., Eisenberg, L., & Good, B. (1978). Culture, illness, and care: Clinical lessons from anthropologic and cross-cultural research. *Annals of Internal Medicine, 88,* 251–256.
8. American Physical Therapy Association Committee on Cultural Competence. (2008). Blueprint for teaching cultural competence in physical therapy education. Retrieved January 26, 2013, from www.apta.org/search.aspx?=Culturalcompetence
9. Boissonnault, J. S., & Boissonnault, W. G. (2010, 1 December). ECHOWS: Development of a physical therapist assessment instrument for competence in patient history-taking. *Journal of Manual & Manipulative Therapy, 18*(4);, 211. 100669817 (Platform Presentation-Accepted Abstract AAOMPT 2010).
10. Goodman, C. C. & Snyder, T. E (2013). *Differential diagnosis for physical therapists screening for referral.* St. Louis, MO: Elsevier.
11. American Physical Therapy Association. (2012). Components of documentation in Patient/Client Management Model. In *Defensible documentation elements.* Retrieved from http://www.apta.org/Documentation/DefensibleDocumentation/

12. Kettenback, G. (2004). *Writing SOAP notes* (3rd ed.). Philadelphia: F. A. Davis.

13. Centers for Medicare and Medicaid Services. (n.d.). *Medicare guidelines.* Retrieved from http://www.cms.hhs.gov/manuals

14. Center for Medicare and Medicaid Services. (n.d.). *Comprehensive Error Rate Testing Program.* Retrieved from https://www.cms.gov/Research-Statistics-Data-and-Systems/Monitoring-Programs/CERT/index.html?redirect=/CERT/

15. Centers for Medicare and Medicaid Services. (n.d.). *Hospital payment monitoring program.* Retrieved from https://www.cms.gov/Regulations-and-Guidance/Guidance/Manuals/downloads/qio110c11.pdf

16. American Physical Therapy Association. (n.d.). *Defensible documentation for patient/client management.* Retrieved from http://www.apta.org/Documentation/DefensibleDocumentation/ updated on an ongoing basis.

17. Weed, L. L. (1970). *Medical record, medical education, and patient care.* Chicago: Yearbook Medical Publishers.

18. Escorpizo, R., Stucki, G., Cieza, A., Davis, K., Stumbo, T., & Riddle, D. L. (2010). Creating an interface between the International Classification of Functioning, Disability, and Health and physical therapist practice. *Physical Therapy, 90*(7), 1053–1063.

19. Escorpizo, R., Davis, K., & Stumbo, T. (2010). Mapping of a standard documentation template to the ICF core sets for arthritis and low back pain. *Physiotherapy Research International, 15*(4), 222–231.

3

Preparation for Patient Care

LEARNING OUTCOMES

Upon completion of this chapter, you will be able to:

1. State who is responsible for properly managing the patient care environment.
2. Describe general guidelines for properly managing the patient care environment.
3. Describe correct body mechanics for safety of both patients and physical therapists/assistants.
4. Describe clinician position when transporting patients on a gurney or in a wheelchair.
5. Discuss the decision-making tree used to incorporate proper body mechanics when treating patients/clients.
6. Describe the purposes of proper draping.
7. Describe proper draping techniques.
8. Describe how to transport patients safely via gurney or wheelchair.

KEY TERMS

Base of support
Body mechanics
Center of gravity
Draping
Isometric muscle contractions
Proper posture
Valsalva maneuver

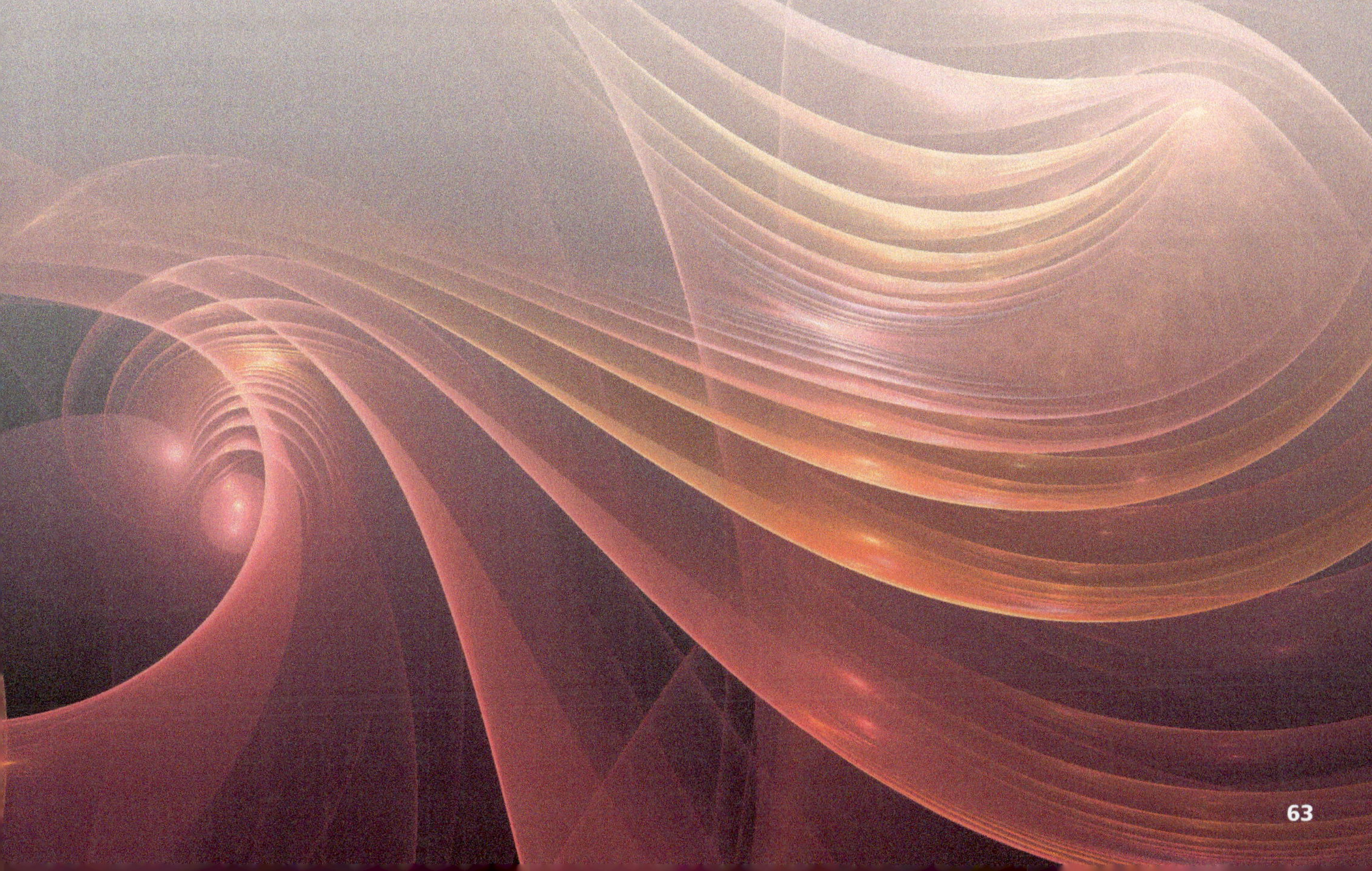

Introduction

Fundamental to all patient care are skills of management of the treatment environment, body mechanics, and communication. By planning and preparing prior to treatment sessions, physical therapists/assistants increase the likelihood of safe, efficient, and effective treatment sessions. Safety of all involved in patient care, both patients and clinicians, must be of paramount consideration at all times.

Management of the Environment

The patient care environment must be organized for protection of patients and clinicians, as well as for efficient use (Figure 3–1 ■). Managing the patient care environment to achieve these goals is a serious responsibility of all clinicians. Physical therapists have the responsibility to ensure that physical therapist assistants and physical therapy support personnel are trained properly in patient care environment management. When tasks are delegated, the physical therapist assistant performing the delegated tasks has responsibility for maintaining a safe and efficient environment for patients and clinicians. The physical therapist delegating the task(s) retains final responsibility for the safe, effective, and efficient performance of those tasks.

Preparation for the next treatment to be given in a patient care area begins at the end of the previous treatment session. Following its use, equipment is cleaned and returned to the proper storage area in a safe, functioning condition. Equipment that is not functioning correctly or is unsafe must be tagged, removed from the treatment area, and reported immediately. Used supplies must be disposed of properly, and unused supplies must be returned to the proper storage area. The person responsible for ordering supplies should be notified in the appropriate manner when consumable supplies are low.

Risk management dictates that all equipment must be inspected to ensure safe function. Annual inspection of all electrical, thermal, and mechanical equipment by a biomedical engineer is required. The physical therapist/assistant is responsible for a simple inspection of equipment, including checking for frayed wiring, worn mechanical parts, and proper function, before each treatment session. Equipment that malfunctions or is determined to be unsafe during any inspection must be removed from use, tagged, and reported at the earliest possible time.

Maintaining clean and orderly environments is part of managing treatment sessions. Some, but not all, tasks to be considered are cleaning of floors, mats, and treatment tables. Proper cleaning of equipment prolongs its life of safe and effective use. Guidelines for safe and clean environments are developed by Centers for Disease Control and Prevention (CDC) and are incorporated into facility policies and procedures. Specifics of some of these procedures are covered in Chapter 4. All facility personnel, not just housekeeping/environmental services personnel, are responsible for following and implementing policies and procedures correctly. Ensuring that the treatment environment is safe and clean is ultimately the responsibility of the supervising physical therapist.

■ Take Note

Everyone is responsible for safe and clean patient care environments.

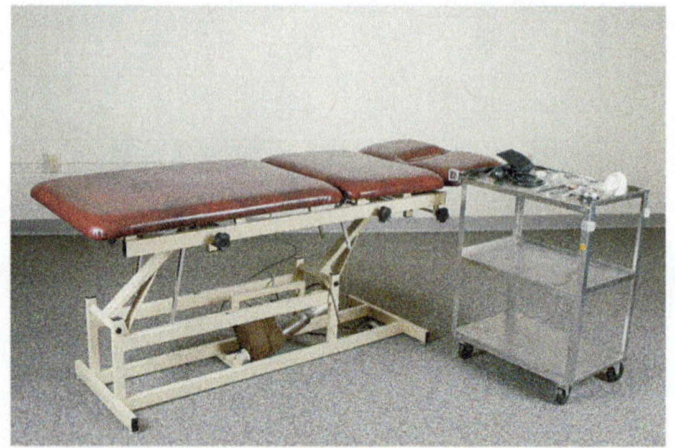

FIGURE 3–1 ■ Preparing a clear patient care environment.

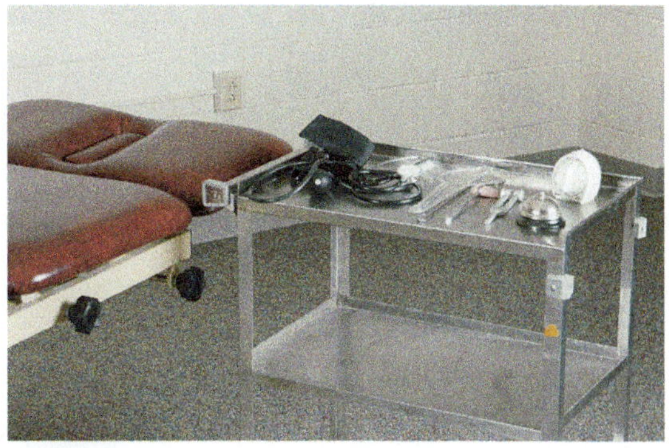

FIGURE 3–2 ■ Equipment and supplies for interventions.

Before initiating any physical therapy patient interaction, the surrounding area is readied. Specific equipment required for a treatment session should be prepared and placed properly prior to escorting a patient into a treatment environment to avoid leaving a patient unguarded or interrupting treatment (Figure 3–2 ■). Treatment tables, mats, chairs, stools, or beds should be prepared before patients arrive in treatment areas. Supplies necessary for treatment areas include linens and pillows. Pillows for patient positioning, comfort, and safety must be within easy reach. Supporting a patient's head while reaching for a misplaced pillow, or leaving a patient in an uncomfortable or unsafe position while equipment is retrieved, is not acceptable patient care. Call bells or patient call buttons must be placed within a patient's reach when patients will be left unattended. Timers, when necessary, must also be available, set properly, and audible to the appropriate personnel. Unneeded equipment and supplies should be removed from any area in which they may interfere with patient care.

■ **Take Note**

Ready treatment areas before bringing the patient into the area.

Adequate room in a treatment environment is necessary for unimpeded movement. Physical therapists/assistants and patients must be able to maneuver in the area without bumping into, or tripping over, equipment. Equipment and furniture not needed during a transport or transfer, such as a mobile stool, should be moved away from the area prior to arrival of patients in treatment areas. Besides getting in the way, many of these pieces of equipment are not stable and become dangerous when patients try to use them as support. When equipment is used in the treatment of a patient/client, you should position the equipment and patient/client to allow easy access to the patient. Improperly positioned equipment may hamper the ability to provide patient assistance quickly.

PROCEDURE 3–1 Body Mechanics

When lifting, lowering, pushing, or pulling, stresses and strains on the musculoskeletal system are increased. Proper **body mechanics** are appropriate adjustments that minimize the unwanted effects of stresses that occur with activity. Proper posture and body mechanics are required to limit stress and strain on musculoskeletal structures of both patients and clinicians. **Proper posture** is appropriate alignment of the musculoskeletal system such that the stresses and strains placed on bones, muscles, ligaments, and cartilage are as minimal as possible. Body mechanics requires strength, range of motion (ROM), and motor control. Proper body mechanics uses these elements to maintain proper skeletal alignment during standing and proper skeletal movement during activity by maintaining the center of gravity within the base of support.

(continued)

PROCEDURE 3–1 Body Mechanics (*continued*)

Although the five cardinal rules of correct body mechanics for lifting are titled for lifting only, they apply to any activity in which a person must lift, lower, push, pull, or carry any object or person. By following these rules, as presented in this procedure, a person can maintain balance and decrease the potential for injury. The five cardinal rules are

1. Keep the load close: Keep the center of gravity of the person or object being lifted/lowered as close as possible to the body of the person performing the lifting/lowering. In this way the center of gravity remains within the base of support. The **center of gravity** is the place in the body on which the force of gravity pulls on the mass of the body.

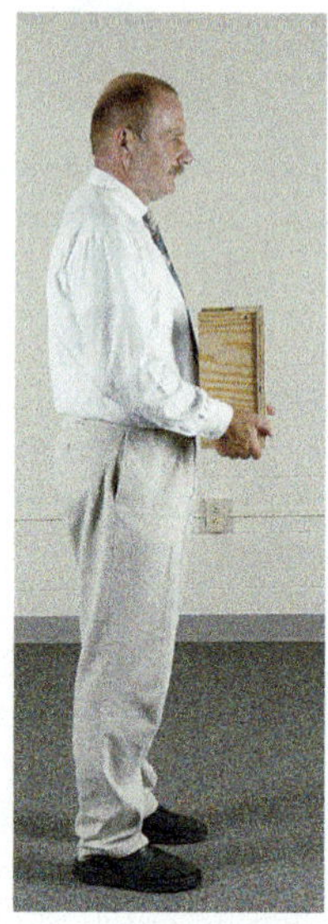

2. Create an appropriate base of support: The **base of support** is defined by the area within the outermost boundaries of a person's contact with the supporting surface. When lifting/lowering, the base of support should be as wide (side to side) and long (front to back) as necessary to maintain balance throughout the lifting/lowering activity. If movement beyond the original base of support is required, an appropriately changing base of support must be maintained. While changing a base of support, avoid awkward positions. When feet must be moved, move in a manner that avoids crossing of the extremities. These strategies decrease the potential for tripping or falling by maintaining an appropriately sized base of support.

3. Use isometric muscle contractions of the trunk (extensor and abdominal muscles): **Isometric muscle contractions** are contractions of skeletal muscle that do not create joint movement. Maintain the trunk in a constant position, preferably erect, during the lifting/lowering activity. Prior to performing the actual lifting/lowering movement, assume a posture of good alignment of the trunk, and perform an isometric contraction of trunk musculature. Creating isometric contractions in the muscles of the trunk prior to lifting can reduce the potential for injury. Although isometric contractions of trunk musculature are used, avoid performing a Valsalva maneuver. A **Valsalva maneuver** is closing of the glottis during heavy exertion resulting in increased intrathoracic and intra-abdominal pressure, which can cause a rapid increase in blood pressure.

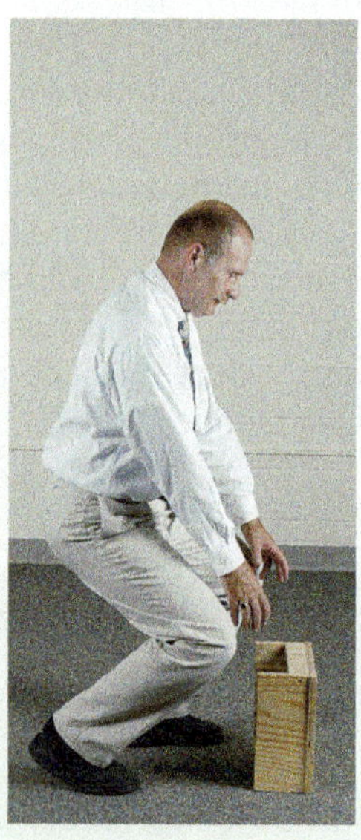

4. Lift with the legs: Lowering yourself by squatting, and raising yourself maintaining an erect trunk, permits use of the large and strong muscles of the legs when lifting and lowering.
5. Do not twist: Avoid rotation of the spine as the lifting/lowering activity is performed. When a change of direction is required, move the feet to achieve the change of direction. Avoid twisting or crossing of the lower extremities, which can decrease the available base of support and interfere with balance, while moving.

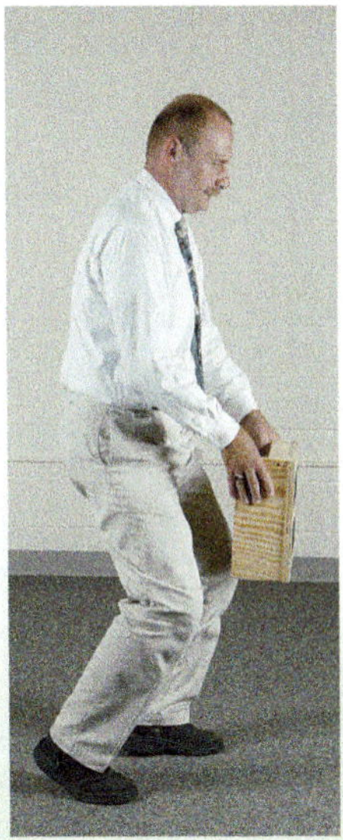

Biomechanics for Lifting, Transfers, and Transport

The initial stance for lifting/lowering requires placing the feet in stride and slightly apart. This stance widens the base of support in both the lateral (side to side) and anterior/posterior (front to back) directions, mitigating the effects of shifts in the center of gravity during lifting/lowering activities. Centering a load within the base of support, and keeping it close to the base of support, aids stability and balance.

The depth of a squat should be sufficient to permit reaching the person or object to be lifted but, if possible, not so deep that the leg muscles are at a disadvantage in regaining the upright position. The person or object is reached by squatting, flexing the hips and knees, rather than flexing the trunk. Trunk position should be set (Rule 3) using isometric contractions. Assuming a position of half-kneeling in preparation for performing a lift is not recommended. When a physical therapist/assistant moves from half-kneeling to standing, an extra step is required to change posture from half-kneeling to squatting. Balance, and thus safety of both the patient and physical therapist/assistant, can be compromised during the maneuver.

■ Take Note

Following rules for proper biomechanics promotes safety of patients and clinicians.

Some transfers require movements that move the center of gravity away from the center of the base of support. These movements have the potential to cause loss of balance as the combined center of gravity moves toward the boundaries of the base of support. Increasing the size of the base of support by setting the feet in stride and slightly apart provides a larger base of support. Proper arrangement of patient and chair, bed, or treatment table reduces the distance to be moved during a transfer. Proper environmental management means that the area is free of unnecessary equipment, allowing room for movement and avoiding interference with free movement of the feet. Avoid crossing the legs (Rule 5) because it decreases the size of the base of support and constrains freedom of foot movement. Specific examples of transfers are presented in Chapter 9.

When guarding a patient during ambulation, position yourself behind the patient, facing in the direction of movement. By positioning yourself behind the patient, you do not obstruct the patient's view and path of movement, and this permits physical therapists/assistants assisting the patient to determine a path free from obstruction and to maintain balance. The same concepts are used when moving large pieces of equipment, such as treadmills or parallel bars. Facing in the direction of movement allows for pushing equipment, rather than pulling it. When pushing equipment, set the trunk muscles by using isometric contractions of the trunk muscles, as when lifting/lowering. Pushing equipment permits use of the strong leg muscles and avoids trunk extension that accompanies a pulling motion.

■ Take Note

The rules for body mechanics apply to gait training.

Specific examples of guarding during ambulation are presented in Chapter 10.

Preparation for Patient Care

For efficient use of treatment time and to limit patient waiting times, preparation of treatment areas should be completed prior to bringing patients into treatment environments. Scheduling patient preparation on the floor and patient transport to physical therapy provides for efficient use of patient and physical therapist/assistant time. When treating patients at the bedside or in private homes, physical therapists/assistants must ensure that environments are safe and ready for activity performance.

Hand hygiene should be done in an appropriate manner before working with each patient and any time that the hands of the physical therapist/assistant become soiled. More information on maintaining hand hygiene and a clean environment is included in Chapter 4.

Appropriate draping for modesty, safety, and effective treatment is the right of every patient and the responsibility of all clinicians. **Draping** is covering a patient appropriately in a manner that maintains patient modesty and comfort. Draping uses a patient's clothing, as well as sheets and towels, to (a) protect patient modesty; (b) provide warmth; (c) protect wounds, scars, and residual limbs; and (d) expose specific body segments for treatment. Secure edges of sheets and towels to avoid shifting of draping material and exposing a patient. Keep sheets, clothing, and draping as smooth as possible to avoid creating pressure points. Planning is necessary to maintain appropriate draping throughout all aspects of treatment sessions.

■ **Take Note**

Maintaining proper draping reassures patients of your concern for them.

Hospital gowns are designed for ease in dressing and access during nursing care and are designed to be donned by the patient with the opening toward the back. Gowns may not provide effective draping during movements, such as transfers, exercise, or gait training. Properly securing the ties of a hospital gown may provide some coverage. Midlength robes or two hospital gowns, with one opening in front and one opening in back, can be used. Long robes may interfere with movement, and their use as draping should be avoided.

Whenever possible, patients should be dressed in slacks or shorts to provide ease of movement without loss of modesty. Shorts are especially useful if a lower extremity must be observed. When slacks or shorts are loose-fitting at the waist, a belt should be worn to prevent slacks or shorts from falling, restricting movement, and posing a safety hazard. A halter top or bra is appropriate when the upper trunk is treated for female patients. Shoes that offer support are required when a patient is to stand, ambulate, or practice transfers. When shoes are worn, socks should be worn for protection, comfort, and sanitation. For nonambulatory patients, slippers may be acceptable, as they are easier to put on and take off. In all situations, decisions concerning dress must be tempered by a patient's needs, safety, a patient's ability to manipulate clothing, and the requirements of treatment.

Gait belts are safety equipment that should be placed on the patient before transfer and gait training. When used properly and under appropriate conditions, gait belts provide a significant margin of safety for patients. Clinical decision making is used to determine how and when a gait belt should be used for safe and effective performance of specific activities. Clinical decision making depends on patient capabilities and the capabilities of the clinician to ensure patient and clinician safety. Decision making about use of gait belts is also based on specific guidelines of each institution.

■ **Take Note**

Ensure that gait belts are properly secured.

Physical therapists/assistants treat patients in a variety of settings. In many settings patients may present with intravenous (IV) lines, chest tubes, urinary catheters, respirators, cardiac monitors, or any combination of these. Take care not to disrupt devices attached to a patient when positioning, transferring, or treating a patient, as these devices are vital to patient well-being. A dislodged chest tube or respirator can be life threatening. When these devices are disrupted, initiate emergency measures properly.

The devices listed limit the amount and ease of movement for patients. Before moving patients or having patients move, check that desired movement can occur without disrupting patient devices. Reposition any devices that may impede safe and effective patient movement. Additional physical therapists/assistants or other clinicians and additional device accessories (such as an IV pole) may be necessary to reposition devices safely. Do not allow tubes or lines to become tangled, pinched, kinked, stretched, or pulled out from their insertion or attachment site. Any of these occurrences will interrupt proper function and can be life threatening. IV drip rates and oxygen flow rates must not be changed without a physician's order. To maintain proper direction of fluid flow, IV fluid containers must remain above the level of the patient's heart, and urinary drainage collection bags must remain below the level of the patient's bladder. Dislodging chest tubes requires replacement of tubes by qualified clinicians. Closing off chest tubes or the chest opening for chest tubes is the immediate action to take when chest tubes are dislodged.

▪ Take Note

Stop, look, listen so proper precautions to manage tubes and lines are taken.

All facilities have policies and procedures for dealing with occurrences of various types of emergencies. Know the policies and procedures for proper implementation of emergency measures. Maintain certification in cardiopulmonary resuscitation, and be capable of providing basic first aid in keeping with institution policies.

Transporting

Transporting is moving patients from one area to another. A gurney (cart) or wheelchair may be required because of patient condition or facility regulations. Patients should be transferred onto/into the required transport device in an appropriate manner while proper draping is maintained throughout transfer and transport. Appropriate methods of selected transfers are covered in Chapter 9.

Physical therapist/assistants often are involved in transporting patients and in teaching patients, families, and caregivers safe methods of transporting. Engage wheel locks on wheelchairs or gurneys before initiating transfers. Adjust patient clothing, draping, and medical devices to avoid the problems discussed previously under *Patient Preparation;* to avoid dragging lines, clothing, or draping on the floor; and to avoid entanglement with wheels during transport. A patient's arms and legs must be within the boundaries of a gurney or wheelchair to avoid injury during transport. Gurneys may have straps or side rails to keep patients within the confines of a gurney, and wheelchairs may have seat belts to keep patients from sliding or falling out of the chair. Additional information with respect to wheelchairs is covered in Chapter 6.

Mattresses on gurneys and cushions on wheelchairs are used for patient comfort and protection. Pillows and padding are positioned for patient comfort and protection as necessary. Appropriate patient positioning is covered in Chapter 7.

PROCEDURE 3–2 Transporting via Gurney

Gurneys have four swivel wheels, making them easier to maneuver from either end. Locks are located on each wheel. Generally there are three positions in which a lock can be set. The three positions in which a lock can be used are (a) to stop wheel swivel, (b) to stop wheel rolling, or (c) to stop both wheel swivel and wheel rolling. Lock locations will vary among different types/brands of gurneys.

1. With the locking lever in a horizontal position, both wheel swivel and wheel rolling movements are permitted.

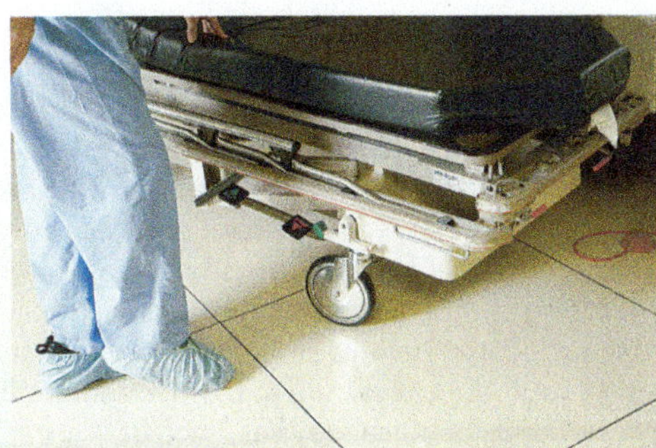

(continued)

PROCEDURE 3–2 Transporting via Gurney (*continued*)

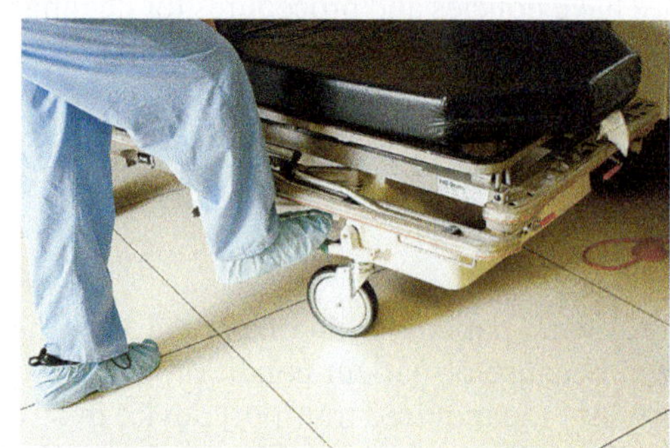

2 When locking levers are tilted in one direction, swivel movements are not possible, and rolling motions are permitted. Tilting locking levers in the other direction locks wheels completely, prohibiting both swivel and rolling movements. Hold the gurney in a stable position, and activate locking levers with your foot.

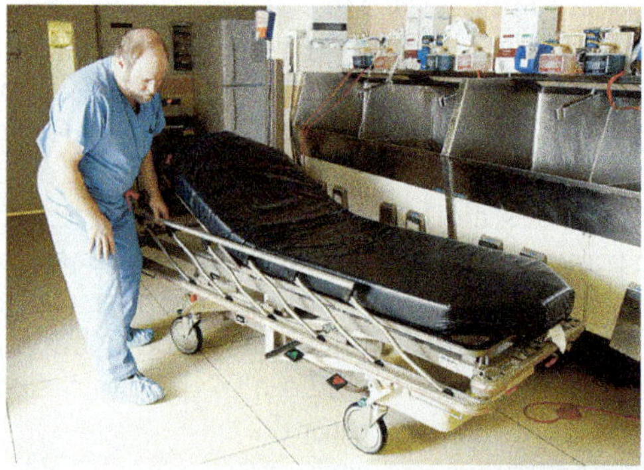

3 Gurney side rails are raised and locked in place before starting transport movement. Gurney side rails are unlocked and lowered for safer transfers once transport movement has stopped.

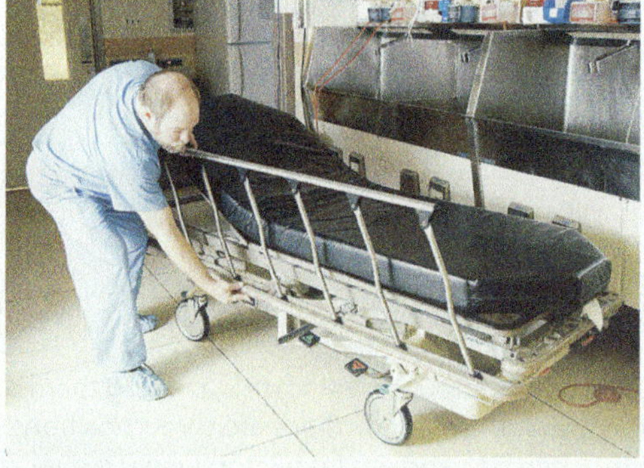

4 Gurney rails have locking mechanisms to secure them in the up position.

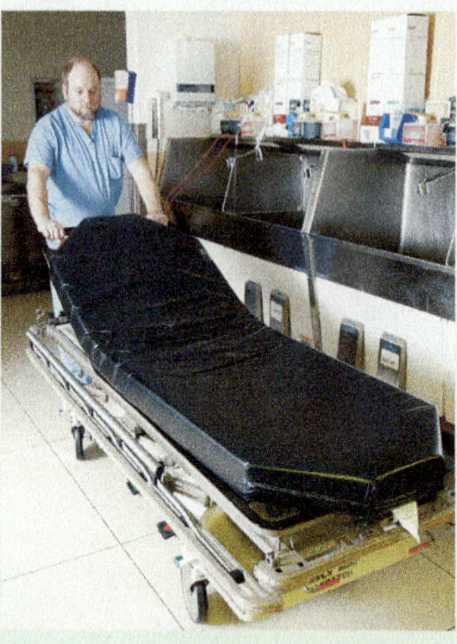

5 Push gurneys from the end at which a patient's head is placed so patients are moving feet first. The pace of transport should be slow and steady. Quick, jerky movements may upset or nauseate patients. Maintain control of gurneys at all times. Turn corners cautiously because of the potential for limited visibility and maneuvering space. Additional clinicians may be needed to maneuver on and off elevators, through doorways, and at blind corners. When necessary, medical devices, such as IVs, can be attached to gurneys at an appropriate height.

PROCEDURE 3–3 Transporting via Wheelchair

Proper patient positioning in a wheelchair includes having patients seated well back on the seat, lower extremities placed on the footrests or leg rests, arms resting on armrests or in laps, and available safety straps or seat belts secured. Push wheelchairs at a slow and steady pace without quick or jerky movements. Maintain control of wheelchairs at all times. When necessary, medical devices such as IVs can be attached to the wheelchair at an appropriate height.

Curbs

The method chosen to ascend and descend curbs depends on the (a) height of the curb, (b) size and weight of the patient and wheelchair, and (c) height and strength of the person transporting the patient. Use proper body mechanics to prevent injury. When descending an average height curb, the backward method places less stress on the person transporting the patient. When ascending an average height curb, the forward method places less stress on the person transporting the patient.

■ Take Note

Check traffic before descending curbs. Go slowly.

Descending Curb—Backward Method

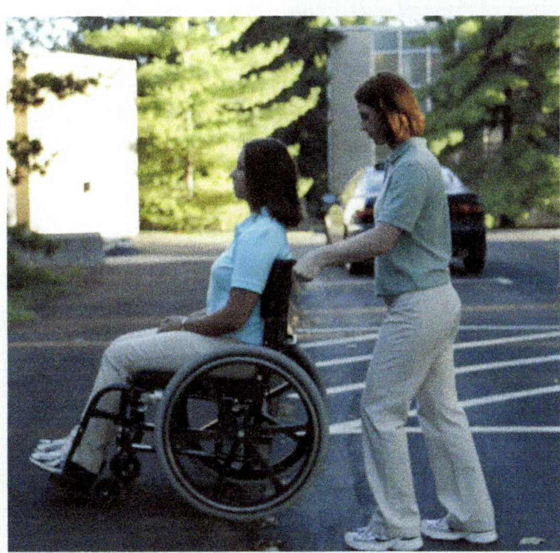

1. To lower a patient in a wheelchair down a curb, position the wheelchair with the patient facing away from the curb. The larger rear wheels are now at the edge of the curb to be descended. Facing the wheelchair from behind, step off the curb backward.

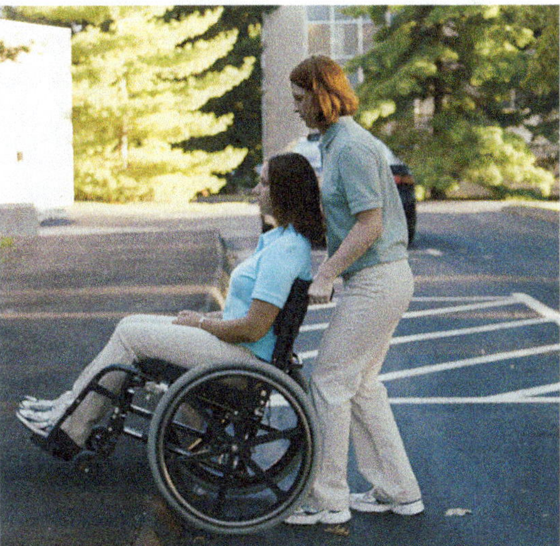

2. Holding onto the wheelchair's push handles, roll the rear wheels of the wheelchair to street level slowly and smoothly.

(continued)

PROCEDURE 3–3 Transporting via Wheelchair (*continued*)

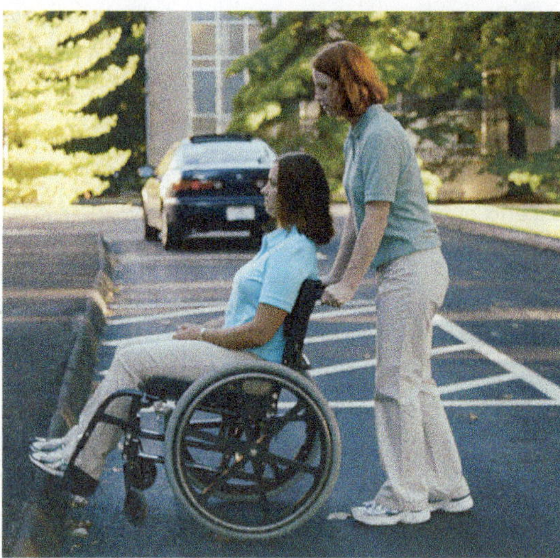

■ **Take Note**

The backward method of descending a curb is the easiest and safest.

3. Securely holding the wheelchair's push handles and maintaining the wheelchair in a tilted position, continue rolling the wheelchair backward until the front wheels and front rigging are clear of the curb. Then lower the front wheels slowly and smoothly until all four wheels are securely on the street level.

Descending Curb—Forward Method

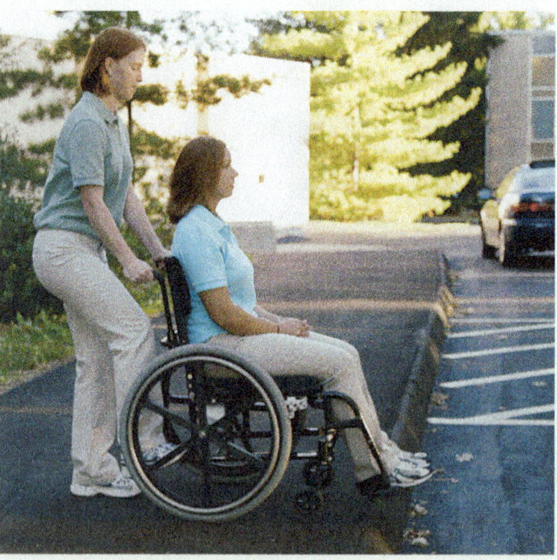

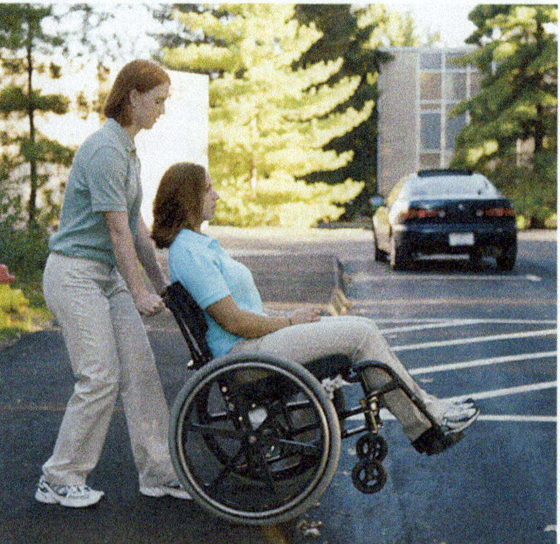

1. Relatively more stress is placed on the person transporting the patient when using this method. The person must maintain backward tilt of the wheelchair while controlling the roll of the wheelchair's rear wheels over the edge of the curb. This method is only recommended for use with low curbs.

2. Position the wheelchair with the front of the wheelchair facing the curb. Face the wheelchair from behind, and tilt the wheelchair backward so the front wheels are approximately 8 inches above the ground. Roll the wheelchair on its rear wheels to the edge of the curb.

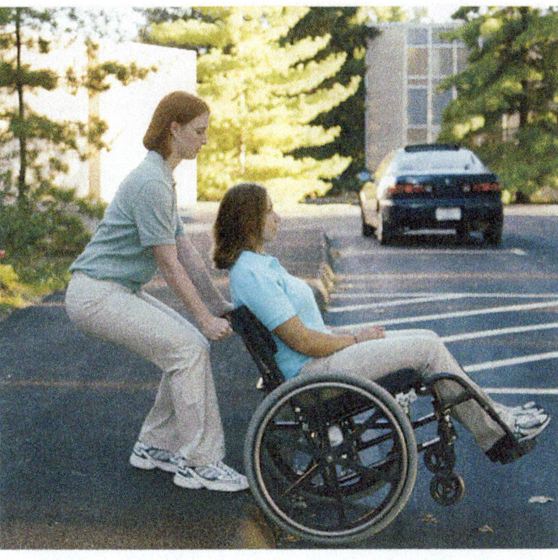

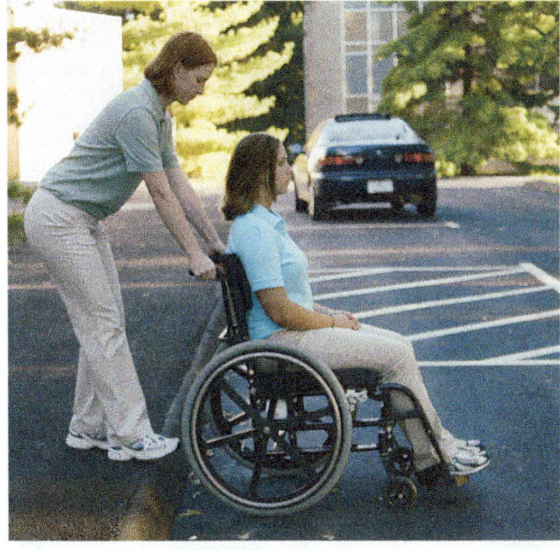

3 The rear wheels of the wheelchair are rolled slowly and smoothly off the curb onto the street level. As the wheelchair rolls over the curb, step forward, flexing the hips and knees to control wheelchair descent.

4 Then slowly lower the front wheels until all four wheels are securely on the street level. Control of the lowering motion may be increased by placing one foot on one of the antitipping bars.

Ascending Curb—Backward Method

This method places relatively more stress on the person transporting the patient. This method is recommended only for use with low curbs.

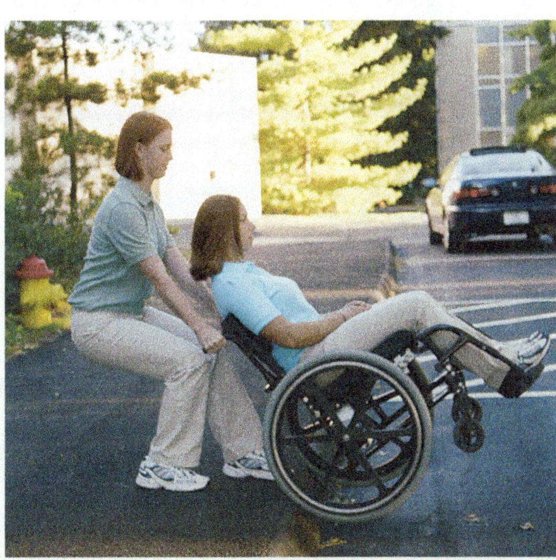

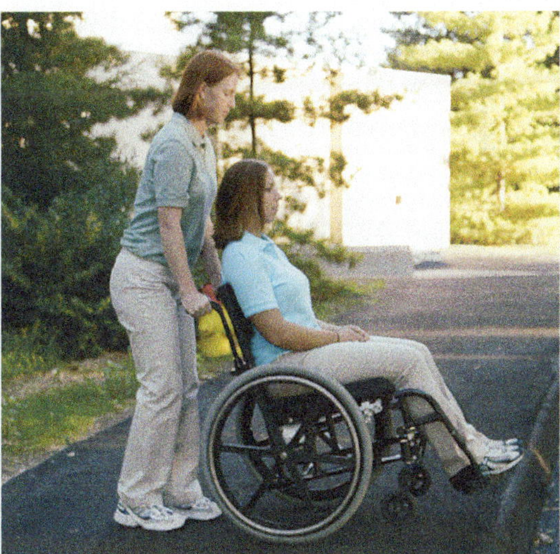

1 Position the wheelchair with the patient facing away from the curb, with the rear wheels of the wheelchair at the edge of the curb. Face the wheelchair from behind, tilt the chair backward, and step backward onto the curb. Position feet on the curb in stride, flex hips and knees, and hold trunk erect. Holding onto the wheelchair's push handles, pull the tilted wheelchair slowly and smoothly up the curb on its rear wheels to sidewalk level.

2 Roll the wheelchair backward until the front wheels are clearly past the edge of the curb and over the sidewalk. Lower the wheelchair slowly and smoothly until all four wheels are securely on the sidewalk. One foot may be placed on one of the antitipping bars to control the rate of lowering the wheelchair onto all four wheels.

(continued)

PROCEDURE 3–3 Transporting via Wheelchair *(continued)*

Ascending Curb—Forward Method

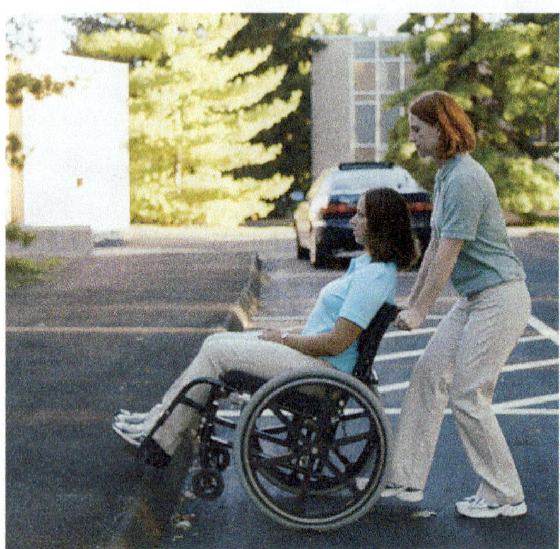

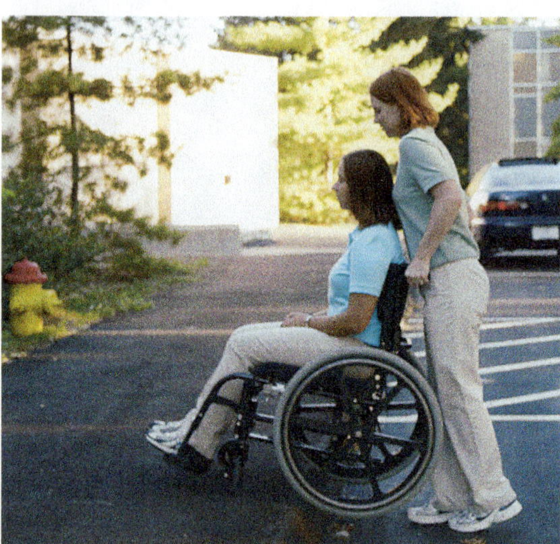

1. Position the wheelchair with the patient facing the curb. Facing the wheelchair from behind, tilt the wheelchair backward so the front wheels are higher than the curb. To assist in tilting the wheelchair safely, one foot may push downward on one of the antitipping bars.

2. Push the wheelchair forward slowly and smoothly until the front wheels are clearly over the sidewalk. The wheelchair is lowered slowly and smoothly until the front wheels are on the sidewalk.

■ Take Note

The forward method of ascending a curb is the easiest and safest.

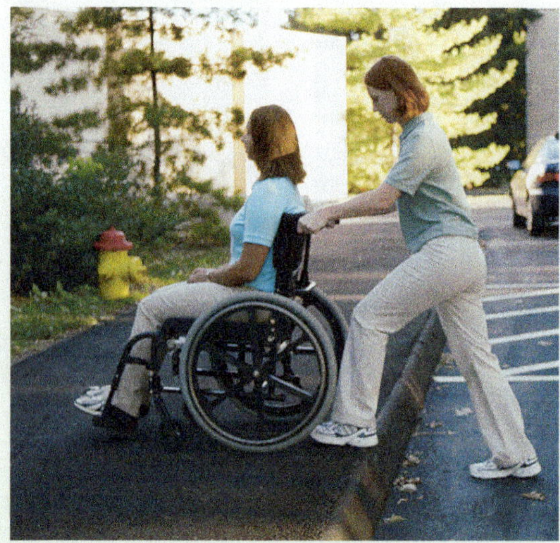

3. Continue to wheel the wheelchair forward until the rear wheels contact the curb. Then push and lift the rear of the wheelchair so the rear wheels roll up and over the curb slowly and smoothly.

Doorways

Most public buildings have automatic doors, both opening and closing, to allow independent access for individuals using ambulation assistive devices. The time an automatic door takes to open or close may vary. There are various degrees of door-closing force on doors with automatic closers. Instruct patients about automatic doors, and encourage them to learn details of opening/closing times and closing forces regarding doors they use frequently. Doors should not be allowed to close and hit either the patient or the wheelchair.

Assisted Progression Through Doorways

Door Opening Away from Patient

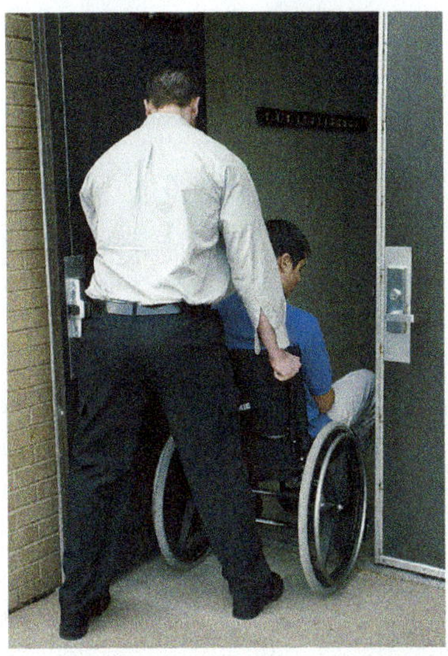

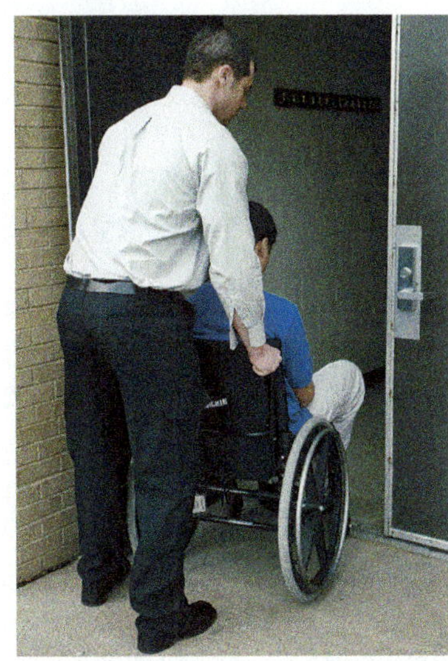

1. To transport patients in wheelchairs through doors opening away from the patient, position the patient facing away from the door. Using the door handles, release the latch of the door. Walk backward through the doorway, pulling the wheelchair backward through the doorway. The person transporting the patient should use his back, shoulder, or foot to open and block the door.

2. As a wheelchair passes the doorjamb, the person transporting the patient uses his body to keep the door open while steering the wheelchair with his hands.

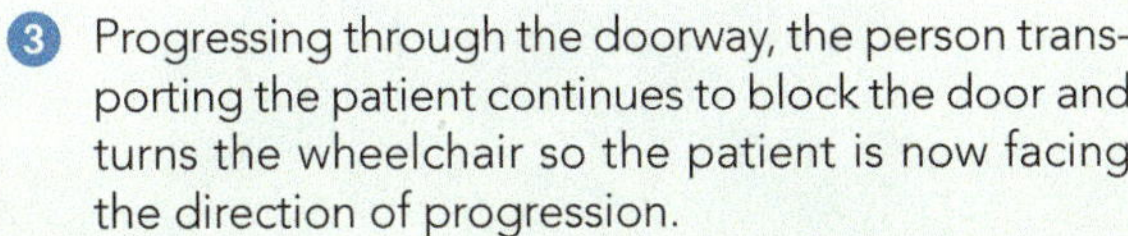

3. Progressing through the doorway, the person transporting the patient continues to block the door and turns the wheelchair so the patient is now facing the direction of progression.

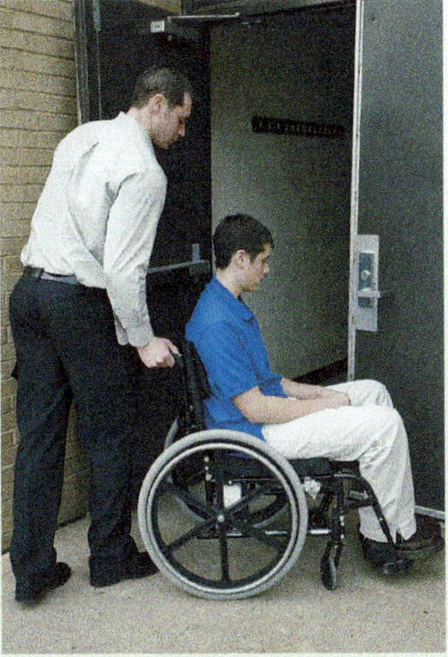

(*continued*)

PROCEDURE 3–3 Transporting via Wheelchair *(continued)*

Door Opening Toward Patient

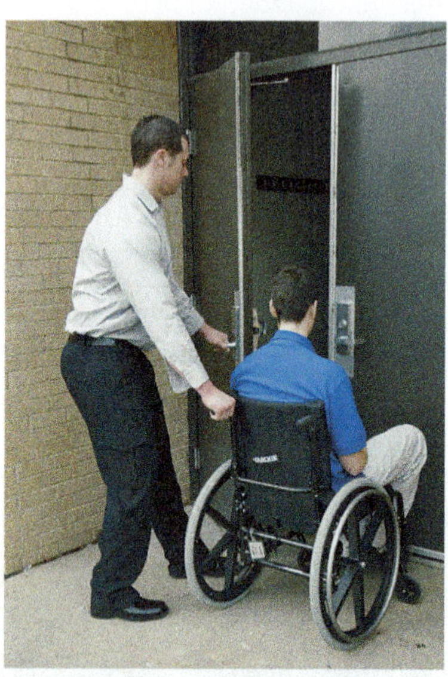

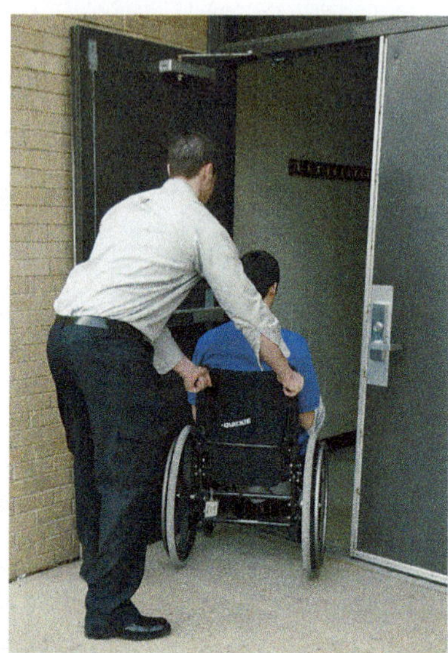

1. Position the patient and wheelchair parallel to the door at the latch side of the door. The person transporting the patient uses one hand to unlatch and pull the door open.

2. Open the door sufficiently for passage of the wheelchair. Block the door open, and align the patient and wheelchair within the doorjamb.

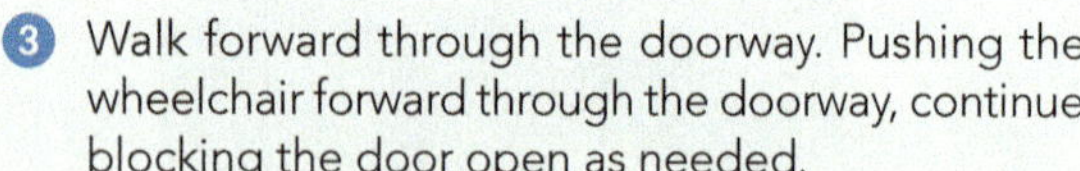

3. Walk forward through the doorway. Pushing the wheelchair forward through the doorway, continue blocking the door open as needed.

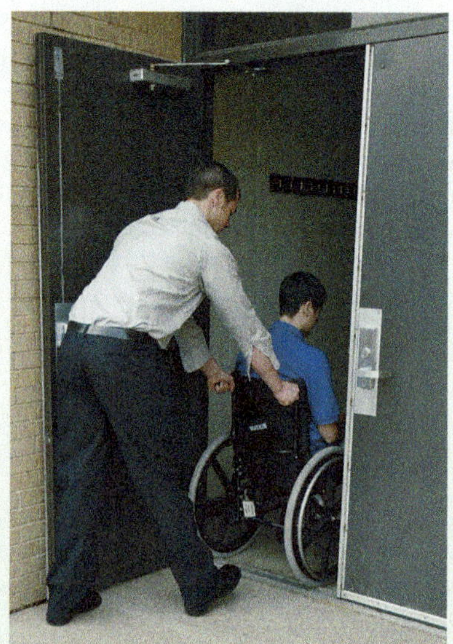

Independent Progression Through Doorways

Techniques for independent wheelchair ambulation through doorways are determined by the (a) abilities of the patient, (b) direction in which doors open, (c) side of doorjamb from which the patient can approach (hinge or latch), (d) available clear space around the doorway, and (e) whether doors are automatic opening/closing doors.

Door Opening Toward Patient (with Automatic Door Closer)

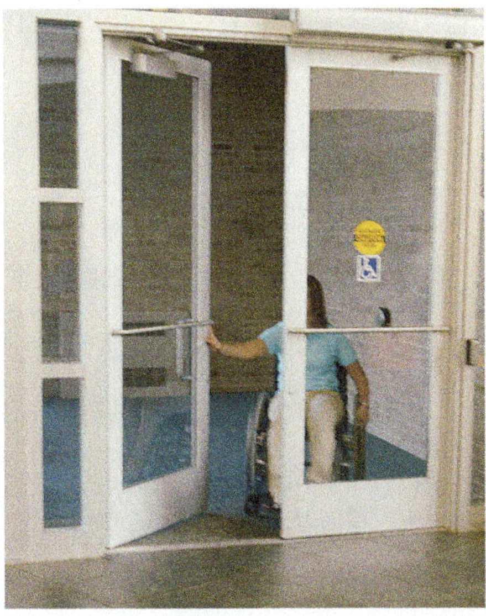

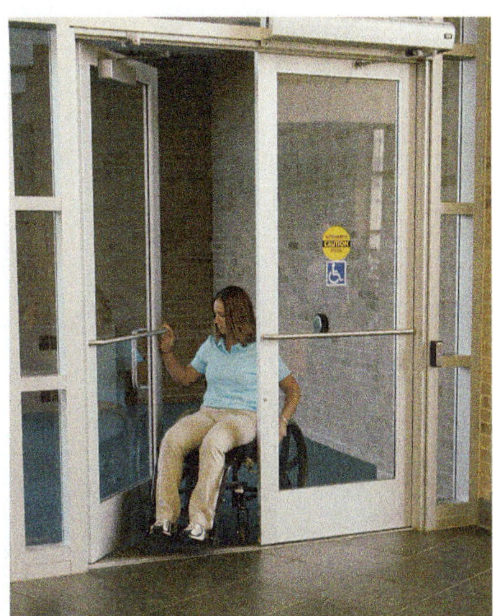

1. The patient wheels to the latch side of the door. When there is ample clear space, the patient stops the wheelchair so that he/she is not in a position that will impede door opening. When there is a lack of clear space around the door, the patient will have to roll the wheelchair up to the handle, and then wheel backward as the door is opened. In either case, the patient's hand on the hinge side of the door grasps the door handle. The patient pulls the door open wider than necessary for progression through the doorway because the door will begin to close prior to the patient completing progression through the doorway.

2. The patient progresses into the doorway quickly to block the closing door. The front rigging of the wheelchair or one of the patient's hands is needed to block open the door. Care must be taken to avoid having closing door strike the patient or hit the wheelchair hard enough to cause a loss of control of the wheelchair and to avoid crushing a patient's fingers between a door and the propulsion wheels as the door is blocked.

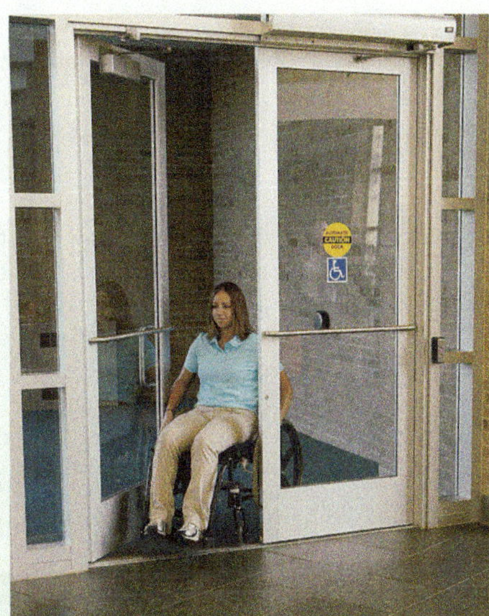

3. Patients may pull on the doorjamb to assist propulsion through the doorway.

(continued)

PROCEDURE 3–3 Transporting via Wheelchair (*continued*)

Door Opens Away from Patient (with Automatic Door Closer)

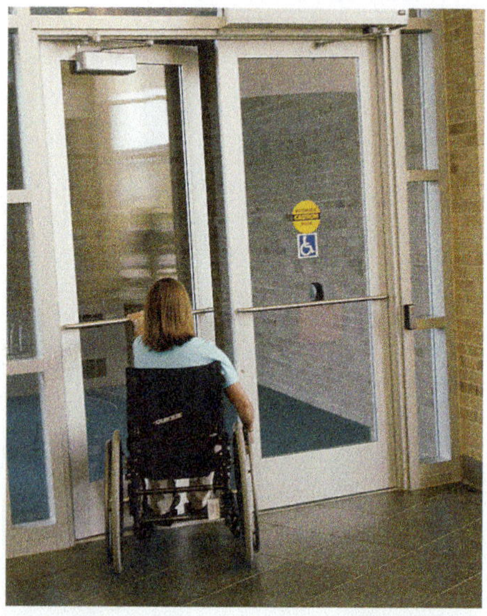

1. The patient approaches the door and grasps the door handle with the hand toward the hinge side of the door.

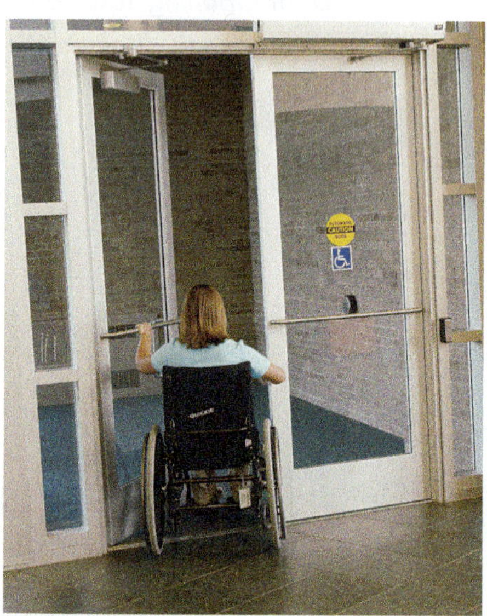

2. Pushing to open the door wide, the patient must enter the doorway before the door closes. While blocking the closing door, propulsion through the doorway may be achieved by (a) rolling though the doorway, (b) pulling on the doorjamb, or (c) using a combination of pulling on the doorjamb and normal propulsion. Take care that the closing door does not strike a patient or hit the wheelchair hard enough to cause a patient to lose control of the wheelchair and to avoid crushing a patient's fingers between a door and the propulsion wheels as the door is blocked.

3. When nearly through the doorway, the door may be given an additional push. The patient then propels the wheelchair quickly out of the arc of the closing door. Then the door is allowed to close behind the patient's wheelchair. When clear space permits, patients can turn their wheelchair around the latch side of the doorjamb to move out of the arc of the closing door more quickly.

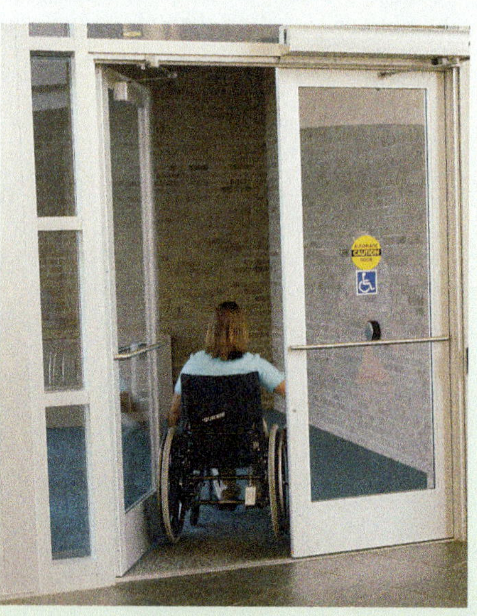

Doors with Patient-Activated Automatic Door Openers (Opening Away/Toward Patient)

Several types of activators are available for automatic door openers. Most commonly, push-plate activators are located along the path to the door at an appropriate height. Alternatively, a pressure activator may be located in the floor in front of the door, or a motion sensor may be used. When doors open toward patients, patients must clear the arc of the opening doors to avoid being struck. The duration a patient-activated automatic door stays open varies. Although doors are usually timed to stay open so patients can progress completely through the doorway prior to closing, patients should not, however, hesitate while progressing through doorways.

Wheelchair Wheelies

Wheelchair wheelies are performed by balancing on the rear wheels of a wheelchair with the (front) caster wheels in the air. Wheelies are used to ascend and descend curbs independently when no curb ramps/cuts are available. Guarding while patients learn to perform wheelies is necessary to prevent injury.

1. Stand behind, and move with, the wheelchair to guard as the patient practices. Position hands beneath or on a wheelchair's push handles, ready to catch the wheelchair if it tilts too far backward.

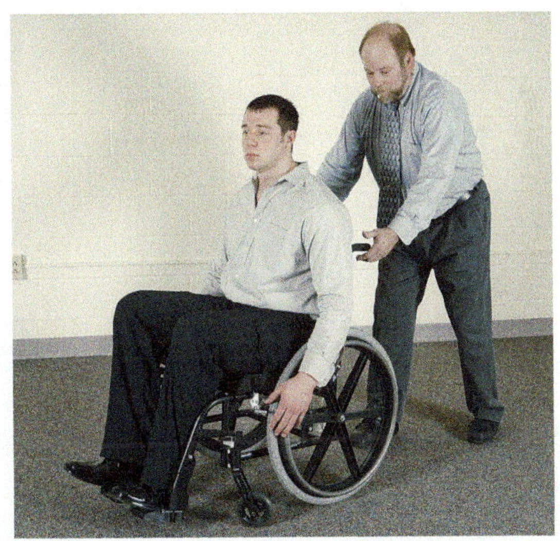

2. The patient begins a wheelie by grasping the anterior portion of the push rims.

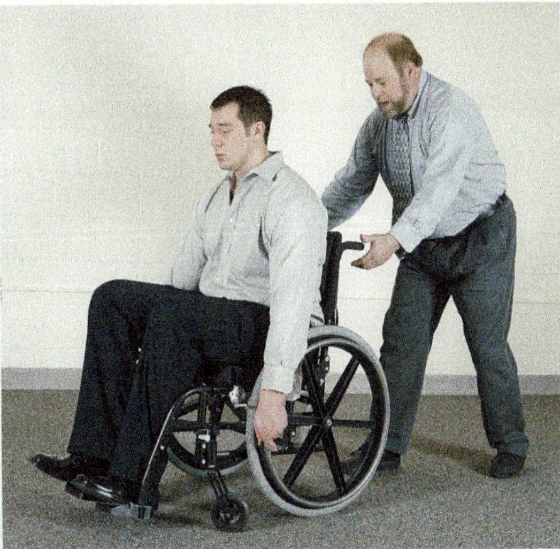

(continued)

PROCEDURE 3–3 Transporting via Wheelchair (*continued*)

3 A quick backward movement equally on both wheels places the patient's hands in position for the forward thrust that achieves the wheelie position.

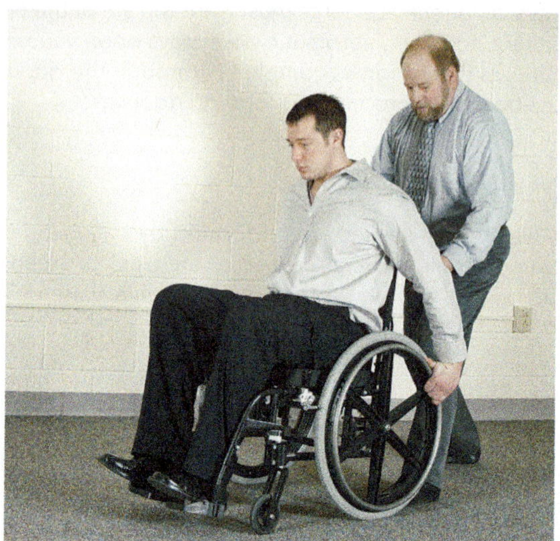

4 The quick backward motion of the wheels is immediately followed by a quick forward thrust on both wheel rims equally. These maneuvers cause the wheelchair to tilt backward, rising onto the rear wheels only.

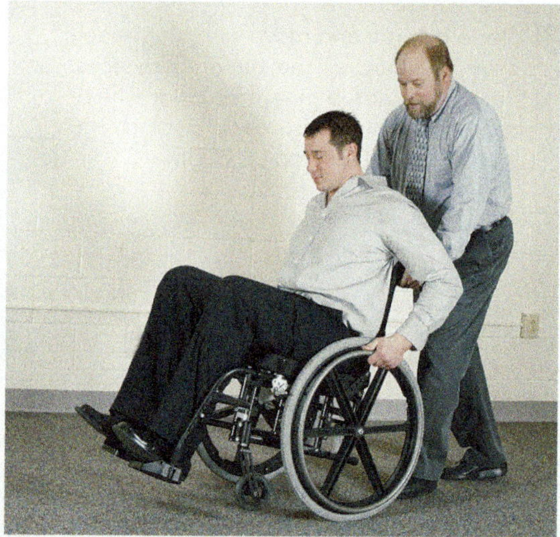

5 Patients control balancing and moving on the rear wheels by forward and backward movements of the rear wheels.

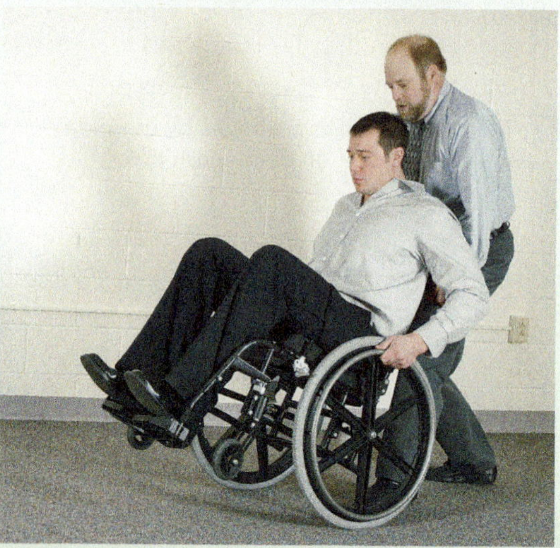

Elevators

When riding in elevators, patients should be positioned facing the elevator door, the position most commonly assumed when riding an elevator. When space is sufficient, a patient may enter an elevator by rolling forward, and then turning around. Patients enter an elevator by rolling backward when space is limited. Facing forward allows patients to monitor floor displays and have access to control panels. Exiting facing forward is usually safer.

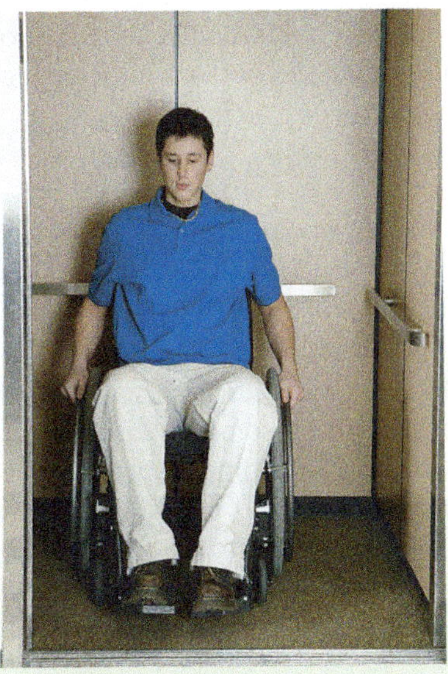

Review Questions

1. Who is responsible for ensuring that patient care environments are safe and efficient?
2. What are the general guidelines for properly managing the patient care environment?
3. What are the five rules of proper body mechanics?
4. How are the rules of proper body mechanics applied in each of the following situations?
   a. When transporting a patient on a gurney
   b. When guarding a patient who is ambulating
   c. When moving large equipment
5. What are the purposes of draping a patient?

Suggested Activities

1. Gurney activities:
   a. Demonstrate correctly locking the wheels of a gurney to permit wheel rolling but not wheel swiveling.
   b. Demonstrate correctly locking the wheels of a gurney prevent both wheel rolling and wheel swiveling.
   c. Demonstrate raising, locking, unlocking, and lowering gurney side rails.
   d. Demonstrate maneuvering a gurney around a corner, alongside a treatment table, and through a doorway.
2. Wheelchair activities:
   a. Demonstrate correctly locking the wheels.
   b. Demonstrate correctly pushing a person in a wheelchair using appropriate body mechanics:
      i. In a hallway and around a corner
      ii. Through a doorway with the door opening toward patient
      iii. Through a doorway with the door opening away from patient
      iv. Down a curb—backward method
      v. Down a curb—forward method
      vi. Up a curb—forward method
      vii. Up a curb—backward method
3. Teach a person to perform a wheelchair wheelie while safely guarding the person.
4. Propel a wheelchair through doorways with automatic closers that:
   a. Open toward patient
   b. Open away from patient
   c. Enter and exit an elevator. While in the elevator determine if all the controls can be reached by a person seated in a wheelchair, including the emergency phone.

5. Discuss experiences in Activities 1–4, including
   a. Perceptions of self when being transported compared to being the person transporting
   b. Perception of the challenges of moving about the environment using a wheelchair
6. Rotate through several stations related to body mechanics. Identify the appropriate principle of body mechanics for safe performance. Suggestions for stations include
   a. Foot Placement: Place foot marks on the floor indicating foot placement. Make some foot placements correct and some incorrect. Students should perform tasks such as lifting boxes from a wheelchair to a mat table, from a wheelchair to a treatment table, and from a table in front to a table behind. Discuss which foot placements are appropriate and why.
   b. Center of Gravity (COG): Carry books in a book bag from the front of a classroom to the rear of a classroom, with the book bag on one shoulder, properly positioned on both shoulders, held in one hand at the side, and held in one hand out in front. Discuss experiences to determine which positions are easier and why.
7. Arrange a treatment area for an initial evaluation of a patient with a fractured tibia post-cast removal.
8. Prepare a patient for treatment by draping to expose the left lower extremity.
9. Document any of the activities using both note formats: SOAP and patient/client management.

Case Studies

1. You are working in a rehabilitation facility with a patient who has a recent complete cervical spinal cord injury. A power wheelchair has been ordered but has not yet been delivered, so transport requires family members to maneuver a manual wheelchair. The patient's family wishes to take her to a restaurant in an older section of town. The family has determined that the restaurant is wheelchair accessible. The parking lot, however, is across the street from the restaurant, and there are no curb ramps on either side of the street. List and describe the transport activities that might be required. Indicate what you would review with the patient and family before their departure for the restaurant.
2. You are to ambulate a patient bedside in an acute care facility. Two patients share the room, resulting in the samll room being crowded. The patient has a history of heart disease, and a cardiac monitor is in place. The patient is receiving oxygen via canula has an IV in the dorsum of the left hand, and has a urinary catheter. List the actions you should take from the time you arrive at the appropriate nurses' station until you actually initiate moving the patient from supine to sitting.

4

Aseptic Techniques

LEARNING OUTCOMES

Upon completion of this chapter, you will be able to:

1. Describe Standard Precautions, who is responsible for implementation, when to implement, and methods of implementation.
2. Describe the requirements and components of a sterile field and guidelines for maintaining sterile fields.
3. Demonstrate proper procedure for donning a sterile gown.
4. Demonstrate proper procedure for donning sterile gloves.
5. Demonstrate proper procedure for removal of contaminated gloves.
6. Describe the purposes and types of wound dressings.
7. List the five major areas of recommendations for isolation precautions.
8. Describe the five modes of transmission of infectious agents.
9. Describe the implementation of selected procedures of isolation precautions.

KEY TERMS

Airborne precautions
Airborne transmission
Antiseptic agent
Aseptic technique
Bacterial barrier
Centers for Disease Control and Prevention (CDC)
Common vehicle transmission
Compression wraps
Contact precautions
Contact transmission
Damp-to-damp dressing
Direct-contact transmission
Disinfection
Droplet precautions
Droplet transmission
Dry-to-dry dressing
Hand antisepsis
Hand hygiene
Handwashing
Hospital Infection Control Practices Advisory Committee (HICPAC)
Indirect-contact transmission
Isolation
Occlusive dressings
Rigid dressings
Shelf life
Spiral wrap
Standard precautions
Sterile field
Sterilization
Transmission-based precautions
Vectorborne transmission

Introduction

Much of the material in this chapter is from publications in the public domain produced by the Centers for Disease Control and Prevention (CDC),[1–4] which is continually updating recommendations for cleaning, disinfecting, and sterile technique based on an increasing body of scientific knowledge. Although the information in this chapter provides a starting point for understanding disease-transmission prevention and practices in aseptic techniques, individuals are strongly advised to become familiar with the specific practices of the institution in which they work and to obtain updated information directly from the CDC on a regular basis. Information can be found at the CDC website by entering a key term such as "Isolation Precautions" in the search box. The contact information for the CDC is

Centers for Disease Control and Prevention

1600 Clifton Rd, Atlanta, GA 30333

800-232-4636/(800-CDC-INFO)

www.cdc.gov

The prevention of disease transmission in healthcare settings is of major concern.[2,3] Each institution is responsible for following up-to-date information from the CDC. Institutions develop information and protocols specific to that institution, which can be obtained from the appropriate department within the institution. It is everyone's job to follow institutional protocols for the benefit of patients and employees. Physical therapists/assistants must recognize situations where patients and healthcare providers are at risk from transmission of microorganisms and implement appropriate measures. The information provided in this chapter is a resource that can assist in developing and reviewing existing policies and procedures. All the guidelines are not appropriate for every healthcare setting. The detail that the CDC provides should impress on all the importance of infection control.

Although the concepts of cleanliness and aseptic technique in patient care have been in use during the past two centuries, changes in these techniques occur from time to time as the result of research on the prevention of disease transmission.

In 1970, the **Centers for Disease Control and Prevention (CDC)** recommended **isolation** procedures that have been updated/revised a number of times. In keeping with the concept of evidence-based practice, CDC established requirements in 1997 that mandated guidelines to (1) have a basis that is epidemiologically sound; (2) emphasize the importance of all body fluids, secretions, and excretions in the transmission of infectious agents; (3) contain adequate precautions for infections transmitted by the airborne, droplet, and contact routes of transmission; (4) be simple to understand and use; and (5) use new terms to avoid confusion with existing systems. CDC guidelines published in 2007 encompass updated recommendations and emphasize that these guidelines cover all healthcare settings, and not just hospitals. Current specific infection control recommendations are contained in the CDC's *Guidelines for Isolation Precautions: Preventing Transmission of Infectious Agents in Healthcare Settings 2007.*

Take Note

Isolation precautions are aimed at preventing disease transmission.

The CDC and its **Hospital Infection Control Practices Advisory Committee (HICPAC)**, operating within the Department of Health and Human Services, are responsible for issuing guidelines related to prevention of disease transmission. The Occupational Safety and Health Agency (OSHA), an agency of the federal government, establishes rules and regulations for the protection of workers. These rules and regulations include the implementation of CDC guidelines for infection control in healthcare facilities.

Definitions

Some, but not all, terms related to *Aseptic Techniques* are defined here.

Alcohol-based hand rub: An alcohol-containing preparation designed for application to the hands for reducing the number of viable infectious agents on the hands. In the United States, such preparations usually contain 60% to 95% ethanol or isopropanol.

Antimicrobial soap: Soap (i.e., detergent) containing an antiseptic agent.

Antiseptic agent: Antimicrobial substances that are applied to the skin to reduce the number of microbial flora. Examples include alcohols, chlorhexidine, chlorine, hexachlorophene, iodine, chloroxylenol (PCMX), quaternary ammonium compounds, and triclosan.

Antiseptic hand rub: Antiseptic hand rub applied to all surfaces of the hands to reduce the number of infectious agents present.

Antiseptic hand wash: Washing hands with water and soap or other detergents containing an antiseptic agent.

Aseptic technique: The methods and procedures used to create and maintain a sterile field.

Bacterial barrier: A barrier that keeps infectious agents from coming in contact with sterile items.

Cleanliness: Three levels of cleanliness—cleaning, disinfection, and sterilization—have been established for equipment use in patient care.

Cleaning: The physical removal of organic material or soil from objects. The process of cleaning is usually performed with water, with or without detergents. Cleaning is the least rigorous of the three levels and is designed to remove infectious agents rather than kill them. Cleaning usually precedes either of the next two levels, disinfection or sterilization.

Disinfection: An intermediate level between cleaning and sterilization. Three levels of disinfection—high, intermediate, and low—have been defined. Disinfection is usually performed using pasteurization or chemical germicides.

Sterilization: The highest level of cleanliness. Sterilization is the destruction of all forms of microbial life by steam under pressure, liquid or gaseous chemicals, or dry heat.

Contaminated: An item, surface, or field that comes in contact with anything that is not sterile.

Decontaminate hands: To reduce bacterial counts on hands by performing antiseptic hand rub or antiseptic hand wash.

Detergent: Compounds that possess a cleaning action. Detergents (i.e., surfactants) are composed of both hydrophilic and lipophilic parts and can be divided into four groups: anionic, cationic, amphoteric, and nonionic detergents. Although products used for handwashing or antiseptic hand wash in healthcare settings represent various types of detergents, the term *soap* is used to refer to such detergents in this guideline.

Hand antisepsis: Either antiseptic hand wash or antiseptic hand rub.

Hand hygiene: A general term that applies to handwashing, antiseptic hand wash, antiseptic hand rub, or surgical hand antisepsis.

Handwashing: Washing hands with plain (i.e., nonantimicrobial) soap and water.

Healthcare infection: Infection acquired in any healthcare environment.

Isolation: Separation and placement of patients in environments that reduce the potential for transmission of infectious agents.

Mask: A nonactive device that filters environmental air.

Nosocomial infection: Infection acquired while hospitalized for treatment of other conditions.

Patient-care equipment categories: Three categories of patient care equipment—critical, noncritical, and semicritical[2,3]—provide a basis for the level of cleanliness deemed necessary.

Critical items: Introduced directly into the circulatory system or other normally sterile areas of the body. Surgical instruments, implants, and the blood compartment of a hemodialyzer are examples of critical items.

Noncritical items: Do not touch the patient or touch the patient in areas that are normally not sterile, such as intact areas of skin. Blood pressure cuffs and crutches are examples of noncritical items.

Semicritical items: Introduced into body cavities not usually considered sterile and include, but are not limited to, endotracheal tubes and fiberoptic endoscopes. There is a lower degree of risk of infection associated with semicritical items.

Plain soap: Detergents that do not contain antimicrobial agents or that contain low concentrations of antimicrobial agents that are effective solely as preservatives.

Recommendations ranking scheme: The CDC's Center for Infectious Diseases has established four categories to indicate the scientific support for their recommendations.[3]

Category IA: Strongly recommended for all hospitals and strongly supported by well-designed experimental or epidemiologic studies.[3]

Category IB: Strongly recommended for all hospitals and reviewed as effective by experts and a consensus of HICPAC, based on strong rationale and suggestive evidence, although definitive scientific studies have not been done.[3]

Category II: Suggested for implementation in many hospitals. Recommendations may be supported or suggested by clinical or epidemiologic studies, a strong theoretical rationale, or definitive studies applicable to some, but not all, hospitals.[3]

No recommendation/unresolved issues: Practices for which insufficient evidence or consensus regarding efficacy exists.[3]

Respirator: A mechanical device that provides a source of air not associated with the immediate environment.

Shelf life: The length of time an unopened sterilized package is considered to remain sterile.

Standard precautions: Precautions designed for the care of all patients, particularly hospitalized patients, regardless of their diagnosis or presumed infection status. This is new terminology to replace the term *universal precautions.*

Sterile: An item or environment free from living infectious agents.

Sterile field: An area considered free from living infectious agents.

Surgical hand antisepsis: Antiseptic hand wash or antiseptic hand rub performed preoperatively by surgical personnel to eliminate transient, and reduce resident, hand flora. Antiseptic detergent preparations often have persistent antimicrobial activity.

Unsterile (nonsterile): Any item or environment that has not been sterilized, has come into contact with an item that is no longer considered sterile, has entered a field that is not sterile, or has exceeded its shelf life.

Waterless antiseptic agent: An antiseptic agent that does not require use of exogenous water. After applying such an agent, the hands are rubbed together until the agent has dried.

Preventing Transmission of Infection

Transmission of infection requires three elements: (1) a source of infecting infectious agents, (2) a susceptible host, and (3) a means of transmission for the infectious agent. Human sources of infecting infectious agents in hospitals may be patients, personnel, or visitors. Included may be persons (1) with acute disease, (2) in the incubation period of a disease, (3) who are colonized by an infectious agent but have no apparent disease, or (4) who are chronic carriers of an infectious agent. Other sources of infectious agents can be the patient's own endogenous flora and contaminated environmental objects, such as equipment and medications. Host factors that may render patients more susceptible to infection include, but are not limited to, (1) age; (2) underlying diseases; (3) certain treatments with antimicrobials, corticosteroids, or other immunosuppressive agents; (4) irradiation; and (5) breaks in the first line of defense mechanisms caused by surgical operations, anesthesia, and indwelling catheters.

Modes of Transmission

Infectious agents are transmitted by several routes, and the same infectious agent may be transmitted by more than one route. The five main routes of transmission are (1) contact, (2) droplet, (3) airborne, (4) common vehicle, and (5) vectorborne. Agent and host factors are less controllable than transmission routes when attempting to avoid infection. Therefore CDC recommendations are based on preventing infection by controlling the route(s) of transmission.

■ Take Note

Modes of transmission include contact, droplet, airborne, common vehicle, and vectorborne.

Transmission-Based Precautions

Transmission-based precautions are designed for use with specific patients who have, or may be susceptible to, infection by epidemiologically important pathogens. Epidemiologically important pathogens are those pathogens that are highly transmissible and for which specific precautions are needed to interrupt transmission. The three types of **transmission-based precautions** are (1) contact, (2) droplet, and (3) airborne. The three types of transmission-based precautions may be used singly or in combination and are used in addition to standard precautions, as described in detail next.

Contact transmission, the most important and frequent mode of healthcare infection transmission, is divided into two subgroups: direct-contact transmission and indirect-contact transmission. **Direct-contact transmission** involves direct body-surface-to-body-surface contact and physical transfer of infectious agents between a susceptible host and an infected or colonized person. This may occur when (1) turning or transferring a patient, (2) performing other patient-care activities that require direct personal contact, or (3) direct contact between patients. **Indirect-contact transmission** involves contact of a susceptible host with a contaminated intermediate object, usually inanimate, such as multiple-use of single-use equipment. Examples are reuse of self-adhesive electrodes on more than one patient and linens or gloves that are not changed between patients.

Droplet transmission is a form of contact transmission in which the mechanism of transfer of infectious agents is quite distinct from either direct- or indirect-contact transmission. Some droplets do not remain suspended in the air, and thus droplet transmission is considered different than airborne transmission. Generation of droplets arises primarily when a source person coughs, sneezes, or talks or during the performance of certain procedures such as suctioning or wound care. Transmission occurs when droplets containing infectious agents generated from the infected person are propelled a short distance through the air and deposited on a host's conjunctivae, nasal mucosa, or mouth.

Airborne transmission occurs through transport of infectious agents as droplet nuclei and on other particles. Droplet nuclei are small residues that remain when fluid from infected hosts evaporates and remain suspended in the air for long periods of time. Particles containing infectious agents are dispersed widely by air currents and inhaled by a susceptible host through the respiratory tract. The distance over which such dissemination may occur is dependent on environmental factors, thus special air handling and ventilation are required to prevent airborne transmission.

Common vehicle transmission applies to infectious agents transmitted by contaminated items such as food, water, medications, devices, and equipment.

Vectorborne transmission occurs when vectors such as mosquitoes, flies, rats, and other vermin transmit infectious agents; this route of transmission is of less significance in hospitals in the United States than in other regions of the world.

Guidelines for Implementing Isolation Procedures

The CDC has defined three crucial areas when outlining guidelines to be used for patients placed in isolation.[3] Implementation and maintenance of isolation measures in healthcare settings requires (1) administrative controls, (2) standard precautions, and (3) transmission-based precautions. Transmission-based precautions include (1) contact, (2) droplet, and (3) airborne transmission. Current CDC recommendations for these areas are at the Category IB level.

▪ Take Note

Category IB recommendations are indicated based on rationale and suggested evidence.

Administrative Controls

Administrative controls entail development of, and adherence to, policies and procedures that govern infection control in healthcare settings. CDC guidelines must be supplemented by policies and procedures for other aspects of infection and environment control, occupational health, and administrative and legal issues in healthcare settings. Information about these policies and procedures should be provided during orientation of newly hired personnel whenever changes are made. Physical therapists/assistants are responsible for knowing and following these policies and procedures. Although physical therapists/assistants are not responsible for some decisions made in care of patients related to infection control, knowing policies and procedures, however, is informative. As an example, for in-patient facilities, patients with an infection or at high risk from infection are placed in private rooms to indicate precautions to prevent transmission of microorganisms are to be implemented.

Examples of administrative controls include, but are not limited to:

Education: Develop a system to ensure that hospital patients, personnel, and visitors are educated about use of precautions and their responsibility for adherence to them.

Personal Protective Equipment (PPE): Provide PPE and education in appropriate use of PPE.

Patient Care Equipment: Develop procedures for cleaning, disinfecting, and sterilization of patient care equipment.

Adherence to Precautions: Evaluate adherence to precautions and use findings to direct improvements.

Standard Precautions

Standard precautions combine the major features of universal precautions (UP) and body substance isolation (BSI) and are based on the principle that all body fluids (blood, secretions, and excretions except sweat), nonintact skin, and mucous membranes may contain transmissible infectious agents. Standard precautions include a group of infection-prevention practices that apply to all patients, regardless of suspected or confirmed infection status, in any setting in which health care is delivered. These include (1) hand hygiene; (2) use of gloves, gown, mask, eye protection, or face shield, depending on the anticipated exposure; and (3) safe injection practices. Also, equipment or items in the patient environment likely to have been contaminated with infectious body fluids must be handled in a manner to prevent transmission of infectious agents (e.g., wear gloves for direct contact, contain heavily soiled equipment, properly clean and disinfect or sterilize reusable equipment before use on another patient). The application of standard precautions during patient care is determined by the nature of the healthcare worker (HCW)–patient interaction and the extent of anticipated blood, body fluid, or pathogen exposure. For some interactions (e.g., performing venipuncture), only gloves may be needed; during other interactions (e.g., wound debridement), use of gloves, gown, face shield or mask, and goggles may be necessary. Education and training on the principles and rationale for recommended practices are critical elements of standard precautions because they facilitate appropriate decision making and promote adherence when HCWs are faced with new circumstances. An example of the importance of the use of standard precautions is wound debridement with a water spray where splashes may spread microorganisms to the practitioner. Standard precautions are also intended to protect patients by ensuring that healthcare personnel do not carry infectious agents to patients on their hands or via equipment used during patient care.

■ Take Note

Standard precautions are to be used with all patients.

Elements of Standard Precautions

Infection control problems that are identified in the course of outbreak investigations often indicate the need for additional recommendations or reinforcement of existing infection control recommendations to protect patients. Because such recommendations are considered a standard of care and may not be included in other guidelines, they have been added to standard precautions. Three such areas of practice that have been added are respiratory hygiene/cough etiquette, safe injection practices, and the use of masks for insertion of catheters or injection of material into spinal or epidural spaces via lumbar puncture procedures (e.g., myelogram, spinal, or epidural anesthesia). Although most elements of standard precautions evolved from universal precautions that were developed for protection of healthcare personnel, these elements of standard precautions focus on protection of patients.

Respiratory Hygiene/Cough Etiquette

The transmission of SARS-CoV in emergency departments by patients and their family members during the widespread SARS outbreaks in 2003 highlighted the need for vigilance and prompt implementation of infection control measures at the first point of encounter within a healthcare setting (e.g., reception and triage areas in emergency departments, outpatient clinics, and physician offices). The strategy proposed has been termed respiratory hygiene/cough etiquette and is intended to be incorporated into infection control practices as a new component of standard precautions. The strategy is targeted at patients and accompanying family members and friends with undiagnosed transmissible respiratory infections and applies to any person with signs of illness, including cough, congestion, rhinorrhea, or increased production of respiratory secretions when entering a healthcare facility. The term *cough etiquette* is derived from recommended source control measures for *Mycobacteria tuberculosis.* The elements of respiratory hygiene/cough etiquette include (1) education of healthcare facility staff, patients, and visitors; (2) posted signs, in language(s) appropriate to the population served, with instructions to patients and accompanying family members or friends; (3) source control measures (e.g., covering the mouth/nose with a tissue when coughing and prompt disposal of used tissues, use of a surgical mask on the coughing person when tolerated and appropriate); (4) hand hygiene after contact with respiratory secretions; and (5) spatial separation, ideally greater than 3 feet, of persons with respiratory infections in common waiting areas when possible. Covering sneezes and coughs and placing masks on coughing patients are proven means of source containment that prevent infected persons from dispersing respiratory secretions into the air. Masking may be difficult in some settings (e.g., pediatrics, in which case the emphasis by necessity may be on cough etiquette). Physical proximity of less than 3 feet has been associated with an increased risk for transmission of infections via the droplet route (e.g., *Neisseria meningitidis* and group A streptococcus) and, therefore, supports the practice of distancing infected persons from others who are not infected. The effectiveness of good hygiene practices, especially hand hygiene, in preventing transmission of viruses and reducing the incidence of respiratory infections both within and outside healthcare settings is summarized in several reviews.

▪ Take Note

Respiratory hygiene/cough etiquette is just like mom says—cover your mouth and nose with a tissue when sneezing/coughing.

Respiratory hygiene and cough etiquette should be effective in decreasing the risk of transmission of pathogens contained in large respiratory droplets (e.g., influenza virus, adenovirus, *Bordetella pertussis,* and *Mycoplasma pneumonia*). Although fever will be present in many respiratory infections, patients with pertussis and mild upper respiratory tract infections are often afebrile. The absence of fever, however, does not always exclude a respiratory infection. Patients who have asthma, allergic rhinitis, or chronic obstructive lung disease also may be coughing and sneezing. Although these patients often are not infectious, cough etiquette measures are prudent.

▪ Take Note

Healthcare workers should protect themselves by using masks and proper hand hygiene when in contact with patients who have respiratory infections.

Healthcare personnel are advised to observe droplet precautions (i.e., wear a mask) and practice hand hygiene when examining and caring for patients with signs and symptoms of a respiratory infection. Healthcare personnel who have a respiratory infection are advised to avoid direct patient contact, especially with high-risk patients. If this is not possible, then a mask should be worn while providing patient care.

Standard Precaution Guidelines

Assume that every person is potentially infected or colonized with an organism that could be transmitted in the healthcare setting, and apply the following infection control practices during the delivery of health care.

A. Hand hygiene

1. During the delivery of health care, avoid unnecessary touching of surfaces in close proximity to the patient to prevent both contamination of clean hands from environmental surfaces and transmission of pathogens from contaminated hands to surfaces.
2. When hands are visibly dirty, contaminated with proteinaceous material, or visibly soiled with blood or body fluids, wash hands with either a nonantimicrobial or antimicrobial soap and water.
3. If hands are not visibly soiled, or after removing visible material with nonantimicrobial soap and water, decontaminate hands in clinical situations. The preferred method of hand decontamination is with an alcohol-based hand rub. Alternatively, hands may be washed with an antimicrobial soap and water. Frequent use of

alcohol-based hand rub immediately following handwashing with nonantimicrobial soap may increase the frequency of dermatitis. Perform hand hygiene:

a. Before having direct contact with patients.

b. After contact with blood, body fluids or excretions, mucous membranes, nonintact skin, or wound dressings.

c. After contact with a patient's intact skin (e.g., when taking a pulse or blood pressure or lifting a patient).

d. If hands will be moving from a contaminated body site to a clean body site during patient care.

e. After contact with inanimate objects (including medical equipment) in the immediate vicinity of the patient.

f. After removing gloves.

4. Wash hands with nonantimicrobial or antimicrobial soap and water if contact with spores (e.g., *Clostridium difficile* or *Bacillus anthracis*) is likely to have occurred. The physical action of washing and rinsing hands under such circumstances is recommended because alcohols, chlorhexidine, iodophors, and other antiseptic agents have poor activity against spores. Steps to proper handwashing:

   a. Hands should be washed using soap and warm, running water.

   b. Hands should be rubbed vigorously during washing for at least 20 seconds with special attention paid to the backs of the hands, wrists, between the fingers, and under fingernails.

   c. Hands should be rinsed well while leaving the water running.

   d. With the water running, hands should be dried with a single-use towel.

   e. Turn off the water using a paper towel, covering washed hands to prevent recontamination.

5. Do not wear artificial fingernails or extenders if duties include direct contact with patients at high risk for infection and associated adverse outcomes (e.g., those in ICUs or operating rooms). As an administrative control, an institution should develop an organizational policy on the wearing of nonnatural nails by healthcare personnel who have direct contact with patients outside the groups specified earlier.

B. PPE

1. Observe the following principles of use:

   a. Wear PPE when the nature of the anticipated patient interaction indicates that contact with blood or body fluids may occur.

   b. Prevent contamination of clothing and skin during the process of removing PPE.

   c. Before leaving the patient's room or cubicle, remove and discard PPE.

2. Gloves

   a. Wear gloves when it can be reasonably anticipated that contact with blood or other potentially infectious materials, mucous membranes, nonintact skin, or potentially contaminated intact skin (e.g., of a patient incontinent of stool or urine) could occur.

   b. Wear gloves with fit and durability appropriate to the task.

      i. Wear disposable medical examination gloves for providing direct patient care.

      ii. Wear disposable medical examination gloves or reusable utility gloves for cleaning the environment or medical equipment.

   c. Remove gloves after contact with a patient and/or the surrounding environment (including medical equipment) using proper technique to prevent hand contamination. Do not wear the same pair of gloves for the care of more than one patient. Do not wash gloves for the purpose of reuse because this practice has been associated with transmission of pathogens.

   d. Change gloves during patient care if the hands will move from a contaminated body site (e.g., perineal area) to a clean body site (e.g., face).

▪ Take Note

Nonsterile examination gloves can be used for most routine patient-care activities.

3. Gowns
   a. Wear a gown that is appropriate to the task to protect skin and prevent soiling or contamination of clothing during procedures and patient-care activities when contact with blood, body fluids, secretions, or excretions is anticipated.
      i. Wear a gown for direct patient contact if the patient has uncontained secretions or excretions.
      ii. Remove gown and perform hand hygiene before leaving the patient's environment.
   b. Do not reuse gowns, even for repeated contacts with the same patient.
   c. Routine donning of gowns on entrance into a high-risk unit (e.g., ICU, NICU, HSCT unit) is not indicated.
4. Mouth, nose, eye protection
   a. Use PPE to protect the mucous membranes of the eyes, nose, and mouth during procedures and patient-care activities that are likely to generate splashes or sprays of blood, body fluids, secretions, and excretions. Select masks, goggles, face shields, and combinations of these according to the need anticipated by the task to be performed.
   b. During aerosol-generating procedures (e.g., suctioning of the respiratory tract [if not using inline suction catheters], endotracheal intubation) in patients who are not suspected of being infected with an agent for which respiratory protection is otherwise recommended (e.g., *M. tuberculosis,* SARS, or hemorrhagic fever viruses), wear one of the following: a face shield that fully covers the front and sides of the face, a mask with attached shield, or a mask and goggles (in addition to gloves and gown).

C. Respiratory hygiene/cough etiquette
1. Educate healthcare personnel on the importance of source control measures to contain respiratory secretions to prevent droplet and fomite transmission of respiratory pathogens, especially during seasonal outbreaks of viral respiratory tract infections (e.g., influenza, RSV, adenovirus, parainfluenza virus) in communities.
2. Implement the following measures to contain respiratory secretions in patients and accompanying individuals who have signs and symptoms of a respiratory infection, beginning at the point of initial encounter in a healthcare setting (e.g., triage, reception, and waiting areas in emergency departments, outpatient clinics, physical therapy clinics/offices, and physician offices).
   a. Post signs at entrances and in strategic places (e.g., elevators, cafeterias) within ambulatory and inpatient settings with instructions to patients and other persons with symptoms of a respiratory infection to cover their mouths/noses when coughing or sneezing, to use and dispose of tissues, and to perform hand hygiene after hands have been in contact with respiratory secretions.
   b. Provide tissues and no-touch receptacles (e.g., foot-pedal-operated lid or open, plastic-lined waste basket) for disposal of tissues.
   c. Provide resources and instructions for performing hand hygiene in or near waiting areas in ambulatory and inpatient settings; provide conveniently located dispensers of alcohol-based hand rubs and, where sinks are available, supplies for handwashing.
   d. During periods of increased prevalence of respiratory infections in the community (e.g., as indicated by increased school absenteeism, increased number of patients seeking care for a respiratory infection), offer masks to coughing patients and other symptomatic persons (e.g., persons who accompany ill patients) on entry into the facility or medical office and encourage them to maintain spatial separation, ideally a distance of at least 3 feet, from others in common waiting areas. Some facilities may find it logistically easier to institute this recommendation year-round as a standard of practice.

D. Patient-care equipment and instruments/devices

1. Establish policies and procedures for containing, transporting, and handling patient-care equipment and instruments/devices that may be contaminated with blood or body fluids.
2. Remove organic material from critical and semicritical instruments/devices using recommended cleaning agents before high-level disinfection and sterilization to enable effective disinfection and sterilization processes.
3. Wear PPE (e.g., gloves, gown) according to the level of anticipated contamination when handling patient-care equipment and instruments/devices that are visibly soiled or may have been in contact with blood or body fluids.

E. Care of the environment

1. Establish policies and procedures for routine and targeted cleaning of environmental surfaces as indicated by the level of patient contact and degree of soiling.
2. Clean and disinfect surfaces that are likely to be contaminated with pathogens, including those that are in close proximity to the patient (e.g., bed rails, overbed tables) and frequently touched surfaces in the patient-care environment (e.g., door knobs, surfaces in and surrounding toilets in patients' rooms) on a more frequent schedule compared to that for other surfaces (e.g., horizontal surfaces in waiting rooms).
3. Use EPA-registered disinfectants that have microbiocidal (i.e., killing) activity against the pathogens most likely to contaminate the patient-care environment. Use in accordance with manufacturer's instructions.
4. In facilities that provide health care to pediatric patients or have waiting areas with child play toys, establish policies and procedures for cleaning and disinfecting toys at regular intervals. *Category IA recommendation.* Use the following principles in developing this policy and procedures:
   a. Select play toys that can be easily cleaned and disinfected.
   b. Do not permit use of stuffed furry toys if they will be shared.
   c. Clean and disinfect large stationary toys (e.g., climbing equipment) at least weekly and whenever visibly soiled.
   d. If toys are likely to be mouthed, rinse with water after disinfection; alternatively, wash in a dishwasher.
   e. When a toy requires cleaning and disinfection, do so immediately or store in a designated labeled container separate from toys that are clean and ready for use.
5. Include multiuse electronic equipment in policies and procedures for preventing contamination and for cleaning and disinfection, especially those items that are used by patients, those used during delivery of patient care, and mobile devices that are moved into and out of patient rooms frequently (e.g., daily).

■ **Take Note**

Select toys that are washable.

F. Textiles and laundry

1. Handle used textiles and fabrics with minimum agitation to avoid contamination of air, surfaces, and persons.
2. If laundry chutes are used, ensure that they are properly designed, maintained, and used in a manner to minimize dispersion of aerosols from contaminated laundry.

Contact Precautions

Contact precautions are intended to prevent transmission of infectious agents, including epidemiologically important infectious agents, that are spread by direct or indirect contact with the patient or the patient's environment. Contact precautions also apply where the presence of excessive wound drainage, fecal incontinence, or other discharges from the body suggest an increased potential for extensive environmental contamination and risk of transmission. A single-patient room is preferred for patients who require contact precautions. When a single-patient room is not available, consultation with infection control personnel is recommended to assess the various risks associated with other patient placement options (e.g., cohorting, keeping the patient with an existing roommate). In multipatient rooms, more than 3 feet of spatial separation between beds is advised to reduce the opportunities for inadvertent sharing of items between the infected/colonized patient and other patients. Healthcare personnel caring for patients on contact precautions should wear a gown and gloves for all interactions that may involve contact with the patient or potentially contaminated areas in the patient's environment. Don PPE before room entry and discard before exiting the patient room to contain pathogens, especially those that have been implicated in transmission through environmental contamination.

■ Take Note

Contact precautions require the use of gowns and gloves, which should be donned before entering the patient's room and removed before exiting the patient's room.

Contact Precaution Guidelines

Use contact precautions for patients with known or suspected infections or evidence of syndromes that represent an increased risk for contact transmission.

A. Use of personal protective equipment
   1. Wear gloves whenever touching the patient's intact skin or surfaces and articles in close proximity to the patient (e.g., medical equipment, bed rails). Don gloves on entry into the room or cubicle.
   2. Gowns
      a. Don gown on entry into the room or cubicle. Remove gown and observe hand hygiene before leaving the patient-care environment.
      b. After gown removal, ensure that clothing and skin do not contact potentially contaminated environmental surfaces that could result in possible transfer of infectious agent to other patients or environmental surfaces.

B. Patient transport
   1. In *acute-care hospitals and long-term care and other residential settings,* limit transport and movement of patients outside the room to medically necessary purposes.
   2. When transport or movement in any healthcare setting is necessary, ensure that infected or colonized areas of the patient's body are contained and covered.
   3. Remove and dispose of contaminated PPE and perform hand hygiene following transport of patients on contact precautions.
   4. Don clean PPE to handle the patient at the transport destination. *Category II recommendation.*

C. Patient-care equipment and instruments/devices
   1. Handle patient-care equipment and instruments/devices according to standard precautions.
   2. In *acute-care hospitals and long-term care and other residential settings,* use disposable noncritical patient-care equipment or implement patient-dedicated use of such equipment. If common use of equipment for multiple patients is unavoidable, clean and disinfect such equipment before use on another patient.
   3. In *home-care settings*
      a. Limit the amount of nondisposable patient-care equipment brought into the homes of patients on contact precautions. Whenever possible, leave patient-care equipment in the home until discharge from home-care services.
      b. If noncritical patient-care equipment (e.g., stethoscope) cannot remain in the home, clean and disinfect items before taking them from the home using a low- to intermediate-level disinfectant. Alternatively, place contaminated reusable items in a plastic bag for transport and subsequent cleaning and disinfection.
   4. In *ambulatory settings,* place contaminated reusable noncritical patient-care equipment in a plastic bag for transport to a soiled utility area for reprocessing.

D. Environmental measures

1. Ensure that rooms of patients on contact precautions are prioritized for frequent cleaning and disinfection (e.g., at least daily) with a focus on frequently touched surfaces (e.g., bed rails, overbed table, bedside commode, lavatory surfaces in patient bathrooms, doorknobs) and equipment in the immediate vicinity of the patient.

Droplet Precautions

Droplet precautions are intended to prevent transmission of pathogens spread through close respiratory or mucous membrane contact with respiratory secretions. Because these pathogens do not remain infectious over long distances, special air handling and ventilation are not required to prevent droplet transmission. A single-patient room is preferred for patients who require droplet precautions. When a single-patient room is not available, consultation with infection control personnel is recommended to assess the various risks associated with other patient placement options (e.g., keeping the patient with an existing roommate). Spatial separation of patients by at least 3 feet and drawing the curtain between patient beds is especially important for patients in multibed rooms with infections transmitted by the droplet route. Healthcare personnel wear a mask for close contact with infectious patients; the mask is generally donned on room entry. Patients on droplet precautions who must be transported outside the room should wear a mask if tolerated and follow respiratory hygiene/cough etiquette.

Droplet Precaution Guidelines

In addition to standard precautions, use transmission-based precautions for patients with documented or suspected infection or colonization with highly transmissible or epidemiologically important pathogens for which additional precautions are needed to prevent transmission.

A. Use droplet precautions as recommended for patients known or suspected to be infected with pathogens transmitted by respiratory droplets (i.e., large-particle droplets greater than 5 μm in size) that are generated when a patient is coughing, sneezing, or talking.

B. In *ambulatory settings,* place patients who require droplet precautions in an examination room or cubicle as soon as possible. Instruct patients to follow recommendations for respiratory hygiene/cough etiquette.

C. Use of personal protective equipment

1. Don a mask on entry into the patient room or cubicle.
2. No recommendation for routinely wearing eye protection (e.g., goggles or face shield), in addition to a mask, for close contact with patients who require droplet precautions.

D. Patient transport

1. In *acute-care hospitals and long-term care and other residential settings,* limit transport and movement of patients outside the room to only medically necessary purposes.
2. If transport or movement in any healthcare setting is necessary, instruct the patient to wear a mask and follow respiratory hygiene/cough etiquette.
3. No mask is required for persons transporting patients on droplet precautions.

Airborne Precautions and Guidelines

Airborne precautions prevent transmission of infectious agents that remain infectious over long distances when suspended in the air (e.g., rubeola virus [measles], varicella virus [chickenpox], *M. tuberculosis,* and possibly SARS-CoV). The preferred placement for patients who require airborne precautions is in an airborne infection isolation room (AIIR). An AIIR is a single-patient room that is equipped with special air handling and ventilation capacity that meet the American Institute of Architects/Facility Guidelines Institute (AIA/FGI) standards for AIIRs (i.e., monitored negative pressure relative to the surrounding area, 12 air exchanges per hour for new construction and renovation and 6 air exchanges per hour for existing facilities, and air exhausted directly to the outside or recirculated through HEPA filtration before return). Some states require the availability of such rooms in hospitals, emergency departments, and nursing homes that care for patients with *M. tuberculosis.* A respiratory-protection program that includes education about use of respirators, fit-testing, and user seal checks is required in any facility with AIIRs. In settings where airborne precautions cannot be implemented due to limited engineering resources (e.g., physicians' offices), masking the patient, placing the patient in a private room (e.g., office examination room) with the door closed, and providing N95 or higher-level respirators or masks if respirators are not available for healthcare personnel will reduce the likelihood of airborne transmission until the patient is either transferred to a facility with an AIIR or returned to the home environment as deemed medically appropriate. Healthcare personnel caring for patients on airborne precautions should wear a mask or respirator, depending on the disease-specific recommendations for respiratory protection, which is to be donned prior to entering the patient's room. Whenever possible, nonimmune healthcare workers should not care for patients with vaccine-preventable airborne diseases (e.g., measles, chickenpox, and smallpox).

Transmission-Based Precautions and Guidelines

In addition to standard precautions, use transmission-based precautions for patients with documented or suspected infection or colonization with highly transmissible or epidemiologically important pathogens for which additional precautions are needed to prevent transmission.

A. In *ambulatory settings:*

1. Develop systems on entry into ambulatory settings (e.g., triage, signage) to identify patients with known or suspected infections that require airborne precautions.
2. Place the patient in an AIIR as soon as possible. If an AIIR is not available, place a surgical mask on the patient, and place him/her in an examination room. Once the patient leaves, the room should remain vacant for the appropriate time, generally 1 hour, to allow for a full exchange of air.
3. Instruct patients with a known or suspected airborne infection to wear a surgical mask and observe respiratory hygiene/cough etiquette. Once in an AIIR, the mask may be removed; the mask should remain on if the patient is not in an AIIR.

B. An administrative control is to restrict susceptible healthcare personnel from entering the rooms of patients known or suspected to have measles (rubeola), varicella (chickenpox), disseminated zoster, or smallpox if other immune healthcare personnel are available.

C. Use of PPE

1. Wear a fit-tested National Institute of Occupational Safety and Health (NIOSH)–approved N95 or higher-level respirator for respiratory protection when entering the room or home of a patient when the following diseases are suspected or confirmed:
   a. Infectious pulmonary or laryngeal tuberculosis or when infectious tuberculosis skin lesions are present and procedures that would aerosolize viable organisms (e.g., irrigation, incision and drainage, whirlpool treatments) are performed.
   b. Respiratory protection is recommended for all healthcare personnel, including those with a documented "take" after smallpox vaccination due to the risk of a genetically engineered virus against which the vaccine may not provide protection or of exposure to a very large viral load (e.g., from high-risk aerosol-generating procedures, immunocompromised patients, or hemorrhagic or flat smallpox).

Apparel

The purposes of apparel have been covered earlier in this chapter. Specific points regarding apparel are presented in this section.

Scrub suits are not sterile. Gowns, whether paper or cloth, should be worn only once, removed properly, and discarded in an appropriate receptacle.

When the use of a mask is indicated, it should be used only once and discarded in an appropriate receptacle. Lowering a mask around the neck and then placing it over the nose and mouth again is the same as reusing a mask and should not be done. Masks should cover both the nose and the mouth.

In most cases, glasses only provide a barrier in front of the eyes. Glasses with side shields provide an additional barrier. When prescription glasses are necessary, shields or goggles should be worn over prescription glasses, providing the best degree of protection. Shields and goggles are usually constructed of clear plastic, providing a barrier in front and on the sides of the eyes.

Nonsterile gloves are worn as a standard precaution. Whether using sterile or nonsterile gloves, handwashing is required after gloves are removed. Used gloves should be removed properly and discarded into an appropriate receptacle.

Additional apparel, including caps, beard covers, and shoe covers, must be worn as necessary to maintain clean or sterile fields.

■ Take Note

Sterile field: There are four requirements for establishment and four requirements for maintenance.

Sterile Field

The primary goal of using aseptic techniques is to prevent infection. One aseptic technique is to provide and maintain a sterile field. A sterile field is most commonly required in an operating room; however, there also may be a necessity for a sterile field in patient-care areas other than the operating room for the performance of minor procedures.

There are eight requirements for providing and maintaining a sterile field. The first four requirements concern creation of a sterile field. The remaining four requirements concern maintenance of the sterile field.

Requirement 1

All items used within the boundaries of a sterile field must be sterile. The items must have been properly sterilized and maintained to preserve their sterile state. Once items have been sterilized, they must be used within the allowable shelf life of the item and sterilization process. The expiration date, or end of shelf life, is marked on each sterile package. Certain types of equipment and different types of packaging may affect the shelf life of a sterile package.

Whenever possible, single-use items are preferred. Because single-use items are discarded after use, there is no concern about contamination because of reuse. This does not mean, however, that single-use items cannot become contaminated before the initial use through improper technique or carelessness.

The shelf-life date of a sterile package is not a guarantee that the package is sterile. Packages are only considered to remain sterile when the

1. Initial packaging was performed properly
2. Package was stored in a proper manner
3. Package was not mishandled during distribution
4. Shelf-life date has not been exceeded

Requirement 2

Once a sterile package has been opened, the edges are not considered sterile. Care in opening sterile packages is required to avoid having the edges touch the contents of the package or having the edges touch the gloved hands or sterile gown. Most sterile packages have enough packaging material around the edges to keep the unsterile edges away from the sterile contents.

Requirement 3

Once donned properly, sterile gowns are considered to be sterile in the front from shoulder level to tabletop level, including the sleeves. For this reason, the hands must be held above tabletop level and in front of the body during and after scrubbing, gowning, and gloving.

Requirement 4

In all cases, only the top surface of a table is considered sterile. Sterile drapes cover the top of a surface and descend on all sides of the surface. Such draping may be covering a patient or on an instrument table. Demarcation of sterile surfaces is fairly easy on tables but more difficult on patients. A guideline to use for demarcation on a patient that is draped is to consider that a surface above the level of the instrument table, or above waist level, whichever is higher, is a sterile surface as long as it is draped properly. Undraped or improperly draped surfaces, or surfaces below the top level of the instrument table or waist, are considered unsterile.

When a sterile field is created using only a sterile towel, a perimeter of 1 inch inside the edges of the towel is not considered sterile.

Requirement 5

Only sterile items and personnel in sterile attire may enter the sterile field or touch items in a sterile area. Personnel considered nonsterile may not touch any item in a sterile area or any item to be placed in a sterile area. Usually, sterile packages are opened by nonsterile personnel, and the contents are released into the sterile area without actually being touched by nonsterile personnel. Transfer of sterile items into a sterile area may also be accomplished by using sterile forceps to hold the item as it is passed into the sterile area. The set of forceps is considered contaminated after a single use and may not be used again until sterilized properly. Nonsterile personnel may not reach across or into a sterile area.

Requirement 6

Activity in a sterile area cannot be allowed to render the area unsterile. Personnel in sterile attire should not sit on or lean against unsterile surfaces. Movement within the sterile area must be measured and careful to avoid contact between sterile and unsterile surfaces.

All personnel, sterile or nonsterile, in or around a sterile area must be aware of the boundaries of a sterile area. Any contamination of a sterile area must be pointed out immediately by any personnel present for protection of the patient.

Requirement 7

Penetration of a sterile covering or barrier is considered to cause contamination of a sterile field. Liquids are the most likely cause of penetration of a sterile barrier. Liquids spilled within a sterile field may cause penetration of a sterile barrier.

A less noticeable but highly potential cause of penetration is air flow. Design of climate control for sterile areas provides for the most purified air possible and a slightly higher gradient of air pressure in the sterile area. Higher air-pressure gradient in the sterile area will cause air flow away from the site of potential infection. Climate-control systems should also be physically separated from other areas of the institution so that airborne infectious agents picked up in sterile areas do not permeate the atmosphere of the entire institution.

Requirement 8

Sterile areas and fields should be prepared as close to the time of use as feasible. They should not be left unattended. Sterile fields should not be prepared and then covered for later use. A delay in using equipment or supplies laid out in a sterile field necessitates the preparation of a new sterile field with new sterile equipment and supplies.

When there is doubt about the sterile quality of an area, a field, or an item, it should be considered unsterile. Improper packaging, sterilization processing, storage, or handling can occur without overt signs. Appropriate use of all items in a sterile environment is the responsibility of the user. Only proper judgement, rigid discipline, and appropriate use provide protection for a patient.

■ Take Note

Everyone is responsible for maintaining a sterile field and ensuring that the sterile field remains uncontaminated.

Scrubbing Versus Handwashing

Handwashing techniques have been presented previously. Handwashing procedures are used prior to donning sterile gloves for procedures other than surgery. Scrubbing is a series of specific steps of hand cleaning using nail cleaners and soap or antimicrobial products prior to donning sterile gloves for surgery. Specific scrubbing procedures are beyond the scope of this text.

PROCEDURE 4–1 Gowning

When necessary for maintaining a sterile environment, don a freshly laundered scrub suit (pants and shirt or gown), scrub cap, and a new mask. Fasten the scrub suit completely and properly. All hair must be covered by a scrub cap. Facial hair, when present, must be covered by a mask and beard cover when necessary. The mask is formed to fit tightly but comfortably over the nose and mouth. Wear eye shields to protect the eyes.

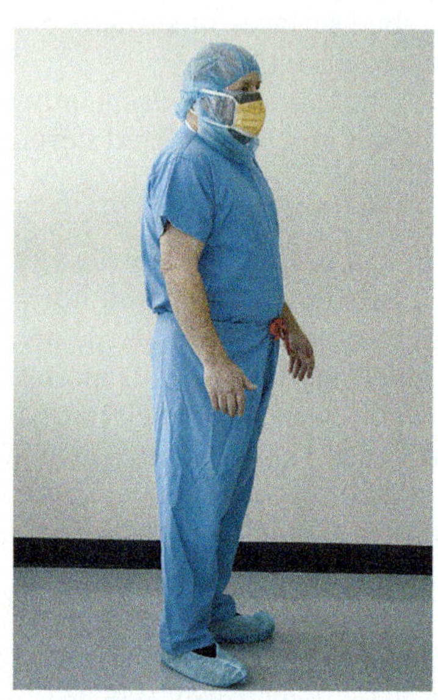

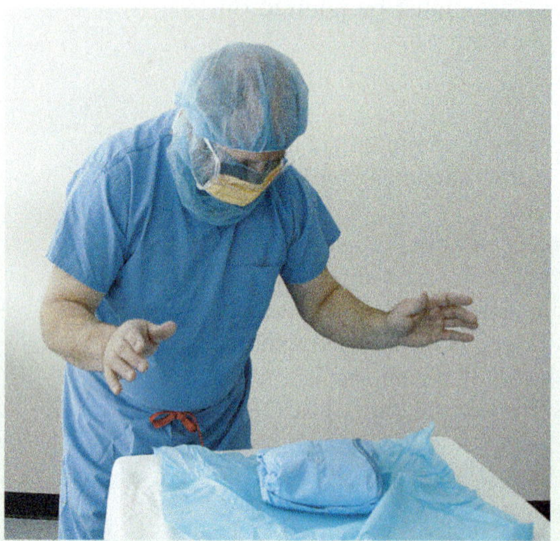

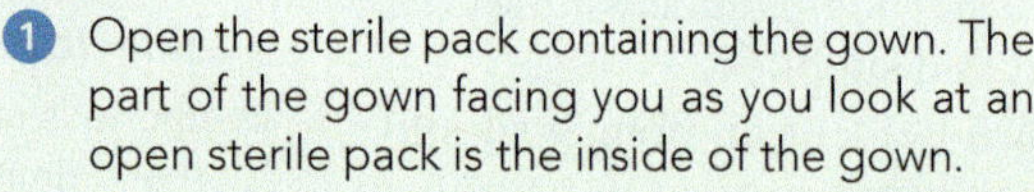
1. Open the sterile pack containing the gown. The part of the gown facing you as you look at an open sterile pack is the inside of the gown.

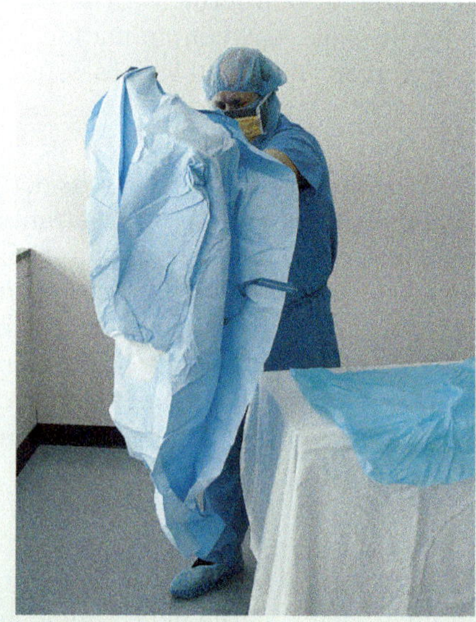

2. Grasp the gown firmly, and lift it up and away from the sterile field. Move away from the table on which the sterile pack rests, keeping hands above waist height at all times. Shake open the gown so it unfolds. Holding the inside of the gown only, locate the neck and armholes of the gown.

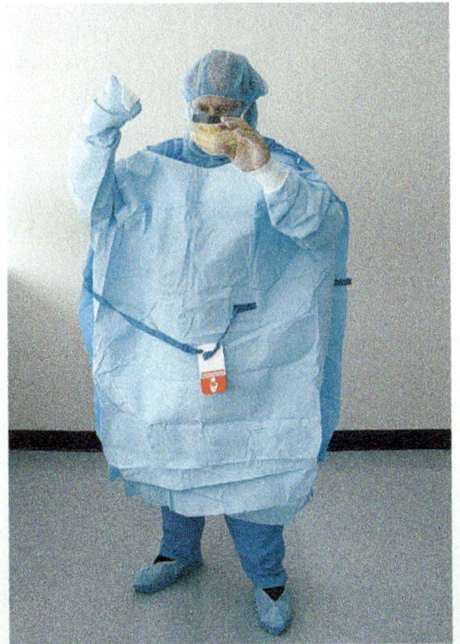

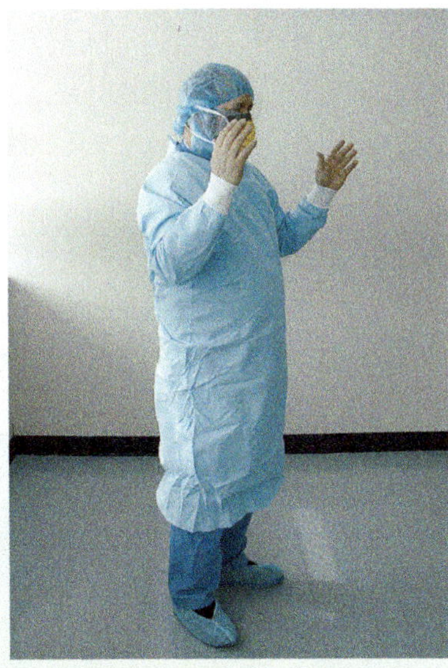

3 Without touching the outside, or sterile side, of the gown, work both arms into the sleeves at the same time. Stop when the hands reach the stockinette cuffs.

4 The gown is tied using back and neck closures by personnel who are not in the sterile field.

PROCEDURE 4–2 Gloving

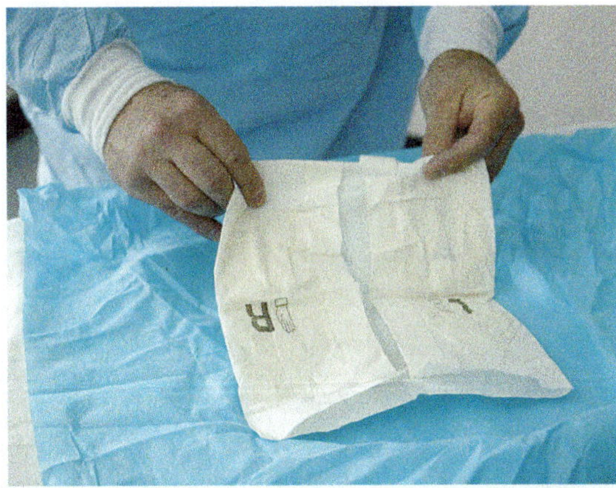

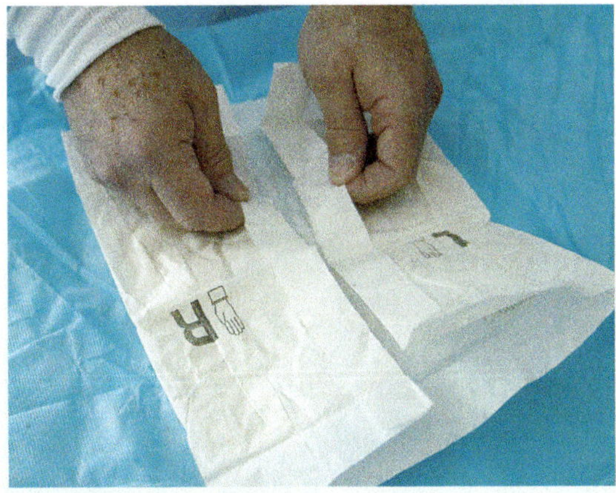

1 Open a glove pack and place the sterile paper enclosure that contains the gloves on a sterile surface with the cuffs toward the person who will be gloving.

2 Open the sterile portion of a glove pack by grasping the folds of the paper enclosing the gloves.

(continued)

PROCEDURE 4–2 Gloving (*continued*)

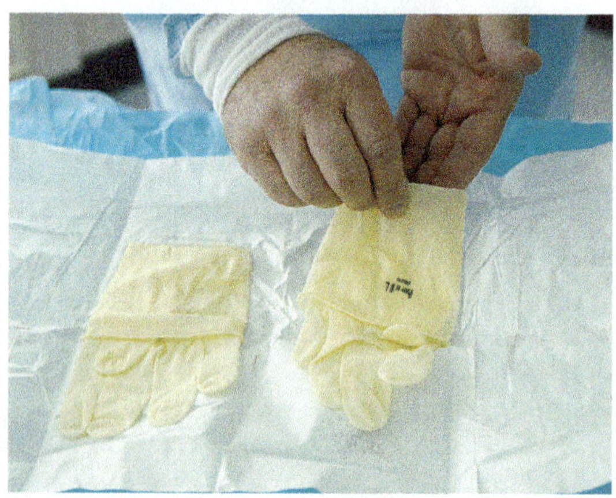

3 The wrist end of each glove has been turned back on itself, creating a cuff where the inside, or unsterile side, is now outward.

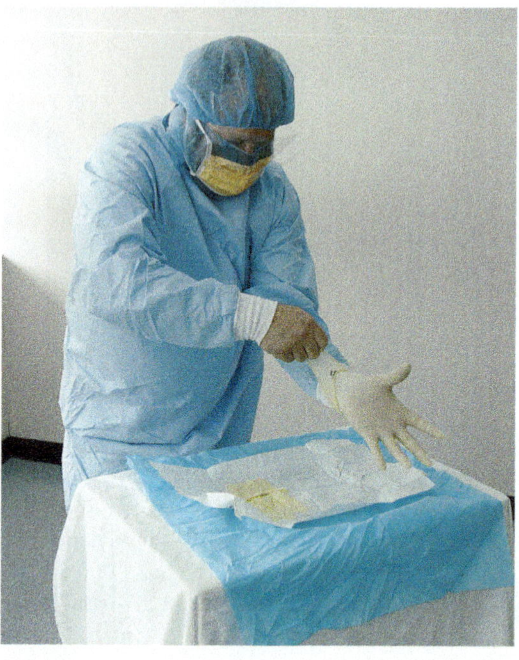

4 Grasping the left glove by its cuff on the nonsterile portion with a bare right hand, work the left hand into the left glove.

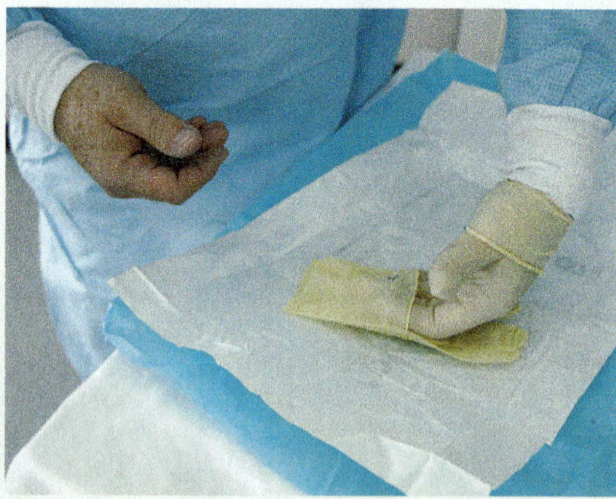

5 Once the left glove is in place, it is now a sterile surface. Slip the first two or three fingers of the gloved left hand down inside the sterile side of the cuff of the right glove, starting at the palm of the right glove and pointing toward the crease of the cuff at the wrist.

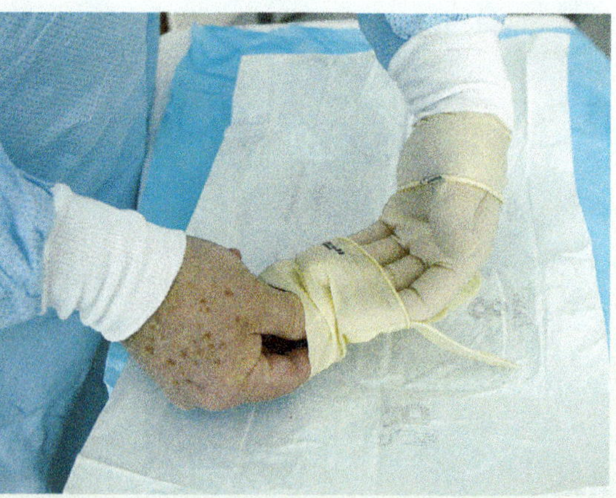

6 Then lift the right glove using the fingers inside the cuff only. The thumb of the gloved left hand cannot be used to grasp the right-hand glove. As the right glove is held by the first two or three fingers on the inside (sterile side) of the cuff, work the right hand into the right glove.

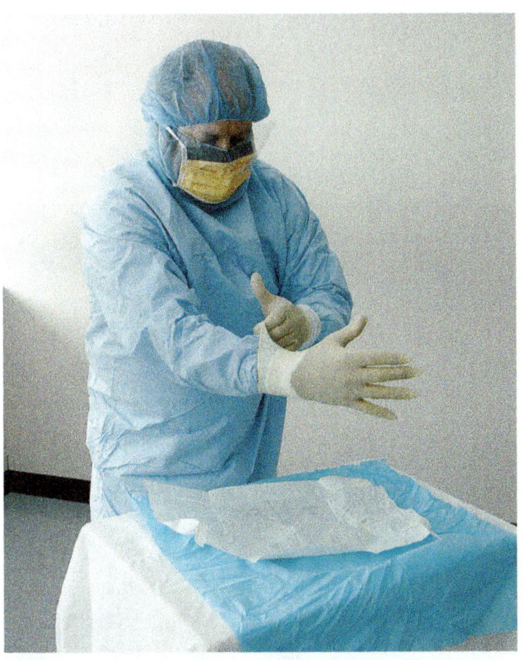

7 Once the right hand is gloved, unfold the cuff by pulling the cuff up over the sleeve of the gown and letting the wrist portion of the glove snap into place.

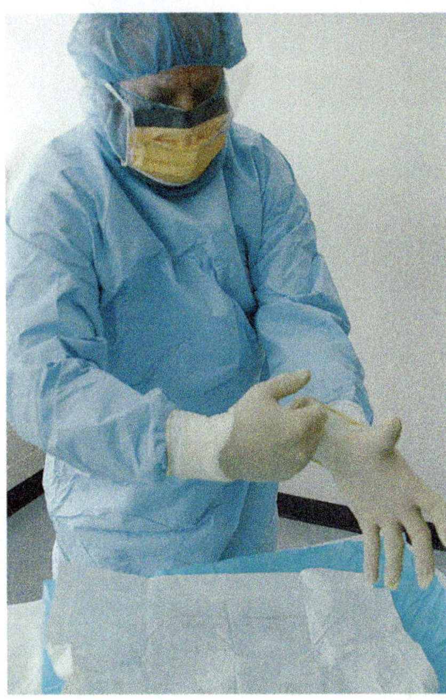

8 Now the fingers of the right hand, now sterile, can be placed on the inside (sterile side) of the left glove cuff. Unfold the left cuff in the same manner as was done for the right glove. If necessary, the gloves can be adjusted on the fingers once both glove cuffs have been properly placed.

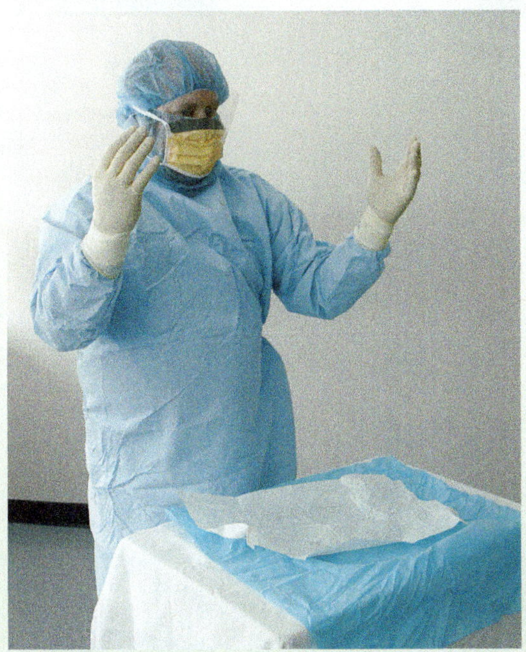

9 Once gloved, both hands must remain above waist level or the level of draping that defines the sterile field, whichever is appropriate.

(continued)

PROCEDURE 4–2 Gloving (*continued*)

Removal of Contaminated Gloves

When a glove becomes torn or punctured during a sterile procedure, it no longer provides proper protection and must be removed and discarded as soon as is feasible, and another sterile glove must be donned. This may require interruption of a procedure provided that the interruption does not threaten the patient's welfare.

1. Remove contaminated gloves in a manner that prevents the spread of contaminants. One hand grasps the cuff of the other glove.

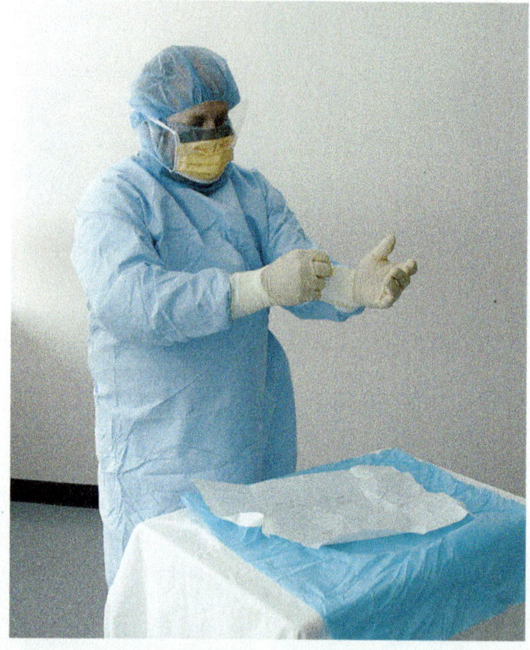

2. The glove that has been grasped at the cuff is turned inside out as it is removed.

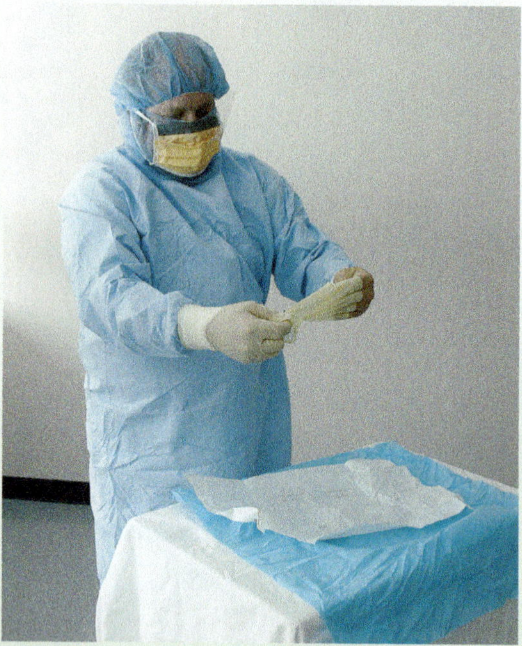

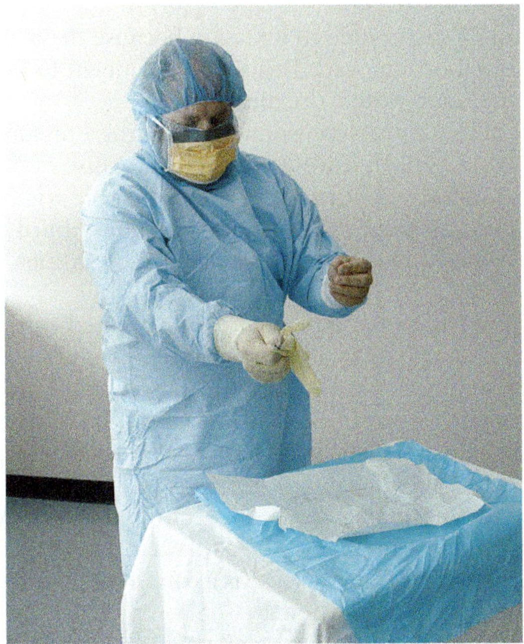

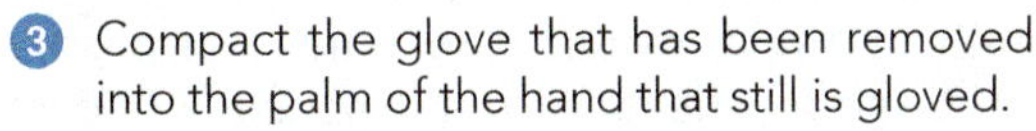

3 Compact the glove that has been removed into the palm of the hand that still is gloved.

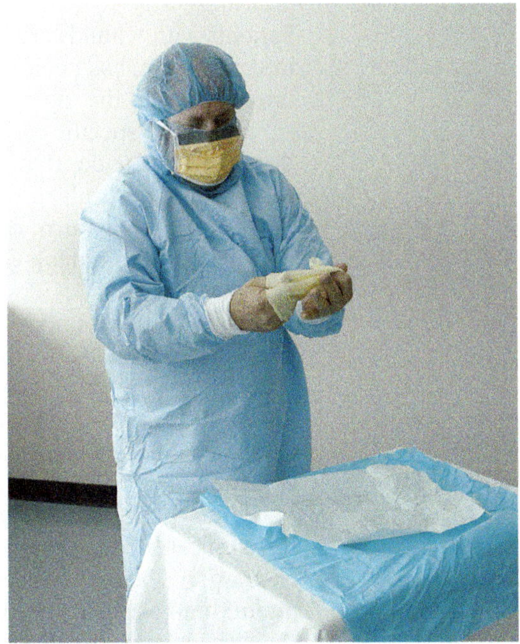

4 Hook the thumb of the ungloved hand inside the remaining glove and pull the remaining glove toward the fingers, turning it inside out over the compacted glove.

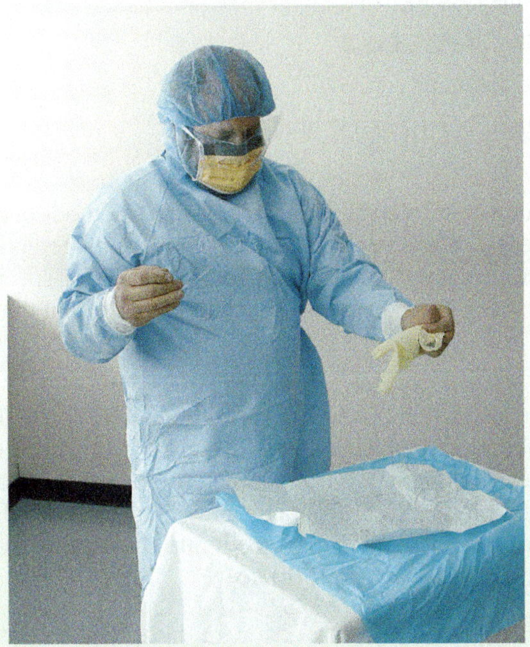

5 Remove both gloves with the contaminated sides inward. When removing gloves, the material should not be permitted to snap in order to avoid dislodging material that has accumulated on the gloves. Dispose of the gloves in an appropriate container, and wash the hands.

Wounds and Wound Dressings

Patients with wounds are extremely susceptible to infection because the major barrier to infection, skin, has been penetrated or removed. This section is meant to be a very brief introduction to the topic of wounds and wound dressings.

There are specific classifications for pressure wounds and burns. Pressure wounds are described by the depth of the wound. Burns are classified by the cause of burn (thermal, electrical, chemical, radiation), depth of burn (superficial or epidermal, superficial partial-thickness burn, deep partial-thickness burn, full-thickness burn), and extent of burn (rule of nines). Other types of wounds are abrasions, lacerations, and surgical incisions.

The location of a wound can dictate the type of dressing applied or the method of application. Wounds over joints may require rigid dressings to prevent joint motion from disrupting the wound, or the dressings may have to be applied in a way that accommodates joint motion. Wounds can require extensive modification of bedding and seating arrangements so sleeping and sitting activities do not disrupt a dressing or put pressure on a wound.

Underlying pathological conditions may have an impact on the dressings chosen and the application of dressings. No dressing should ever be applied in a manner that impedes circulation. The existence of peripheral vascular disease is a condition that requires special attention to avoid further impairment of circulation.

When long-term care of a wound is required, care may be provided outside an institutional setting. When noninstitutional care is appropriate, a patient or patient's family must be instructed carefully in proper wound care. Whenever possible, use simple procedures. Give careful evaluation and consideration to the patient's, or family's, ability to understand and carry out specific instructions. A wound site that cannot be seen easily by the patient may not be well cared for by a patient. A physical impairment, such as a stroke, or mental impairment, such as Alzheimer's disease, may prohibit a patient from providing wound care. Provide supervision to ensure that proper techniques are followed.

Purpose

The purposes of wound dressings are to

1. Provide physical protection of the wound
2. Prevent contamination of a wound
3. Prevent transmission of infection from a wound
4. Promote healing

Many institutions and healthcare professionals have preferred methods of caring for specific types of wounds, and there is increasing evidence to support several methods. This section presents basic information concerning wound dressings. Information for a specific institution should be sought from the appropriate departments or practitioners within the institution.

Evaluation

Examination of wound characteristics is necessary for appropriate selection of dressing materials and protective agents. A physical therapist performs the initial examination and evaluates the results using the clinical decision-making process to determine a plan of care. A plan of care may be implemented by a physical therapist/assistant where permitted by state law. Documentation of wound characteristics and management must be explicit and precise.

Evaluation of the wound is necessary to determine

1. The cause of the wound
2. The location, area, and depth of the wound
3. Whether the wound is wet or dry
4. Whether the wound is infected and, if infected, the source, mechanism, and infectious agent

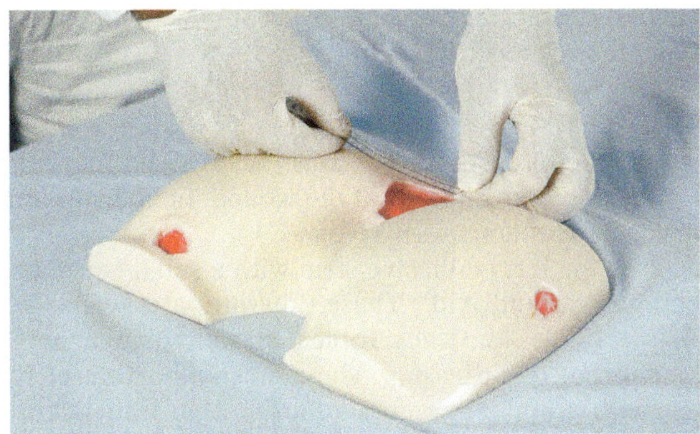

FIGURE 4–1 ■ Measuring a wound using a ruler.

Measurement of a wound can be performed using a ruler (Figure 4-1 ■). In addition to regular rulers, there are specialized clear plastic circular rulers. The ruler should not make contact with the wound itself and should be limited to single-patient use. Measurements should include width, length, and depth. Another method of documenting the extent of a wound is by photographing the wound.

Types of Dressings

Four methods of dressing applications generally used for wound management are

1. Dry to dry
2. Damp to damp
3. Occlusive
4. Rigid

A **dry-to-dry dressing** is the application of a dry absorbent or nonabsorbent dressing to cover the wound. A **damp-to-damp dressing** is the application of a gauze pad moistened with normal saline solution or another similar solution before application. Remoistening a damp dressing is performed while the dressing remains in place. This prevents the dressing from drying out and becoming embedded in the eschar. The damp-to-damp dressing assists in softening the eschar in preparation for removal. A dressing should not be allowed to dry and become embedded in the eschar, as it debrides the wound nonselectively when the dressing is removed. **Occlusive dressings** are applied to provide a semipermeable barrier to air and moisture penetration. **Rigid dressings** provide physical protection to a wound and the adjacent area.

Choice of materials for, and method of application of, dressings may depend on

1. The cause of the wound
2. Whether the wound is clean or infected and if infected, the infectious agent causing the infection
3. The type of dressing (damp, dry)
4. The type, if any, of antimicrobial agent to be applied
5. The site, area, and depth of the wound
6. Whether a trained professional, the patient, or the patient's family will be responsible for monitoring and changing the dressing

Identification of the specific infectious agent responsible for infection is beneficial in treating any wound. Specific antimicrobial agents may require specific types of dressing materials to ensure that the antimicrobial agent is applied properly to the wound.

When a wound is draining, absorption of exudate can be a consideration requiring a dry dressing. When a wound tends to be dry and the dryness impedes healing, a damp

■ Take Note

Wet wound—dry dressing. Dry wound—moist dressing.

dressing would be required. Limiting exposure to air or maintaining a moist environment within the wound can require an occlusive dressing.

Materials

The size of dressings, whether prepackaged or constructed, should cover a wound site, plus some portion of healthy tissue on all sides of the wound. In no case should the adhesive portion of a dressing come in contact with a wound.

The most basic dressing is an adhesive strip with a small gauze center, commonly known by the brand name Band-Aid®. These dressings are available from a number of companies in various shapes and sizes. Topical antimicrobial agents may be applied under the gauze portion of this dressing. The adhesive portion of the dressing may be plastic or paper, with a hypoallergenic adhesive that limits skin reaction to the adhesive.

Dressings with nonadhering pads that do not stick to wounds or the exudate from wounds are also available. These dressings, commonly known by the brand name Telfa® pads, are available from a number of companies in various shapes and sizes. These basic dressings are usually best for small wounds, although self-made dressings of the same nature can be constructed in any size when the necessary material is available.

Gauze is the most common material used for dressings and is available in pads and rolls. Sterile and nonsterile gauze is available in several sizes. If sterile gauze is to be used, perform proper aseptic handling techniques during opening and application. Dressings constructed from gauze can be used with topical antimicrobial agents under the dressing when required.

Compression wraps are applied to control edema in a limb segment or to provide some support for a joint. Compression wraps are constructed of an elastic material and are commonly known by the brand name Ace® wrap. Common sizes are 2-, 3-, 4-, 5-, and 6-inch widths.

Edges of lacerations can be approximated using thin adhesive strips, commonly known by the brand name Steri-Strips™. The edges of a wound are placed together, and the adhesive strips are placed across the wound. The number of strips required is determined by the open length of the wound.

Tape used to secure a dressing can be cloth adhesive tape or paper tape that has a hypoallergenic adhesive. Tape can be cut to the required length with scissors or torn from the roll. Tear tape by unrolling the desired amount and firmly grasping the tape between the pad of the thumb and the side of the index finger of each hand, with the hands approximately 1 inch apart. Take care not to roll the edges of the tape over because this makes the tape harder to tear. A quick movement of one hand away from the body and the other hand toward the body will cause the tape to tear between the two hands. Even cloth adhesive tape can be torn in this manner as long as the edges have not been rolled.

Preparation

Necessary supplies, such as gauze pads, roll gauze, tape, and topical agents, must be easily accessible during the procedure. Sterile fields, when required, must be prepared appropriately. Protection of the wound from contamination requires the appropriate application of aseptic techniques. Proper preparation for personnel includes handwashing or scrubbing and masking, gowning, and gloving, when required.

Tape for securing dressings may need to be prepared before starting the application of a dressing because tearing or cutting tape usually takes two hands. The pieces can be hung from the edge of a table, cabinet, or bed frame by sticking only a small portion of one end to the object and letting the remainder of the piece hang free. The pieces should be hung in an accessible place because one hand is usually required to secure the dressing or wrap while tape is applied. When tape is applied circumferentially on a limb segment, the ends should not overlap. Adhesive and paper tape do not have enough elasticity to avoid impairment of circulation if the ends overlap in this situation.

PROCEDURE 4–3 Application of Dressings and Wraps

Packing a Wound

1. Depending on the depth of a wound, it may be packed with gauze to ensure that deeper layers of a wound heal before surface layers, avoiding development of an unhealed cavity.

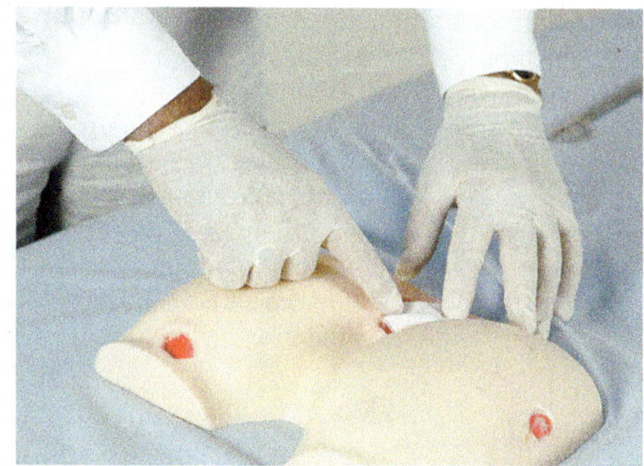

2. Once packed, the wound and packing are covered with additional dressing that is secured with roll gauze or tape.

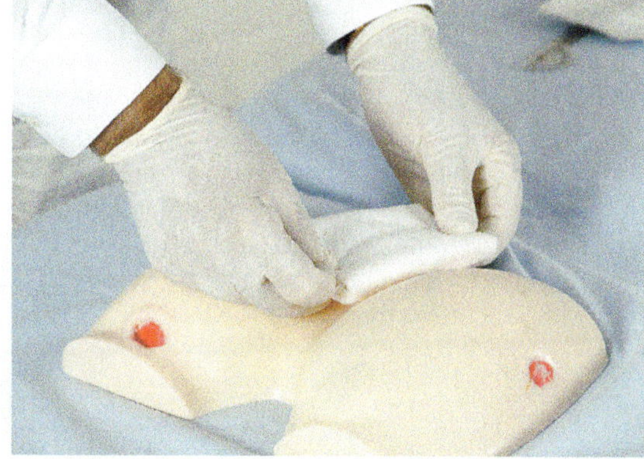

Applying a Gauze Wrap

Gauze pads are secured by tape or a gauze roll. Gauze rolls are applied in a spiral wrap or in a "figure-of-eight" wrap. To avoid impairing circulation, the amount of pressure applied when using gauze wraps should not be excessive.

1. To apply a **gauze wrap**, lay the portion of the gauze roll that is unwrapping against the limb segment, with the still-rolled gauze away from the limb.

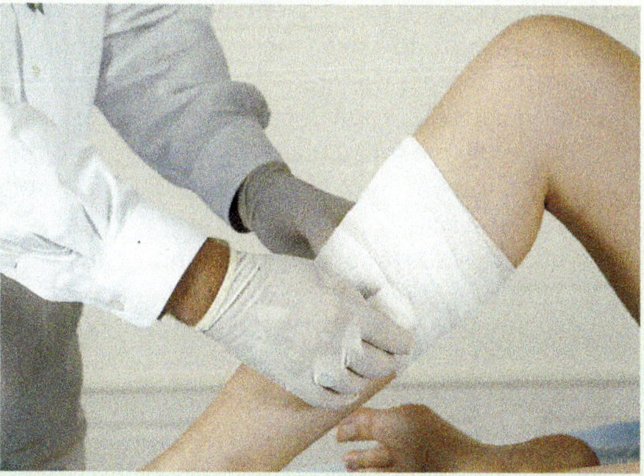

(continued)

PROCEDURE 4–3 Application of Dressings and Wraps (*continued*)

2 A **spiral wrap** is applied by wrapping gauze in a continuous manner around the limb segment. The roll of gauze is angled slightly to accommodate for the sloping contour of the limb segment to be wrapped and to avoid creating a tourniquet. The roll of gauze is unrolled around the limb segment, with each successive wrap overlapping the previous wrap by half. When the wrap is completed, secure the gauze with tape.

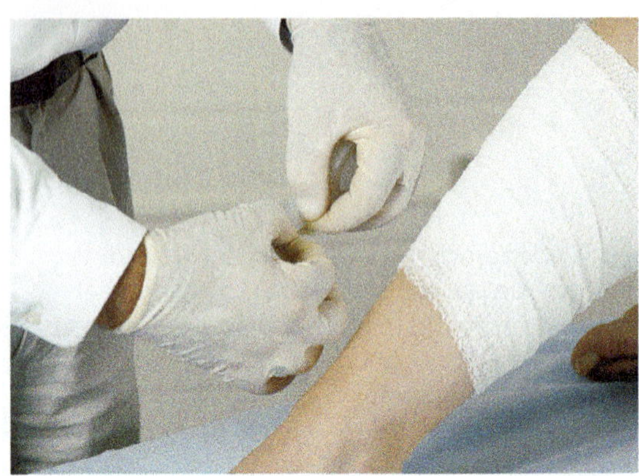

3 Removal of gauze wraps secured with tape requires careful cutting to avoid injuring patients; use bandage scissors (scissors with one flat arm). The flat arm slides under the wrap and next to the skin, permitting the wrap and tape to be cut without cutting the skin.

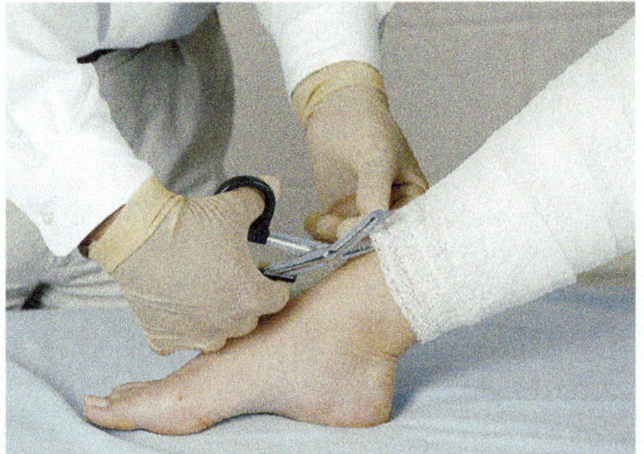

Applying a Compression Wrap

Compression wraps may be applied in spiral or figure-of-eight wraps. When applying compression wraps to control edema, use a spiral wrap, with more pressure applied distally than proximally. This provides for compression on edematous segments without constricting the flow of fluid toward the core of the body for subsequent elimination. When controlling edema, use the wrap with approximately graded pressure to cover the entire limb segment distal to the proximal edge of the wrap. When applying compression wraps for joint support, a figure-of-eight or spiral wrap may be used. When providing support, apply a compression wrap with even pressure from distal to proximal. Applying a compression wrap for support does not require the entire limb segment distal to the proximal edge of the wrap to be covered. In no case should a wrap be applied with the proximal pressure greater than the distal pressure.

The technique for applying a compression wrap is the same as for applying a gauze wrap. Frequent examination of compression wraps is necessary to ensure that the amount of compression applied is appropriate and that the wrap remains in place.

Start a figure-of-eight wrap in the same manner as a spiral wrap. Rather than a continuous wrap in the same direction, however, change the direction of wrapping each time the wrap completes one loop of the figure-of-eight. The illustrations for this section demonstrate application of a compression wrap of the ankle for support.

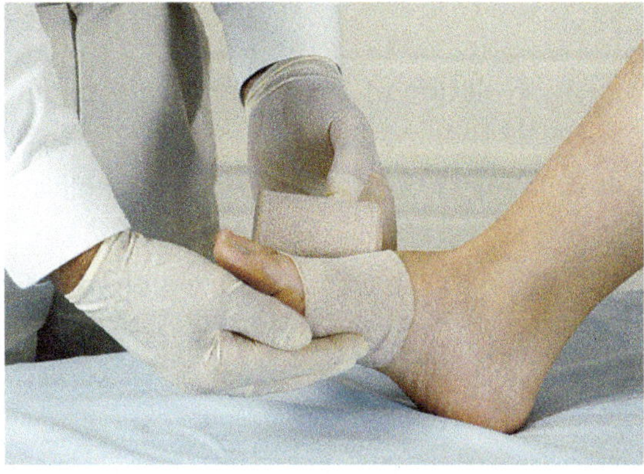

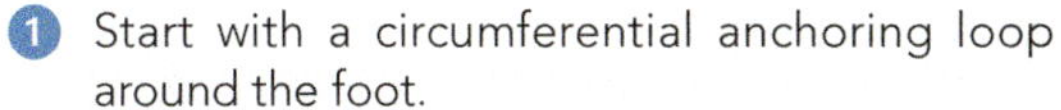

1 Start with a circumferential anchoring loop around the foot.

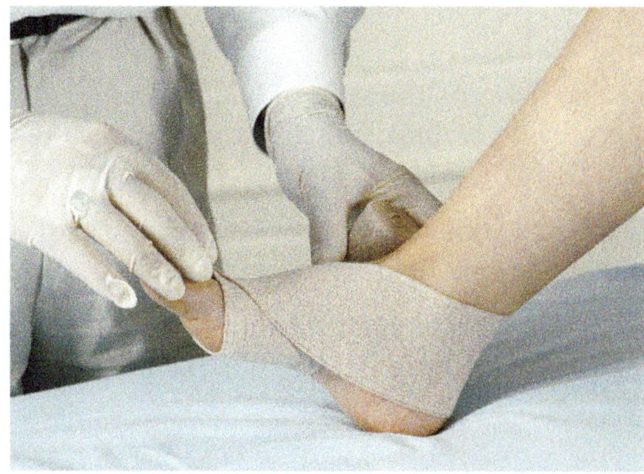

2 Wrap from lateral to medial around the ankle.

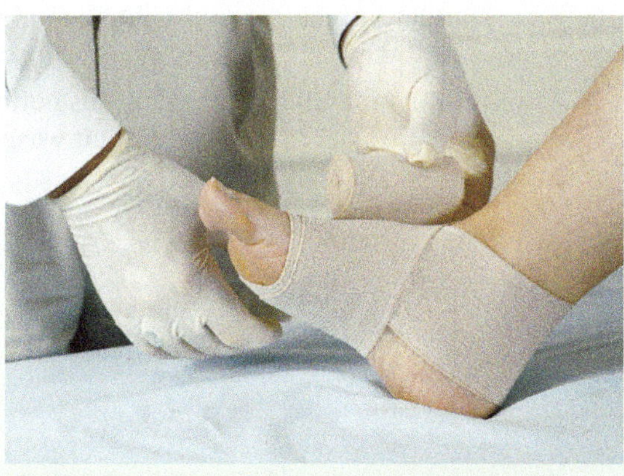

3 Wrap from medial to lateral around the foot.

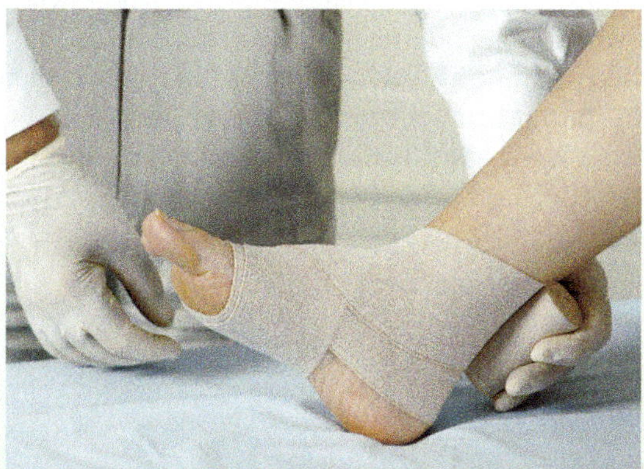

4 Wrap from lateral to medial around the ankle (second time) with an angle that will permit continuing a spiral wrap up the ankle from distal to proximal. Secure the end of the compression wrap with adhesive tape.

Review Questions

1. Which federal agency is responsible for developing and issuing guidelines for aseptic techniques and isolation systems?
2. What are the eight guidelines for providing and maintaining a sterile field? Describe each.
3. What apparel is necessary for aseptic techniques?
4. What is the most important procedure for preventing transmission of nosocomial infections?
5. What are the four purposes of wound dressing?
6. What are four types of wound dressings? Describe the purpose of each.
7. What six factors affect selection of wound-dressing materials?
8. What are the five main routes of microorganism transmission?
9. Who is responsible for implementing and monitoring isolation and sterile procedures?
10. What is the usual level of infection control practiced for contact with all patients?
11. What is the difference between standard precautions and transmission-based precautions?
12. What are the five major areas of recommendations for isolation precautions?

Suggested Activities

1. Practice and describe the skills of handwashing, gowning, gloving, wound assessment, and application of wound dressings.
2. Establish a sterile field, and describe guidelines for maintaining a sterile field.
3. Observe other students performing wound dressings using a sterile field, and make note of any violation of the guidelines for maintaining a sterile field.
4. Role-play wound assessment and application of dressings.
5. Document wound assessment and wound-dressing procedures performed during Activity 3.

Case Study

Mrs. Shimizu is an 80-year-old female admitted to the hospital 9 days ago for treatment of cirrhosis of the liver. On admission she was placed in a semiprivate room with a roommate with kidney failure. Because of her age, she has a compromised immune system and has begun to show signs, by auscultation and radiograph, of lung infiltrate. Physical therapy services, specifically respiratory care, and bed mobility have been ordered for Mrs. Shimizu.

1. Would you expect that Mrs. Shimizu will remain in her semiprivate room?
2. What infection-control guidelines should be followed in providing care?
3. What standard precautions should be implemented by physical therapists/assistants providing care?
4. As part of overall management of this patient, when should the physical therapist/assistant wash their hands?

References

1. Boyce, J. M., & Pittet, D. (2002). *Guideline for hand hygiene in health care settings.* Atlanta, GA: Centers for Disease Control and Prevention, Healthcare Infection Control Practices Advisory Committee and the HICPAC/SHEA/APIC/IDSA Hand Hygiene Task Force.
2. Department of Health and Human Services. (1997). *Part I: Evolution of isolation practices.* Atlanta, GA: Centers for Disease Control and Prevention, Hospital Infection Control Practices Advisory Committee.
3. Department of Health and Human Services. (1997). *Part II: Recommendations for isolation precautions in hospitals.* Atlanta, GA: Centers for Disease Control and Prevention, Hospital Infection Control Practices Advisory Committee.
4. Schulster, L., & Chinn, R. Y. W. (2003). *Guidelines for environmental infection control in health care facilities.* Atlanta, GA: Centers for Disease Control and Prevention, Healthcare Infection Control Practices Advisory Committee.

5

Vital Signs and Anthropometrics

LEARNING OUTCOMES

Upon completion of this chapter, you will be able to:

1. Describe the purposes, methods, and norms for the measurement of the vital signs of pulse, blood pressure, respiration, temperature, and pain.
2. Describe the purposes and methods for the subjective measurement of pain levels perceived by a patient.
3. Indicate the sites at which measurements of vital signs of pulse, blood pressure, respiration, and temperature are usually taken.
4. Measure pulse, blood pressure, respiration, and temperature correctly and accurately.
5. Measure patient pain levels correctly and accurately.
6. Use correct terms to describe vital sign measurements outside normal ranges.
7. Identify vital sign measurements that are below, within, or above normal ranges.
8. Document vital sign measurements correctly and accurately.
9. Document pain measurements correctly and accurately.
10. Describe the use of the anthropometric measures of height and weight and how they relate to body mass index.

KEY TERMS

Afebrile
Anthropometric measures
Auscultation
Basal heart rate
Blanching
Blood pressure
Body mass index (BMI)
Bradycardia
Diastolic pressure
Doppler
Febrile
Hyperthermia
Hypothermia
Maximal heart rate
Pain
Patency
Pulse
Red flag
Regularity
Respiratory rate
Resting heart rate
Systolic pressure
Tachycardia
Target heart rate
Temperature
Trophic
Visual analog scale

Introduction

■ **Take Note**

Vital signs: heart rate, blood pressure, respiration rate, SpO_2 temperature, pain.

Physical therapists/assistants should be aware of, and be able to perform, objective measurements of physiological functions known as vital signs. Vital signs are used to monitor a patient's status before, and at any given time during, patient care. Vital signs consist of heart rate (HR) or pulse (P), blood pressure (BP), respiratory rate (RR), oxygen saturation (SpO_2), and temperature (T). Oxygen level is a measure that is now frequently included with vital signs. These are objective measures of physiological activity.

Although historically not considered a vital sign, perception of pain is now included when measuring vital signs. Measurements of pain are self-reported and are subjective measurements. **Anthropometric measures** of height and weight are also not traditional vital signs but are used in assessing patient health. Anthropometric measurements are objective measures. Heart rate (or pulse), blood pressure, respiratory rate, oxygen saturation, temperature, pain, and anthropometric measures are all considered in developing a safe and effective plan of care.

When vital signs are assessed, the lack of an expected change or an unexpected change may occur. Changes in vital signs may create no flag, a "yellow flag," or a "red flag" (see Chapter 2). The determining factors that may raise a flag are related to the specific vital sign, the degree to which the specific vital sign changes, and the overall response of the patient. Based on vital signs, a determination is made to (1) continue treatment, (2) halt treatment, or (3) halt treatment and refer to an appropriate healthcare provider immediately. Thus the examination and evaluation of vital signs is basic to patient safety.

Pulse

Purpose

Pulse rate, regularity, and amplitude, as well as patency, provide information concerning cardiovascular status.

Pulse Rate

Pulse (in beats per minute) is a measurement of heart rate. **Basal heart rate** is the pulse rate measured after an extended period of rest and is one indication of cardiovascular function in the absence of physical stress. **Resting heart rate** is a measurement of heart rate without imposed stress.

Pulse rates are measured before, during, and following an imposed physiological or physical stress. Determination of when pulse rate is measured during physical therapy patient/client management is contingent on a patient's condition. When measured during imposed physiological or physical stress, such as physical therapy interventions, pulse rate is one measurement of the cardiovascular system's capacity to provide blood flow under conditions of stress. Measured after stress, pulse rate is a measure of the cardiovascular system's recovery capability.

The range of normal resting heart rate for adults is 60–100 bpm. Resting heart rate in adults can vary greatly, due to the state of physical conditioning of each individual. Individuals who maintain a high level of physical training may have a resting heart rate between 40 and 60 bpm. Individuals who maintain a moderately sedentary lifestyle may have a resting heart rate between 60 and 85 bpm. A resting heart rate greater than 85 bpm is usually indicative of either deconditioning or a medical condition. The normal resting heart rate for infants and children under the age of 10 is between 70 and 160 bpm. A child's height and weight as well as age must also be considered when reviewing heart rate.

A very slow resting heart rate, or **bradycardia**, is a heart rate of less than 60 bpm. A very fast heart rate, or **tachycardia**, is a heart rate greater than 100 bpm. Bradycardia or tachycardia at a resting state may be indicative of disease or side effects of medication. Table 5–1 ■ presents the usual ranges of resting heart rate.

Measuring pulse rate also allows examination of the regularity of heartbeat. **Regularity** refers to the evenness of pulse rate. This measure of regularity is subjective.

Table 5–1 ■ Usual ranges of resting heart rate	
Newborn to 6 months	100–160 bpm
Infant of 1 year	90–150 bpm
Child of 3 years	80–125 bpm
Child of 5 years	70–115 bpm
Child of 10 years up and adult normal range	60–100 bpm
Bradycardia	<60 bpm
Tachycardia	>100 bpm

Amplitude of a pulse is rated on a subjective scale of 0–4+. This scale includes the measures of

0 = absent
1+ = thready, weak
2+ = normal
3+ = strong
4+ = full bounding

A pulse that varies from normal in rate, regularity, or amplitude may be indicative of deconditioning, disease, or injury.

■ **Take Note**
Characteristics of pulse: rate, regularity, amplitude.

Methods

The most common clinical method of measuring pulse is manual palpation with mechanical devices used in specific situations. **Auscultation** of the heart, which is monitoring of the heart using a stethoscope, is also used to obtain heart rate. **Doppler** measurements, which use frequency changes during blood flow, are used to examine patency (Figure 5–1 ■).

A pulse oximeter is a small device, attaching to either the distal end of an index finger or an earlobe, that measures pulse rate and blood oxygen concentrations (Figure 5–2 ■). When using a pulse oximeter on a finger to obtain oxygen saturation levels, fingernails must be free of nail polish or crèmes. Nail polish and crèmes block absorption of light, which impedes accurate readings of oxygen saturation levels. Results are provided by digital display. This is an easy method of monitoring both pulse rate and blood oxygen saturation during both rest and activity. These devices are used more and more to measure important vital signs, allowing patient response to activity to be monitored in real time.

■ **Take Note**
Means of measuring pulse: palpation, auscultation, EKG, Doppler.

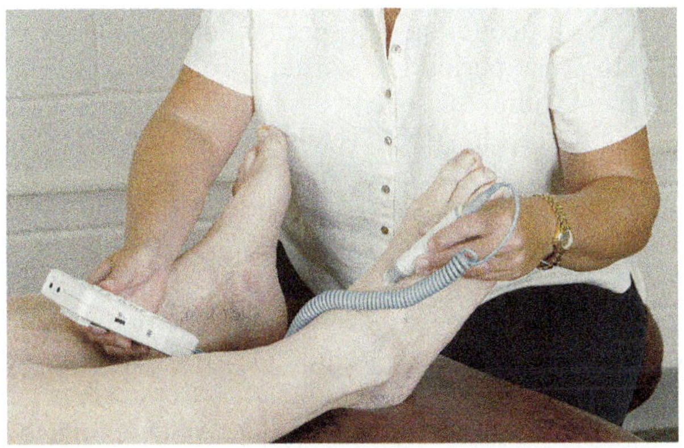

FIGURE 5–1 ■ Doppler sonography.

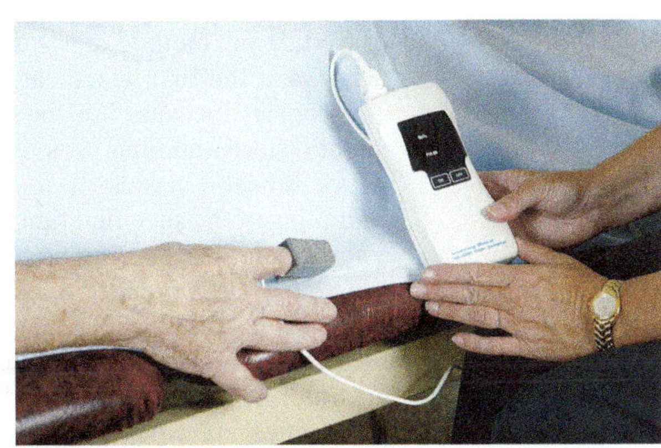

FIGURE 5–2 ■ Pulse oximeter.

Oxygen saturation (SpO_2) levels are not the same as arterial blood gases (PaO_2). SpO_2 measurements indicate the amount of saturation of oxygen-carrying hemoglobin. The normal range of SpO_2 is 95% to 100%.[1] An SpO_2 reading below normal may indicate conditions that must be considered when providing physical therapy interventions. Initial SpO_2 readings are taken with vital signs before initiating interventions. SpO_2 readings should be monitored during physical therapy interventions to assess the effect of interventions on oxygen saturation. Readings below 90% are considered low[1] and should be considered a yellow or red flag.

To palpate a pulse manually, place the pads of the index and middle fingers of one hand lightly over the site where the pulse is to be measured. The thumb is not used for palpation when measuring pulse because there is an artery in the pad of the thumb, which may cause one's own pulse to be mistaken for the patient's pulse. Take care not to press too hard while palpating pulses. Excessive pressure during palpation can obliterate the pulse, impede blood flow, or cause arterial spasm. Obliterating a pulse prevents measurement, and impeding blood flow or causing arterial spasm can be dangerous to a patient. This is especially true when examining distal pulses, most commonly palpated when measuring peripheral vascular patency. These pulses are reported as present or absent.

▪ Take Note

Use index and middle fingers to palpate pulses.

Heart rate is measured in beats per minute (bpm). To obtain a heart rate, use a watch or clock that displays time in seconds. Once a pulse is palpated, count beats within a specified interval of time. The most accurate method is to count beats for a period of 60 seconds. The count is reported without additional calculation. A period of at least 30 seconds is recommended.

Alternative methods require less time to monitor the pulse but require additional calculation. Counting beats for a 10-second time period and multiplying by six or using a 15-second time period and multiplying by four are the most common shortcuts used. Using a shorter sampling period may result in a measurement that is less precise. Many times, a whole number of beats does not occur within a shorter period of time. An estimate of a fractional heart rate is not as accurate as an exact count. Irregularities in heart rate are not detected as readily when a shorter sampling period is used. The necessity of additional calculation provides a potential source of error. Sometimes one beat in a time period is missed. Using a shortcut may increase the error either sixfold or fourfold, respectively.

▪ Take Note

It is most accurate to count a pulse for 60 seconds.

As an example, an error of one beat during measurements taken over a 60-second period of time and over a 10-second period will provide two very different results. For a patient with an actual heart rate of 72 bpm, missing one beat during the 60-second count produces an error of 1/72 or 1.4%. Using a 10-second count, the same heart rate should yield 12 beats. If one beat is missed during the 10-second count, only 11 beats will be counted. This is multiplied by six, resulting in a calculation of 66 bpm for the same patient, an error of 6/72, or 8.3%. Although shortcut methods are used routinely, and results are recorded without question, take care to provide an accurate and valid measurement.

▪ Take Note

Calculating pulse:

- Count for 60 seconds.
- Count for 30 seconds and double (multiply by 2).
- Count for 15 seconds and quadruple (multiple by 4).

There are two methods of timing when counting heart rate. The key factor in counting heart rate is that the number of heartbeats within a given time period is counted. The first, or traditional, method starts the time period of counting at a specific time on a clock or watch, and the first heartbeat felt after the time period has started is considered beat 1. This is beat 1 because it is the first heartbeat within the specified time period. The second method starts the time period of counting when a heartbeat is felt; that heartbeat is beat 0. This is beat 0 because it does not occur within the specified time period but marks the beginning of the specified time period. Whichever method is used will provide an accurate count when attention is paid to the basis for when the interval begins and the number of counts that fall *within* the specified interval.

Maximal heart rate is the highest heart rate a person should achieve on exertion with respect to age and medical condition. The following guidelines for determining maximal heart rate are based on the absence of cardiovascular pathology. Maximal heart rates are calculated for each individual patient based on age, subtracting the patient's age from 220. For a 43-year-old individual, the maximal heart rate is 220 – 43, or 177.

PROCEDURE 5–1 Measuring Heart Rate

The radial and carotid arteries are the most commonly used sites for measuring pulse, an indicator of heart rate.

The radial pulse is most easily palpated on the distal volar surface of the wrist, just lateral to the tendons of the finger flexors.

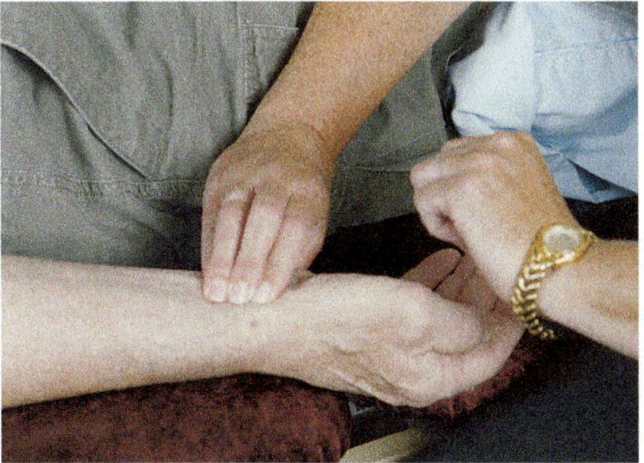

■ Take Note

The best sites for monitoring heart rate are the radial and carotid arteries.

The carotid pulse is most easily palpated on the lateral aspect of the neck, inferior to the angle of the mandible.

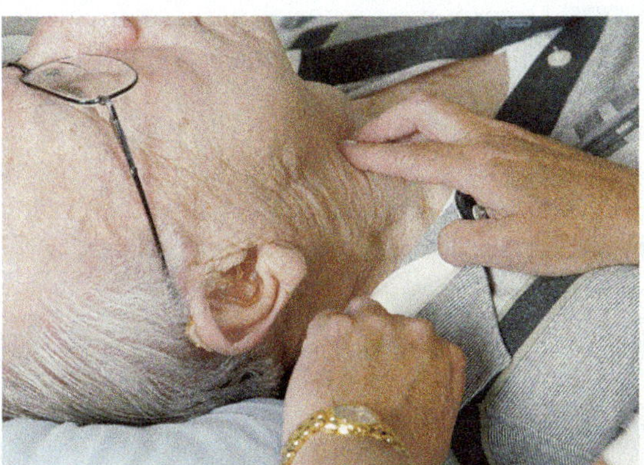

Palpate the carotid pulse carefully and without reaching across the patient's throat. Placing a hand across the patient's throat creates the potential for compromising a patient's airway. Baroreceptor reflexes produce decreased heart rate and strength of heart contractions. "Massage" to the carotid artery can elicit this reflex, so accuracy in placement and type of palpation is necessary when measuring carotid artery pulses.

The site used to obtain a pulse via auscultation is medial to the midclavicular line at the level of the fifth intercostal space.

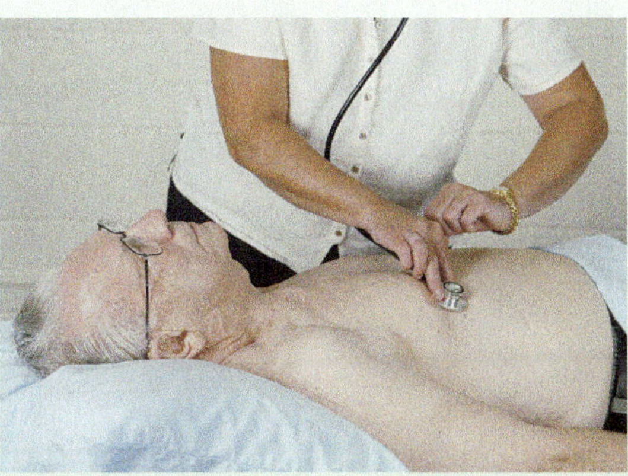

■ **Take Note**

Example maximum heart rate calculation:
220 − 60 = 160

Example target heart rate calculations:

- X% (maximum heart rate)
- 50% × 160 = 80 (*deconditioned patient*)
- 80% × 160 = 128 (*fit patient*)

Target heart rate is the heart rate that an individual should achieve during exercise for cardiovascular conditioning with respect to age and medical condition. For a patient without contraindications, the target heart rate must fall between 60% and 80% of the maximal heart rate. Target heart rates for patients with cardiovascular pathology are adjusted by physicians based on clinical findings for individual patients. Thus, the formula used to determine a target heart rate for cardiovascular exercise for the 43-year-old person presented earlier is between 106 and 142 bpm.

80% max target heart rate

$$\begin{aligned} &(0.80) \times (220 - \text{age}) \\ &= (0.8)(220 - 43) \\ &= (0.8)(177) \\ &= 142 \text{ bpm} \end{aligned}$$

60% max target heart rate

$$\begin{aligned} &(0.60) \times (220 - \text{age}) \\ &= (0.6)(220 - 43) \\ &= (0.6)(177) \\ &= 106 \text{ bpm} \end{aligned}$$

■ **Take Note**

Other factors to monitor while taking a pulse:

- Loss of hair
- Dry or flaky skin
- Muscle atrophy
- Skin temperature
- Skin color

Arterial Patency

Palpation of pulses is also used to determine **patency** of arteries. Although not traditionally considered a vital sign, examination of patency is commonly included when assessing circulation. Patency indicates the presence or absence of blood flow at the point of pulse palpation. A lack of patency, absence of a pulse, is an indication of arterial occlusion resulting from physical blockage or peripheral vascular disease. The presence of edema makes the determination of patency difficult. Precautions and contraindications associated with decreased or obstructed blood flow must be taken into account when developing a plan of care.

METHODS Determining arterial patency includes three major methods: observation, palpation of pulses, and rate of capillary refill. A lack of arterial patency is one sign of peripheral arterial disease. Observe the extremities for **trophic** changes, such as loss of hair, dry or flaky skin, and muscle atrophy. A decrease in skin temperature is often noted in areas of decreased patency. Skin temperature may be determined by palpation or measured with a skin thermometer. Pallor, the loss of normal coloring of the skin, may also result from decreased circulation.

PROCEDURE 5–2 Determining Arterial Patency: Palpation of Pulse

Common sites for palpation of pulses to determine vascular patency are the brachial, femoral, popliteal, posterior tibial, and dorsal pedal pulses.

The pulse of the brachial artery is palpated on the medial aspect of the arm midway down the shaft of the humerus.

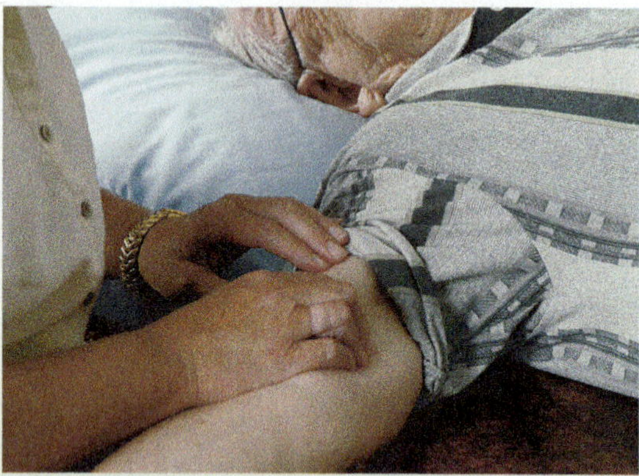

■ **Take Note**

The best sites to monitor patency are the brachial, popliteal, posterior tibial, and dorsal pedal arteries.

The pulse of the femoral artery is palpated in the femoral triangle. Although a strong pulse, the femoral artery lies close to several large muscles, making palpation difficult. When preparing to palpate the femoral artery, explaining to patients what you are about to do will decrease surprise and reduce risk of embarrassment. Palpation of the femoral artery that is too firm can cause pain.

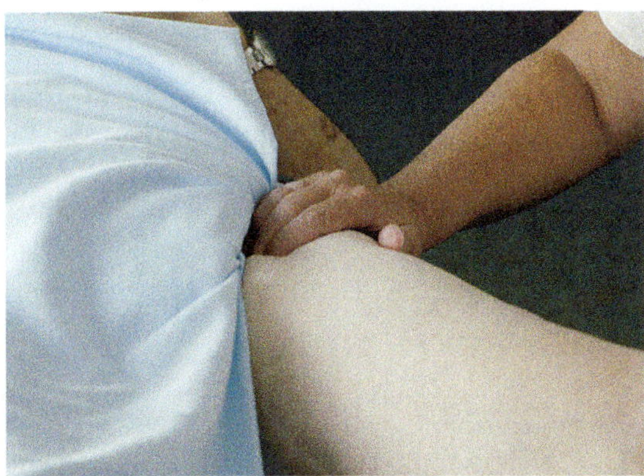

Location of the popliteal, posterior tibial, and dorsal pedal arteries, and avoiding obliteration of their pulse with excessive pressure, can be difficult, even in healthy patients. These pulses are commonly susceptible to degradation of strength in patients with peripheral vascular insufficiency.

The pulse of the popliteal artery is palpated at, or just above, the posterior aspect of the knee.

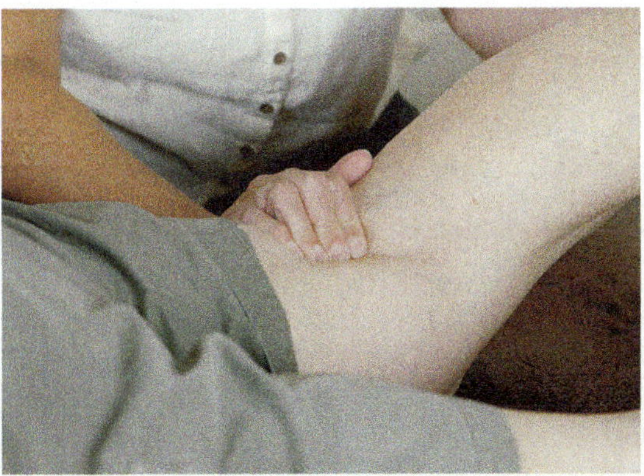

The pulse of the posterior tibial artery is palpated posterior or inferior to the medial malleolus.

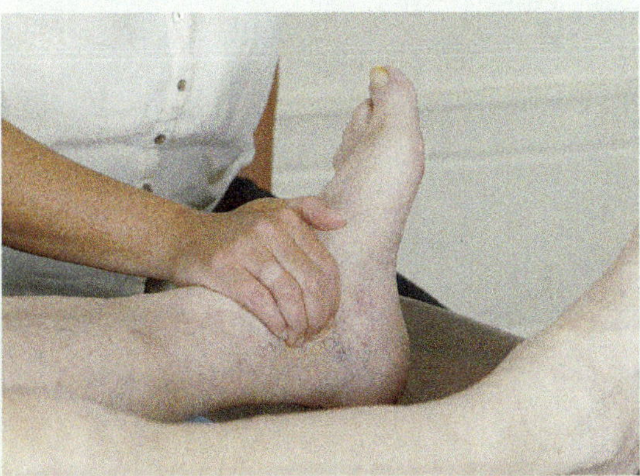

(continued)

PROCEDURE 5–2 Determining Arterial Patency: Palpation of Pulse (*continued*)

The dorsal pedal pulse is palpated on the dorsum of the foot over the cuboid bones.

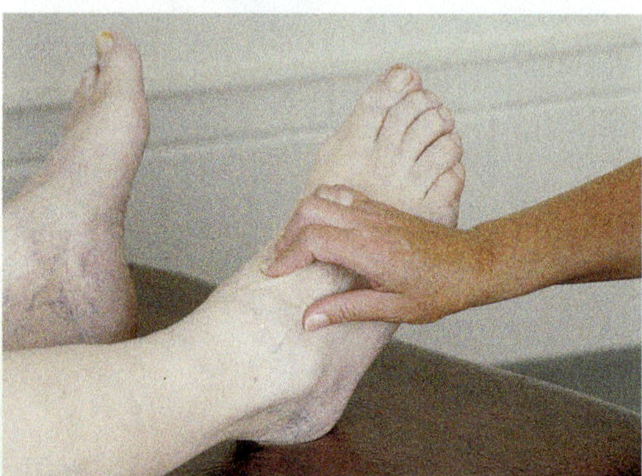

PROCEDURE 5–3 Determining Arterial Patency: Refill Tests

Additional noninvasive tests to determine arterial patency include a capillary refill test and a reactive hyperemia test, such as the rubor of dependency test. To perform the capillary refill test, observe the color and the nail bed, and then compress the nail bed.

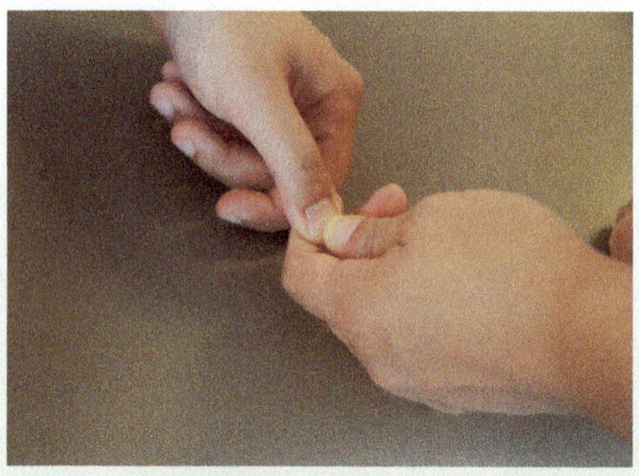

Quickly release the pressure on the nail bed. **Blanching** is noted immediately, followed by return of color in the nail bed within seconds. A delay of the return of color indicates a loss of arterial patency.

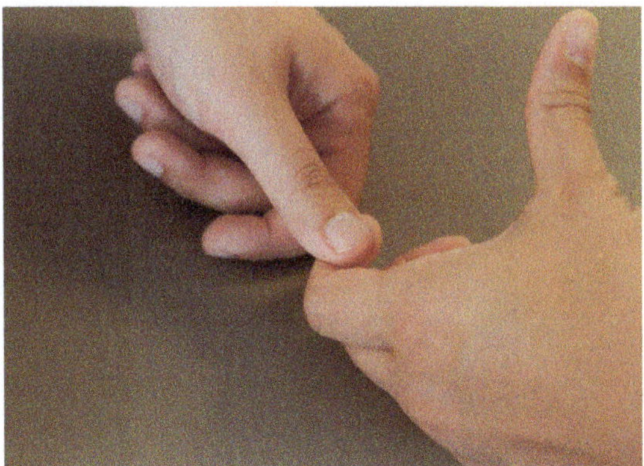

Changes of skin color associated with the interruption of capillary circulation may be induced by raising an extremity above the level of the heart. This is the basis of the reactive hyperemia test. To perform the rubor of dependency test, place the patient in a supine position.

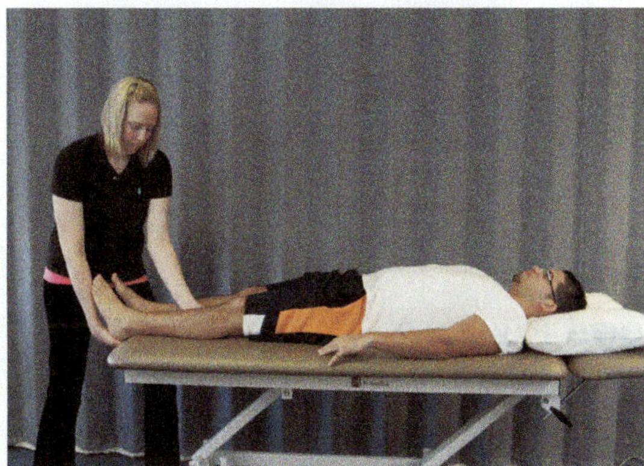

Raise one lower extremity, with the knee straight, to a 45-degree angle from the bed or table. Maintain this position for approximately 1 minute. Pallor will occur when decreased patency is present.

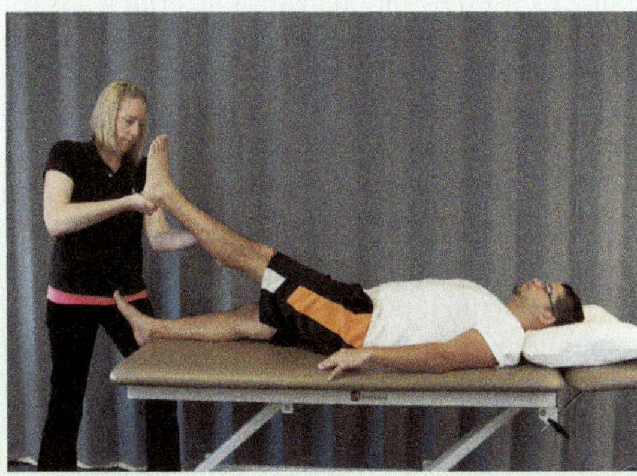

(continued)

PROCEDURE 5–3 Determining Arterial Patency: Refill Tests (*continued*)

Then lower the limb and assist the patient to sitting with the feet over the side of the bed or table. Within seconds color should begin to return to the limb. Shortly after sitting with the feet over the side of the bed or table, hyperemia (rubor) may occur.

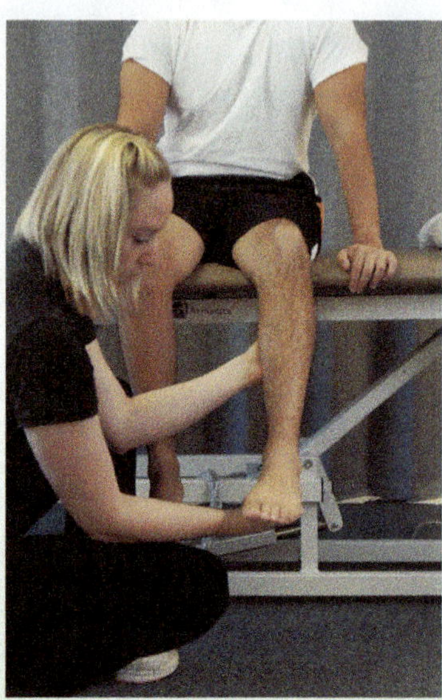

Blood Pressure

Purpose

Blood pressure is a measure of vascular resistance to blood flow. The primary purposes for measuring blood pressure are to determine vascular resistance to blood flow and the effectiveness of cardiac muscle in pumping blood to overcome vascular resistance.

■ Take Note

Blood pressure numbers:

- Systolic: pressure when heart is contracting
- Diastolic: pressure when heart is at rest

BLOOD PRESSURE COMPONENTS Two values are reported as a measurement of blood pressure. The first value represents the component of **systolic pressure**, a measure of pressure exerted by blood against arterial walls when the heart is contracting. The second value represents the component of **diastolic pressure**, a measure of the pressure exerted by arterial walls against blood when the heart is not contracting.

Blood pressure is measured using a sphygmomanometer, or blood pressure cuff, by listening for Korotkoff sounds. As pressure in the cuff falls to the level of the systolic pressure, blood flows through the artery during systole (contraction phase) but not during diastole (noncontraction phase). The first sounds heard through the stethoscope are usually described as tapping sounds. Initially, the tapping sound may be difficult to hear, as these sounds may be faint or soft and may not occur evenly. As cuff pressure falls, tapping sounds become more clear and distinct. The tapping nature of the sound is a result of the start of blood flow during systole and the stopping of blood flow during diastole. The tapping sounds occur because at this level of cuff pressure, arterial flow can occur only during systole. When the first tapping sounds are heard, a pressure reading is noted. This reading represents the value of systolic blood pressure.

As more air is evacuated from a cuff, pressure falls toward the diastolic level. When cuff pressure is at a diastolic pressure level, the distinct and clear tapping becomes muffled and usually disappears after an additional drop of 5 to 10 mm Hg. Muffled sounds occur at this level of cuff pressure because blood flows through the artery during both systole and

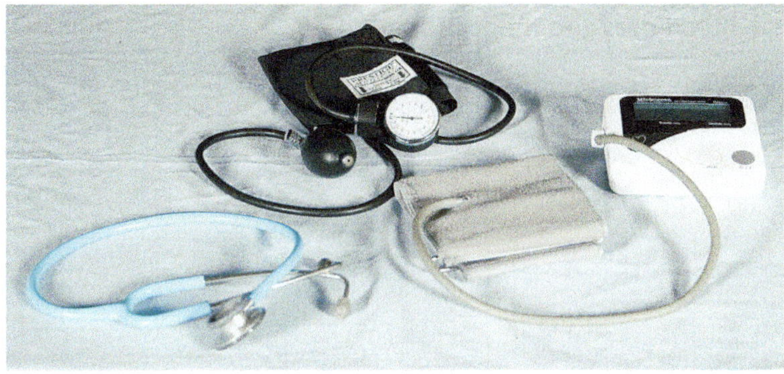

FIGURE 5–3 ■ Examples of sphygmomanometers.

diastole. When tapping sounds become muffled, a pressure reading is noted. This reading represents the value of diastolic blood pressure.

Blood-pressure readings are reported as the systolic pressure over the diastolic pressure. A systolic pressure of 120 mm Hg and a diastolic pressure of 80 mm Hg is documented as 120/80 mm Hg and verbally reported as "120 over 80."

■ **Take Note**

$$\text{Blood pressure} = \frac{\textit{Systolic}}{\textit{Diastolic}}$$

Method

Measure blood pressure by auscultation of an artery using a stethoscope while a sphygmomanometer is applied over the artery being auscultated. A sphygmomanometer consists of an air bladder inside a cuff, a device for inflating the bladder, and a device for measuring the pressure in the bladder (**Figure 5–3** ■). Blood-pressure measurements are actually measurements of the cuff's air bladder pressure. The pressure corresponds to arterial pressure as arterial blood flows, or attempts to flow, past the restricting cuff.

Blood-pressure measurements were originally based on the pressure required to raise a column of mercury in a glass tube. Therefore, blood-pressure measurements continue to be reported in mm Hg (millimeters of mercury). Sphygmomanometers may provide output using a mechanical gauge or a digital readout. A stethoscope is used to auscultate the sounds of arterial blood flow through the brachial artery as it passes through the antecubital fossa. Blood-pressure sounds monitored by auscultation are called Korotkoff sounds. Some electronic methods of blood-pressure measurement do not require auscultation.

Site

The most common site for measuring blood pressure is the left upper arm. This site corresponds closely to the level of the tricuspid valve of the heart, which is considered the "reference level for pressure measurement." Although body position may change blood pressure, such changes are accurately measured when using the left upper arm as the reference. Initially, blood-pressure measurements should be taken in both arms, and subsequent blood pressure measurements should be taken in the arm with the highest reading. Documentation should include the arm in which measurement was taken and the position of the patient.

In certain cases, or for specific reasons, blood-pressure readings may be taken at sites other than the upper arm. Taking blood pressure readings other than the upper arm are necessitated for a patient without arms or with a cast, lymphodema, or open wounds. Taking blood pressure readings in the lower extremity may be used in such cases.

Norms

As a reference point for blood pressure, 120/80 mm Hg has been considered ideal. New guidelines emphasize a range of values rather than set numbers. **Table 5–2** ■ presents ranges of normal and abnormal blood pressures for an adult.[2] Blood pressure will change with stress, physical activity, and age. Lower levels are considered to indicate the existence of hypotension. Clinical decision making based on the values presented in Table 5-2 must also include consideration of age and medical status and should take into account all available data concerning patient status. Clinical decision making with respect to the impact of

Table 5–2 ■ Blood pressure ranges for adults

	Systolic (mm Hg)	Diastolic (mm Hg)
Normal	<120	<80
Prehypertension	120–139	80–89
Stage 1 hypertension	140–159	90–99
Stage 2 hypertension	≥160	≥100

medical status on patient-care intervention is in the realm of the physical therapist. Physical therapists are to provide the acceptable range of blood pressure changes when directing physical therapist assistants in administering patient care.

Changes from resting blood pressure can result as patients change position or increase activity. Red flags, which are indications to stop activity and examine cardiac status, include (1) failure of systolic pressure to rise in proportion with increased intensity of activity, (2) a decrease in systolic pressure greater than 10 mm Hg, (3) a systolic pressure greater than 240 mm Hg, or (4) an increase greater than 20 mm Hg for diastolic pressure during activity.

Interpretation of pediatric blood pressure is based on a child's age and height percentile on standard growth charts. Generally, the prehypertension range is considered to be 120/80 mm Hg. Detailed tables for blood pressure for infants and children by age, gender, and height percentile are available at http://www.cc.nih.gov/ccc/pedweb/pedsstaff/bp.html.

PROCEDURE 5–4 Measuring Blood Pressure

1. Before placing a cuff around a patient's left upper arm, consider the size of the cuff. Inaccurate readings will be obtained if the wrong size cuff is used. Cuff sizes range from pediatric to large adult. The bladder of a cuff should cover approximately 80% of the circumference of the upper arm, and the width should be approximately 40% of the circumference of the upper arm.[3]

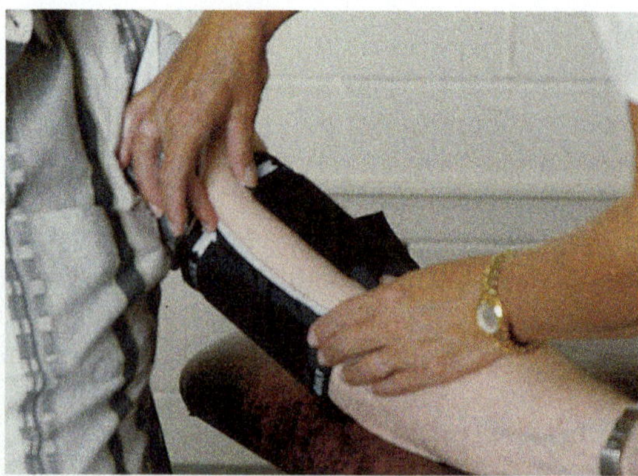

2. A blood pressure cuff is placed snugly around the upper arm with the bladder centered over the anterior surface and with the lower border approximately 2–3 cm above the antecubital fossa.
3. Support the patient's arm, either on a table or by resting on the physical therapist's/assistant's arm, so the cuff is at the patient's heart level.
4. Hold the inflation bulb and its attaching tube, and the stethoscope and its tubing, so that the tubes do not touch each other. When the respective tubes touch each other, sounds can be distorted.

5. With the patient's arm supported, locate the brachial artery on the anterior medial surface of the elbow as the artery crosses the antecubital fossa.
6. Palpate the pulse as the bladder is inflated. Note the pressure when the pulse can no longer be palpated.
7. Deflate the cuff.
8. Place the stethoscope drum or bell over the artery, and inflate the cuff to about 30 mm Hg greater than that noted when the pulse could no longer be palpated. When a cuff is inflated beyond the systolic blood pressure, the artery is totally occluded. Therefore, no sounds of blood flow come from the artery.

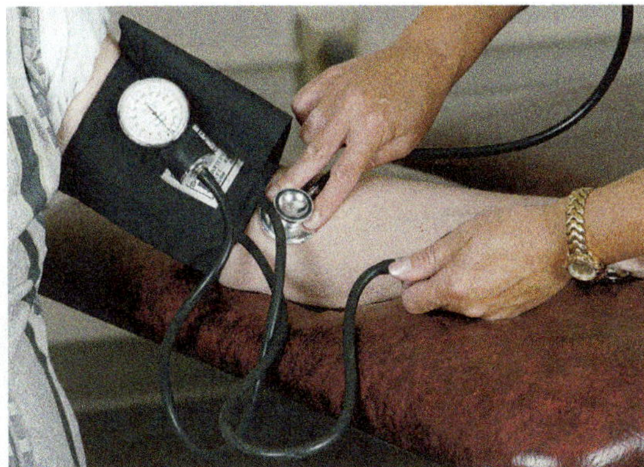

9. Evacuate air from the cuff slowly by opening the pressure-relief valve.
10. Note the pressure reading when the Korotkoff sounds start—usually a tapping sound. This is the systolic pressure.
11. Note the pressure reading when the Korotkoff sound of tapping becomes muffled. This is the diastolic pressure.
12. Release the remainder of the pressure in the cuff by opening the pressure relief valve rapidly and completely.
13. Remove the stethoscope and cuff from the patient.
14. Document both the systolic and diastolic values as blood pressure.

Throughout this procedure, take care not to maintain pressure on the artery for more than 2 or 3 minutes without relief. If cuff occlusion occurs for more than 2–3 minutes without relief, patients may experience symptoms of tingling or numbness, such as when an arm or leg "falls asleep."

Respiration

Purpose

Respiratory rate (RR) is the rate of breathing. Each respiratory cycle includes one inspiration and the subsequent expiration. RR can be measured, and the quality of respiration can be observed. While performing auscultation for respiratory rate, the nature of breath sounds can also be determined.

Methods

Methods of measuring respiratory rate are auscultation and observation. Auscultation is auditory, performed with a stethoscope. Observation is performed visually, by palpation, or by hearing without a stethoscope. Unobtrusive visual and auditory observations can be made just before, or just after, taking a pulse. In situations where shallow or quiet breathing patterns make visual or auditory observation difficult, auscultation with a stethoscope may improve auditory observation.

Take Note

Methods of measuring respiration rate:

- Auscultation with a stethoscope
- Observation of chest-wall movement
- Palpation of chest-wall movement
- Palpation of breath flow

RR is measured as the number of breathing cycles per minute. To measure respiratory rate, use a watch or clock that displays time in seconds. Count respiratory cycles for a set period of time. Only complete respiratory cycles, those consisting of both complete inspiratory and expiratory phases, are counted. Measurements may be over a 60-second time period, or shorter time periods may be used. Problems of accuracy noted previously for determining heart rate when using shortcut methods also apply to measurements of respiratory rate. Respiration is measured as cycles per minute but is reported without the use of units. A respiration rate of 12 respirations per minute is reported as 12 RR.

Duration of inspiratory and expiratory phases is observed, with expiratory phases usually of longer duration than inspiratory phases. Depth of inspiration, regularity of inspiration, and use of accessory muscles of respiration can also be observed as indicators of the quality of respiration. The importance of these observations varies with the diagnosis and condition of the patient. When documenting specific measurements of respiratory rate, also document information concerning these additional observations when pertinent.

PROCEDURE 5–5 Measuring Respiratory Rate

Palpation of a patient's thorax permits determination of the rise and fall of the chest during respiration.

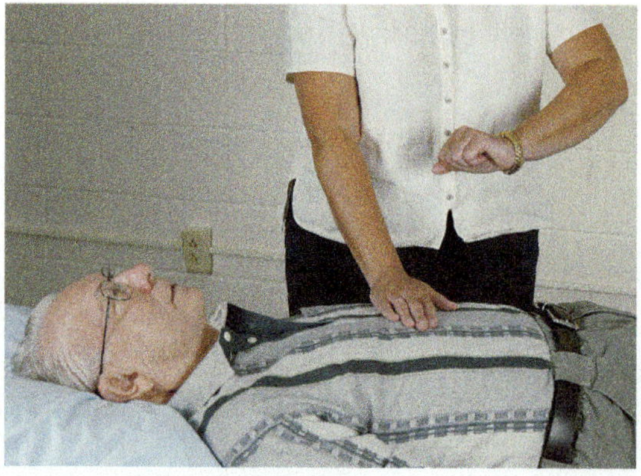

An alternative method of palpation requires placing the dorsum of one's hand close to, but not touching or occluding, a patient's mouth and nose. Changes in the direction of air flow during respiration can be felt as slight changes in pressure or temperature on the dorsum of one's hand.

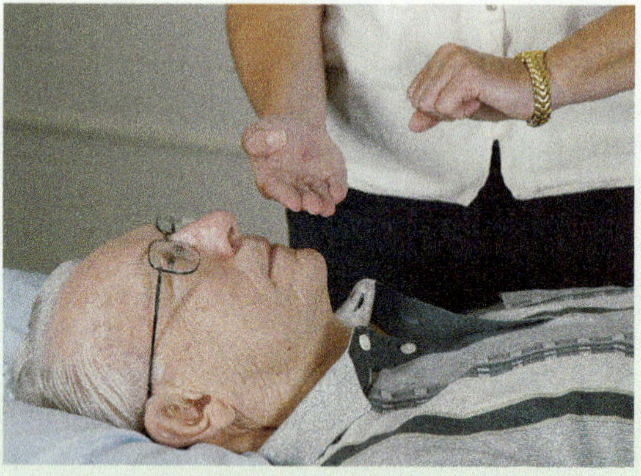

Norms

Normal cycle-to-cycle breathing patterns are even, are relatively quiet, and have a slight pause between the end of expiration and the initiation of inspiration. Only a very low-level hiss of air movement through the nose or mouth should be evident. Small variations may be noted, depending on an individual's level of physical training and state of anxiety. The range of normal resting respiratory rate for adults is considered 12–20 breaths per minute. The ratio of inspiratory time to expiratory time within one respiratory cycle (I/E ratio) is normally 1:2. Resting respiratory rates of less than 10 breaths per minute or more than 20 breaths per minute are considered abnormal.

Normal resting respiratory rate of infants and children varies by age. Newborn normal resting respiratory rate is 30–60 breaths per minute. At 6 months of age the normal resting respiratory rate is 24–38 breaths per minute. The rate for children decreases gradually to about 20–24 breaths per minute by age of 5, 16–22 breaths per minute by age of 10, and 14–20 breaths per minute by age of 14.

Following periods of exercise, or during respiratory distress, respiration may increase to 25 to 35 breaths per minute for short periods of time. With increased respiratory rates, breathing will be shallower, and accessory muscles of respiration are more likely to be involved.

■ Take Note

Normal respiratory rates: Adults 12, children 20.

■ Take Note

Inspiratory time is less than expiratory time.

Temperature

Purpose

Body **temperature** provides information concerning basal metabolic state, potential presence of infection, and metabolic response to exercise. Physical therapists/assistants may not routinely measure a patient's body temperature but need to know the methods and norms. Skin temperature provides information concerning circulatory status and local inflammatory responses.

Methods

A variety of devices are available for measuring patient temperatures. Primary sites for taking temperatures are tympanic (ear) and oral.

Electronic thermometers with disposable probes or probe covers produce a reading of the temperature. A new probe cover must be used each time a new temperature is to be taken, even for the same patient. Temperature measurements may be recorded in degrees Fahrenheit or degrees Celsius. Documentation must indicate which temperature scale was used.

Palpation of skin temperature is performed using the dorsal surface of the hand. Place the dorsum of the hand lightly on the site to be examined. Move the hand slowly from distal to proximal, noting temperature changes. Comparison of one extremity to another, such as left arm to right arm, may provide information concerning differences in temperature.

■ Take Note

Methods for temperature measurement: thermometers (electronic, heat-sensitive strips) or palpation.

Norms

Normal ranges of body temperature are centered at 98.6°F or 37°C. An individual's temperature will fluctuate throughout a 24-hour period. These fluctuations should not be more than a few degrees, depending on time of day, site of measurement, and level of activity. Normal body temperatures vary within general ranges. Therapeutic treatments of heat and cold will cause variations of local site temperatures of several degrees Fahrenheit. Table 5–3 ■ presents temperature ranges for various situations.

Patients with a normal body temperature of 98.6°F are considered to be **afebrile** when oral temperature remains below 100°F (37.8°C). When oral temperature in these patients exceeds 100°F, they are considered to be **febrile. Hyperthermia** is defined as a rectal temperature greater than 106°F (41.1°C). **Hypothermia** is defined as a rectal temperature less than 94°F (34.4°C).

Table 5-3 ■ Temperature ranges for different activities

Situation	Oral	
	°F	°C
Usual normal range	98.6–99.5	36.0–37.5
Morning/cold weather	95.0–96.8	35.0–36.0
Hard work/emotion/a few normal adults/many active children	99.7–101.0	37.6–38.3

Pain

Pain is a subjective perception described by patients and, thus, is difficult to measure. Although not traditionally considered a vital sign, determination of pain sites, levels, and characteristics are commonly included when assessing patient vital signs. Perceptions of pain are unique to each individual and may depend on previous experiences, type of injury or disease (laceration, crush, burn, migraine headaches, arthritis, etc.), body part affected, age, time since onset, and ethnic background. There may also be situations in which pain is expressed when an injury or disease does not truly present pain. Because pain is a subjective symptom, assessment is difficult.

Purpose

The purposes of measuring perceptions of pain are to determine (1) diagnosis, (2) prognosis, (3) appropriate interventions, and (4) responses to interventions. Measurements of perceptions of pain that assist in diagnosis seek to determine type of pain (burning, tingling, sharp, dull, etc.), location (specific joint or limb), extent of painful location, intensity, duration, and frequency.

Method

The most commonly used method of measuring pain is an adaptation of a **visual analog scale (VAS)**. A VAS is a straight horizontal printed line, with 0 at the left side and 10 at the right side. The left side, 0, represents a complete absence of pain. The right side, 10, represents the worst pain a patient can imagine. Patients are asked to mark on the horizontal line the point that corresponds with their perception of their current pain. A common adaptation of the visual analog scale is for patients to be asked to provide a number between 0 and 10 that represents where they rank their current perception of pain, rather than being asked to mark an actual scale.

■ Take Note

Visual analogy scale (VAS)
0 = no pain
1, 2, 3 = minimal pain
4, 5, 6 = moderate pain
7, 8, 9, 10 = severe pain

Young children can have difficulty with the concept of ranking pain perceptions. Often a series of faces, from very happy to very unhappy, is used (Figure 5-4 ■). Children are asked to select the face that represents their perception of pain. This is analogous to selecting a number that represents a perception of pain.

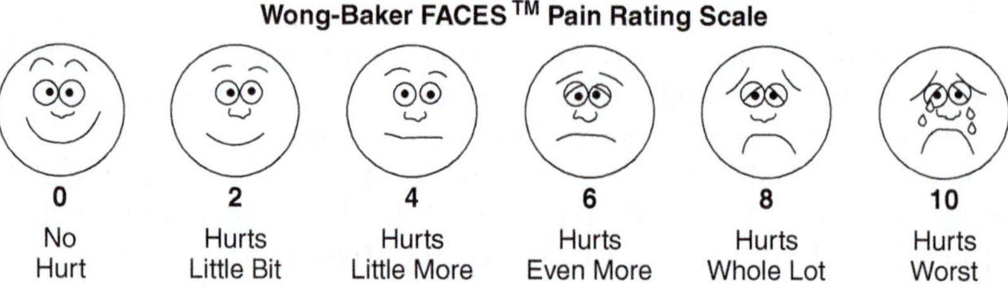

FIGURE 5-4 ■ Wong-Baker FACES Pain Rating Scale.

Site

Body diagrams can be used to document the site of pain. Document each site in which pain is perceived, including type, intensity, duration, and frequency. Each site of pain is marked. Types of pain may be noted by different markings (e.g., x, #), and intensity may be noted by different colors or numbers.

Norms

Normally, pain is not present. A commonly accepted interpretation of pain scale patient reports considers 0 as nonexistent, 1–3 as minimal, 4–6 as moderate, and 7–10 as severe pain.

Anthropometrics

Anthropometry is the science that deals with the measurements of the human body. Anthropometrics indicate the size, weight, and proportions of the human body that are measured.[4]

Purpose

Changes of weight or height, either increases or decreases, can indicate changes in health status. Differences in limb length, limb girth, or the expected relationship of limb length and torso length may indicate pathology. Measurements of adult height are monitored over time to determine if the degree of change in height is of expected magnitude or indicative of pathology.

Childhood physical growth is monitored by changes in height and weight. Rates of change of height and weight are also monitored. Height and weight are correlated with age and percentile and presented in height and weight charts.

Body mass index (BMI) is used to classify a person's weight and height relationship with respect to being underweight, normal, overweight, and obese. BMI results can be misleading. A person with significant muscular development can have a high BMI but may not be overweight or obese because the source of weight (muscle or fat) is not a factor when calculating BMI.

Methods

Side-to-side comparisons of limb length and girth are performed by measurements using consistent and documented landmarks as reference points. Differences in side-to-side limb length and limb girth measurements indicate further examination or evaluation is necessary. The timeline for differences and changes occurring in these measurements is an important aspect of documentation.

To determine physical development of a child, height, weight, and head circumference are measured using tape measures and scales. Measured height, weight, and head circumference and age are compared to height and weight charts.[5]

BMI is calculated in two different manners, depending on whether U.S. units or metric units are used.[6] When U.S. units are used, the formula is (703.1)(weight in pounds)/(height in inches). When metric units are used, the formula is (weight in kilograms)/(height in meters).

Norms

Government websites are available that provide information on anthropometrics and the calculation of certain anthropometric values. Tables of correlations of height and weight for child development may be found at the Centers for Disease Control and Prevention website, www.cdc.gov/. Calculators and tables related to BMI may be found at www.nhlbi.nih.gov/. NHLBI is the acronym for the National Heart Lung and Blood Institute, a component of the Department of Health and Human Service's (DHHS) National Institutes of Health (NIH). Nongovernmental websites may also be found that provide this information. Current norms used by the CDC for BMI are presented in Table 5–4 ■.

Table 5–4 ■ BMI Classifications

Underweight	BMI of <18.5
Normal	BMI between 18.5 and 24.9
Overweight	BMI between 25.0 and 29.9
Obese	BMI >30

Review Questions

1. What are the purposes for taking vital signs routinely as part of patient care?
2. What is pulse rate, and list the common sites at which pulse rates are measured?
3. What are the purposes for determining pulse rates and quality of pulses?
4. What are the normal and abnormal ranges, and the appropriate descriptive term, of heart rate?
5. What is target heart rate, and how is it determined?
6. What is respiratory rate, and what are the common methods for measuring respiratory rate?
7. What are the normal and abnormal ranges, and appropriate descriptive term, of respiratory rate?
8. What is blood pressure, and what are the usual sites at which blood pressure is measured?
9. What are the normal and abnormal ranges, and the appropriate descriptive term, for blood pressure?
10. What is body temperature, and what are the common sites at which body temperature is measured?
11. What are the normal and abnormal ranges of body temperature?
12. What are the units used when documenting heart rate, respiratory rate, blood pressure, and temperature?
13. What are the commonly used methods for measuring pain?
14. What are the four categories and their ranges of body mass index?

Suggested Activities

1. Demonstrate the proper methods to measure pulse, arterial patency, respiratory rate, blood pressure, and temperature.
2. Practice measuring vital signs of classmates in the proper position of sitting or lying quietly and during walking.
3. Properly document the results from Activity 2.
4. Compare results from Activity 2 to norms to determine if the values obtained are in the normal range.
5. Practice assessing vital signs of classmates before, during, and after activities such as riding a stationary bike, running on a treadmill, or lifting weights.
6. Were changes in vital signs with activity compared to those taken prior to activity what you expected?
7. Properly document the results from Activity 5.
8. Visit a skilled nursing facility to practice taking vital signs.

Case Studies

1. Mr. Rangarajan is a 47-year-old construction worker. Four days ago he fell from the roof framing of a two-story house under construction. His fall was through the unfinished floor/ceiling framing to the first floor, landing on a pile of used lumber with nails. Upon admission to the hospital, Mr. Rangarajan was diagnosed with two fractured ribs on his right side, a fractured left radius, puncture wounds to his right chest and forearm, a dislocated right shoulder, and a Grade 2 concussion. A referral for physical therapy services has been forwarded to the Physical Therapy Department.
   - For your first visit, what vital signs would you measure and record?
   - What methods and sites would you use to perform the measurements?
   - What method of measurement of pain perception would you use?
2. Emma May Jones, age 78, is 3 days post left total hip replacement. She has hypertension and a history of asthma. Before initiating a plan of care that includes strengthening exercises, transfer training, and gait training, you are to determine her maximum heart rate and calculate what her exercise heart rate should be. Provide a rationale for your answers.
3. Carl White, age 24, a computer programmer, was referred to physical therapy for a wellness program. His height is 5'6", and his weight is 255 lb for a BMI of 41. He is concerned about developing hypertension and diabetes like his father. Determine his maximum heart rate and calculate what his exercise heart rate should be (BMI chart: http://www.nhlbi.nih.gov/guidelines/obesity/bmi_tbl.pdf).

References

1. Mayo Clinic. (2013). *Hypoxemia (low blood sugar)*. Retrieved March 16, 2013 from http://www.mayoclinic.com/health/hypoxemia/MY00219
2. National Heart, Lung, and Blood Pressure Institute. (2003). *The seventh report of the Joint National Committee on Prevention, Detection, Evaluation, and Treatment of High Blood Pressure* (JNC 7). Retrieved from www.nhlbi.nih.gov/guidelines/hypertension/index.htm
3. Bickley, L. S. (2003). *Bates' guide to physical examination and history taking* (8th ed.). Philadelphia, PA: Lippincott Williams & Wilkins.
4. *Dorland's Medical Dictionary* (28th ed.). (1994). Philadelphia, PA: W. B. Saunders.
5. Centers for Disease Control (CDC). (2000). *Growth training chart.* Retrieved April 27, 2008, from www.cdc.gov/nccdphp/dnpa/growthcharts/
6. National Heart, Lung, and Blood Institute (NIH). (n.d.). *Calculate your body mass index.* Retrieved April 27, 2008, from www.nhlbisupport.com/bmi/

6

Wheelchairs

LEARNING OUTCOMES

Upon completion of this chapter, you will be able to:

1. Identify different types of wheelchairs, including
   - Amputee-frame
   - Fixed frame
   - Folding
   - One-arm drive
   - Reclining-back
   - Standard
   - Tilt-in-space
2. Identify different components of a wheelchair, including:
   - Anti-tipping components
   - Armrests
   - Front rigging
   - Pelvic positioners
   - Wheels
   - Wheel locks
3. Describe the purpose or function of wheelchair components and types.
4. Describe and demonstrate how wheelchair components and types are manipulated.
5. Describe activities of basic wheelchair maintenance.
6. Describe and demonstrate how to measure an individual to determine correct size and components required for a wheelchair.

KEY TERMS

Anti-tipping devices
Armrests
Caster wheels
Drive wheels
Fixed frame
Folding-frame wheelchair
Footrest
Front rigging
Heel loops
Legrest
One-arm drive
Pelvic positioners
Reclining back wheelchair
Sacral sitting
Tilt-in-space wheelchair
Wheel locks

Introduction

In situations when an individual will use a wheelchair as the primary means of mobility, a wheelchair is usually fabricated specifically for that individual. Healthcare providers, in consultation with patients and caregivers, contribute to development of a wheelchair prescription. Careful measurement of an individual, and the selection of appropriate components with respect to specific needs, provides the user of a wheelchair with a piece of equipment that allows that individual to function with the most independence and safety possible. Guidelines for selection of a wheelchair design indicate that wheelchairs should have a short wheelbase and be as light and narrow as possible. These features make propulsion and maneuvering easier for the user.

Wheelchairs have many common components. However, a variety of mechanisms can be selected to operate some components. This chapter presents selected components, selected types of wheelchairs, and other mobility devices and illustrates how to measure a patient for a wheelchair.

Wheelchair Components

Wheel Locks

One of the most important safety features on a wheelchair is the wheel-lock system (Figure 6–1 ■). **Wheel locks** are devices that stabilize the wheels of a wheelchair *after* the wheelchair has been stopped. Wheel locks usually employ a cam and lever system. In some situations, a slot-locking mechanism is used rather than a cam-locking mechanism. Previously, wheel locks were referred to as brakes. Some patients understood that to mean that wheel locks functioned as braking devices, such as on an automobile, which is not correct.

A general safety rule is that wheel locks must be engaged whenever an individual is moving into, or out of, a wheelchair. Engaging wheel locks on the rear wheels prevents forward and backward movement of a wheelchair. Wheel locks on front caster wheels minimize side-to-side movement. Although wheel locks are available for front caster wheels, they are not typically placed on wheelchairs. Therefore, slight side-to-side movement of a wheelchair may result as an individual moves into or out of a wheelchair when front caster wheels are not secured.

■ **Take Note**

Safety: Engage wheel locks before moving in or out of a wheelchair.

To work properly, wheel locks must make secure contact with tires to prevent movement of the wheels. An example of inadequate wheel-lock contact may occur is when pneumatic tires are not inflated sufficiently or when entire wheel-lock mechanisms become loose or slide forward on the wheelchair frame.

The direction of the force needed to engage or release wheel locks can be selected during wheelchair ordering to match a patient's abilities. Wheel locks are usually engaged by pushing forward a lever on each side (Figure 6–2 ■), whereas pulling the levers backward releases the wheel lock (Figure 6–3 ■). The reverse mechanism, engaging wheel locks by pulling levers backward, and releasing them by pushing levers forward, is an option. A decision on which method to use is made by a physical therapist and patient, with respect to the

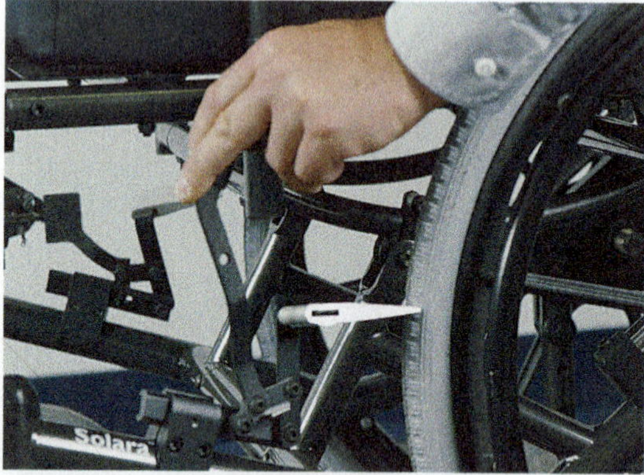

FIGURE 6–1 ■ Wheel lock.

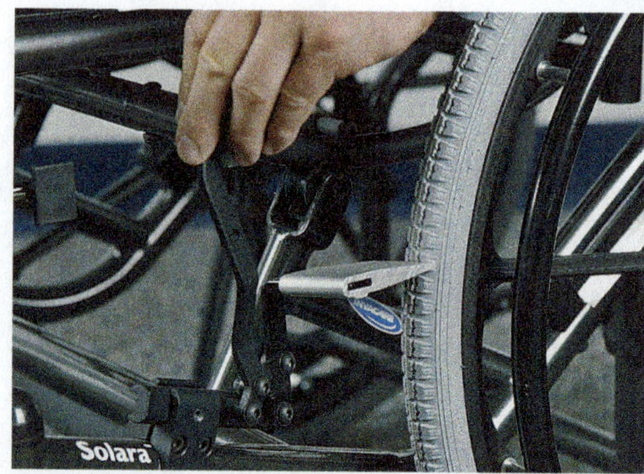

FIGURE 6–2 ■ Engaging wheel locks.

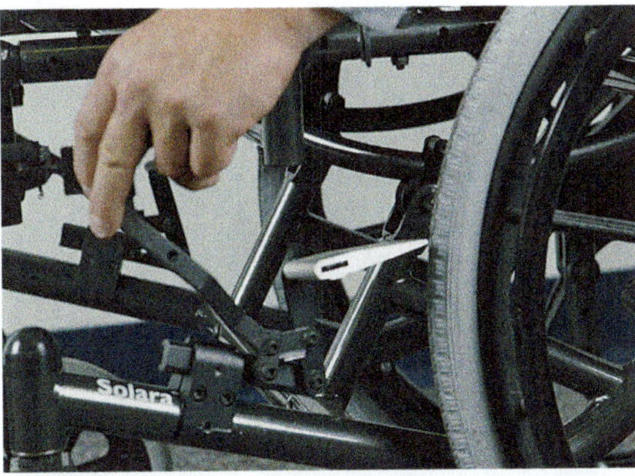

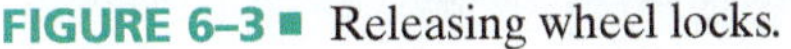

FIGURE 6–3 ■ Releasing wheel locks.

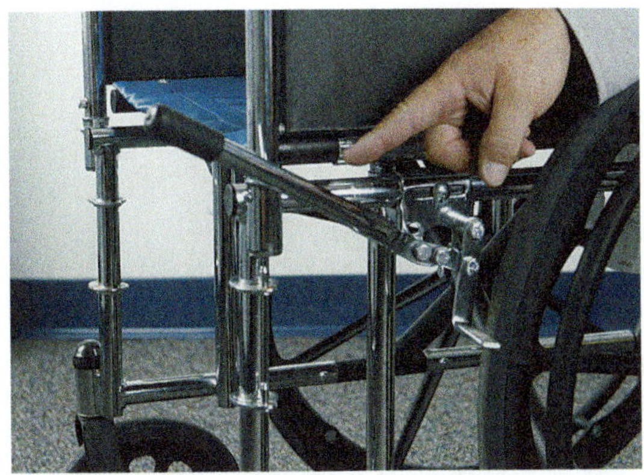

FIGURE 6–4 ■ Wheel-lock handle extension.

patient's strength and balance. The direction of a patient's greatest strength is the direction of movement that should engage the wheel locks.

Extensions for wheel-lock levers are available (Figure 6–4 ■). Extensions increase the mechanical advantage of a wheel-locking mechanism by increasing the length of the wheel-lock lever. Increasing the length of a wheel-lock lever increases the length of the force arm with respect to the resistance arm of the cam. This increase in mechanical advantage decreases the force required of a patient to engage or disengage the wheel lock. Wheel-lock extensions are usually removable or hinged to allow them to be moved out of the way when a patient must transfer laterally over the wheelchair wheel.

On some reclining-back wheelchairs, the anterior/posterior dimension of the wheelbase increases when the back is reclined. When the wheelbase is enlarged as the back reclines, the relationship of the wheel lock and the tire is altered, resulting in an ineffective wheel lock because wheel-lock contact with the tire is decreased. An additional wheel lock is necessary for these wheelchairs. The additional lock is attached to the back upright of the wheelchair so it is effective when the wheelchair is in the reclined position. Such locks, however, cannot be operated by the person using the wheelchair.

Pelvic Positioners

Pelvic positioners are devices that stabilize a patient's pelvis in the proper position while seated in a wheelchair (Figure 6–5 ■). Pelvic positioners are not intended to be used to prevent a patient from falling out of a wheelchair. Rather they are part of a positioning system designed to provide proper positioning of a patient in a wheelchair. Pelvic positioners are often thought of as seatbelts, but are not intended to be used as restraints to keep patients from getting, or falling, out of a wheelchair.

Three mechanisms are used for fastening pelvic positioners: Velcro straps; latching buckles, such as those used for seat belts in airplanes; and push-button buckles, such as those used for seat belts in automobiles.

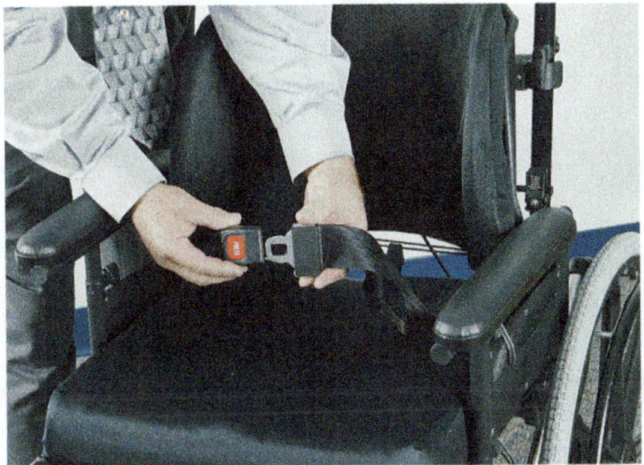

FIGURE 6–5 ■ Pelvic positioner.

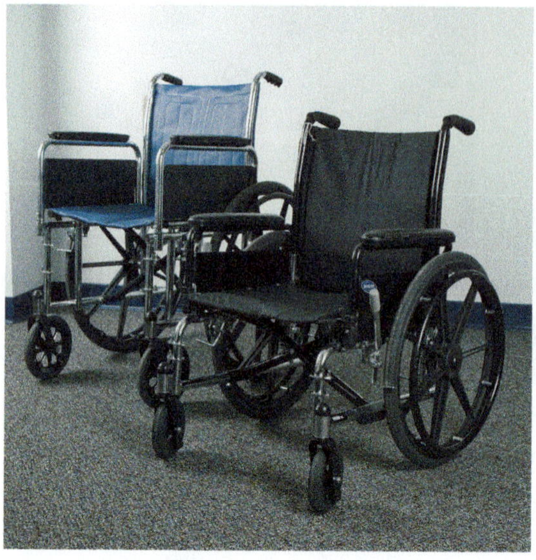

FIGURE 6–6 ■ Pneumatic caster wheels.

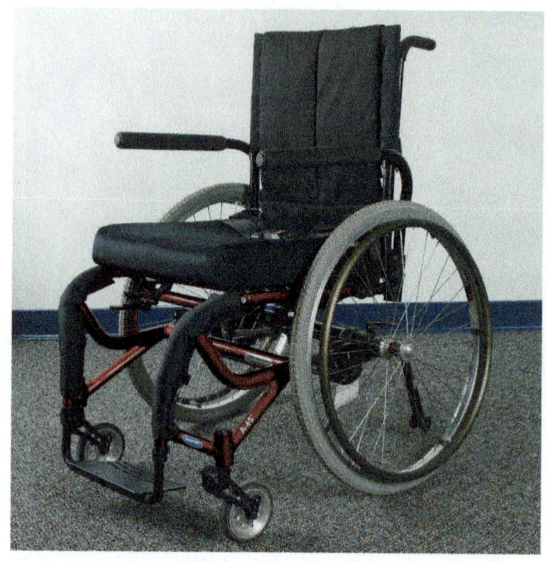

FIGURE 6–7 ■ "Rollerblade" caster wheels.

Caster Wheels

Caster wheels are the small front wheels of a wheelchair. Two basic styles of tires are available—standard solid rubber and pneumatic. Pneumatic tires are filled with air, providing some shock absorption, and thus a smoother ride (Figure 6–6 ■). Pneumatic tires are wider than standard solid rubber tires, making travel easier on soft or uneven surfaces such as sand or gravel. Some wheelchair owners use "rollerblade" wheels for front caster wheels (Figure 6–7 ■). Typically these are users of ultralight, or sport, wheelchairs. Because of their construction and materials, rollerblade wheels are small, are very durable, and have excellent quality bearings. A trade-off, however, is that these smaller wheels may become caught in sidewalk cracks.

■ **Take Note**

Discuss with patients the pros and cons of tire options for the drive wheels.

Drive (Push) Wheels

Drive wheels are the large rear wheels of a wheelchair, which are used for propulsion. Rear tires may be one of two basic types—standard solid rubber or pneumatic. Pneumatic tires may or may not have tread (Figure 6–8 ■). Tires with treads may be used on wheelchairs that are often used outdoors, providing more traction than smooth tires. Pneumatic tires have been modified to reduce the potential for flat tires, and may be called "flat-free" tires.

■ **Take Note**

Hand rim projections may be horizontal, angled, or vertical.

Drive wheels have inner and outer rims. The inner rim is for mounting tires. The outer, or hand, rim is used for propelling the wheelchair. Adaptations of the outer rim, such as projections, are available for use by individuals who do not have sufficient ability to grasp (Figure 6–9 ■). Projections add weight and width to the wheelchair and may make maneuvering in small spaces difficult. Nonslip coatings, rather than projections, are more commonly used on hand rims to assist propulsion.

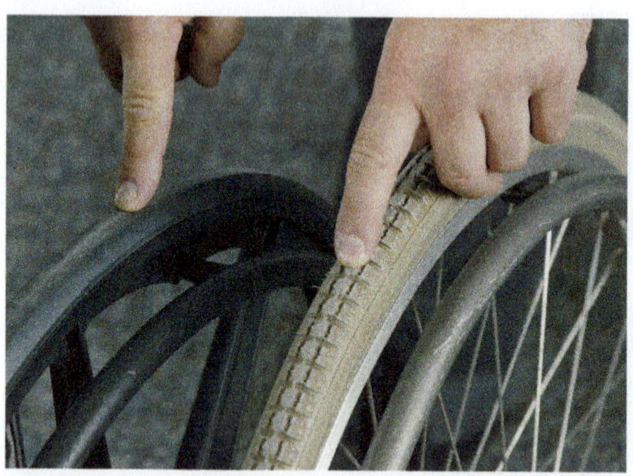

FIGURE 6–8 ■ Drive wheels—smooth (left), tread (right).

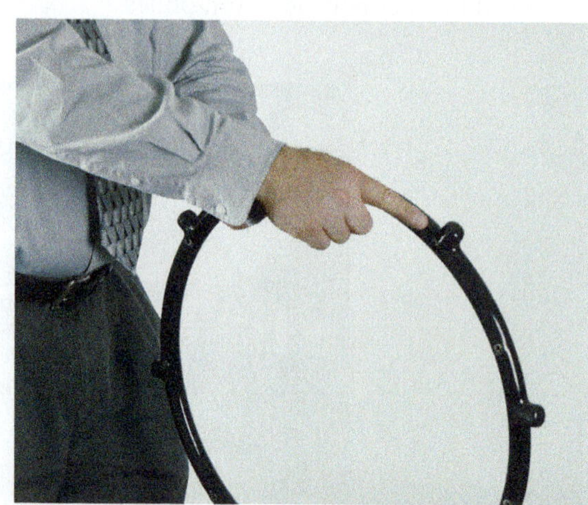

FIGURE 6–9 ■ Drive wheel rim with projections.

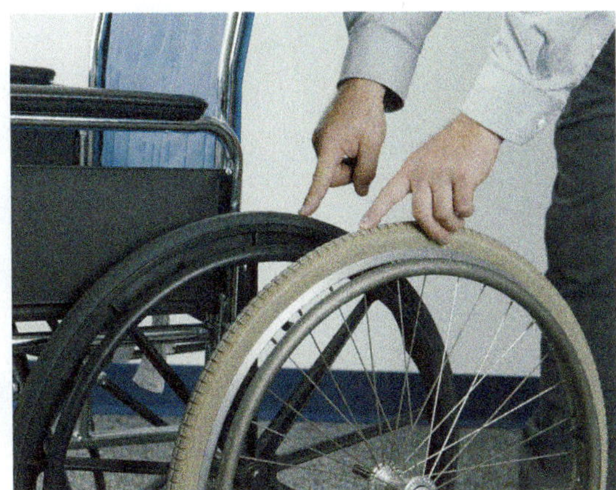

FIGURE 6–10 ▪ Drive wheels—mag (left), spoke (right).

Drive wheels come in two types—standard or "mags" (Figure 6–10 ▪). Standard wheels are fabricated with multiple steel or aluminum spokes. Spokes are thin and individually adjustable to maintain proper alignment of a wheel. Mag wheels do not use spokes but usually have eight thicker struts that connect the outer rim to the hub. Mag wheels are so-named because they are fabricated from magnesium, a very strong, lightweight metal. The material strength of magnesium is sufficient to maintain original alignment and eliminates the need for multiple adjustable spokes. Because of their design and material, maintenance of mag wheels is easier than that of standard wheels.

Drive wheels on some chairs are easily removable (Figures 6–11 ▪ and 6–12 ▪), making the chair lighter and smaller. Removable wheels increase the ease of maneuvering the wheelchair into and out of a vehicle.

Armrests

Several configurations of **armrests** are available. Armrests are either full length or desk length (Figure 6–13 ▪). The height of full-length armrests is the same along the entire length of the armrest. Desk-length armrests have two heights. In a standard setup, the front portion of the armrest is lower than the rear portion, permitting a wheelchair to be rolled under a table or desk. Most desk-length armrests can be removed and reversed, placing the higher part of the armrest toward the front of the wheelchair. Reversing a desk armrest provides a higher support for patients when pushing to standing or when performing other transfers. Both types of armrests have an option for adjustable height with respect to the top of the seat (Figures 6–14 ▪ and 6–15 ▪). Proper adjustment of armrest height permits the person sitting in the wheelchair to rest his or her forearms on the armrest with the elbow flexed to approximately 90 degrees.

▪ Take Note

Desk armrests allow a person to get close to tables and desks.

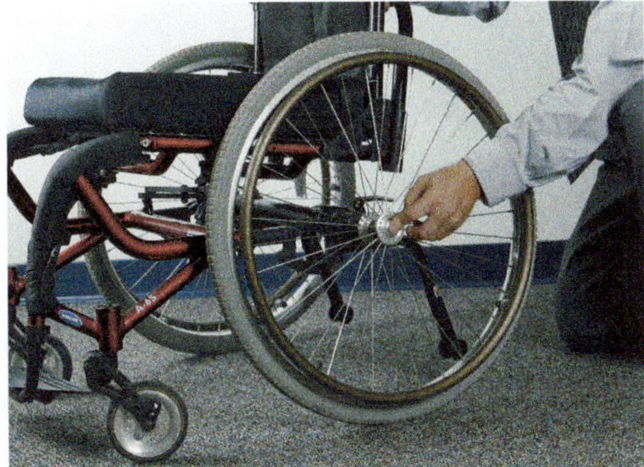

FIGURE 6–11 ▪ Releasing quick-release drive wheels.

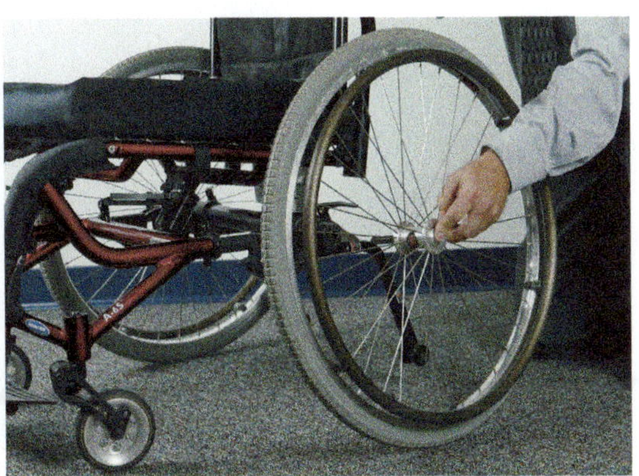

FIGURE 6–12 ▪ Removing quick-release drive wheels.

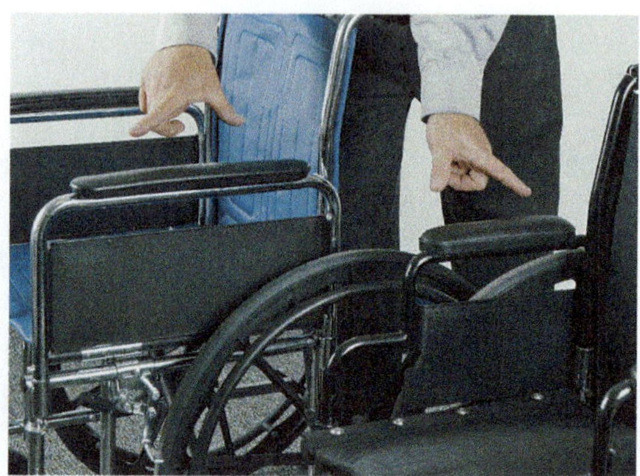

FIGURE 6–13 ■ Full-length (left) and desk-length (right) armrests.

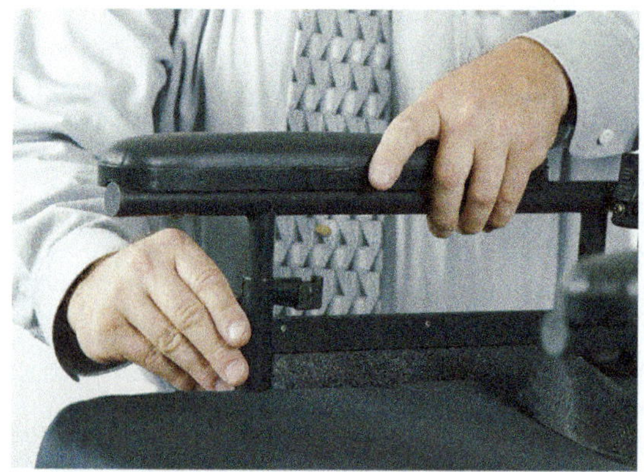

FIGURE 6–14 ■ Lowered elevating armrest.

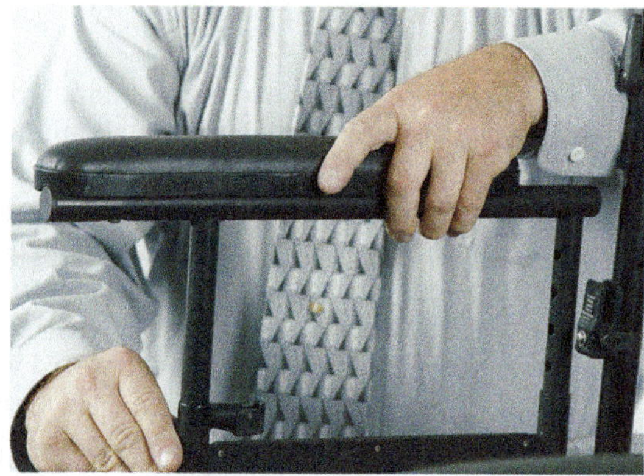

FIGURE 6–15 ■ Raised elevating armrest.

Armrests, both full length and desk length, can be either removable or fixed. Removable armrests often allow easier performance of transfers and permit a patient to sit even closer to a table or desk than desk-length armrests allow. Nonremovable armrests usually result in a lighter and narrower wheelchair. Removable armrests may be designed so that they wrap around the back uprights of the wheelchair, decreasing wheelchair width (Figure 6–16 ■). When a wraparound design is used, the posterior upright of the armrest

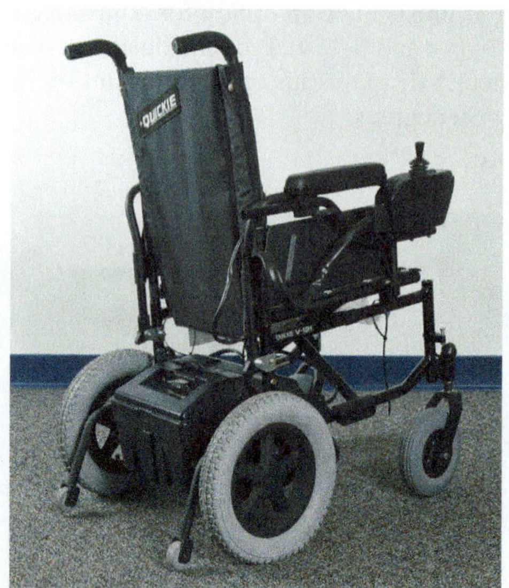

FIGURE 6–16 ■ Removable wraparound armrest.

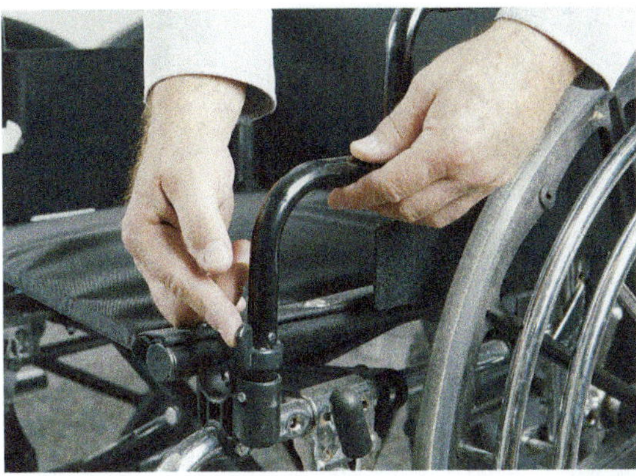

FIGURE 6–17 ■ Removable armrest lock.

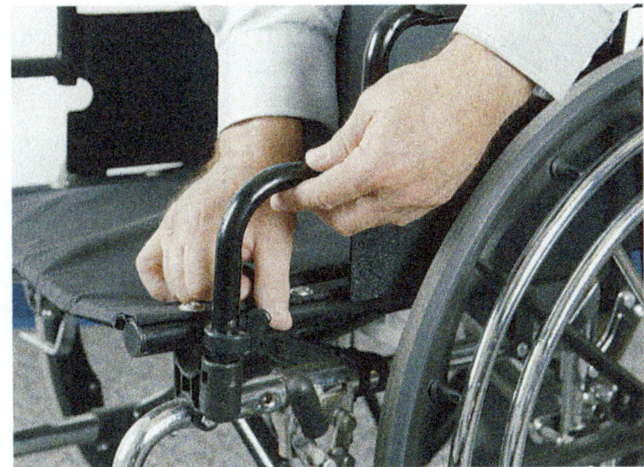

FIGURE 6–18 ■ Releasing removable armrest.

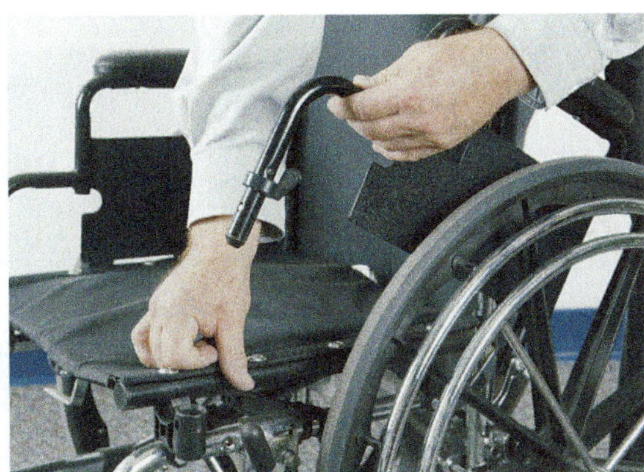

FIGURE 6–19 ■ Armrest being removed.

is directly behind the upright of the wheelchair back. Wraparound desk-length armrests cannot be reversed to place the higher portion toward the front of the wheelchair.

Several types of mechanisms are used to lock armrests in place for patient safety. Both the location and type of armrest-locking mechanisms vary. A common type of lock is operated by a lever that is either pushed down or rotated to release the lock (Figures 6–17 ■ and 6–18 ■). Once released, the lever remains in the released position. Thus, only one hand is required to unlock and then remove the armrest (Figure 6–19 ■).

Lap trays, when used, are secured to or rest on armrests. Full-length armrests offer greater support for lap trays than desk-length armrests.

Front Rigging

Front rigging on a wheelchair consists of a footplate attached to either a footrest or an elevating legrest. The purpose of front rigging is to provide support for the lower extremities. Front rigging with a footplate only is called a **footrest**. Front rigging with a footplate and calf pad support is called a **legrest**.

■ **Take Note**

Proper foot support is important for comfort and function.

FOOTPLATES Patients' feet rest on footplates, which are available in several sizes to accommodate feet of different sizes. **Heel loops** constructed of strapping or webbing, attach to footplates and prevent a patient's feet from sliding off the footplates and under the wheelchair (Figure 6–20 ■). Ankle and toe loops, also constructed of strapping or webbing, may also be used to maintain a patient's feet on the footplates.

Footplates are raised to allow patients to transfer safely into and out of a wheelchair (Figures 6–21 ■ and 6–22 ■). When raising footplates, push heel loops forward to allow the footplates to be raised completely. Doing this prolongs the life of heel loops by preventing heel loop material from being crushed and allows the footplate to be folded completely so it does not interfere with patient movements.

The distance from seat to footplate for both footrests and legrests can be adjusted to match a patient's lower leg length and to provide proper support for the entire lower

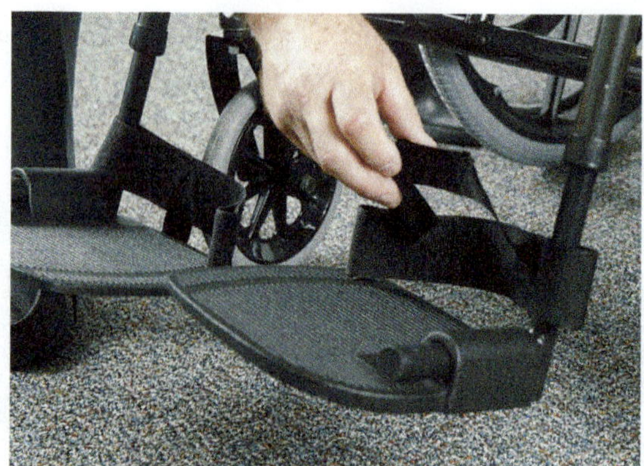

FIGURE 6–20 ■ Heel loop on footrest of front rigging.

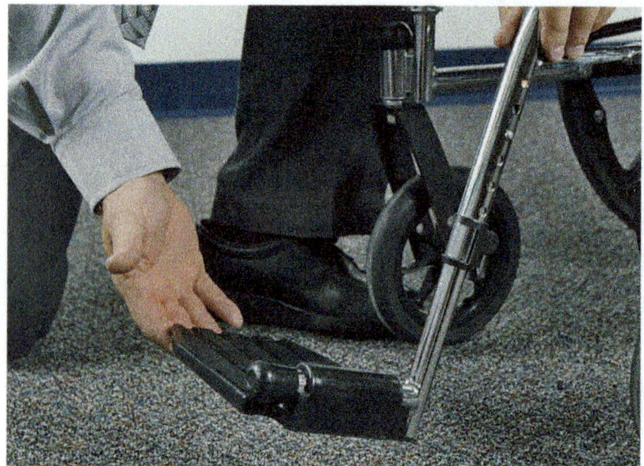

FIGURE 6–21 ■ Footplate in down position.

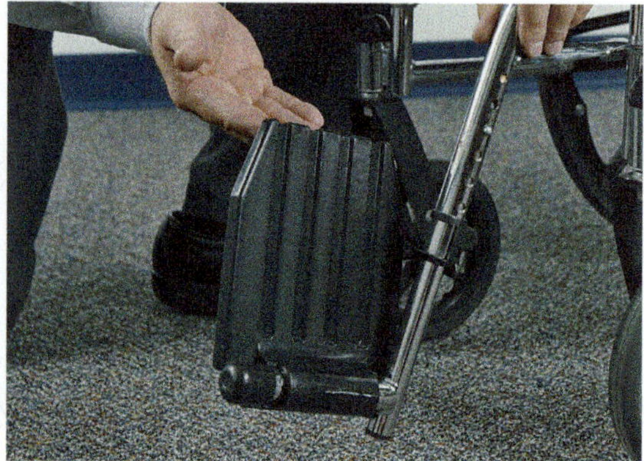

FIGURE 6–22 ■ Footplate in up position.

extremity. There are several mechanisms for making this adjustment. The method illustrated uses a push-button release and a clamp to ensure that the desired position is achieved and maintained (Figures 6–23 ■ and 6–24 ■).

Other types of mechanisms use clamps, or tension-adjustment screws, located inside the footrest or legrest tube. The adjustment screws are accessible from the underside of the footrest or legrest.

Footrests can be fixed or removable. Fixed footrests are usually less expensive and result in a lighter wheelchair. Fixed footrests are part of a unitized construction design in standard wheelchairs. In this design, footplates can be raised, but the footrest itself cannot be removed. The footrests can be adjustable in length, however.

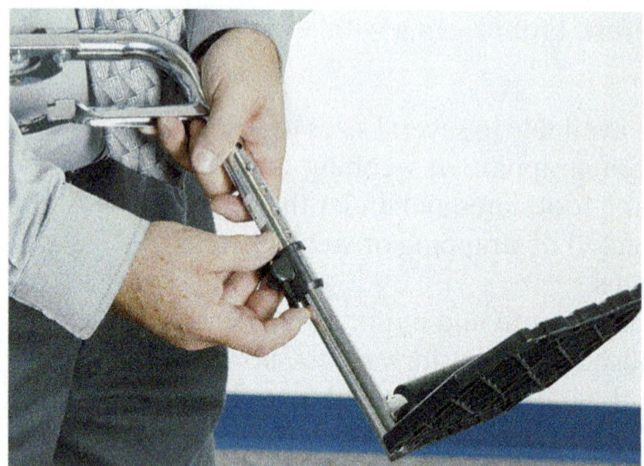

FIGURE 6–23 ■ Preparing to lengthen front rigging—securing lever and button adjustment.

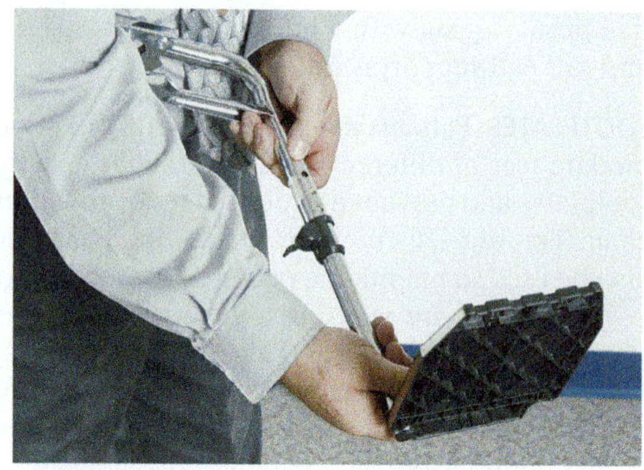

FIGURE 6–24 ■ Adjusting front rigging length—lengthening while holding button.

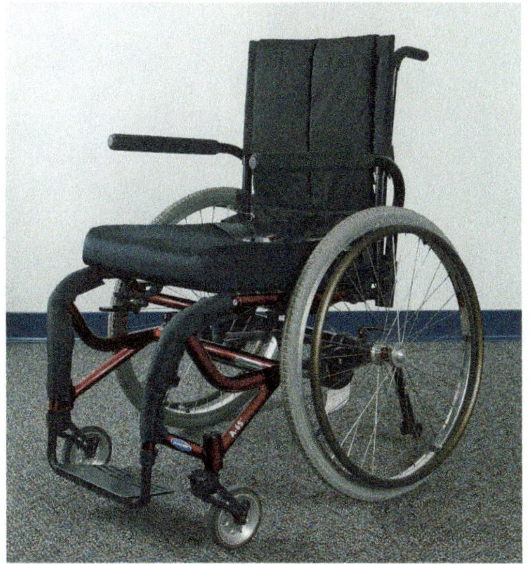

FIGURE 6–25 ■ Fixed-frame wheelchair—unitized footrest construction.

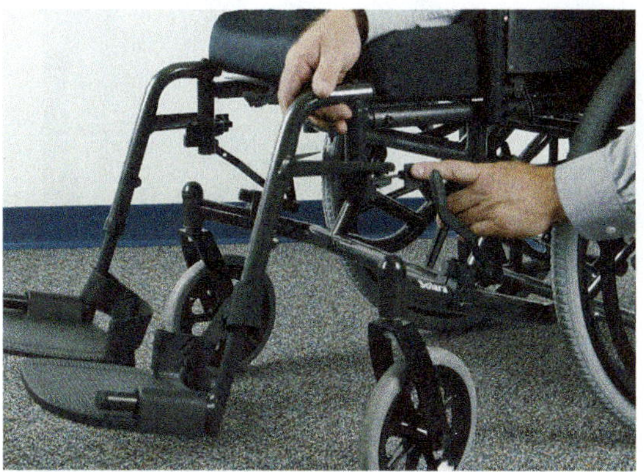

FIGURE 6–26 ■ Preparing to release pivoting footrest.

Footrests for fixed-frame wheelchairs (wheelchairs that cannot be folded) are also part of a unitized construction design, but cannot be adjusted to accommodate differences in leg length (Figure 6–25 ■). In fixed-frame wheelchair design, footplates are typically bolted to a bar that is positioned so the knees are flexed 90 degrees or more. This results in a shorter overall dimension for the wheelchair. Fixed-frame wheelchairs are usually ultra lightweight sport models.

Removable footrests typically pivot to the sides of wheelchairs, where they can be removed. Several types of locks are used to secure pivoting footrests (Figure 6–26 ■).

Pivoting footrests use pivot pins as the center of rotation. To remove a pivoting footrest, the footrest is unlocked or released, pivoted to the side, and then lifted from the pivot pins (Figures 6–27 ■ and 6–28 ■).

ELEVATING LEGRESTS Elevating legrests are necessary when a patient is unable to flex his or her knee, when a dependent position of the leg contributes to swelling, or with a reclining-back wheelchair. A calf pad support provides a cushion for the calf and support for

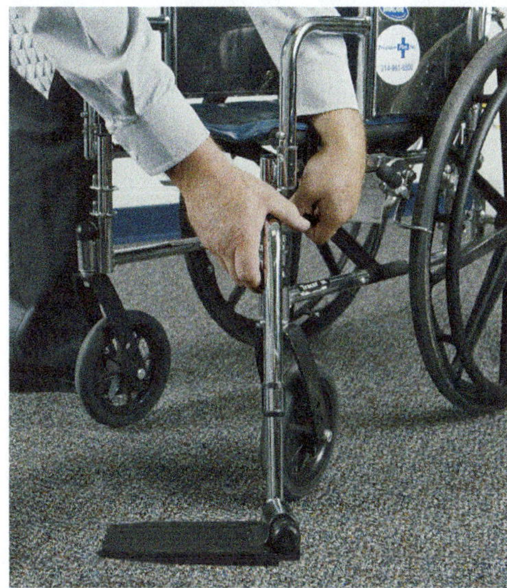

FIGURE 6–27 ■ Pushing lever to release pivoting footrest.

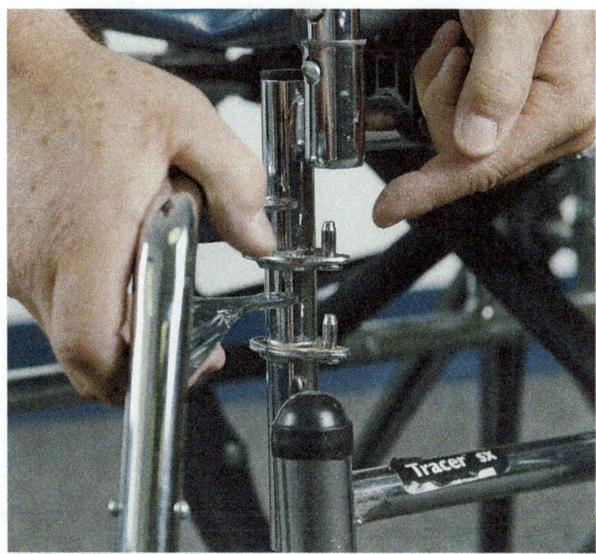

FIGURE 6–28 ■ Pivoting footrest.

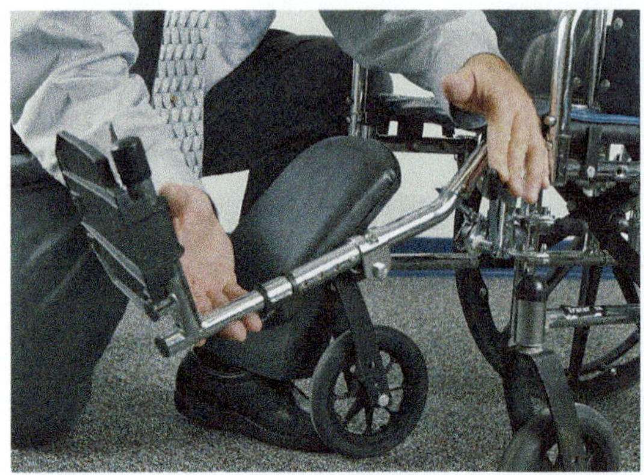

FIGURE 6–29 ■ Preparing to raise elevating legrest by pushing lever.

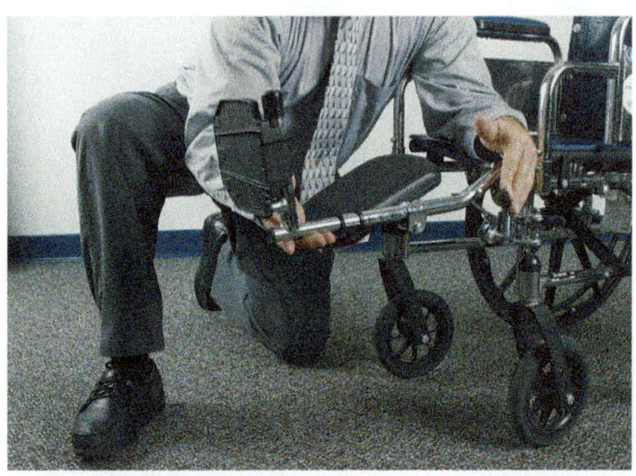

FIGURE 6–30 ■ Elevating legrest in up position.

the leg. The height of the legrest position is adjustable. Legrest height position is maintained by a locking mechanism. The lock is released and activated by a lever. The legrest position is adjusted by releasing the lock with one hand while raising or lowering the legrest with the other hand (Figures 6–29 ■ and 6–30 ■). Swing-away removable elevating legrests are removed in a similar manner as swing-away removable footrests.

To permit a patient to move safely into and out of a wheelchair with elevating legrests, the footplate and calf pad must be moved out of the way. The calf pad support must be pivoted before the footplate is raised (Figures 6–31 ■ through 6–33 ■) to ensure that the footplate can be raised completely.

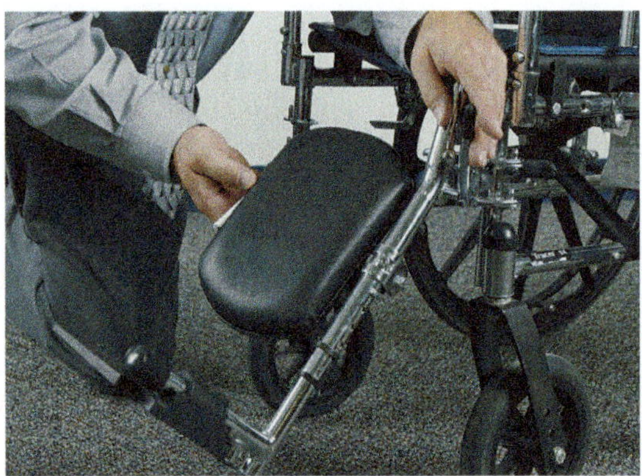

FIGURE 6–31 ■ Calf pad support in down position.

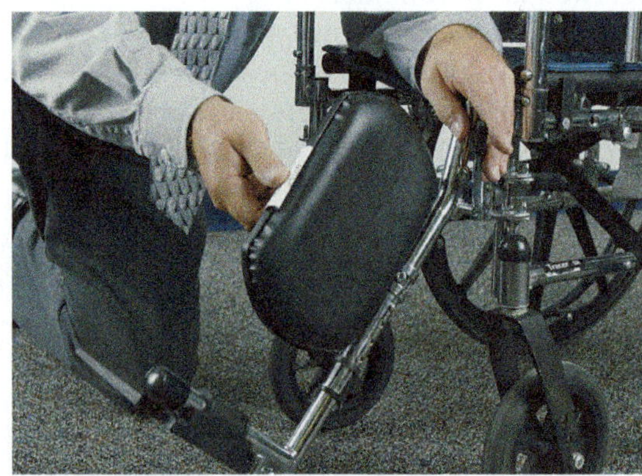

FIGURE 6–32 ■ Calf pad support pivoted to up position.

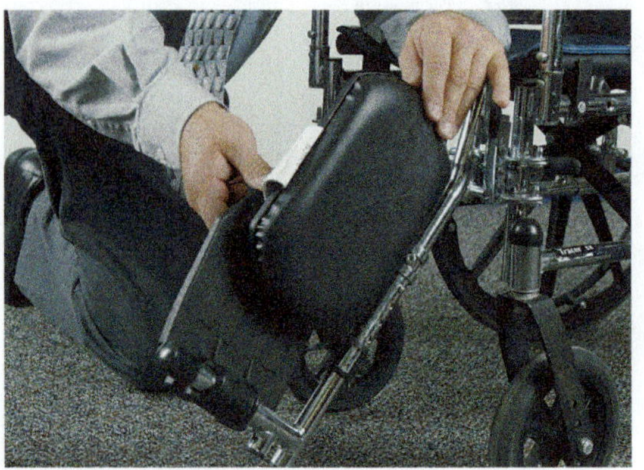

FIGURE 6–33 ■ Raising footplate with calf pad support in up position.

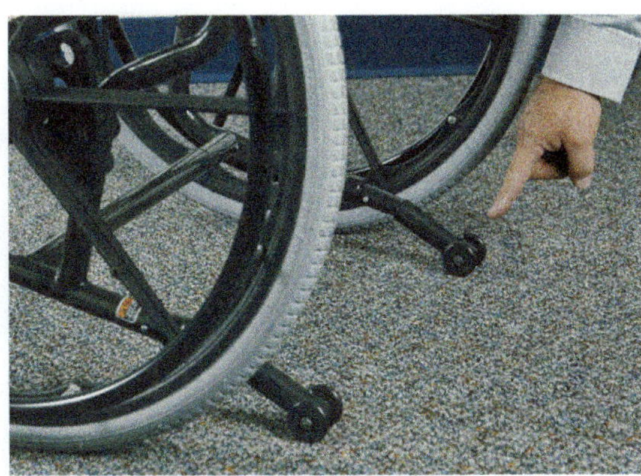

FIGURE 6–34 ■ Anti-tipping device.

ANTI-TIPPING DEVICES **Anti-tipping devices** (Figure 6–34 ■) are small extensions, with or without wheels, attached to the rear lower horizontal support bars of a wheelchair. These devices are used to prevent accidental backward tipping of the wheelchair. Anti-tipping devices must permit some tipping of the wheelchair so front casters can roll up and over doorsills, curbs, or other low obstructions. Anti-tipping devices often can be removed once a patient can use the wheelchair safely without them.

Wheelchair Types

Different styles of wheelchairs have been developed to meet specific patient needs. Some styles are minimal modifications of standard wheelchairs. Other styles required extensive reengineering of basic wheelchair design. Designs such as those that move from a seated to standing position, or stair-climbing wheelchairs, are beyond the scope of discussion of wheelchair types included in this text. The emphasis in this section is on standard and most-often-used types of wheelchairs.

Standard Wheelchair

A standard wheelchair comes with basic features of front rigging and armrests, which can be either fixed or removable. This wheelchair is durable and is the standard for facility use. Standard wheelchairs are available in several sizes to fit patients ranging from pediatric to adult to bariatric. Seat-to-floor height can be varied, with a lower seat height facilitating propulsion for individuals who propel the wheelchair with their feet (Figure 6–35 ■).

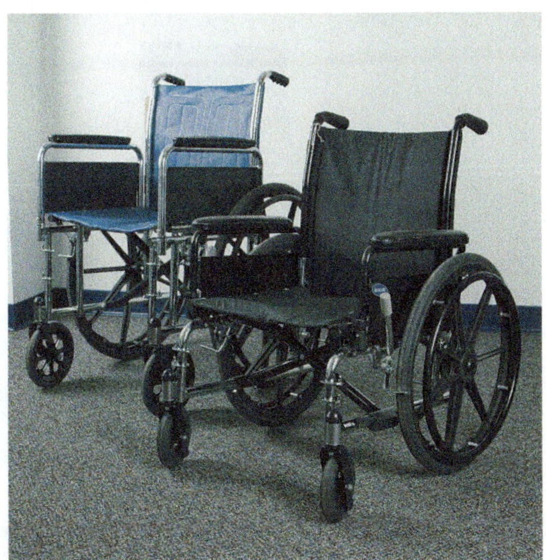

FIGURE 6–35 ■ Seat height—standard (left), low (right).

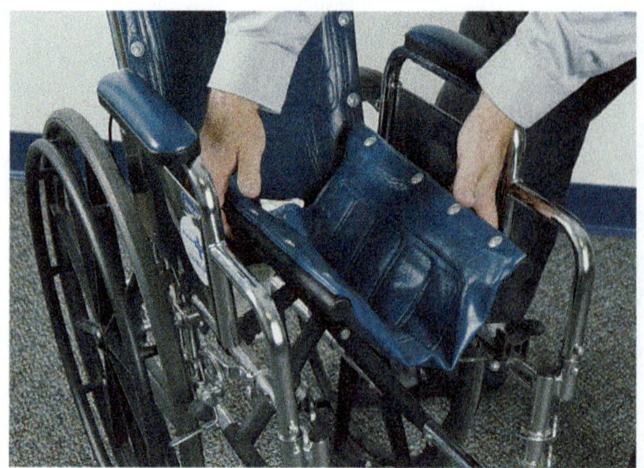

FIGURE 6–36 ■ Mid-position of folding a wheelchair.

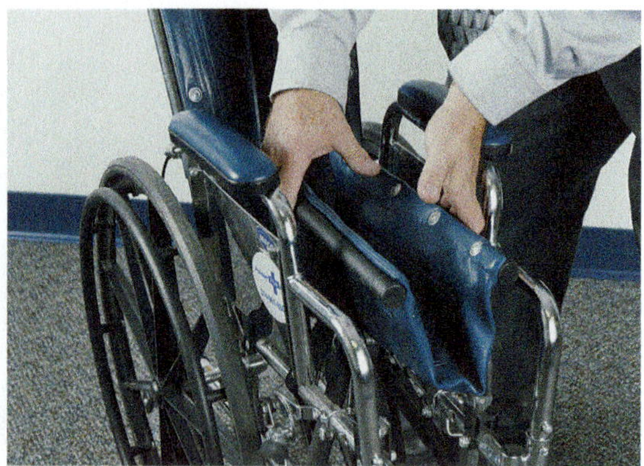

FIGURE 6–37 ■ End position of folding a wheelchair.

■ **Take Note**

Wheelchairs should be folded by pulling up on the handles at the edges of the seat.

Folding Wheelchair

Folding-frame wheelchairs that can be folded or collapsed for storage or transport use a similar method for folding (Figures 6–36 ■ and 6–37 ■). Raising footplates and pulling up on the bars to which the seat upholstery is attached will fold most wheelchairs. Pulling up on the middle of the wheelchair seat upholstery to fold a wheelchair will weaken the upholstery, and eventually the seat upholstery will tear. Push down on the horizontal bars of the seat to unfold the wheelchair.

Fixed-Frame Wheelchair

A **fixed frame** means the wheelchair frame is of unitized construction and cannot be folded (Figure 6–38 ■). Front rigging is part of the frame and not always removable. The wheelchair back may be able to fold onto the seat. Back height is often lower than on a standard wheelchair. On sport models of fixed-frame wheelchairs, armrests are not used typically. Overall frame length in fixed-frame wheelchairs is reduced because the front rigging is an integral part of the frame, and the front rigging is placed farther back on the frame. This improves maneuverability, which is important in small spaces. There are fewer components, and the materials used to construct them are lighter than on standard wheelchairs. Thus fixed-frame wheelchairs are usually ultra lightweight. One disadvantage of the fixed frame is reduced shock absorption because unitized frame design is rigid.

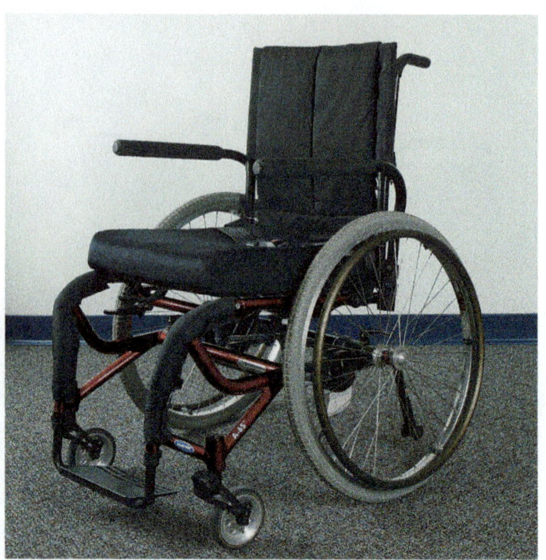

FIGURE 6–38 ■ Unitized, fixed-frame, ultralight wheelchair construction.

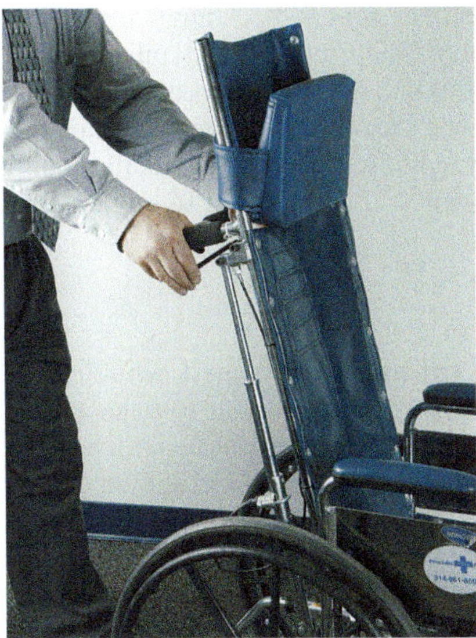

FIGURE 6–39 ■ Reclining-back wheelchair in upright position.

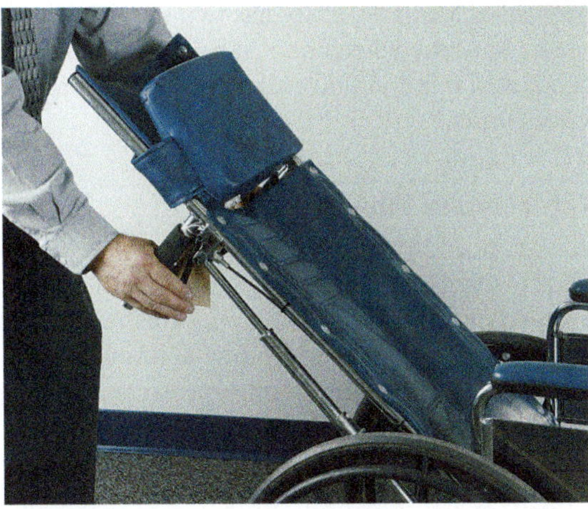

FIGURE 6–40 ■ Reclining-back wheelchair in reclined position.

Reclining-Back Wheelchair

Reclining-back wheelchairs are indicated when a patient is unable to sit erect for long periods of time or not at all. There are two variations of reclining-back wheelchairs—those that recline completely and those that recline only partially. An extended back is used with both types of reclining-back wheelchairs. An extended back provides support for the upper body when the wheelchair back is in a reclined position. Head support is also required when the back is reclined. Reclining-back wheelchairs usually have elevating legrests, permitting patients to be in a mostly supine position when the back is reclined. A reclining-back wheelchair takes much more space to maneuver when reclined because of the increase in overall length (Figures 6–39 ■ and 6–40 ■).

There are several types of mechanisms for unlocking and adjusting the angle of inclination of the wheelchair back. To change the wheelchair's back angle, the locking mechanism is released, the angle of the back is adjusted, and the locking mechanism is activated.

A bar across the back of a reclining-back wheelchair provides support and stability. Several different methods of securing the support bar exist. To fold a reclining-back wheelchair, the back support bar must be removed (Figures 6–41 ■ and 6–42 ■). Then a reclining-back wheelchair can be folded following the same steps used when folding a standard wheelchair.

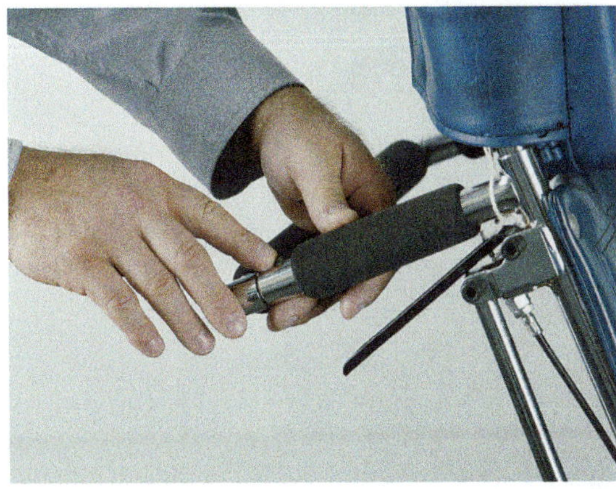

FIGURE 6–41 ■ Releasing support crossbar to fold reclining-back wheelchair.

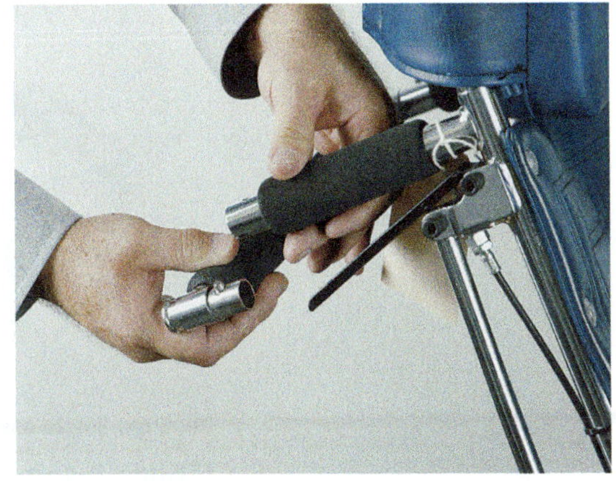

FIGURE 6–42 ■ Lowering support crossbar on reclining-back wheelchair.

When a reclining-back wheelchair's back is lowered, the seat-to-back angle increases. As the seat-to-back angle increases, the wheelbase increases to maintain stability. Traditionally placed wheel locks will not engage the tires in this situation. Therefore, a reclining-back wheelchair typically has two sets of wheel locks. The second set is usually located on the back of the wheelchair to be able to engage the tires and for easy use by an attendant because the individual using a reclining-back wheelchair will not be able to engage the wheel locks.

Tilt-in-Space Wheelchair

A variation of a reclining-back wheelchair is a **tilt-in-space** framed wheelchair (Figures 6–43 ■ through 6–45 ■). A tilt-in-space wheelchair has a fixed seat-to-back angle, even when reclined. Maintaining this relative seat-to-back angle is useful for individuals who require customized seating systems on their wheelchair. The tilt-in-space frame permits changes of orientation for pressure relief, or for different activities, while maintaining the postural control provided by the customized seating system.

One-Arm Drive Wheelchair

A patient with only one functional upper extremity and not able to use lower extremity propulsion adequately may achieve self-propulsion using a one-arm drive wheelchair.

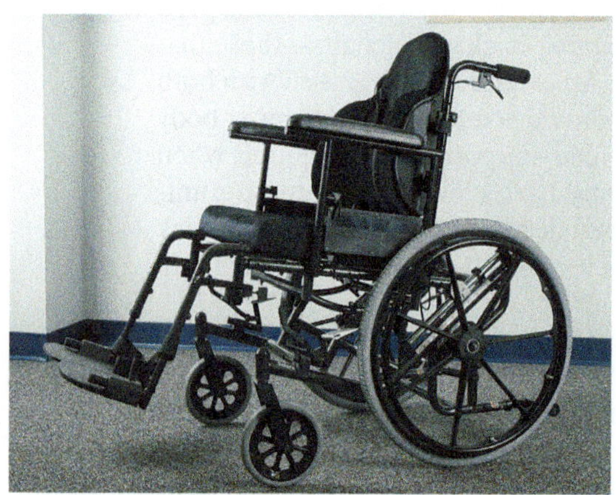

FIGURE 6–43 ■ Tilt-in-space wheelchair in upright position.

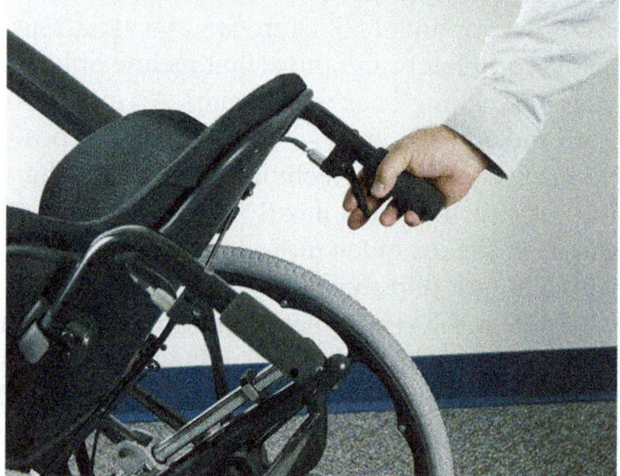

FIGURE 6–44 ■ Releasing mechanism to reposition tilt-in-space wheelchair.

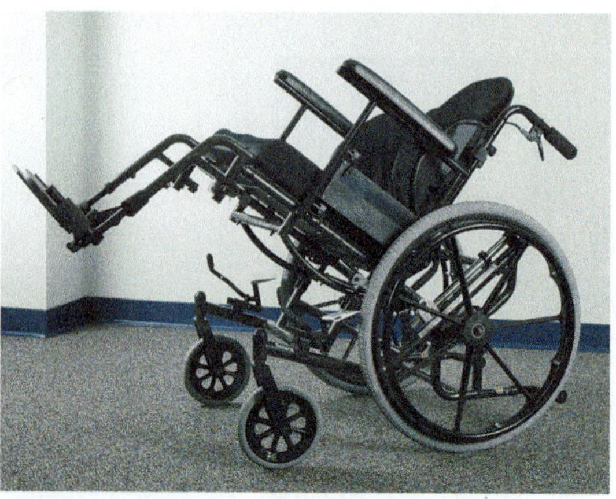

FIGURE 6–45 ■ Tilt-in-space wheelchair in a reclined position.

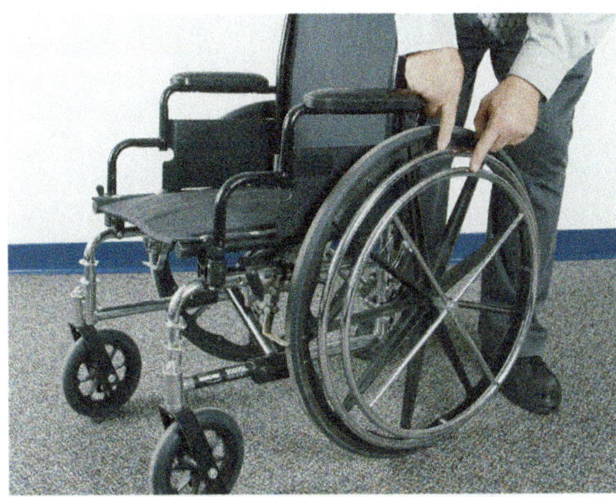

FIGURE 6–46 ■ One-arm drive wheelchair.

One-arm drive wheelchairs have two hand rims on one drive wheel (Figure 6–46 ■). A linking mechanism between the drive wheels provides control for both drive wheels using one upper extremity. With both hand rims on one drive wheel, the two hand rims are used simultaneously to achieve forward or backward propulsion. Applying force to one rim at a time turns the wheelchair.

Amputee Wheelchair

An amputee wheelchair frame has the drive wheels set behind the vertical back supports (Figure 6–47 ■). This configuration moves the posterior boundary of the base of support farther to the rear to accommodate the loss of mass of the amputated lower extremities. Lower extremity amputations move the patient's center of mass posterior when seated in a wheelchair, necessitating a change in the wheelchair's base of support. If the wheelchair's base of support is not moved posterior with respect to the patient, the wheelchair will be less stable and more likely to tip backward, especially when moving up a ramp or curb. This type of wheelchair is most necessary for patients with bilateral lower extremity amputations.

Propulsion by a patient is more difficult with the drive wheels placed farther to the rear. Rather than using a wheelchair with an amputee frame to avoid tipping to the rear, two other methods can be used. Anti-tipping devices can be added to a standard frame, or weights can be added to the front of the wheelchair frame.

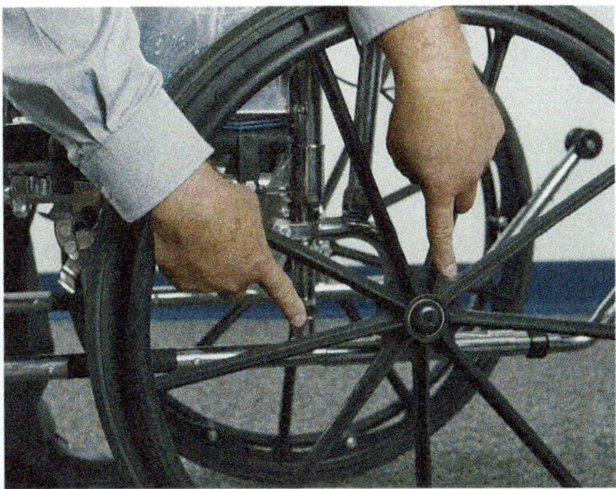

FIGURE 6–47 ■ Backset drive wheels on frame of amputee wheelchair.

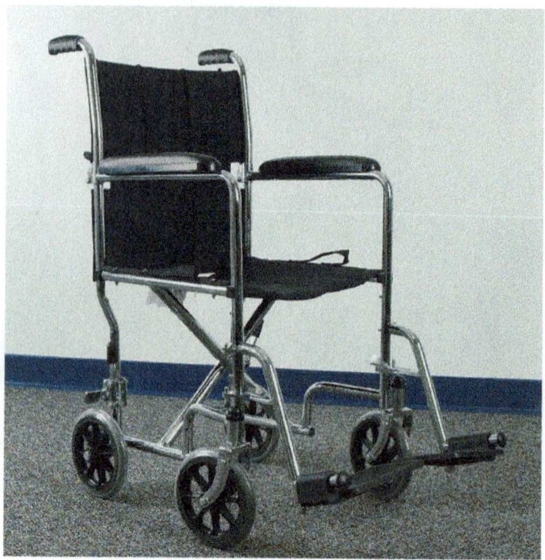

FIGURE 6–48 ■ Lightweight travel or companion wheelchair.

Companion Wheelchair

A companion chair, also called a travel chair, is a lightweight wheelchair that does not have drive wheels (Figure 6–48 ■). The rear wheels are the size of caster wheels, so all four wheels are the same size. Smaller wheels, and the use of lightweight components, reduce the weight of a companion wheelchair with respect to a standard wheelchair. A companion pushes the wheelchair. The person using the wheelchair may also be able to propel it using his or her feet. Footrests are detachable for safety and ease of movement during transfers. Detachable footrests also make lifting and storage of companion wheelchairs easier.

Motorized Wheelchairs and Scooters

A variety of motorized or power devices are increasingly available (Figures 6–49 ■ and 6–50 ■). Although expensive, motorized devices offer individuals with minimal or limited functional abilities an opportunity to have independent mobility. There are a large number of choices and complexities in making decisions concerning motorized devices. In addition to determining available components, such as armrests, headrests, and front rigging, the method of power activation must be determined. Given the number of choices, and the complexity involved in making choices for specific patients, a discussion of the types of, and indications for, various methods of power activation and the various configurations of power devices is beyond the scope of this text.

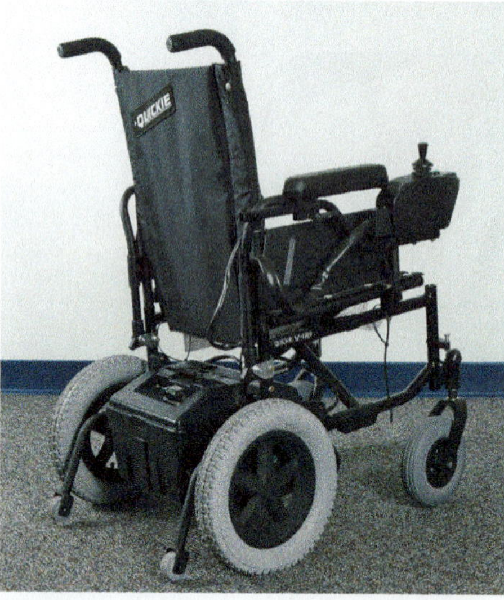

FIGURE 6–49 ■ Standard power wheelchair.

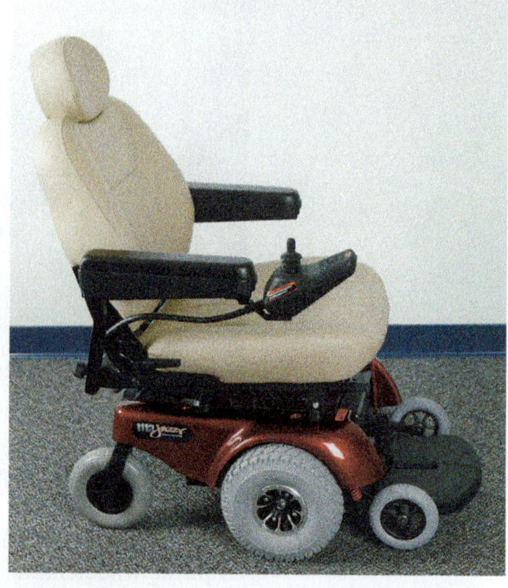

FIGURE 6–50 ■ Power wheelchair with reclining back.

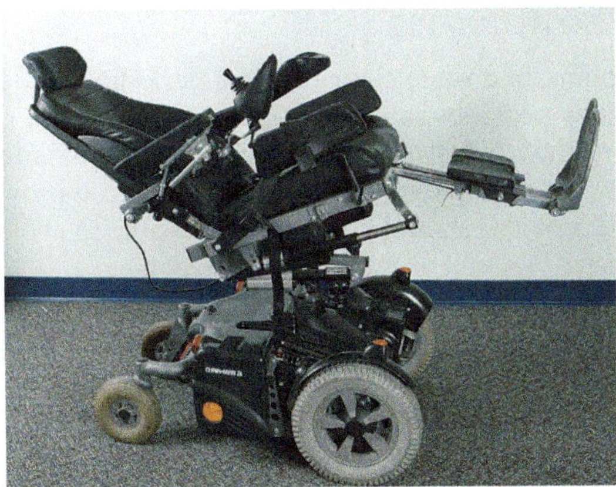

FIGURE 6–51 ■ Power wheelchair with reclining back in reclined position.

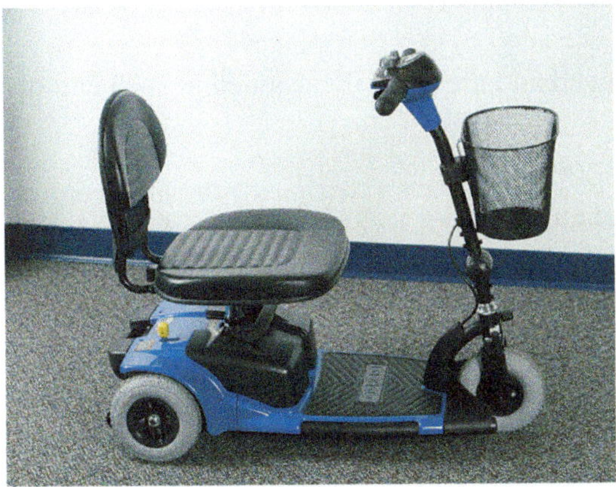
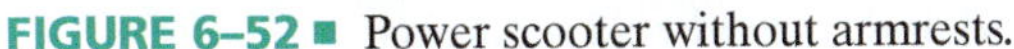

FIGURE 6–52 ■ Power scooter without armrests.

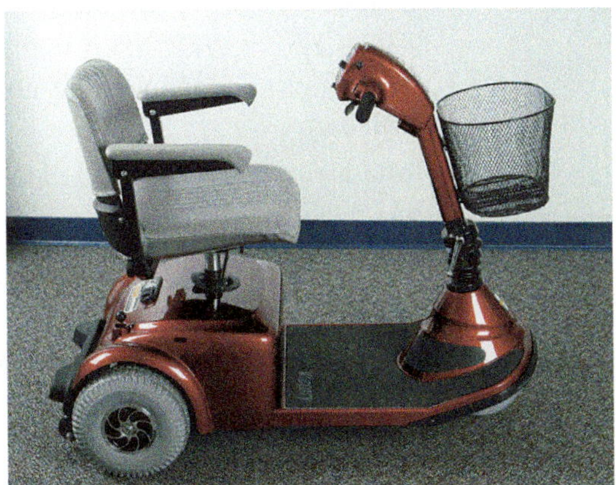

FIGURE 6–53 ■ Power scooter with armrests.

Some motorized wheelchairs also have the capability to use a power mechanism to recline the back of the wheelchair (Figure 6–51 ■). This permits patients to change position for different activities and provides for pressure relief.

Power scooters are an alternative to power wheelchairs for individuals with the ability to ambulate short distances (Figures 6–52 ■ and 6–53 ■). Power scooters may be of three- or four-wheel design. Four-wheel scooters have greater stability and are recommended for patients who will use them primarily outdoors on uneven terrain.

Power-Assist Wheelchair

A power-assist wheelchair is a hybrid power–manual wheelchair (Figure 6–54 ■). The individual propels the wheelchair using the drive wheels. The power-assist mechanism provides additional propulsion, increasing the duration or distance that may be attained.

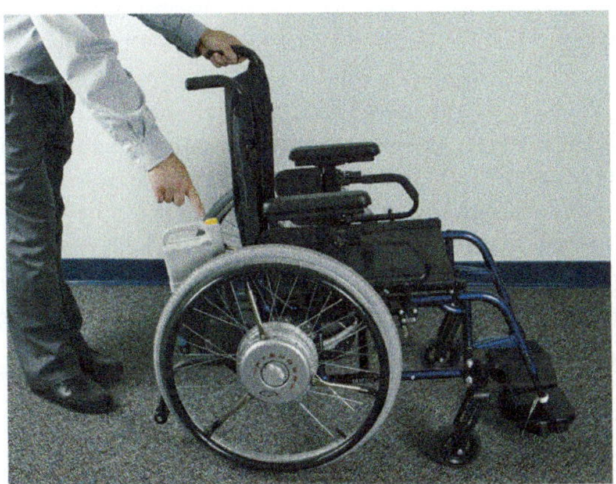

FIGURE 6–54 ■ Hybrid power–manual wheelchair.

Wheelchair Maintenance

Ensuring safe functioning of a wheelchair requires periodic maintenance. Periodic maintenance of a wheelchair provides safety and ease of use for the patient and caregivers. Patients and caregivers must be instructed in basic wheelchair maintenance, as well as being aware of requirements for periodic servicing by an authorized provider. Contact information for an authorized provider should be readily accessible to avoid delays in servicing or repairing wheelchairs.

Cleaning a wheelchair appropriately is necessary to maintain hygiene. Upholstery, seating inserts, armrests, and wheelchair tubing must be cleaned frequently according to the manufacturer's directions. The tool kit that comes with a new wheelchair should be maintained properly and kept accessible.

Activities of basic maintenance include checking and maintaining that:

- Axle hubs are secure and free of debris (hair, string, grease, etc.)
- Batteries for powered devices are properly charged
- Electrical connections and control mechanisms for powered devices function properly
- Heel loops and toe loops are not damaged and are securely fastened at each end of each loop
- Inflatable wheels are inflated to proper pressure
- Physical connectors, such as screws and nuts, are fastened securely
- Removable arm rests and removable front rigging are not damaged and are easily manipulated
- Seat belts and other components of specialized seating are not damaged, are securely attached, function properly, and are adjusted for proper size with regard to patient size
- Upholstery is not cracked or torn
- Wheel locks (brakes) can be fully applied and lock wheels securely
- Wheel spokes are straight and have appropriate tension

PROCEDURE 6–1 Measuring to Determine Wheelchair Size

Selection of the type, size, and components of a wheelchair for a patient depends on a variety of information. Discussion with the patient and caregivers and determination of the environments in which the device will be used are critical to successful decision making. The decision-making process is the responsibility of a physical therapist. Taking measurements may be delegated to physical therapist assistants.

Wheelchair size is determined by selected measurements of the individual. Using proper equipment and reading a tape measure or ruler accurately are essential. Accurate measurement requires assuming a position in which the tape measure or ruler is at eye level when measurements are taken. The optimal patient position for obtaining accurate measurements is to have the patient sit on a solid flat surface with solid flat back support. Wood inserts can be used in a wheelchair or straight-back chair to ensure accuracy when measuring. Note that in some of the accompanying photographs, the position of the person performing measurements is altered to allow the tape measure to be seen clearly.

Seat cushions and back supports are for comfort and to promote function. Inserts for seats and backs may be custom made or off-the-shelf. Some inserts for seats and backs may require modification of the following methods of determining size.

Measuring for Seat Depth

Seat depth is one of the two most important measurements for determining wheelchair size. Proper seat depth provides support for the pelvis and thigh. The front edge of the seat should end 2 to 3 inches from the lower leg or knee when the knee is in a position of 90 degrees of flexion.

When seat depth is too short, the thighs are not supported properly, which affects weight distribution and comfort adversely. Seat depth that is longer than appropriate may affect circulation or lead to "sacral sitting" by a wheelchair user. **Sacral sitting** occurs when an individual slouches, sliding the buttocks forward and tilting the pelvis posteriorly. Sacral sitting places the posterior aspect of the sacrum on the seat of the chair, resulting in improper postural alignment. This position increases pressure on the posterior aspect of the sacrum and may lead to skin breakdown. In addition, a sacral-sitting position is not optimal for efficient propulsion.

One measurement and one calculation are necessary to determine seat depth.

1. During measuring, patients are to sit with proper alignment—hips and knees flexed to 90 degrees and the back in contact with the flat back support while avoiding posterior pelvic tilt.
2. Measure the horizontal distance from the flat back support to the posterior aspect of the lower leg parallel to, and at the level of, the solid seat surface.
3. Subtract two or three inches from this measurement.
4. The result of this measurement and calculation provides the desired seat depth.
5. *CAUTION:* When a back cushion or other back insert is used, seat depth measurements must be calculated by adding the anterior/posterior thickness of the back insert.

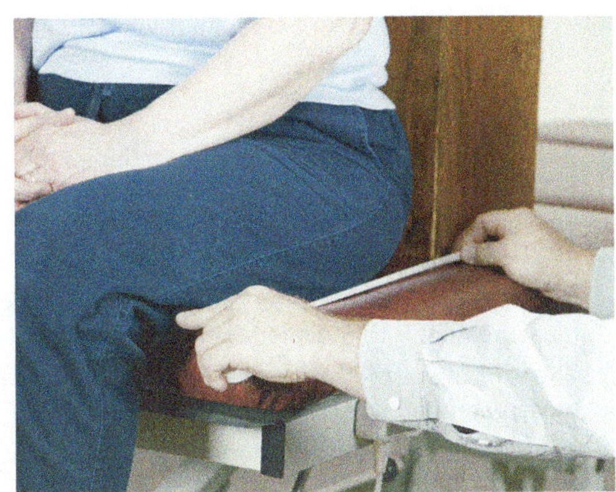

Measuring for Seat Width

The second of the two most important measurements for determining wheelchair size is seat width. Accurate measurement of seat width results in comfort and properly positioned drive wheels and armrests for easy and efficient wheelchair use. Ease of movement within the wheelchair must also be considered.

When a wheelchair is too wide, a patient may have difficulty reaching the drive wheels for effective propulsion. Proper use of armrests is impeded when wheelchair width is too great. When a wheelchair is too narrow, excessive pressure on the lateral aspects of the pelvis and thighs may occur, causing discomfort or skin breakdown. In addition to body width, accommodation is necessary for clothing, such as winter coats, and prosthetic or orthotic devices.

One measurement and one calculation are necessary to determine seat width.

1. With the individual sitting in proper alignment on the solid flat seat, measure the widest aspect of the patient's hips or thighs, whichever is wider, parallel to the solid flat seat.
2. Add two inches to this measurement.
3. The result of this measurement and calculation provides the desired seat width.

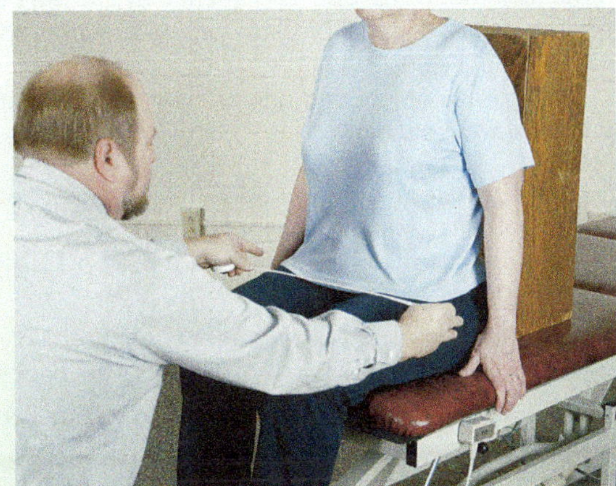

(continued)

PROCEDURE 6–1 Measuring to Determine Wheelchair Size (*continued*)

Measuring for Back Height

The amount of back height required depends on how much back support is needed by the patient. A back height that is too high may restrict a patient's movement. A back height that is too short for a patient's needs may not provide adequate support. Wheelchair users with adequate sitting balance may choose a low back height. Low back height decreases wheelchair weight and improves mobility within the wheelchair. Some wheelchair users also prefer the low back height for esthetic reasons, as it reduces the visual impact of the wheelchair.

One measurement and one calculation are necessary to determine back height.

1. Back height is measured with the patient sitting on the solid flat seat in proper alignment, with the back flat against the solid back support.
2. Vertical distance, parallel to the back support, is measured from the top of the seat. For standard back height, measurement is to the inferior angle of the scapula.
3. The thickness of the seat cushion is added to this measurement.
4. The result of this measurement and calculation provides the desired back height.

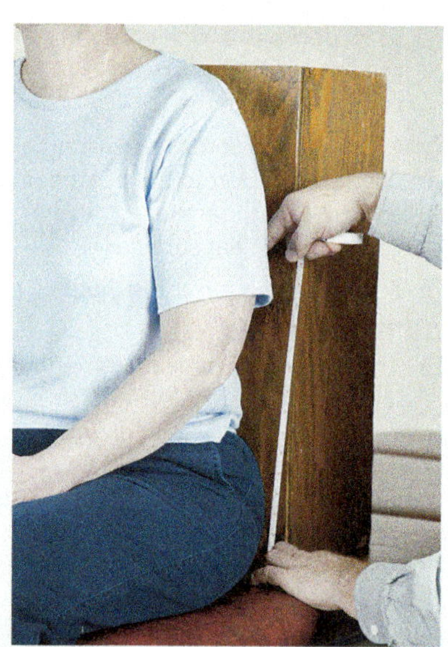

Measuring for Armrest Height

Proper armrest height promotes proper positioning and alignment. When armrests are set appropriately, and with the patient sitting with proper alignment, a patient's forearms rest comfortably on the armrests. Some patients may elect not to use armrests if their sitting balance is adequate. Eliminating armrests decreases the weight of the wheelchair; allows patients to sit close to surfaces such as sinks, desks, and tables; and reduces the visual impact of the wheelchair.

When set at an improper height, a patient will be unable to rest the forearms comfortably on the armrests and maintain proper alignment. Improper alignment may cause a patient to be subjected to unequal pressure on the forearms and ischia and may affect spinal curvature.

One measurement and one calculation are necessary to determine armrest height.

1. Armrest height is measured with the patient sitting on the solid flat seat in proper alignment, the upper arm is held against the chest wall, and the elbow is flexed to 90 degrees.
2. Measure the vertical distance between the solid seat surface and the patient's forearm, parallel to the back support.
3. Add the thickness of the seat cushion to be used to this measurement.
4. The result of this measurement and calculation provides the desired armrest height.

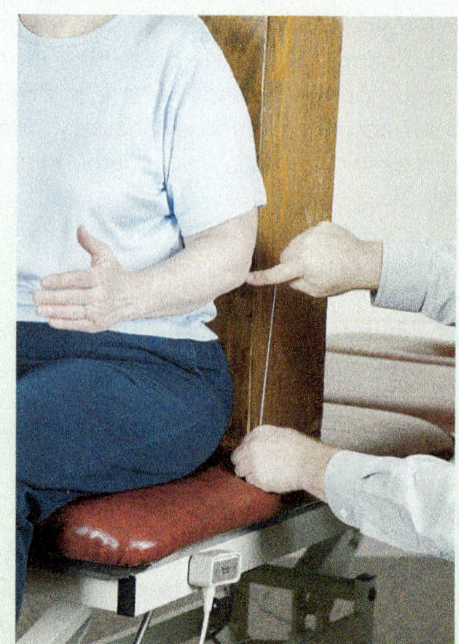

Measuring for Seat-to-Footplate Length

Appropriate seat-to-footplate length contributes to proper alignment and support of the lower extremities. When seat-to-footplate length is too great, an individual may sacral sit to rest the feet on the footplate. When the length is too short, pressure distribution along the thighs is reduced and uneven, forcing excessive weight bearing on the ischia and coccyx. Excessive pressure on the ischia or coccyx may result in skin breakdown.

Seat-to-footplate distance and footplate clearance height must be determined in combination with the type of front rigging to be chosen. Seat-to-footplate length is a factor when considering the seat-to-floor height of a wheelchair. A minimum of 2 inches between the floor and the undersurface of the footplate are necessary to provide clearance over thresholds and other small obstacles. The distance from the footplate to the floor is measured from the lowest point of the footplate.

One measurement is used to determine seat-to-footplate length.

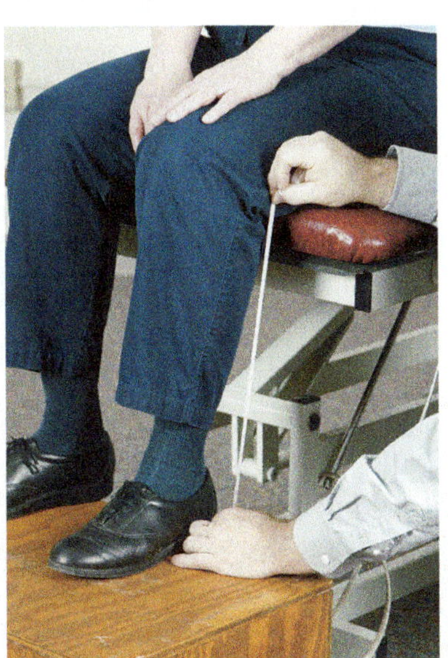

1. With the patient sitting on a hard surface, the knee flexed to 90 degrees, and the foot resting on the floor or stool, measure the length of the patient's lower leg and foot, from the posterior aspect of the thigh at the popliteal fossa to the sole of the foot at the heel.
2. To adjust the seat-to-footplate length when using a cushion, ensure that the seat-to-footplate length measured in step 1 is now measured from the top of the seat cushion (not just the seat itself) to the footplate.
3. *CAUTION:* If this adjustment does not permit 2 inches of clearance between the footplate and floor, the angle or type of front rigging or seat-to-floor distance must be adjusted.

Measuring for Footplate Size

Footplate size is determined by the length of the patient's foot. Supporting the foot provides proper support of the lower extremity and assists in preventing development of deformities of the foot and ankle. Although a significant portion of the foot must be supported, footrest length should be kept to a minimum to avoid interference with wheelchair maneuverability.

Footplates for fixed-frame sport wheelchairs are often smaller than those used on other frame styles. When patients are positioned with the knee in 90 degrees or more of flexion, more of the forefoot than the hindfoot and heel is on the footplate.

One measurement is necessary to determine footplate size for standard front rigging.

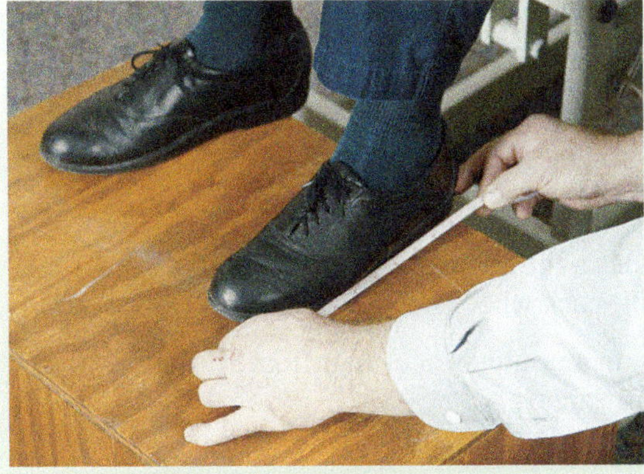

1. The portion of the foot that must be supported by a footplate extends from the calcaneus to the heads of the metatarsals.
2. With the foot supported and the ankle in neutral, measure the horizontal distance from the posterior aspect of the foot (calcaneus) to the head of the first metatarsal.
3. The result of this measurement provides the desired footplate size.

Table 6–1 ■ Standard wheelchair sizes

Size	Seat Depth (inches)	Seat Width (inches)	Seat Height (inches)
Adult	16.0	18.0	20.00
Narrow adult	16.0	16.0	20.00
Slim adult	16.0	14.0	20.00
Tall adult	17.0	18.0	20.00
Hemi or low seat[1]			17.50
Preschool	8.0	10.0	19.50
Tiny tot	11.5	12.0	19.50
Child	11.5	14.0	18.75
Junior	16.0	16.0	18.50

[1] Hemi or low seat can be any adult-size chair with respect to depth and width.

Standard Wheelchair Sizes

Table 6–1 ■ provides standard measurements for wheelchairs of different sizes. When a standard-sized wheelchair appropriately fits an individual, the wheelchair is usually less costly and available in a shorter period of time. Custom fabrication is used to provide wheelchairs most appropriate for each patient.

Review Questions

1. When are wheel locks used?
2. What are the indications for the following variations of wheelchair components?
   a. Desk-length armrests
   b. Full-length armrests
   c. Adjustable-height armrests
   d. Elevating legrests
   e. Footrests
3. How does a tilt-in-space wheelchair differ from a reclining-back wheelchair?
4. How is an amputee wheelchair frame different from a standard frame?
5. How is an individual measured for a wheelchair, including seat width, seat depth, seat-to-footplate length, back height, and armrest height?
6. How do wheelchair cushions affect measurements used to determine wheelchair fit?
7. What are the effects of inappropriate seat depth, seat width, or armrest height on sitting posture?
8. What is the effect of inappropriate footplate-to-seat distance on sitting posture?
9. What are the standard wheelchair sizes?

Suggested Activities

1. Examine available wheelchairs.
   a. Measure to determine size.
   b. Describe the components.
   c. Discuss the impairments and activity limitations of individuals likely to use the wheelchairs as configured.
2. Measure several classmates, and compare findings with standard wheelchair size measurements to determine an appropriate size of wheelchair. Document the results of the measurements in an appropriate format.
3. Role-play teaching patients and families how to manipulate the various components of a wheelchair.

Case Studies

1. An 8-year-old boy with a diagnosis of cerebral palsy presents with spastic quadriplegia. He is nonambulatory, has difficulty adjusting position and maintaining head alignment, and has the ability to grasp a pencil. Patient and parents desire independent mobility. Make appropriate recommendations for:
   a. Type of mobility device
   b. All components the device will need
2. A 17-year-old female is 10 weeks after a complete T10 spinal cord injury. Before her injury, she participated on several elite sport teams. She has indicated that she will use a wheelchair rather than ambulate with crutches and orthosis.
   a. List the measurements necessary to determine wheelchair size.
   b. Recommend appropriate type of mobility device and components.
3. A 67-year-old male with right hemiplegia following left CVA presents with slight spasticity and minimal voluntary control over both right extremities. Recommend:
   a. Appropriate type of wheelchair and components.
   b. What other type of wheelchair would be appropriate?
4. A 46-year-old female with a 20-year history of rheumatoid arthritis has significant involvement of all four extremities. She is able to walk only a few steps and to stand for short periods. Recommend:
   a. Appropriate type of mobility device and components.
   b. Appropriate type of wheelchair and components.

7

Turning and Positioning

LEARNING OUTCOMES

Upon completion of this chapter, you will be able to:

1. Describe the purposes of proper positioning.
2. Determine the amount of time a patient can spend in a position.
3. Implement a decision-making algorithm to determine the amount of assistance required for positioning a patient.
4. Use the Braden Scale to predict the likelihood of a patient developing skin ulceration.
5. Describe the stages of pressure ulcers.
6. Describe general procedures used to properly turn and position a patient.
7. Perform specific procedures used to turn a patient to, and to position in, supine, prone, sidelying, and sitting positions.

KEY TERMS

Long sitting
Orthostatic hypotension
Prone
Sidelying
Supine

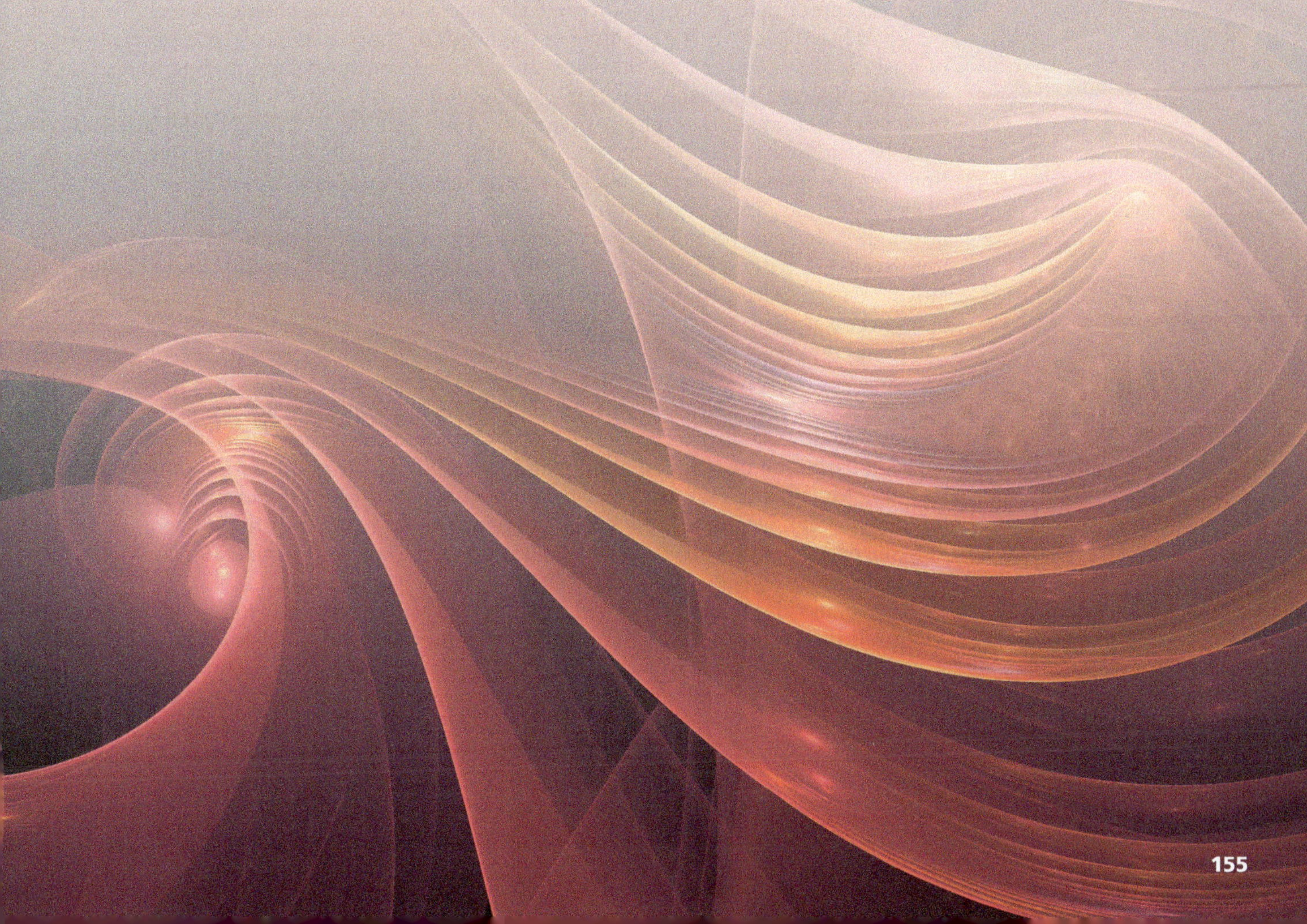

Introduction

Proper positioning is a valuable tool to maintain patient function. Physical therapists/assistants work with other healthcare professionals to determine optimal positions for patients. Physical therapists/assistants are responsible for positioning patients properly for physical therapy interventions and for function within a patient's environment. For patients unable to change position independently, proper positioning is essential for increasing function and preventing complications.

Goals

The goals of proper positioning are to

1. Ensure patient comfort.
2. Maintain integumentary integrity by preventing development of ulceration resulting from pressure or friction.
3. Maintain musculoskeletal integrity by preventing loss of range of motion.
4. Maintain neuromuscular integrity by preventing peripheral nerve impingement resulting from pressure.
5. Maintain cardiovascular/pulmonary integrity by using changes in position to assist secretion elimination, breathing patterns, and vascular flow.
6. Provide patient access to the environment.
7. Provide proper positioning for specific interventions.

To achieve these goals, patients and environments must be managed properly. Proper positioning includes moving patients into and out of desired positions in a safe and effective manner. These goals are appropriate for both short- and long-term positioning.

All healthcare providers who have contact with a patient have a responsibility to maintain appropriate patient positioning. Short-term positioning should not compromise the goals listed earlier. One example of the need for short-term positioning is changes of position required for tests and measures. Because of the minimum time in a given position, however, some modifications of positioning and support may be appropriate. In the example of short-term positioning for tests and measures, particular attention must be paid to accurate patient positioning for reliable and valid testing. During positioning for tests and measures, considerations of long-term effects on musculoskeletal or integumentary integrity are not as critical as for long-term positioning. Aspects of positioning that may be modified are a patient's position and supports (pillows, blankets, towels, etc.). A patient's position should be one from which the patient can move or be moved readily. Placement of supports should allow movement with the least rearrangement necessary.

Long-term positioning is prolonged periods in one position, which may affect musculoskeletal structures. Loss of range of motion, compromised joint nutrition, decreased joint stress, and loss of strength will occur if changes in position are not performed. Tissue (muscle, tendon, ligament, capsule) may be affected in two ways. There may be shortening of tissues on one side of a joint, and lengthening may occur on the other side of the joint. Musculoskeletal structures respond positively to appropriate stresses resulting from movement. Decreased movement eliminates these beneficial stresses, contributing to tissue degeneration and compromised function, such as bone demineralization, loss of sarcomeres, and degeneration of cartilage.

■ Take Note

Prolonged periods without repositioning may cause changes in tissues other than just skin.

Neuromuscular tissue, nerves and receptors, may be affected by prolonged periods in one position. Pressure on peripheral nerves will interfere with function. Pain, decreased sensation, and loss of tissue mobility may result. Decreased sensation may contribute to integumentary problems.

Circulation may be reduced by prolonged periods in one position. Decreased blood flow resulting from pressure on vascular structures may exacerbate integumentary problems, cause pain, and decrease nutrition to all tissues distal to the site of compression. **Orthostatic hypotension**, the inability of the cardiovascular system to adapt to upright postures after prolonged horizontal positioning, can be avoided if changes in position include an upright position in the positioning schedule. Breathing is also easier in an upright position. Frequent changes of position aid a patient's capability to excrete lung secretions.

Braden Scale

The Braden Scale[1] is a scale used to identify the risk level of a patient developing pressure ulcers. Completed when a patient is admitted to inpatient care, the Braden Scale (**Figure 7–1** ■) is a basis for patient management to prevent integumentary ulceration. Components of the Braden Scale include sensory perception, moisture, activity, mobility, and nutrition; are all scored on a scale of 1 to 4. Friction and shear are scored on a scale of 1 to 3. Lower scores indicate greater risk of integumentary ulceration. Improving patient activity and mobility are goals of physical therapy that assist in reducing complications of integumentary ulceration, poor circulation, and decreased respiratory function.

■ Take Note

Pressure ulcer risk assessment scales are used by many healthcare professionals.

RATING PRESSURE ULCERS Skin breakdown results from pressure interrupting circulation and friction that causes tissues to be torn. Interruption of circulation can occur when a patient does not or is not moved sufficiently. Friction can occur when patients move, or are moved, without adequate clearance or assistance. Pressure ulceration is rated on a scale of 1 to 4,[2] as presented in **Table 7–1** ■.

BRADEN SCALE FOR PREDICTING PRESSURE SORE RISK

Patient's Name ______________ Evaluator's Name ______________ Date of Assessment

SENSORY PERCEPTION ability to respond meaningfully to pressure-related discomfort	**1. Completely Limited** Unresponsive (does not moan, flinch, or grasp) to painful stimuli, due to diminished level of consciousness or sedation. OR limited ability to feel pain over most of body.	**2. Very Limited** Responds only to painful stimuli. Cannot communicate discomfort except by moaning or restlessness. OR has a sensory impairment which limits the ability to feel pain or discomfort over ½ of body.	**3. Slightly Limited** Responds to verbal commands, but cannot always communicate discomfort or the need to be turned. OR has some sensory impairment which limits ability to feel pain or discomfort in 1 or 2 extremities.	**4. No Impairment** Responds to verbal commands. Has no sensory deficit which would limit ability to feel or voice pain or discomfort.				
MOISTURE degree to which skin is exposed to moisture	**1. Constantly Moist** Skin is kept moist almost constantly by perspiration, urine, etc. Dampness is detected every time patient is moved or turned.	**2. Very Moist** Skin is often, but not always moist. Linen must be changed at least once a shift.	**3. Occasionally Moist** Skin is occasionally moist, requiring an extra linen change approximately once a day.	**4. Rarely Moist** Skin is usually dry, linen only requires changing at routine intervals.				
ACTIVITY degree of physical activity	**1. Bedfast** Confined to bed.	**2. Chairfast** Ability to walk severely limited or non-existent. Cannot bear own weight and/or must be assisted into chair or wheelchair.	**3. Walks Occasionally** Walks occasionally during day, but for very short distances, with or without assistance. Spends majority of each shift in bed or chair.	**4. Walks Frequently** Walks outside room at least twice a day and inside room at least once every two hours during waking hours.				
MOBILITY ability to change and control body position	**1. Completely Immobile** Does not make even slight changes in body or extremity position without assistance.	**2. Very Limited** Makes occasional slight changes in body or extremity position but unable to make frequent or significant changes independently.	**3. Slightly Limited** Makes frequent though slight changes in body or extremity position independently.	**4. No Limitation** Makes major and frequent changes in position without assistance.				
NUTRITION usual food intake pattern	**1. Very Poor** Never eats a complete meal. Rarely eats more than ⅓ of any food offered. Eats 2 servings or less of protein (meat or dairy products) per day. Takes fluids poorly. Does not take a liquid dietary supplement. OR is NPO and/or maintained on clear liquids or IV's for more than 5 days.	**2. Probably Inadequate** Rarely eats a complete meal and generally eats only about ½ of any food offered. Protein intake includes only 3 servings of meat or dairy products per day. Occasionally will take a dietary supplement. OR receives less than optimum amount of liquid diet or tube feeding.	**3. Adequate** Eats over half of most meals. Eats a total of 4 servings of protein (meat, dairy products) per day. Occasionally will refuse a meal, but will usually take a supplement when offered. OR is on a tube feeding or TPN regimen which probably meets most of nutritional needs.	**4. Excellent** Eats most of every meal. Never refuses a meal. Usually eats a total of 4 or more servings of meat and dairy products. Occasionally eats between meals. Does not require supplementation.				
FRICTION & SHEAR	**1. Problem** Requires moderate to maximum assistance in moving. Complete lifting without sliding against sheets is impossible. Frequently slides down in bed or chair, requiring frequent repositioning with maximum assistance. Spasticity, contractures or agitation leads to almost constant friction.	**2. Potential Problem** Moves feebly or requires minimum assistance. During a move skin probably slides to some extent against sheets, chair, restraints or other devices. Maintains relatively good position in chair or bed most of the time but occasionally slides down.	**3. No Apparent Problem** Moves in bed and in chair independently and has sufficient muscle strength to lift up completely during move. Maintains good position in bed or chair.					
				Total Score				

FIGURE 7–1 ■ The Braden Scale for Predicting Pressure Sore Risk. Reprinted with the permission of Barbara Braden.

Table 7–1 ■ Stages of pressure ulcers

Stage I	Skin intact with nonblanchable redness
Stage II	Partial thickness loss of skin—may be either a blister or open ulcer with red or pink wound bed
Stage III	Full-thickness tissue loss—subcutaneous fat exposed if present. May have undermining and tunneling.
Stage IV	As in Stage III with exposure of bone, muscle, or tendon.
Unstageable	Full-thickness tissue loss with slough and/or eschar in wound bed.

"National Pressure Ulcer Advisory Panel and European Pressure Ulcer Advisory Panel. Pressure Ulcer Prevention and Treatment: Clinical Practice Guideline." Washington, DC: National Pressure Ulcer Advisory Panel, 2009.

Time in Positions

The time in any one position is determined by the condition of all patient systems and any necessary precautions. Following chart review, interview, and systems review, a physical therapist determines positioning to be used during tests and measures. After a physical therapy evaluation and in consultation with other healthcare providers when appropriate, a plan for a patient's positioning is established. Physical therapist assistants may implement the positioning plan. All healthcare providers, including physical therapist assistants, have a responsibility to observe, report, and document changes that may require modification of a positioning plan.

The first time a patient is placed in a new position, the patient's skin, particularly over bony prominences that are pressure sites, should be examined after 5 to 10 minutes and frequently thereafter. Observation over time allows determination of tolerance for the position. A general rule is to reposition a patient at least every 2 hours initially to maintain integrity of all four movement systems (integumentary, musculoskeletal, neuromuscular, cardiovascular/pulmonary). Repositioning in less than 2 hours may be required for patients who have additional problems, such as poor circulation, fragile skin, decreased sensation, easily compromised peripheral nerves, difficulty breathing or excreting secretions, or inability to move.

When a patient is repositioned, skin over the area on which the patient was lying should be inspected and observed for color and integrity. Pay special attention to areas of skin that cover bony prominences, such as the greater trochanter or sacrum. Allow skin redness to resolve before putting pressure on that area of skin again. When recovery from pressure is delayed, modification of the positioning plan is required, such as changes in position, supports, and time in position. Excessive or prolonged redness indicates tissue damage (Stage 1 ulcer).

■ Take Note

Redness of skin must resolve before positioning on the area again.

When sitting, a patient must relieve pressure on the buttocks and sacrum at least every 10 minutes. Sitting push-ups using the arm rests of a chair, leaning first to one side and then to the other, and leaning forward, are methods to relieve pressure on the buttocks in the sitting position. Specialized wheelchairs, such as tilt-in-space and reclining-back wheelchairs, are used to provide pressure relief to patients who are unable to use other methods to relieve pressure on their own.

To determine the level of assistance patients require for repositioning, algorithms can be used. An algorithm for repositioning a patient in bed is presented in Figure 7–2 ■, and an algorithm for repositioning a patient in a chair is presented in Figure 7–3 ■.

In the following procedures, activities of turning and positioning are presented as if the patient cannot assist in the activity. When patients can assist in activities of turning and positioning, they should be encouraged to do so.

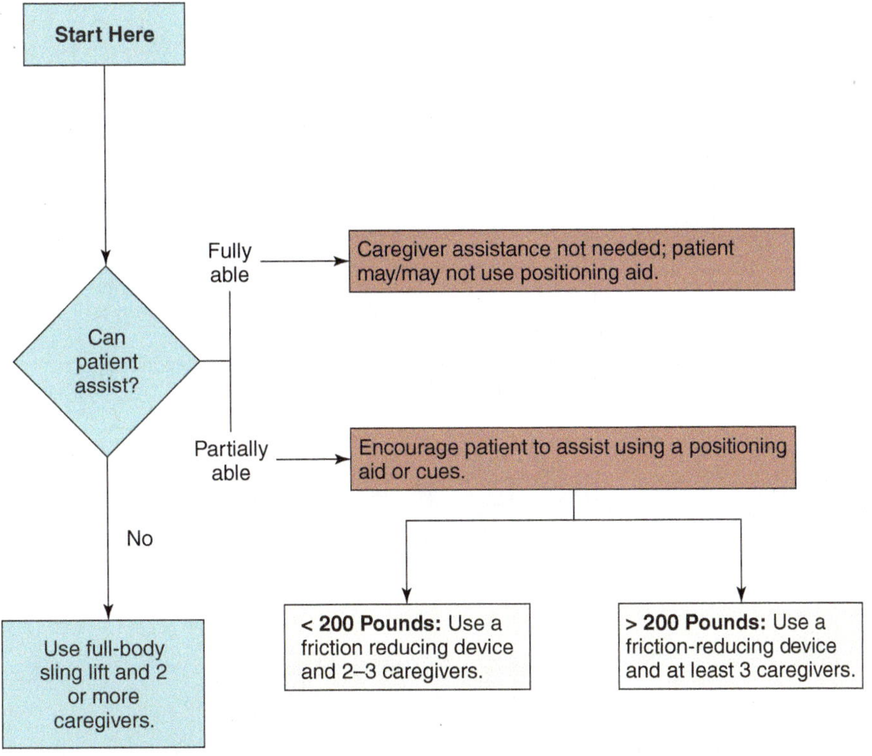

FIGURE 7–2 ■ An algorithm for repositioning a patient in bed. Reproduced from *Patient Care Ergonomics Resource Guide: Safe Patient Handling and Movement.* This was developed by the Patient Safety Center of Inquiry (Tampa, FL), Veterans Health Administration, and Department of Defense.

The procedures presented demonstrate the most difficult performance of these activities. Knowing the sequence and techniques to turn and position a patient passively permits a physical therapist/assistant to perform those portions of the activities a patient cannot perform. As the level of patient participation increases, the level of assistance provided by physical therapists/assistants can be decreased. Patients benefit from increasing their participation during activities of turning and positioning.

A specific example of increasing patient participation is the activity of turning from supine to prone (**Procedure 7–2**). Rather than a physical therapist/assistant moving a passive patient to the edge of a bed, the patient can be taught and encouraged to assume a hook-lying position and use bridging to lift the buttocks and move to the edge of the bed. Any of the other portions of the activity, such as moving extremities, can be patient-assisted movements rather than just passive movement performed by a physical therapist/assistant. Following practice of the procedures as presented, consider how to modify and practice these modifications in a manner that encourages and permits patient participation.

Illustrations in this chapter demonstrate a patient on a treatment table or mat. The same procedures are used when turning or positioning a patient in bed. Procedures and positions are modified to accommodate specific needs of each individual patient.

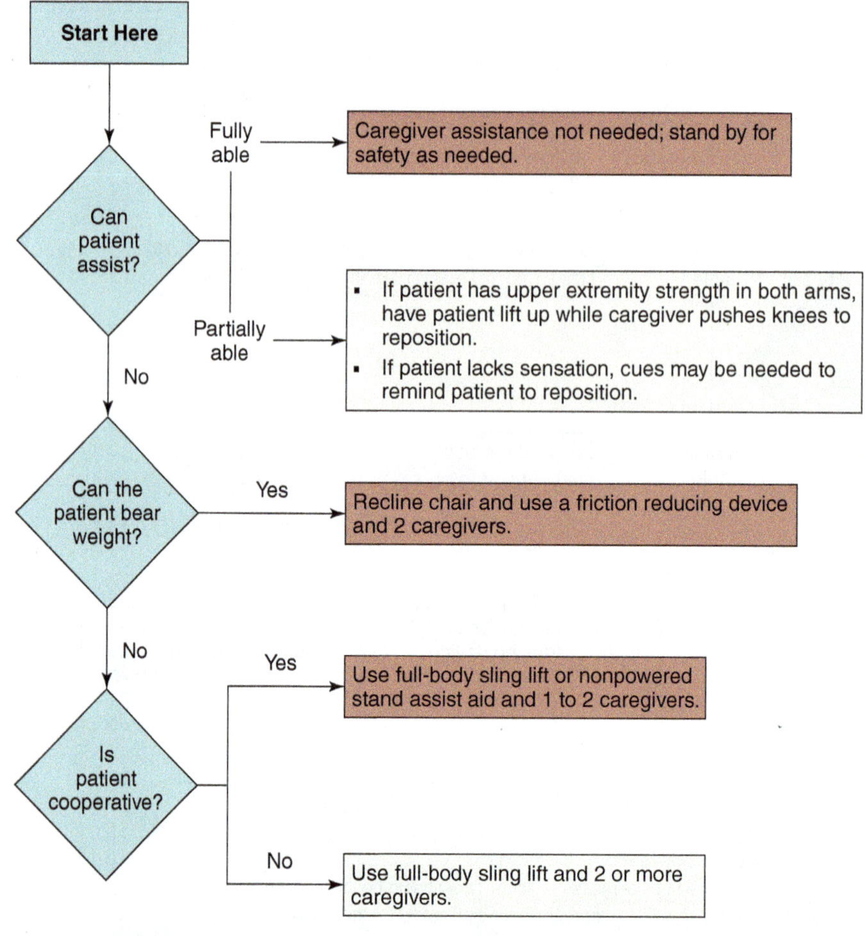

FIGURE 7–3 ■ An algorithm for repositioning a patient in a chair. Reproduced from *Patient Care Ergonomics Resource Guide: Safe Patient Handling and Movement.* This was developed by the Patient Safety Center of Inquiry (Tampa, FL), Veterans Health Administration, and Department of Defense.

PROCEDURE 7–1 General Procedures

Preparing the environment assists in safe and effective turning and positioning. Preparing the environment means having a clear area for movement and having all necessary supplies, including sheets, pillows, and towels, available within easy reach. A sufficient number of appropriately trained personnel must be available. Following these general procedures reduces the risk of harm to the patient and personnel. Before moving a patient, check carefully for tubes, lines, and monitor leads to avoid disconnecting or compromising them accidentally. The safety and well-being of patients with respect to positioning is the responsibility of all healthcare providers who have contact with the patient.

1. *Smooth all undersheets, towels, and patient clothing.* Avoid wrinkles in the sheets, blankets, and personal clothing because they increase pressure on a small area of skin and cause skin irritation. Such pressure points are uncomfortable for patients with sensation, especially when unable to move independently.

2 *Pillows, blankets, and towels may be used to support body parts and to avoid strain or pressure on ligaments, nerves, and muscles.* A sufficient quantity of these items must be available and within reach before beginning positioning. Pillows or towels are used to provide relief to bony prominences or areas most susceptible to ulceration. When patients must be positioned in a specific way for a procedure, be sure to relieve sensitive areas of pressure. Supporting the body segment just proximal and distal to, but not under, a sensitive area relieves pressure on sensitive areas. This type of positioning is shown in **Figure 7–4 ■**. Place pillows or towels close to the involved area to prevent contact of the involved area with the supporting surface. In these circumstances, reduce time in the position, as pressure may increase at the site of the pillows or towels, thereby compromising circulation.

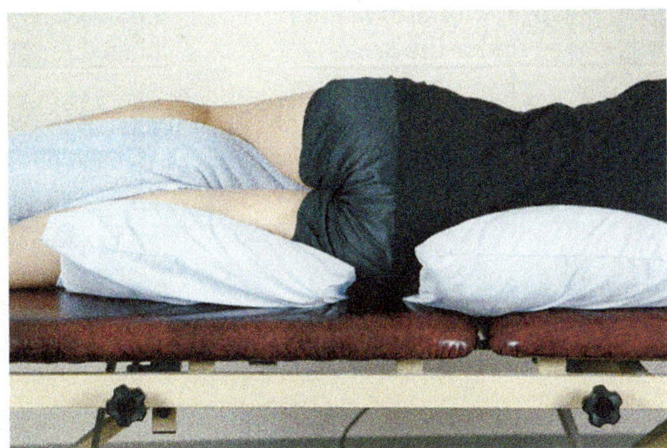

FIGURE 7–4 ■ Position to relieve pressure on bony prominences.

3 *Ensure that enough clear area exists and equipment is ready for moving patients safely.* A clear area allows all personnel involved in moving and positioning a patient sufficient space to move without impediment and without bumping into walls, chairs, and other equipment. Make sure all beds, gurneys, wheelchairs, and other movable equipment are locked or secured prior to initiating moving a patient.

4 *Ensure sufficient personnel trained in moving and positioning patients are present.* When turning and positioning patients, patients must be lifted, rather than dragged, across the sheets. Dragging may result in skin irritation as a result of friction.

5 *Draping should allow appropriate positioning while maintaining patient modesty and warmth.* Sheets or blankets are used for draping or covering the patient. Covers tucked tightly at the foot of the bed force the ankle into a position of plantar flexion. This should be avoided to reduce the risk of developing contractures.

6 *Whenever possible, patients should participate actively during moving and positioning.* For simple procedures, give explanations and directions before initiating a procedure. Give cues throughout the procedure. For procedures with many steps, give a general explanation prior to the start of a procedure and then individual cues prior to each step of the procedure. Give additional directions as needed. Providing directions and cues as a complex procedure progresses assists patients who may not be able to remember all steps for an entire procedure while concentrating on the first few steps.

Supine Position

A **supine** position is one in which a person lies on his or her back on a supporting surface. In the supine position, a patient is positioned with shoulders parallel to hips and a straight spine. Many people require a small pillow to support the head for comfort. A pillow can be placed under the knees to relieve strain on the lower back (**Figure 7–5 ■**). Positioning with a pillow under the knees, however, can lead to decreased hip and knee extension range of motion as a result of prolonged positioning in hip and knee flexion. A pillow placed lengthwise under the legs will reduce knee flexion and relieve pressure on the heels (**Figure 7–6 ■**).

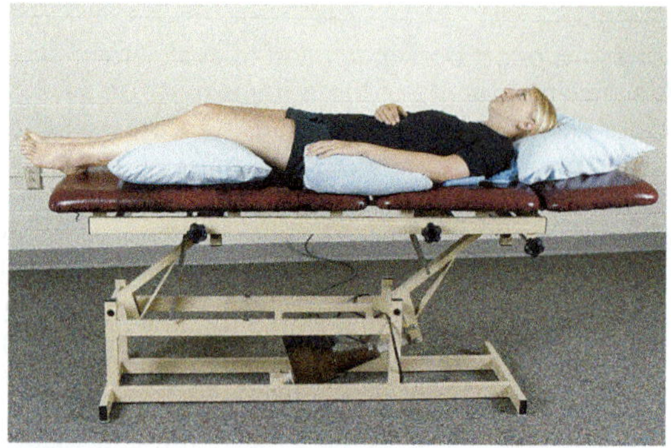

FIGURE 7–5 ■ Supine position with arm support and a pillow placed crosswise under the knees.

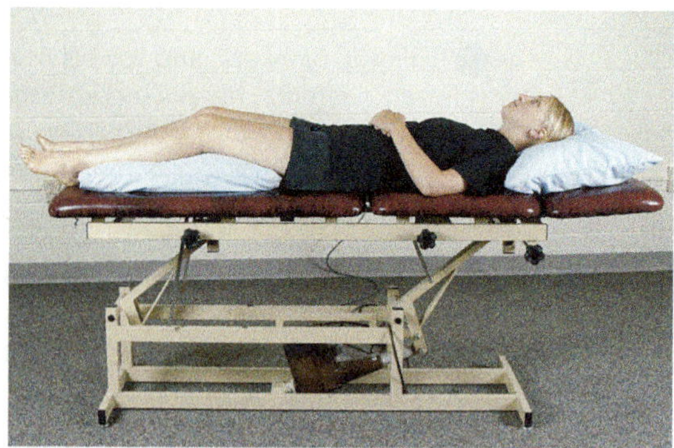

FIGURE 7–6 ■ Supine position with a pillow placed lengthwise under the legs.

PROCEDURE 7–2 Turning from Supine to Prone

The patient's initial position is supine. Move the patient far enough to one side of the treatment table to allow a full turning movement to the prone position without coming too near the opposite edge on completion of the turning movement. To turn to the left, first move the patient to the right side of the treatment table. When segmental movement of the trunk and lower extremities is possible, move the patient in stages. When a patient cannot tolerate such movement, more than one person, or specialized beds, will be needed.

To turn a patient from supine to prone, the following steps occur in sequence.

■ Take Note

Safety first—Prepare environment before starting to move patient.

1. Move the patient's upper trunk and head to the right side of the treatment table.

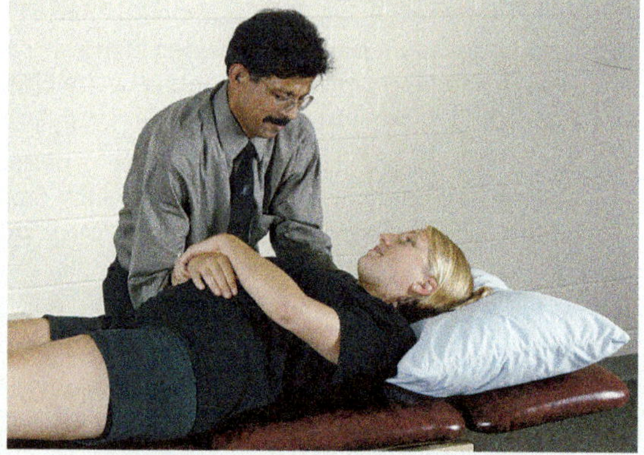

2. Move the patient's lower trunk to the right side of the treatment table.

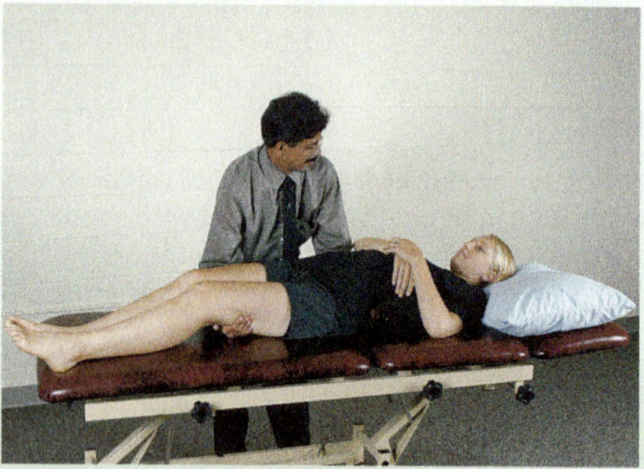

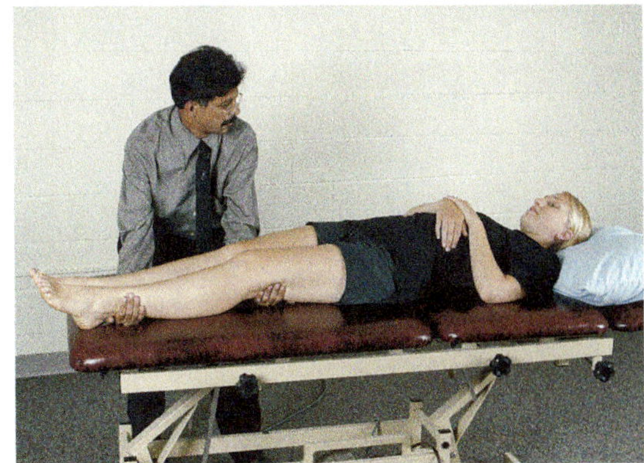

3 Move the patient's lower extremities to the right side of the treatment table.

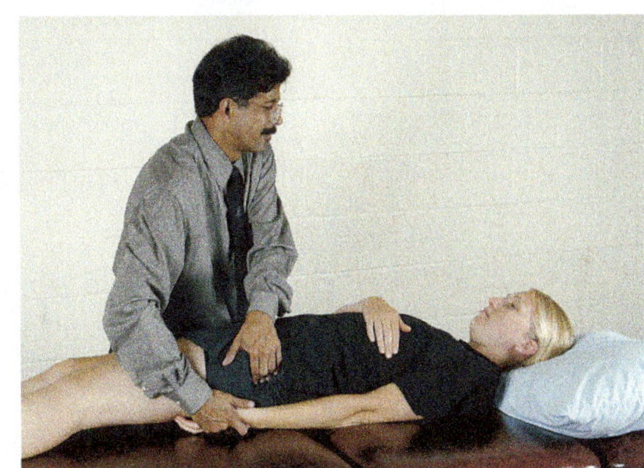

4 Cross the patient's right lower extremity over the left lower extremity, with the right ankle resting on top of the left ankle. The patient's left upper extremity is adducted, placing the hand under the left hip, palm against the hip. This positioning of the extremities applies when a patient is being turned to the left, as presented in these figures. In situations where turning is to the right, the positioning movements must be mirror images of these positions.

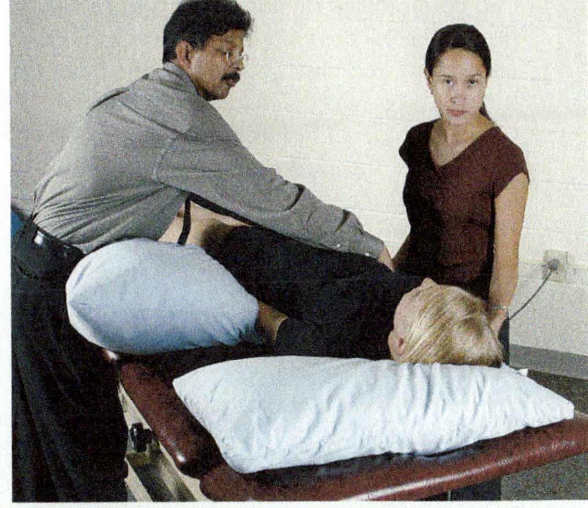

5 Position yourself on the side to which the patient is being turned. Personnel assisting in turning a patient should stand next to the patient on the side from which the patient is being turned, to prevent the patient from falling while the physical therapist/assistant moves from one side of the treatment table to the other. Personnel assisting in turning a patient can help with positioning of pillows and turning the patient.

When a pillow will be under a patient while the patient is in the prone position, position the pillow in the proper orientation before the patient is rolled.

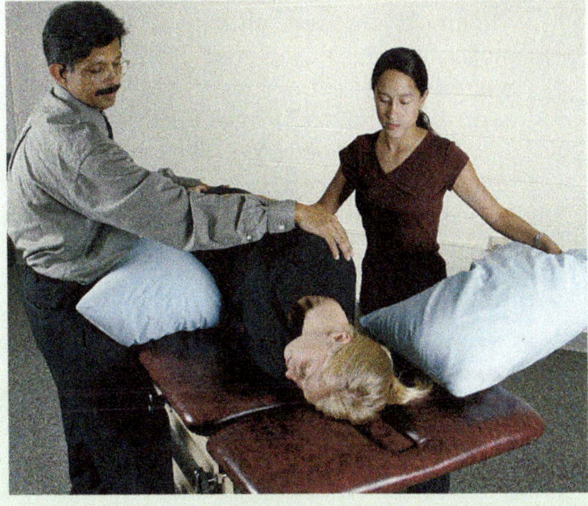

6 When patients have head and neck control, they can assist in turning their head and neck in the direction of the roll as turning is initiated. When patients do not have head and neck control, be aware that a patient's face may be subject to some rubbing on the mattress or mat during turning. When ready to begin the turning movement, ask the patient and any assisting personnel if they are ready. After receiving an affirmative reply, a preparatory count is given, followed by a specific verbal cue to initiate turning.

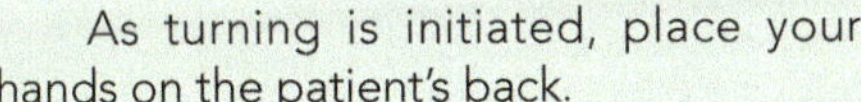

As turning is initiated, place your hands on the patient's back.

(continued)

PROCEDURE 7–2 Turning from Supine to Prone *(continued)*

7 When a patient reaches the halfway point, gravity can complete the movement, but will do so in an uncontrolled manner. Therefore rotate and reposition your hands as the patient reaches the midpoint of the turn. Reposition your hands to the anterior surface of the patient to control the second half of the turning movement.

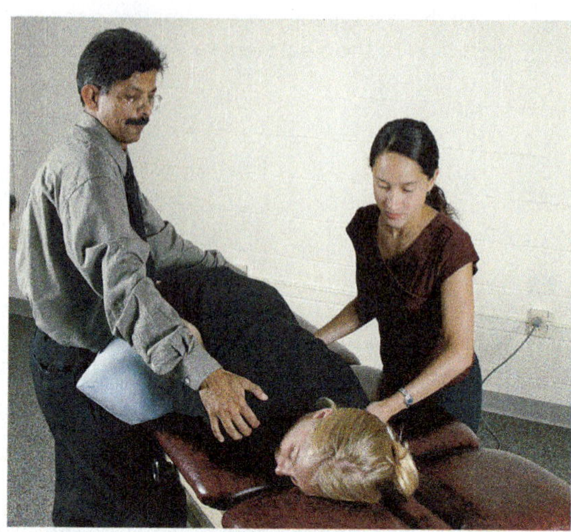

8 When a turn is completed, a patient's head and neck are the first body segments to be repositioned. Place the patient's head in a comfortable position facing the side that will allow best interaction with others and the environment. Positioning the head turned to one side eliminates pressure on the eyes, nose, or mouth but may increase pressure on the external ear. Place a small towel under the temple to relieve pressure on the external ear. In some situations the head may be maintained in the midline, using a small pillow or towel under the forehead to relieve pressure on the eyes, nose, and mouth and to permit unimpeded respiration.

Adjust the position of the pillow under the trunk as needed. Place the patient's arms in a position of slight abduction. Finally, uncross the patient's feet if they remained crossed after the turning movement was completed. Position the patient's lower extremities so the feet are approximately 6 to 8 inches apart.

To turn supine to prone to the right, the previous procedure is used, with the designation of left side becoming right side and the designation of right side becoming left side.

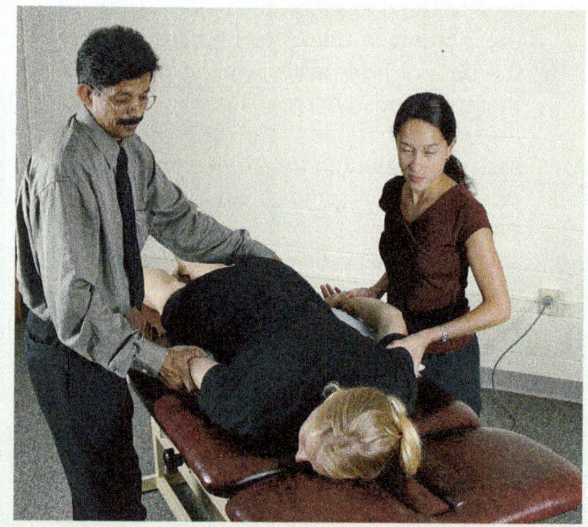

Prone Position

A **prone** position is a position in which a person lies on his or her stomach on a supporting surface. When in a prone position, patients are positioned with shoulders parallel to hips and with a straight spine. The patient's head may be turned to either side or maintained in the midline, as described in the Procedure 7–2. A patient's upper extremities may be positioned alongside the trunk or alongside the head. For some patients, circulation in the upper extremities may be compromised when a patient's arms are placed alongside the head. Position upper extremities alongside the head only when a patient has sensation in the upper extremities and can communicate reliably if a problem arises. When a patient's upper extremities are positioned alongside the head, you should question the patient frequently to determine if the patient is experiencing numbness or tingling.

A pillow may be placed lengthwise or crosswise under the trunk to ensure that spinal curvature is not excessive at any segment. A lengthwise position may be more comfortable when patients have limited neck mobility. The lumbar region's lordotic curve is reduced by crosswise positioning of the pillow. Therefore, that position may be more comfortable for patients with low back pain. Patients with tender or large breasts may also be more comfortable with the pillow in a crosswise position, distal to the breasts. A pillow under the lower legs can also be used to avoid positioning the ankles in plantar flexion (Figure 7–7 ■). A pillow under the lower legs places the knees in slight flexion, however, and may promote loss of knee extension range of motion. A patient's feet can be positioned over the end of a treatment table to avoid positioning the ankles in plantar flexion (Figure 7–8 ■).

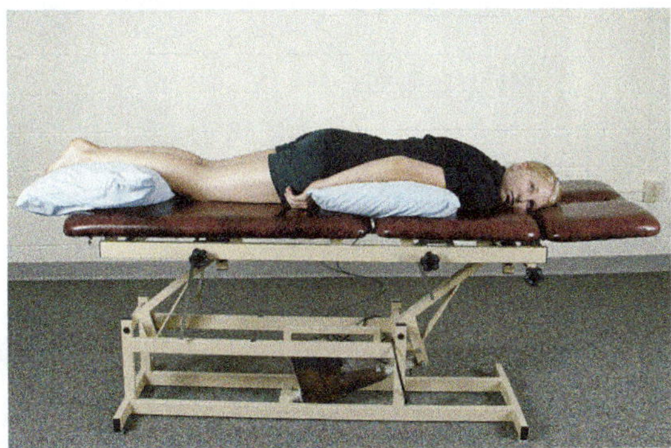

FIGURE 7–7 ■ Prone position with pillows under the trunk and lower legs.

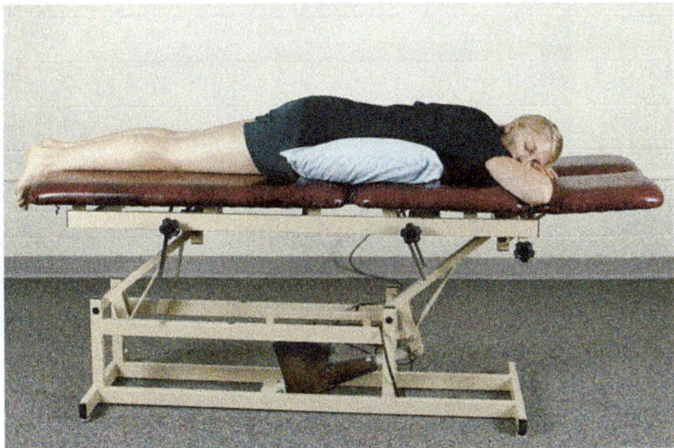

FIGURE 7–8 ■ Prone position with a pillow under the trunk and feet positioned over the end of the treatment table.

PROCEDURE 7–3 Turning from Prone to Supine

Turning a patient from prone to supine is similar to turning a patient from supine to prone. Because the patient's initial position is prone, move the patient far enough to one side of the treatment table to allow a full turning movement to the supine position without coming too near the opposite edge on completion of the turning movement. To turn to the right, move a patient to the left side of the treatment table. When segmental movement of the trunk and lower extremities is possible, move the patient in stages. When a patient cannot tolerate such movement, more than one person or specialized beds will be needed.

To move a patient from prone to supine, the following steps occur in sequence.

1. Move the patient's upper trunk and head to the side of the treatment table.
2. Move the patient's lower trunk to the side of the treatment table.
3. Move the patient's lower extremities to the side of the treatment table.

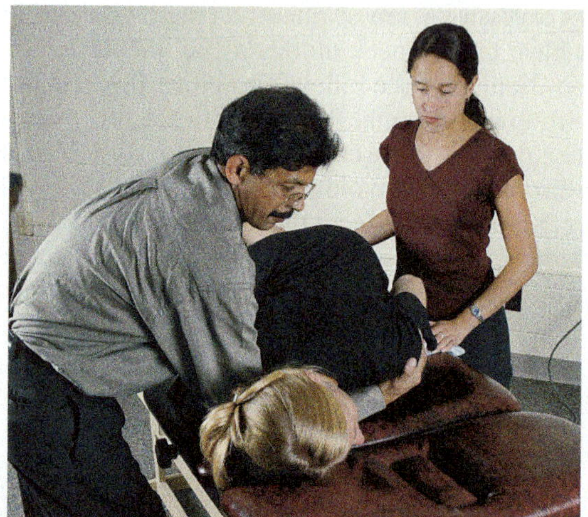

4. Position yourself on the side to which the patient is being turned. Personnel assisting in turning a patient should stand next to the patient on the side from which the patient is being turned to prevent the patient from falling as you move from one side of the treatment table to the other. Personnel assisting in turning the patient can help with positioning of pillows and turning the patient.

   When a patient does not have head and neck control, rubbing of the patient's face on the mattress or mat can be avoided by having the patient start by facing away from you. A patient with head and neck control can assist by looking up and over the shoulder while being turned toward you.

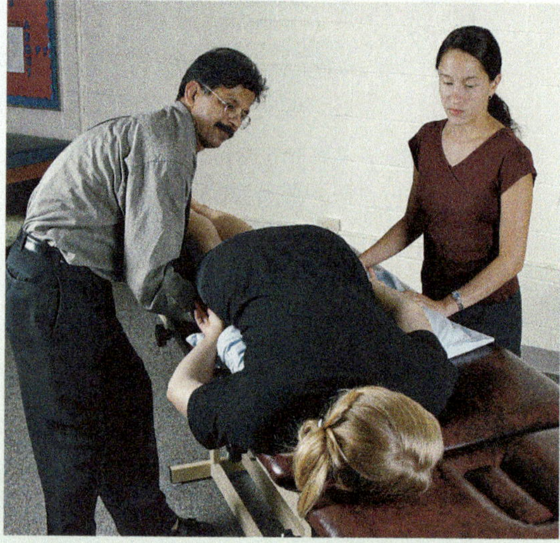

5 The patient's left upper extremity is adducted, placing the hand at the hip, palm against the hip. Support the right upper extremity against the patient's body as the patient is turned.

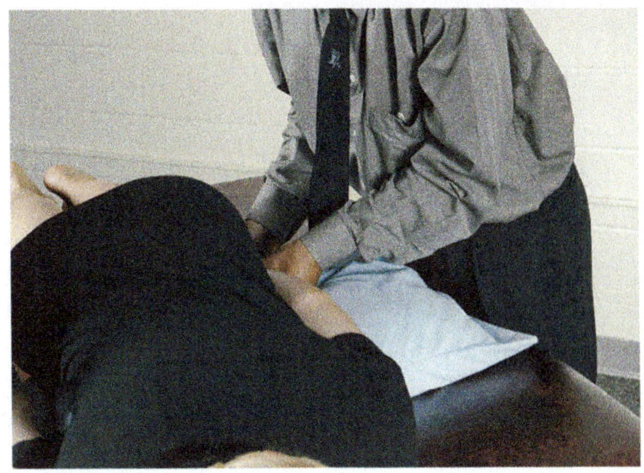

6 As in turning from supine to prone, control both phases of the turning motion. Initially, reach over the patient, placing your hands on the patient's anterior surface.

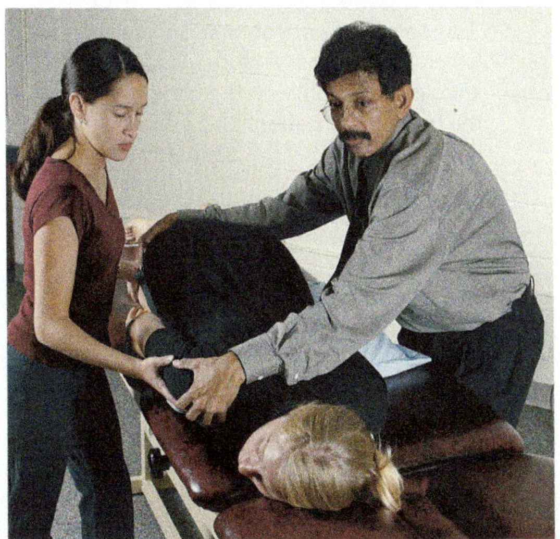

7 When a patient reaches the halfway point, gravity can complete the movement but will do so in an uncontrolled manner. Therefore rotate and reposition your hands as the patient reaches the midpoint of the turn. Reposition your hands to the posterior surface of the patient to control the second half of the turning movement.

8 When a turn is completed, a patient's head and neck are the first body segments to be repositioned. The extremities are then positioned as in the supine position.

To turn from prone to supine to the left, the previous procedure is used, with the designation of left side becoming right side and the designation of right side becoming left side.

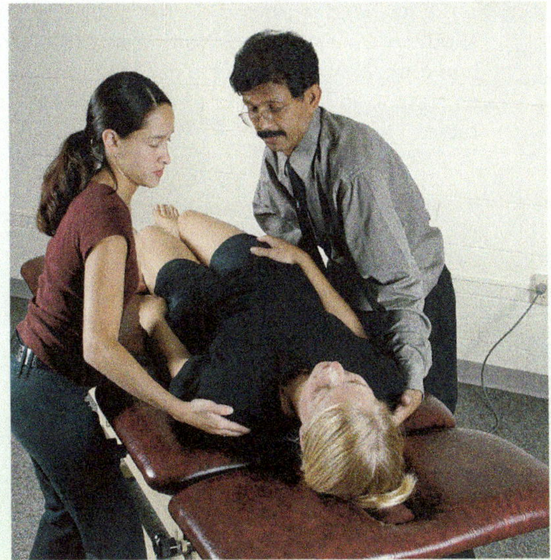

PROCEDURE 7–4 Turning on a Floor Mat

When turning a patient on a floor mat, the same steps and sequence are followed as when turning a patient on a treatment table. Proper body mechanics become more important in preventing injury to physical therapists/assistants when turning a patient on a floor mat.

To turn a patient on a floor mat, the following steps occur in sequence.

■ Take Note

Be safe by being aware of your body mechanics.

1. After a patient is moved to one side of the mat, position yourself on the side to which the patient will turn. Assume a half-kneeling position, with the "down" knee at the level of the patient's hips and the "up" knee at the level of the patient's shoulders.

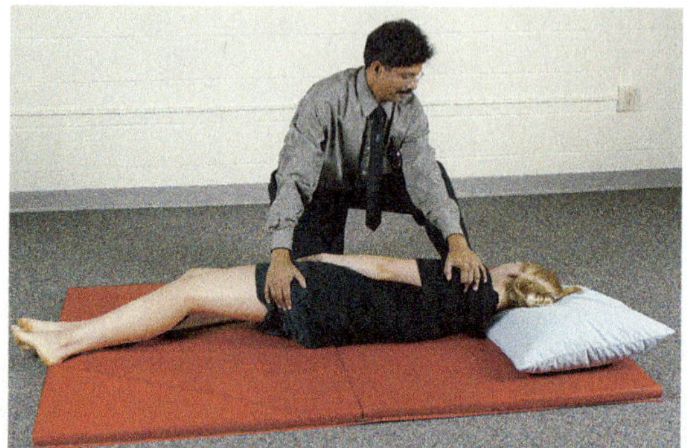

2. Place the hand over which the patient will roll against the hip on the same side, with the palm facing the hip.
3. Place the hand that will be on top during the roll against the hip on the same side, with the palm facing the hip. Using the hand closest to the patient's hips, hold the patient's hand in place against the patient's hip. Your hand that is closer to the patient's head is placed on the patient's shoulder. Your hand position must rotate and reposition at the midpoint of the turn, as described for turning on a treatment table.

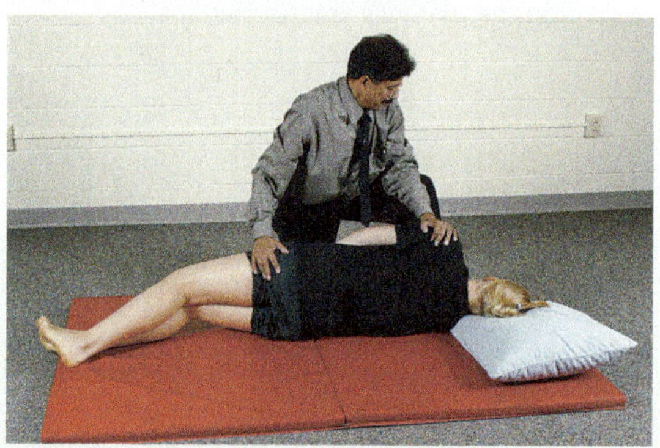

4. Move out of the patient's way as the turn is completed, allowing the patient to complete the turn without rolling into your body.

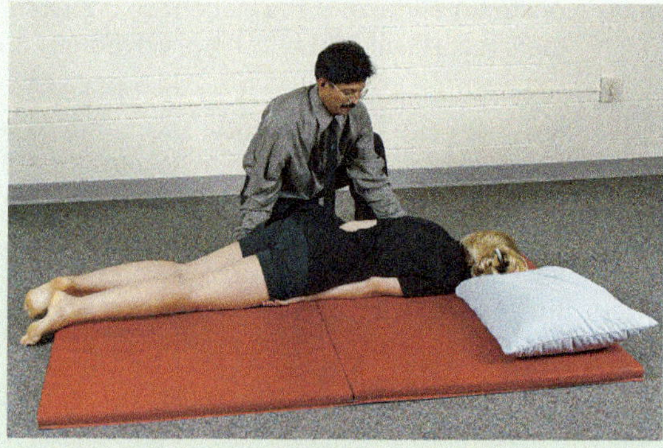

Sidelying

A **sidelying** lightface is a position in which a patient is lying on one side. The positions of the upper extremities and lower extremities will vary, depending on whether the patient's upper trunk is rotated forward or backward while in a sidelying position.

In a sidelying position in which a patient's upper trunk is rotated forward (Figure 7–9 ■), the lowermost upper extremity is slightly flexed at the shoulder so the patient is not lying on the humerus, the uppermost upper extremity is flexed at the shoulder and supported by a pillow, the lowermost lower extremity is relatively extended, and the uppermost lower extremity is flexed at the hip and knee and supported on pillows. The uppermost lower extremity should be supported by enough pillows so that it is not lowered into adduction. To avoid excessive pressure on the lowermost lower extremity, the uppermost lower extremity should not lie directly on top of the lowermost lower extremity.

In a sidelying position in which a patient's upper trunk is rotated backward (Figure 7–10 ■), the lowermost upper extremity shoulder girdle is protracted, and the shoulder is slightly flexed so the patient is not lying on the humerus, the uppermost upper extremity is extended and supported by pillows behind the patient, the lowermost lower extremity is flexed at the hip and knee, and the uppermost lower extremity is relatively extended and supported on pillows. The uppermost lower extremity should be supported by enough pillows so that it is not lowered into adduction. To avoid excessive pressure on the lowermost lower extremity, the uppermost lower extremity should not lie directly on top of the lowermost lower extremity.

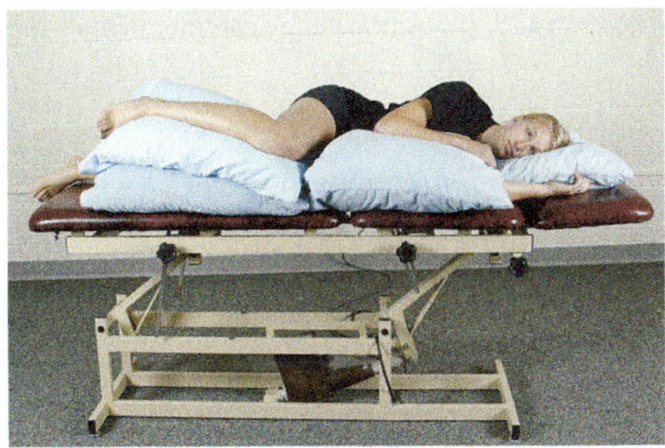

FIGURE 7–9 ■ Sidelying position with upper trunk rotated forward.

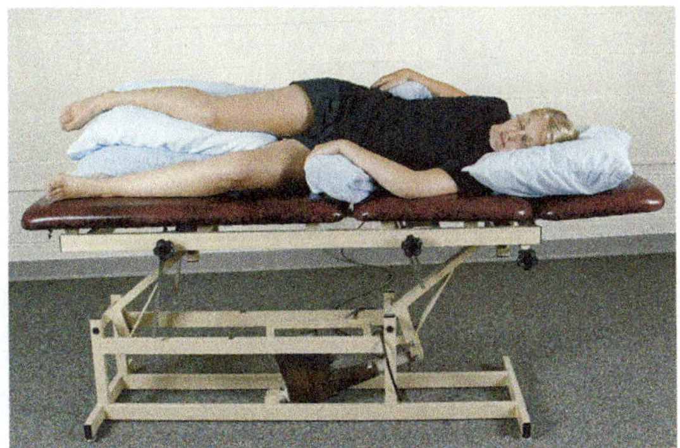

FIGURE 7–10 ■ Sidelying position with upper trunk rotated backward.

PROCEDURE 7–5 Turning from Supine or Prone to Sidelying

A patient can be turned to a sidelying position from either the supine or prone position. The steps in turning a patient from supine to sidelying are similar to those for turning a patient from supine to prone, with the movement stopping when the patient reaches the midpoint of the turn. The patient is then positioned in the chosen one of the two sidelying positions.

The steps in turning a patient from prone to sidelying are similar to those for turning a patient from prone to supine, with the movement stopping when the patient reaches the midpoint of the turn. The patient is then positioned in the chosen one of the two sidelying positions.

PROCEDURE 7–6 Moving from Supine to Sitting

There are various methods for assisting a patient to assume a sitting position. The method chosen will depend on a patient's functional abilities, medical problems, and starting position. Whichever method is chosen, patients should not be left unguarded in a sitting position if they cannot maintain the position independently in a safe manner.

Supine to Long Sitting

Long sitting is a position in which a person sits with hips flexed to 90 degrees and knees fully extended on a supporting surface. When patients have sufficient strength, they can assume a long-sitting position by doing a sit-up from supine to sitting. To assist a patient in moving from supine to long sitting, the following steps occur in sequence.

1. When minimal assistance is needed, as for patients with generalized weakness, a trapeze bar can be used. In some situations patients can perform a sit-up or use a trapeze bar while assistance is provided. You can place an arm behind a patient's back to assist the patient in changing position. When a trapeze bar is not available, you can stabilize an arm in front of the patient in lieu of a trapeze bar.

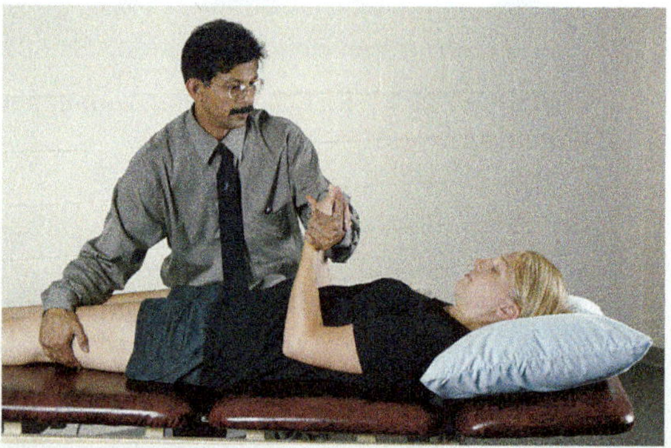

2. A patient can pull up by pulling on your arm. You may add additional assistance for the sit-up movement by placing an arm across the patient's thighs to stabilize the patient's lower extremities.

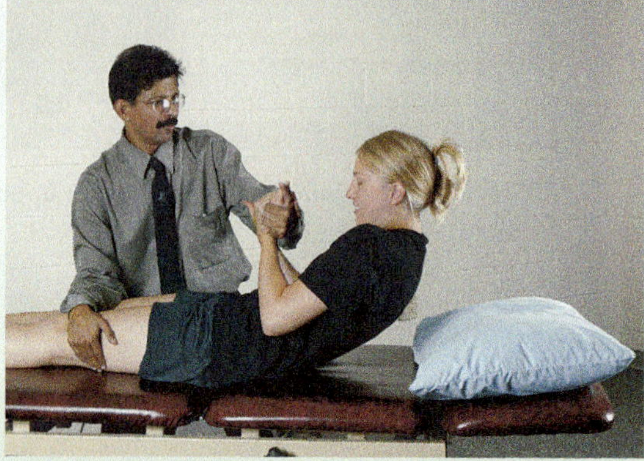

3 You should not move the arm and do the patient's work of pulling up into a sitting position. As necessary, you should move toward the patient's feet to permit the patient to assume a long-sitting position.

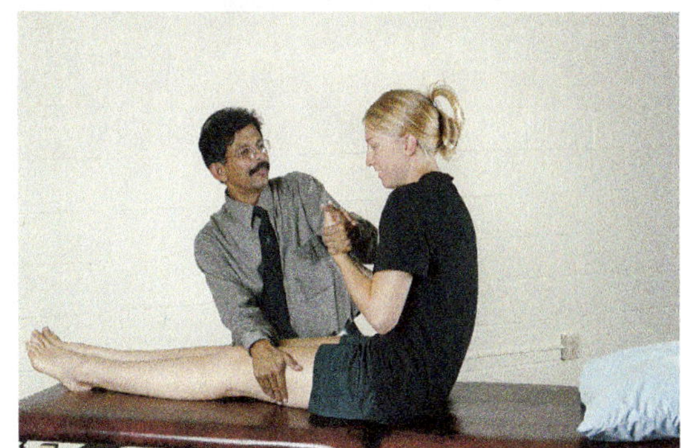

Sidelying to Sitting on Side of Table

To assist a patient in moving from sidelying to sitting, the following steps occur in sequence.

1 The patient assumes a sidelying position to the side of the treatment table on which the patient wishes to sit.

The patient's hips and knees are flexed 60 degrees to 90 degrees, and the patient's lower legs are moved over the edge of the treatment table to act as counterweight to the patient's trunk and upper extremities.

You can assist the patient in assuming a sitting position by placing one arm under the patient's thighs to control the rate of lowering the patient's lower extremities and one arm under the patient's shoulder to assist in coming to the sitting position.

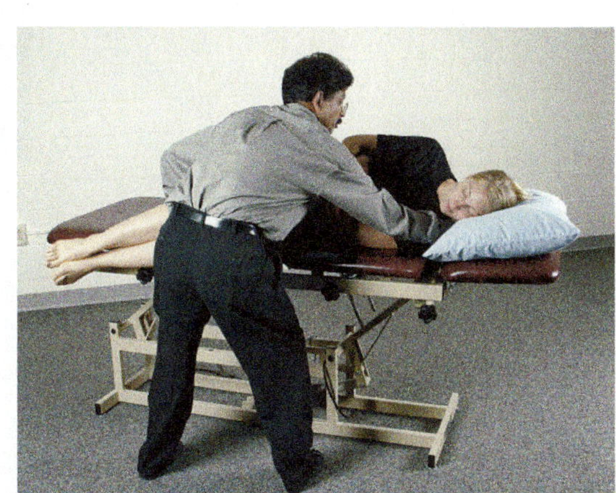

2 With the lower extremities acting as counterweights, the patient uses the upper extremities to push to sitting.

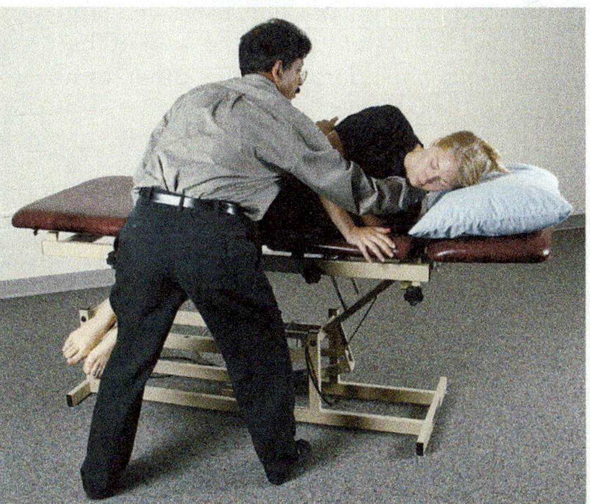

(continued)

PROCEDURE 7–6 Moving from Supine to Sitting (*continued*)

3 You can assist by controlling lowering of the patient's lower extremities and lifting the upper trunk as necessary.

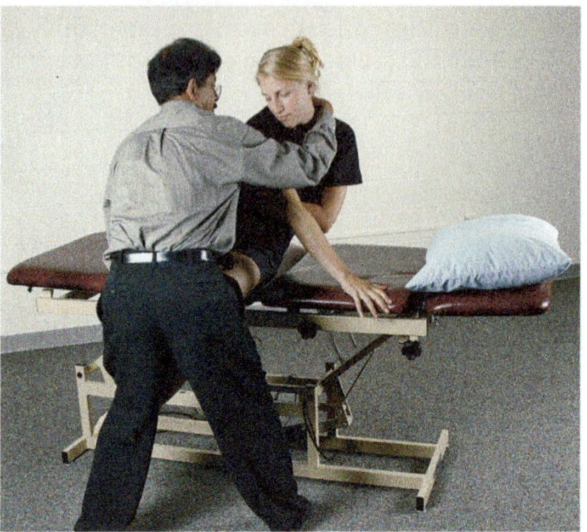

Supine to Sitting on Side of Table

When patients are dependent on higher levels of assistance, you can use the lower extremities as counterweights to provide additional assistance. To move a patient from supine to sitting, the following steps occur in sequence.

1 Starting in supine position, place one arm around the upper trunk at the level of the patient's shoulders and the other arm under the patient's thighs.

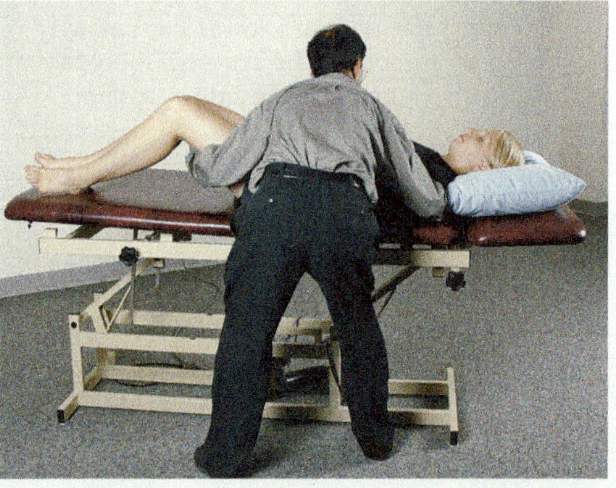

2 At the same time, lift the patient's trunk and lower the patient's lower extremities over the side of the table.

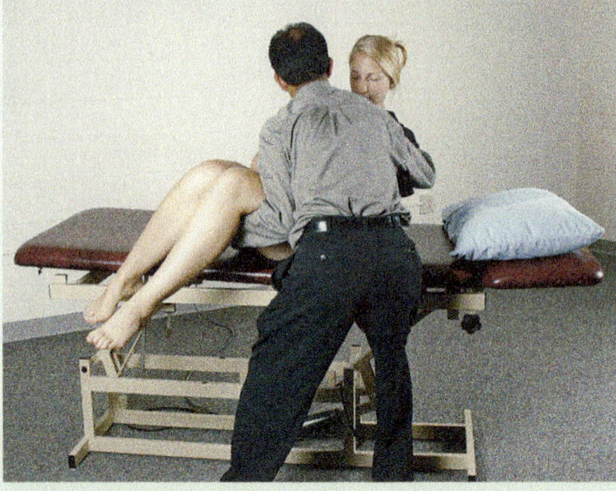

3 Lift the patient into a sitting position and pivot to sitting over the side of the table.

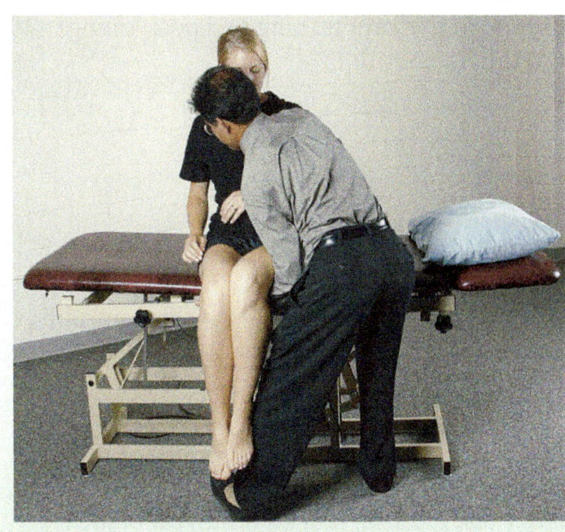

Review Questions

1. What are the purposes for proper positioning for the four practice patterns: integumentary, musculoskeletal, neuromuscular, and cardiovascular/pulmonary?
2. How do physical therapists determine the proper amount of time a patient can be in a position?
3. How is a patient positioned when properly positioned in the supine, prone, and sidelying positions?
4. How is a patient properly turned from supine to prone, supine to sidelying, sidelying to prone, sidelying to supine, and prone to supine?
5. How is a patient assisted to sitting from supine?
6. What are the components of the Braden Scale, and how are the components scored?
7. What are the characteristics of ulcers in each stage of pressure ulcers?
8. Upon examination of an elderly patient 3 days after a cerebral vascular accident, redness is noted over the left greater trochanter. What would be an appropriate positioning schedule for this patient?
9. How should a family be instructed to properly position a patient with a recent complete cervical spinal cord injury?
10. A patient recovering from a myocardial infarction has comorbidities of diabetes and peripheral vascular disease. What precautions should be taken to prevent pressure ulcers while the patient is in bed because of restricted activity?

Suggested Activities

1. Demonstrate the specific procedures presented in this chapter.
   - Practice specific procedures working in groups of at least three, rotating through the roles of patient, physical therapist, and physical therapist assistant.
   - Take vital signs of the patient once in new position.
   - Practice performing turning and positioning while partners role-play diagnoses (see following case studies). The student role-playing the patient can add "character" to the role by employing behaviors such as being cooperative, noncooperative, in pain, hard of hearing, or faint. The "patient" must role-play the diagnosis and character consistently, so the students must have researched the diagnosis, signs, and symptoms.
   - The student role-playing the physical therapist/assistant should document the "intervention."
2. Review the Braden Scale. Use the Braden Scale for the patients in the case studies that follow to determine their risk for developing pressure ulcers.

3. Practice teaching family, patient, and other healthcare providers how to perform turning and positioning. Document the intervention.
4. Implement a decision-making algorithm to determine the amount of assistance required for positioning the patients described in the following case studies.

Case Studies

For the following case study situations:

- Select and describe and/or demonstrate appropriate turning and positioning procedures.
- Provide an appropriate rationale for choices.
- Document interventions provided.

1. The patient is a 59-year-old male with right hemiplegia 1 day after surgery to remove a blood clot. He presents with mild spasticity in both right extremities, minimal active movement of the right extremities, and expressive aphasia.
2. The patient is a 21-year-old with T12 complete spinal cord injury who has loss of muscle performance and sensation in the lower extremities.
3. The patient is a 12-year-old with moderate spastic quadriplegic cerebral palsy who is hospitalized for management of pneumonia.
4. The patient is a 75-year-old with a fractured right hip 1 day after total hip replacement.

References

1. Braden Scale. http://www.bradenscale.com/images/bradenscale.pdf
2. National Pressure Ulcer Advisory Panel. http://www.npuap.org/

8

Range of Motion Exercise

LEARNING OUTCOMES

Upon completion of this chapter, you will be able to:

1. Describe anatomical position.
2. Define terms used to describe movements in anatomical planes.
3. Distinguish between joint range of motion (ROM) and muscle length ROM.
4. Indicate when passive ROM (PROM), active-assisted ROM (AAROM), or active ROM (AROM) intervention is appropriate.
5. Describe different joint end feels.
6. Describe differences in movement when patients have normal muscle tone, spasticity, rigidity, and pain.
7. Describe general methods used to perform ROM exercises properly.
8. Describe the benefits of using diagonal patterns of motion.
9. Describe combining components of motion used in Proprioceptive Neuromuscular Facilitation (PNF) patterns.
10. Describe specific procedures used to perform ROM exercises in anatomical planes and diagonal patterns of motion.

KEY TERMS

Active-assisted range of motion (AAROM)
Active range of motion (AROM)
Anatomical planes of movement
Anatomical position
Combining components
Diagonal patterns of movement
End feel
- Bony (hard) end feel
- Capsular (firm or leathery) end feel
- Empty end feel
- Soft end feel

Frontal (coronal) plane
Joint range of motion
Midsagittal plane
Multiarticular
Muscle length (muscle range of motion)
Passive range of motion (PROM)
Proprioceptive Neuromuscular Facilitation (PNF)
Range of motion (ROM)
Rigidity
Sagittal plane
Spasticity
Tenodesis
Transverse (horizontal) plane
Uniarticular

Introduction

Range of motion (ROM) is movement of each joint and muscle through its available arc of motion. Measurements of ROM are a part of tests and measures that contribute to the evaluation component of the physical therapy patient/client management process (Chapter 2). ROM exercises are part of interventions within the plan of care component of the physical therapy patient/client management process (Chapter 2). ROM exercises are used to prevent development of contractures, muscle shortening, and tightness in capsules, ligaments, and tendons, all of which can limit mobility. Additional benefits of ROM interventions may include sensory stimulation and enhanced circulation when performed as active or active-assisted ROM.

Joint ROM is moving a joint in all planes of motion appropriate for the specific joint. Limitations of joint ROM may result from bony structure of joint surfaces, internal derangement of joint structures, lack of length of soft tissue (capsule, cartilage, ligament, muscle, skin, or tendon) surrounding the joint, or pain. Examples include decreased joint ROM resulting from deterioration of joint surfaces, meniscal tears, ligament adhesions, or shortness of single-joint (**uniarticular**) muscles.

■ **Take Note**
Joint ROM: Movement to maintain mobility of joints.

Muscle length, **or muscle ROM**, is lengthening a muscle through its available length for all appropriate joint motions. To lengthen muscle, joints must be moved in the direction opposite the shortening action of the specific muscle. This affects both single-joint (uniarticular) and multijoint (**multiarticular**) muscles. When joints are moved through all available ROM, lengthening of muscles that cross only that joint (uniarticular muscles) is also achieved. To lengthen muscles that cross more than one joint (multiarticular muscles), all joints crossed by the multiarticular muscles must be moved in a manner that achieves full elongation of the multiarticular muscles as a final result. An example of decreased muscle length occurs when the biceps brachii muscle, a multiarticular muscle that flexes the shoulder, flexes the elbow, and supinates the forearm, becomes shortened following prolonged immobilization. To lengthen the biceps brachii muscle to its greatest available length, the shoulder and elbow must be extended and the forearm pronated. These movements may occur simultaneously or in sequence, provided that the end result is having all joint movements at their greatest limit at the same time.

■ **Take Note**
Muscle ROM: Movement to maintain mobility of multijoint muscles.

In certain circumstances, a goal of treatment is to allow multiarticular muscles to become shortened. When multiarticular muscles are shortened, they are not able to be lengthened over all the joints they cross at once. Functional use of muscle shortening is called **tenodesis**. An example of tenodesis producing function is when shortened long finger flexors cause grasp as the wrist is extended and release as the wrist is flexed. Patients with quadriplegia use this tenodesis action to hold and release utensils, such as a fork, toothbrush, or writing implement.

When developing a plan of care, physical therapists must differentiate between ROM exercises, which use only the available range of motion, and stretching exercises. Stretching exercises are designed to increase the available range of motion. Physical therapist assistants may provide both interventions, ROM and stretching, under the supervision of a physical therapist.

Joint ROM and muscle length interventions may be performed as passive range of motion (PROM), active-assisted range of motion (AAROM), and active range of motion (AROM) exercises. **Passive range of motion** exercise is performed with the patient relaxed and a physical therapist/assistant moving a patient's body segment without patient assistance. Passive range of motion is used when determining range of motion, both joint ROM and muscle length ROM, as part of tests and measures. Passive range of motion is examined prior to testing muscle performance (strength). **Active-assisted range of motion** is performed by assisting patients in performing movements. **Active range of motion** exercises are performed independently by patients, although they may be supervised to ensure correct and safe performance. Table 8–1 ■ indicates the different types of joint ROM and muscle lengthening interventions and the impairments patients may have, for which specific types of range of motion exercises are indicated.

■ **Take Note**
Types of ROM: passive ROM, active-assistive ROM, and active ROM.

The limit of ROM is achieved when a body segment cannot be moved further because of restriction by joint structure or soft tissues or because of patient reports of pain. When a limit of motion is reached, the quality of restriction felt by the clinician is described as

Table 8–1 ■ Types of range of motion and indications for use

Type	Use
Passive	Paralysis, paresis, weakness, pain, increased muscle tone
	When active assisted or active, would cause excessive cardiopulmonary stress
	When a patient lacks safe control of movement
	Maintain joint and soft tissue mobility
	Maintain joint and tissue nutrition
	Increase kinesthetic awareness
Active assisted	Paresis, weakness, pain, cardiopulmonary problems, abnormal tone
	Maintain joint and soft tissue mobility
	Maintain joint and tissue nutrition
	Increase kinesthetic awareness
Active	Patient can move correctly without causing undue stress on any body system
	Maintain joint and soft tissue mobility
	Maintain joint and tissue nutrition
	Increase kinesthetic awareness

end feel. Normal end feels vary depending on the structures limiting further movement. When further motion is limited by bone abutting bone, the end feel is hard and is called **bony**, or **hard, end feel**. An example of a nonpathological bony end feel occurs when complete elbow extension is attained. At this point, movement is halted by contact between the olecranon process of the ulna and the olecranon fossa of the humerus. When further motion is limited by a soft tissue approximation, there is a **soft end feel**. An example of nonpathological soft end feel occurs when elbow flexion is limited by forearm soft tissue approximating the muscle bulk of elbow flexors on the anterior surface of the upper arm. An end feel with minimal give is a result of a taut capsule or ligament. This is known as a **capsular**, or **firm**, or **leathery end feel**. An example of nonpathological capsular end feel occurs when a nonpathological knee is stress-tested for varus (adduction) and valgus (abduction) strain. When further motion is limited by pain, there is no tissue limitation to motion, and the end feel is described as an **empty end feel**.

■ Take Note

End feel: the "feel" the clinician perceives when a joint reaches the end of its motion.

Patients with upper motor (central nervous system) lesions may have involuntary muscle contractions. Muscle tone is altered in the presence of upper motor neuron lesions, presenting as spasticity or rigidity. **Spasticity** presents as increased resistance to movement, especially as the velocity of movement increases. When spasticity is present, a point in the range of motion may be reached where further muscle lengthening is temporarily prevented. Maintaining a force in same direction of motion may result in a sudden reduction in tone, permitting movement through the remaining range of motion. This is referred to as the *clasp-knife phenomenon.* Spasticity usually occurs in antigravity muscles. **Rigidity** presents as resistance to passive movement that is not affected by movement velocity. Both antigravity and progravity muscles may present with rigidity. In the presence of spasticity or rigidity, slow maintained movement usually permits movement through the complete range of motion without eliciting interference of involuntary muscle contractions.

Methods

To maintain proper posture and body mechanics, physical therapists/assistants should use a table or bed of appropriate height. Preparing treatment areas, and the use of proper body mechanics, is covered in Chapter 3.

The exact frequency, number of repetitions, and sets of repetitions of PROM exercises needed to maintain tissue extensibility is not known and likely varies for each patient and the need for such exercises. Passive ROM (PROM) exercises during rehabilitation are performed twice each day. Family members can be taught to perform selected ROM exercises to increase frequency of exercise. A frequently chosen number of repetitions for each movement is ten; however, fewer repetitions still provide benefits. In many cases, one or two sets of repetitions are sufficient. When a patient can perform active-assisted or active ROM exercises, physical therapists determine the frequency of treatment periods and the number of repetitions for each movement.

ROM exercises are performed by moving the body segments through each **anatomical plane of movement**, either separately or by combining components of motion. When using anatomical plane movements, multiple joints may be exercised simultaneously. Examples include combinations of hip and knee flexion with ankle dorsiflexion and hip and knee extension with ankle plantar flexion. **Combining components** of motion occurs when more than one plane of joint motion is performed simultaneously. **Diagonal patterns of movement**, described by **Proprioceptive Neuromuscular Facilitation (PNF)**,[1] are combining components of motion at one joint, as well as at all the joints of an extremity.

Physical therapists determine whether anatomical planes of movement or diagonal patterns of movement are to be performed. Anatomical planes of movement allow more specific isolation of joint motions and involved musculature. Complete joint motion is more easily accomplished using anatomical planes of movement. Diagonal patterns of movement simulate functional joint movement more closely than do anatomical planes of motion.

Gentle, but secure, manual contacts provide support when performing range of motion exercises. Hand placement should allow movement of body segments through complete ROM and provide support with minimal hand repositioning. Velocity of movement should be slow to moderate. Joint ROM exercises should encompass all planes of motion available in a joint. Muscle length exercises must result in lengthening multiarticular muscles across all joints crossed simultaneously.

■ Take Note

Anatomical planes of motion—flexion/extension, abduction/adduction, and medial/lateral rotation.

Anatomical Planes of Movement

All motions of the body are described in terms of starting from the anatomical position. The **anatomical position** is described as that position in which a person is standing upright, eyes looking straight ahead, arms at the sides with palms facing forward, and the feet approximately 4 inches apart at the heels, with the toes pointing forward (Figures 8–1 ■ and 8–2 ■).

Three anatomical, or cardinal, planes are defined with respect to the anatomical position. The ***sagittal* plane** divides the body into two sides—left and right. The ***midsagittal* plane** divides the body exactly into left and right halves. Motions of flexion and extension occur in the sagittal plane. The ***frontal,* or *coronal,* plane** divides the body into front and back portions. Motions of abduction and adduction occur in the frontal plane. The only motions of flexion/extension and abduction/adduction that do not occur in their respective planes of motion are motions of the thumb. Thumb flexion and extension occur in the frontal plane, and thumb abduction and adduction occur in the sagittal plane. The ***transverse, or horizontal,* plane** divides the body into upper and lower portions. All movements of rotation, and horizontal abduction and adduction of the shoulders, occur in the transverse plane.

The following definitions assume the starting position is the anatomical position:

Flexion: Except for the thumb, flexion is movement in a sagittal plane. For the neck, trunk, upper extremities, and lower extremities except knees and toes, flexion results in approximation of anterior surfaces of the limb segment. For knees and toes, flexion results in approximation of the posterior and plantar limb segment

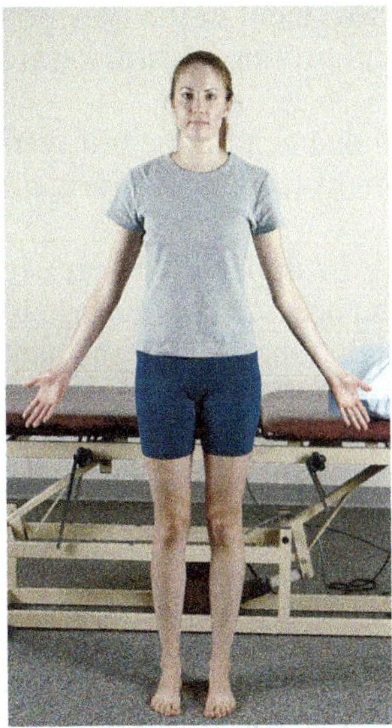

FIGURE 8–1 ■ Anterior view of anatomical position

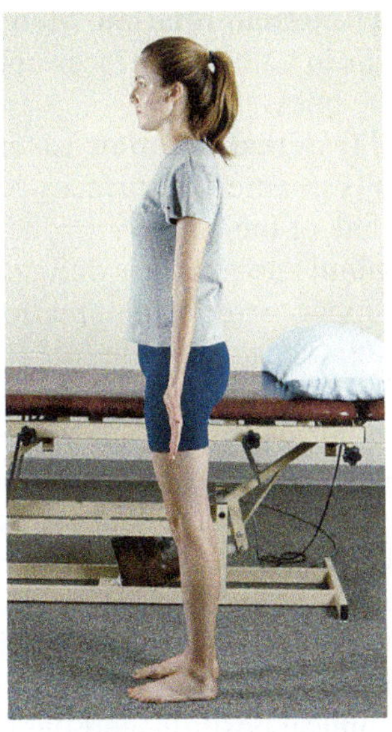

FIGURE 8–2 ■ Lateral view of anatomical position

surfaces, respectively. Dorsiflexion, moving the foot upward, is the movement of the ankle considered flexion. Thumb flexion is movement of the thumb across the palm toward the fifth digit, and occurs in the frontal plane.

Extension: Except for the thumb, extension is movement in the sagittal plane. For the neck, trunk, upper extremities, and lower extremities other than knees and toes, extension results in anterior surfaces of the limb segment moving away from each other. For knees and toes, extension results in posterior and plantar limb segment surfaces moving away from each other, respectively. Plantar flexion, moving the foot downward, is the movement of the ankle considered extension. Thumb extension is moving the thumb across the palm away from the fifth digit and occurs in the frontal plane.

■ **Take Note**

Exceptions for flexion and extension are thumbs, knees, and toes.

Abduction: Except for the thumb, abduction is movement in the frontal plane and is the result of the limb segments moving away from the midline of the body. Thumb abduction is movement of the thumb away from the palm of the hand and occurs in the sagittal plane. When the wrist is moved such that the hand moves away from the midline of the body, the movement is labeled **radial deviation**.

Adduction: Except for the thumb, adduction is movement in the frontal plane and is the result of the limb segments moving toward the midline of the body. Thumb adduction is movement of the thumb into the palm of the hand and occurs in the sagittal plane. When the wrist is moved such that the hand moves toward the midline of the body, the movement is labeled **ulnar deviation**.

Horizontal abduction: Horizontal abduction is movement of the upper extremity posteriorly when the shoulder has already been abducted to 90 degrees in the frontal plane.

Horizontal adduction: Horizontal adduction is movement of the upper extremity anteriorly when the shoulder has already been abducted to 90 degrees in the frontal plane.

Protraction: Protraction is multiplanar movement of the scapula around the lateral aspect of the ribs toward the anterior aspect of the thorax. This motion is often termed scapular abduction.

Retraction: Retraction is multiplanar movement of the scapula around the lateral aspect of the ribs as the scapula moves toward the spine. This motion is often termed scapular adduction.

Opposition: Opposition is multiplanar movement of the carpometacarpal joint of the thumb that results in approximation of the tip of the thumb and the tip of a finger of the same hand. There is no term that describes the opposite motion.

Medial (internal) rotation: Medial rotation is movement in the transverse plane that results in anterior surfaces of the limb segment turning inward, toward the midline of the body.

Lateral (external) rotation: Lateral rotation is movement in the transverse plane that results in anterior surfaces of the limb segment turning outward, away from the midline of the body.

Supination: Supination is defined differently for the upper and lower extremities. For the upper extremity, supination of the forearm occurs when the arm is stabilized in the anatomical and the forearm is rotated so that the palm of the hand faces anteriorly. This is a uniplanar movement occurring in the transverse plane when in the anatomical position. Supination of the forearm is the position of the forearm in the anatomical position. For the lower extremity, supination of the foot occurs when the leg is stabilized and the foot is rotated about the oblique axis of the subtalar and other midfoot joints. This is a triplanar motion that incorporates plantar flexion, forefoot adduction, and inversion of the foot.

Pronation: Pronation is defined differently for the upper and lower extremities. For the upper extremity, pronation of the forearm occurs when the arm is stabilized in the anatomical position, and the forearm is rotated so that the palm of the hand faces posteriorly. This is a uniplanar movement occurring in the transverse plane when in the anatomical position. For the lower extremity, pronation of the foot occurs when the leg is stabilized and the foot is rotated about the oblique axis of the subtalar and other midfoot joints. This is a triplanar motion that incorporates dorsiflexion, forefoot abduction, and eversion of the foot.

Inversion: Inversion is movement of the foot that occurs in the frontal plane about the long axis of the foot. Inversion occurs when the foot is rotated about the long axis of the foot such that the plantar surface of the foot faces toward the midline of the body.

Eversion: Eversion is movement of the foot that occurs in the frontal plane about the long axis of the foot. Eversion occurs when the foot is rotated about the long axis of the foot such that the plantar surface of the foot faces away from the midline of the body.

Confusion exists concerning the use of the terms *supination/pronation* and *inversion/eversion* when describing motion at the ankle and foot. The definitions provided earlier are those used by clinicians. The clinical definitions are based on the writing of Root, Orien, and Weed.[2] Using clinical definitions, *supination* and *pronation* are terms describing triplanar movements, of which inversion and eversion are uniplanar components. Anatomists Warwick and Williams,[3] however, describe these terms of ankle and foot motion in the opposite manner. Under the anatomical definitions, *inversion* and *eversion* are terms describing triplanar movement, of which supination and pronation are uniplanar components. In the text, these terms are used in accordance with the clinical definitions presented by Root et al.[2]

Diagonal Patterns of Movement

Two diagonal patterns of movement, presented as part of Proprioceptive Neuromuscular Facilitation (PNF), have been described for the upper extremities and the lower extremities, respectively.[1,4] Diagonal patterns of movement are achieved by combining simultaneously components of all three cardinal planes of motion and of multiple joints of an extremity. Figure 8–3 ■ illustrates the difference between two successive cardinal planes of motions and the simultaneous combining of three cardinal planes of motion into a diagonal pattern.

Specific diagonal patterns of motion are described by the combination of motions performed by either the shoulder or hip joints (Figures 8–4 ■ through 8–12 ■). Each basic diagonal pattern is modified by varying position or movement of the elbow or knee, providing the ability to perform both joint ROM and muscle length exercises. The two diagonal PNF patterns are commonly referred to as D1 and D2, where *D* stands for diagonal, and *1* and *2* refer to specific PNF diagonal patterns.

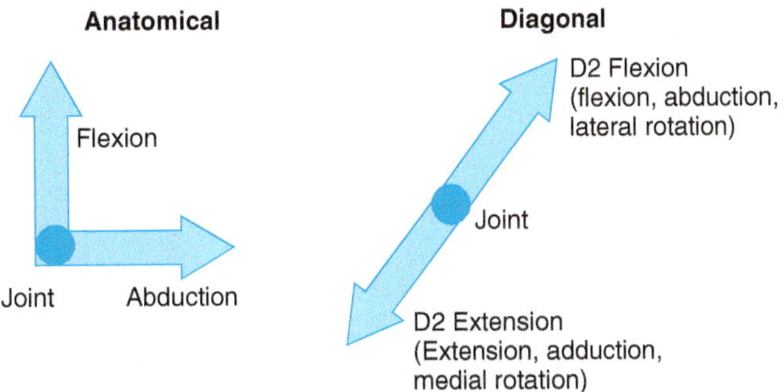

FIGURE 8–3 ■ Anatomical vs. diagonal patterns of movement

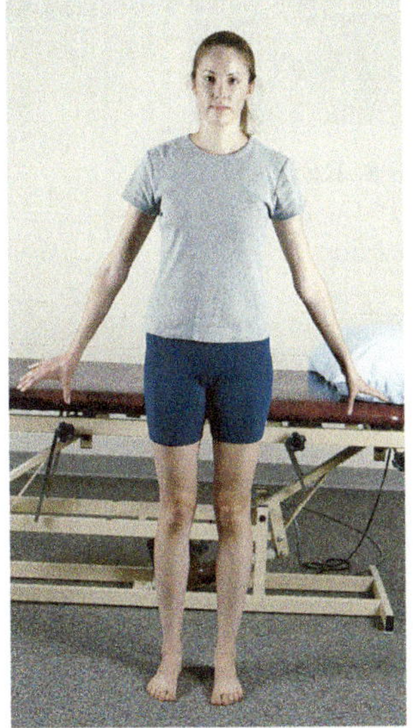

FIGURE 8–4 ■ Bilateral upper extremity D1 extension

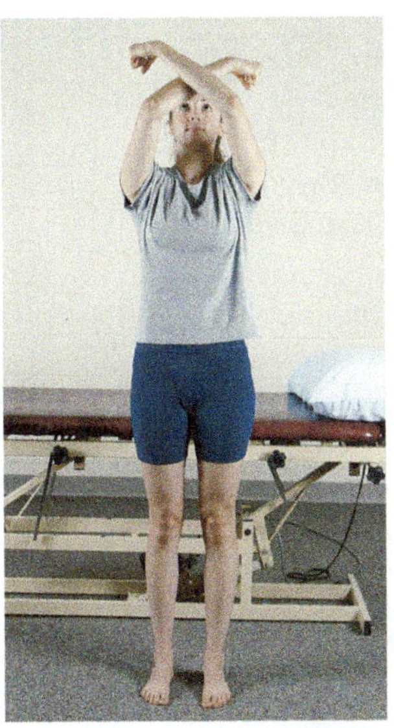

FIGURE 8–5 ■ Bilateral upper extremity D1 flexion

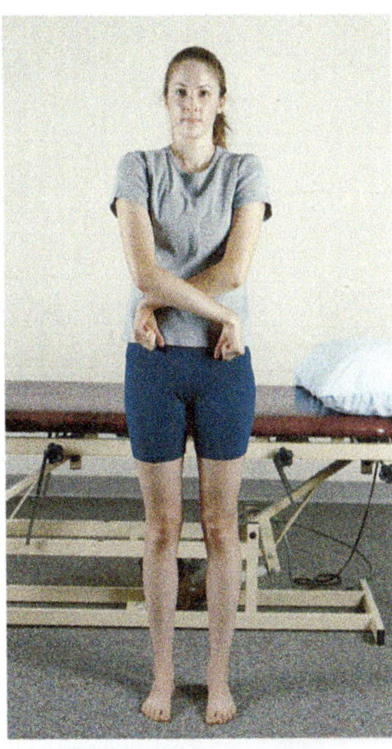

FIGURE 8–6 ■ Bilateral upper extremity D2 extension

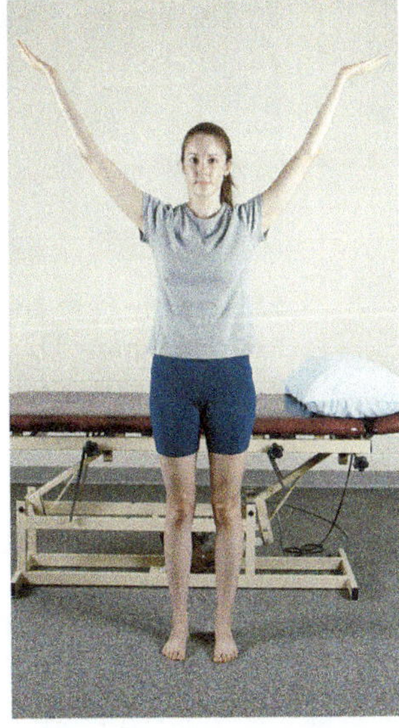

FIGURE 8–7 ■ Bilateral upper extremity D2 flexion

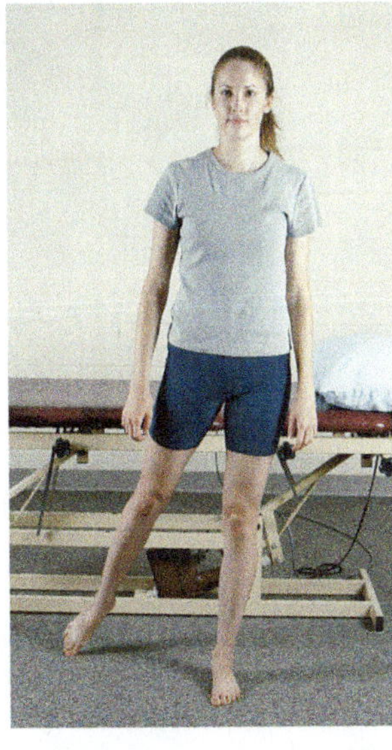

FIGURE 8–8 ■ Right lower extremity D1 extension with knee extension

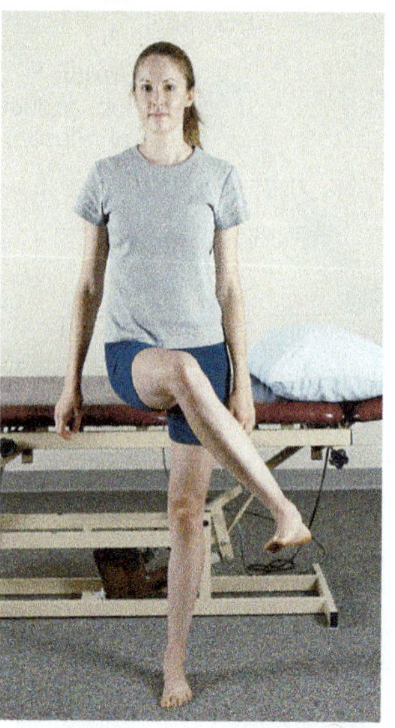

FIGURE 8–9 ■ Right lower extremity D1 flexion with knee flexion

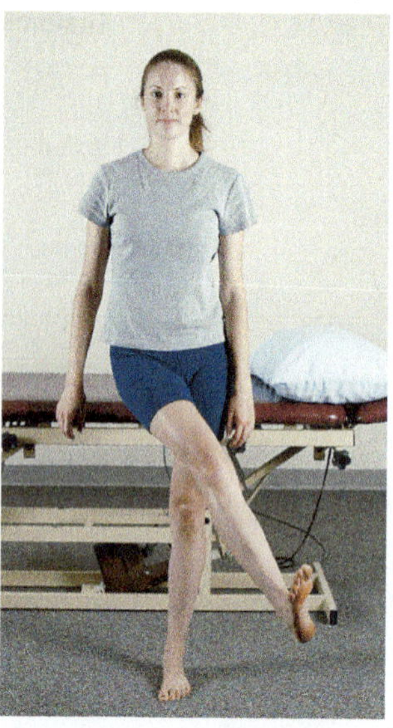

FIGURE 8–10 ■ Right lower extremity D1 flexion with knee extension

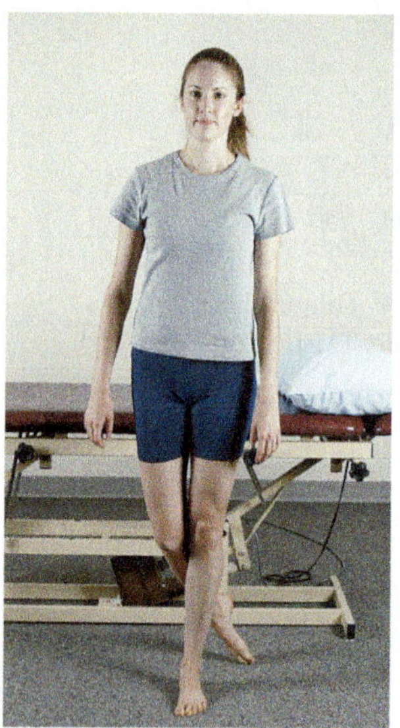

FIGURE 8–11 ■ Right lower extremity D2 extension with knee flexion

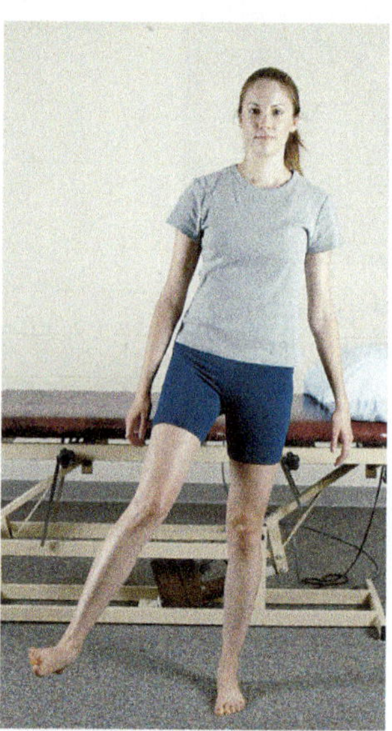

FIGURE 8–12 ■ Right lower extremity D2 flexion with knee extension

When combined components of motion are performed, joint movements and muscle lengthening may not occur through as much ROM as when anatomical planes of motion are performed. The mobility that is necessary for function, however, is maintained by use of diagonal patterns. Sensory feedback from movement in diagonal patterns is thought to be closer to the sensory feedback provided by normal active movement than movement in individual anatomical planes.

Table 8–2 ■ lists the combining components of motion defined as diagonal patterns.

Table 8–2 ■ Combining components of motion in PNF diagonals

	Diagonal 1 Upper Extremity			Diagonal 1 Lower Extremity	
Segment	**Flexion**	**Extension**	**Segment**	**Flexion**	**Extension**
Scapula	Elevation	Depression			
	Abduction	Adduction			
	Upward rotation	Downward rotation			
Shoulder	Flexion	Extension	Hip	Flexion	Extension
	Adduction	Abduction		Adduction	Abduction
	Lateral rotation	Medial rotation		Lateral rotation	Medial rotation
Elbow	Straight or flexion or extension	Straight or extension or flexion	Knee	Straight or flexion or extension	Straight or extension or flexion
Forearm	Supination	Pronation			
Wrist	Flexion	Extension	Ankle	Dorsiflexion	Plantar flexion
	Radial deviation	Ulnar deviation		Inversion	Eversion
Fingers	Flexion	Extension	Toes	Extension	Flexion
	Adduction	Abduction			
Thumb	Flexion	Extension			
	Diagonal 2 Upper Extremity			**Diagonal 2 Lower Extremity**	
Segment	**Flexion**	**Extension**	**Segment**	**Flexion**	**Extension**
Scapula	Elevation	Depression			
	Adduction	Abduction			
	Upward rotation	Downward rotation			
Shoulder	Flexion	Extension	Hip	Flexion	Extension
	Abduction	Adduction		Abduction	Adduction
	Lateral rotation	Medial rotation		Medial rotation	Lateral rotation
Elbow	Straight or flexion or extension	Straight or extension or flexion	Knee	Straight or flexion or extension	Straight or extension or flexion
Forearm	Supination	Pronation			
Wrist	Extension	Flexion	Ankle	Dorsiflexion	Plantar flexion
	Radial deviation	Ulnar deviation		Eversion	Inversion
Fingers	Extension	Flexion	Toes	Extension	Flexion
	Abduction	Adduction			
Thumb	Extension	Opposition			

Instructions

Illustrations in this chapter present ROM performed as passive ROM exercises. Presented are the joint(s) for which the exercise is being performed, joint motion, patient position, and hand placement of the physical therapist/assistant. Notes provide additional information about the exercise and its correct performance. For procedures specifically involving multijoint muscles, the multijoint muscles are listed. Movements required to *lengthen* multijoint muscles, *not* movements produced by the muscles, are presented.

■ Take Note

Before performing ROM, ensure that lines and tubes will not be compromised.

PROCEDURE 8–1 Lower Extremity ROM Exercises: Anatomical Planes

Joint Range of Motion

Joint(s):	Hip and knee
Motion:	Extension and flexion
Position:	Supine
Hand placement:	Heel and posterior knee
Notes:	Hip motion is complete when pelvic rotation starts to occur.
	Anterior pelvic rotation with hip extension, posterior pelvic rotation with hip flexion.
	Do not allow pelvic rotation to occur as hip motion is performed.

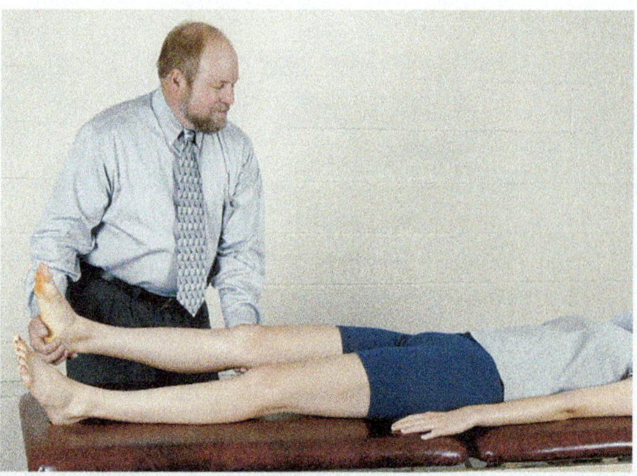

Hip and knee extension.

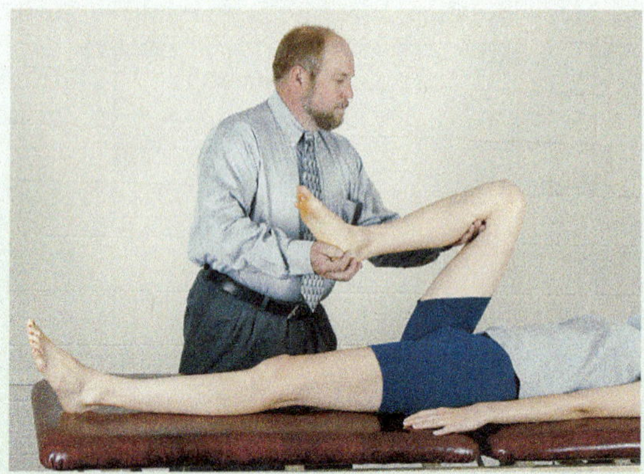

Hip and knee flexion.

Joint(s):	Hip
Motion:	Extension
Position:	Sidelying
Alternative Position:	Prone
Hand placement:	Place one hand on the pelvis for stabilization. The other hand and forearm support the patient's lower extremity in the anatomical position.
Notes:	Maintain the knee in extension. The end of hip extension is achieved when the pelvis starts to rotate anteriorly.

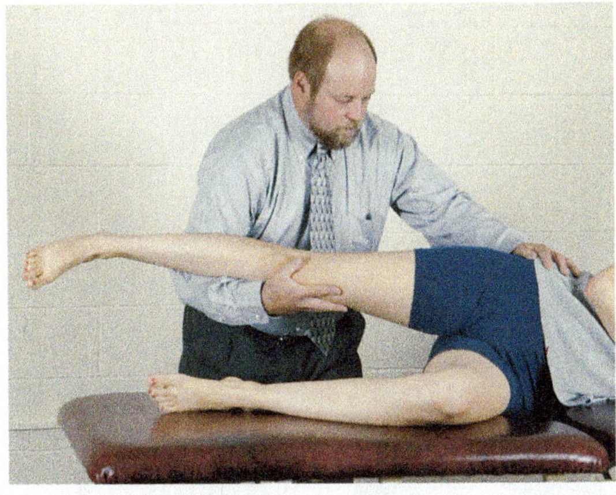

Hip extension in sidelying position.

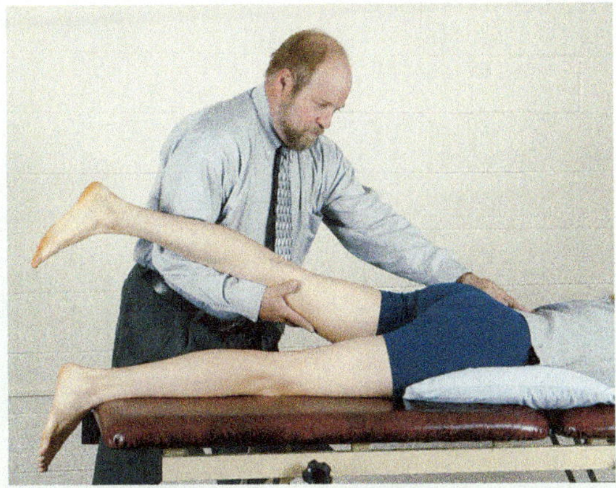

Hip extension in prone position.

(continued)

PROCEDURE 8–1 Lower Extremity ROM Exercises: Anatomical Planes (*continued*)

Joint(s):	Hip
Motions:	Abduction and adduction
Position:	Supine
Hand placement:	Heel and posterior knee
Notes:	To perform adduction beyond neutral, abduct the opposite lower extremity. Avoid hip flexion, hip rotation, and pelvic motion.

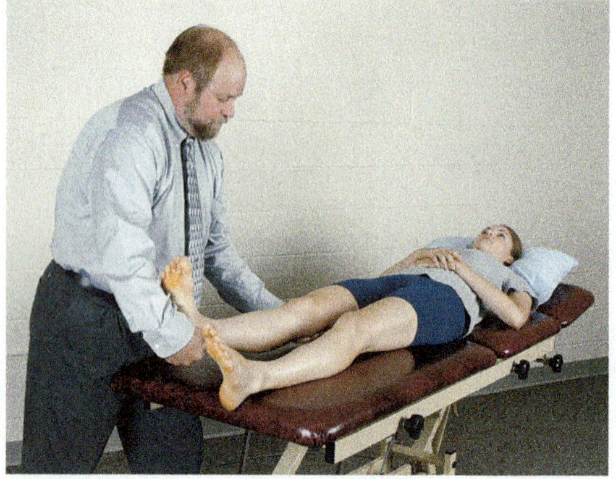
Starting position for hip abduction.

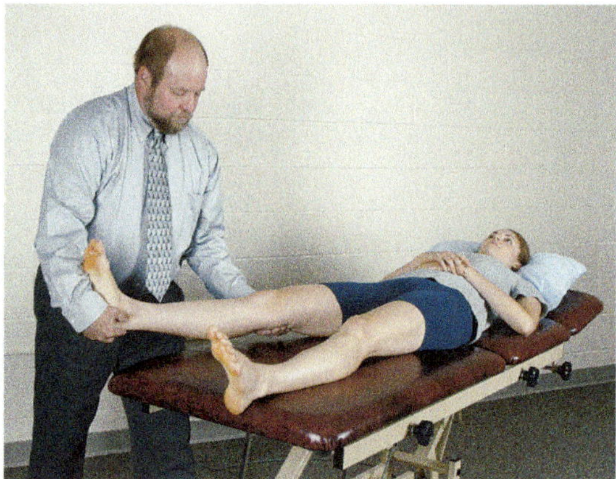
End position for hip abduction.

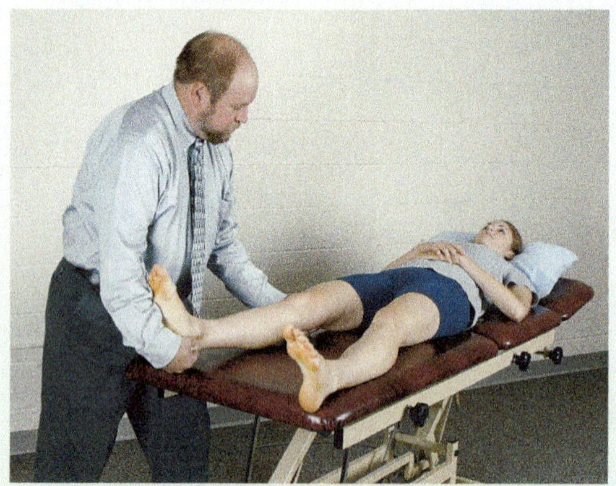
Starting position for hip adduction.

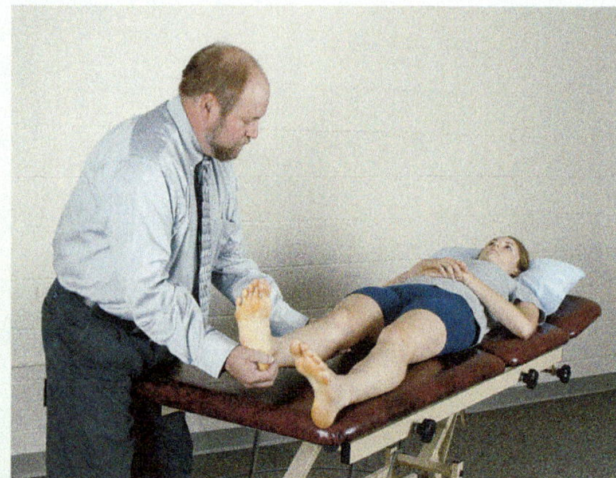
End position for hip adduction.

Joint(s):	Hip
Motions:	Medial and lateral rotation
Position:	Sitting
Hand placement:	One hand stabilizes the femur. The other hand grasps the distal leg.
Notes:	During medial rotation of the hip, the femur rotates medially causing the foot to move laterally. During lateral rotation of the hip, the femur rotates laterally causing the foot to moves medially.

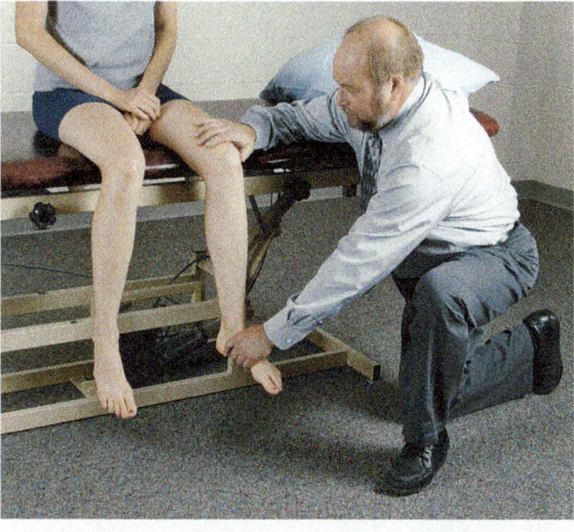

Starting position for hip medial rotation in sitting.

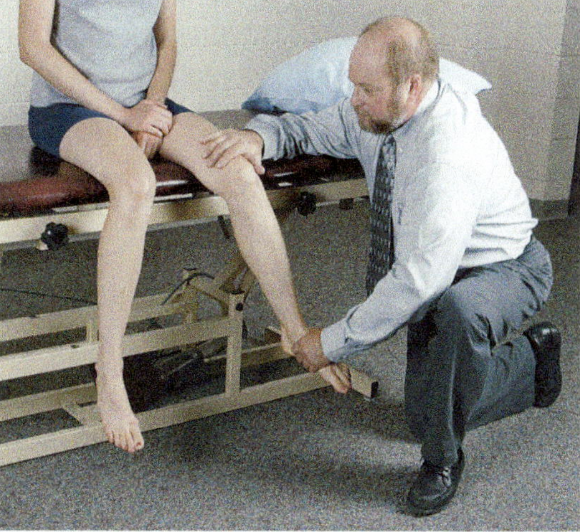

End position for hip medial rotation in sitting.

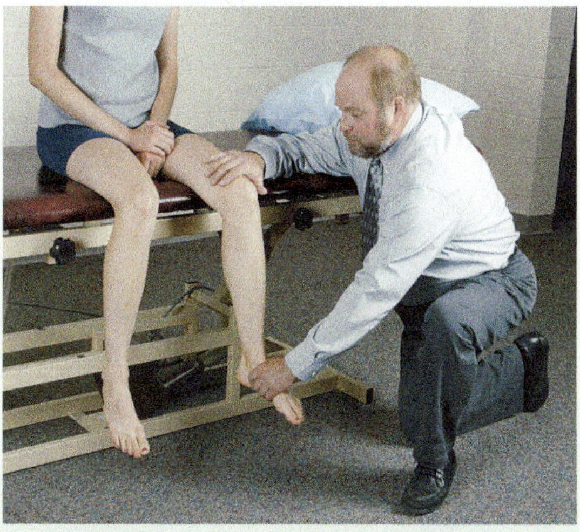

Starting position for hip lateral rotation in sitting.

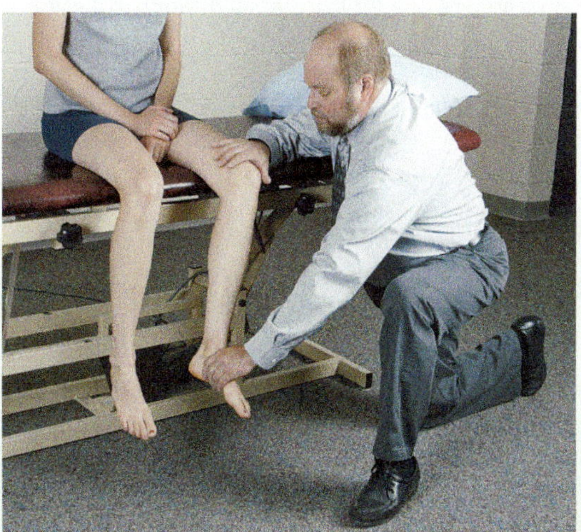

End position for hip lateral rotation in sitting.

(continued)

PROCEDURE 8–1 Lower Extremity ROM Exercises: Anatomical Planes (*continued*)

Joint(s):	Hip
Motions:	Medial and lateral rotation
Position:	Supine, with hip and knee flexed to 90 degrees
Hand placement:	Heel and anterior knee
Alternative placement:	Heel and posterior thigh
Notes:	Avoid excessive stress on the medial and lateral structures of the knee. Maintain the pelvis flat on the supporting surface.

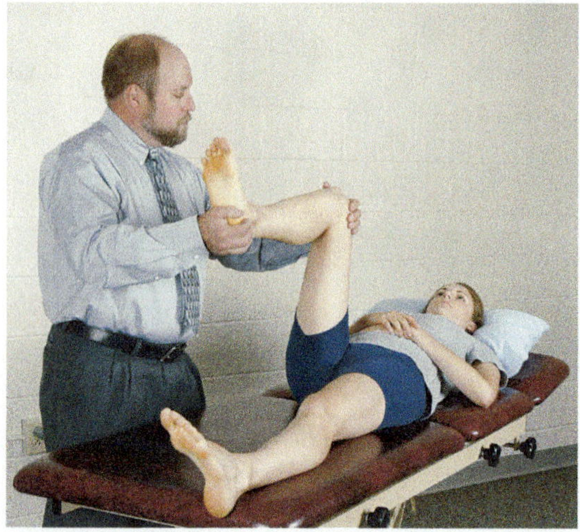

Starting position for hip medial rotation in supine with hip flexion.

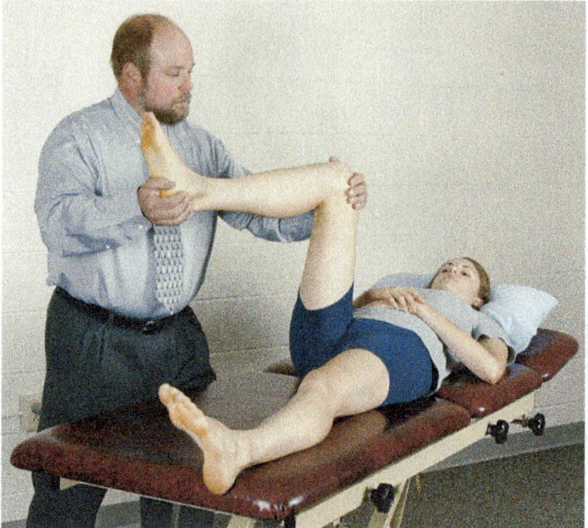

End position for hip medial rotation in supine with hip flexion.

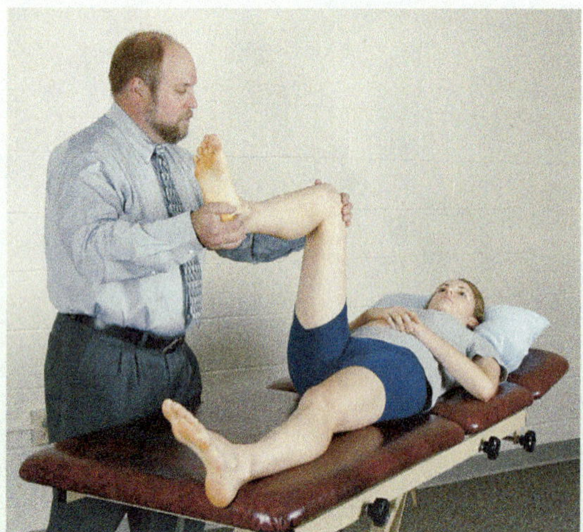

Starting position for hip lateral rotation in supine with hip flexion.

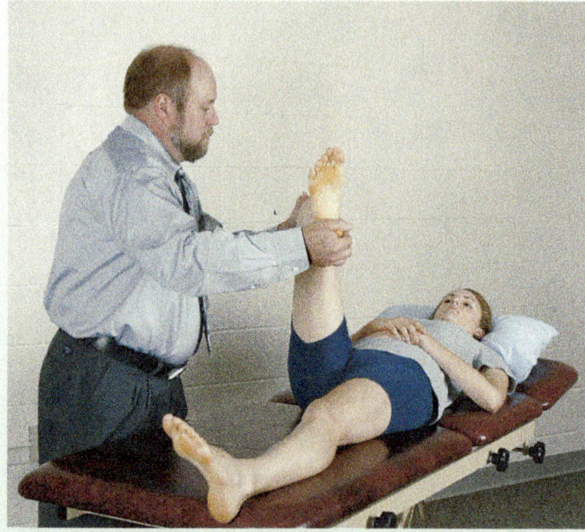

End position for hip lateral rotation in supine with hip flexion.

Joint(s):	Hip
Motions:	Medial and lateral rotation
Position:	Supine, with hip and knee extended
Hand placement:	Heel and posterior knee
Notes:	Avoid excessive stress on the medial and lateral structures of the knee. Maintain the pelvis flat on the supporting surface.

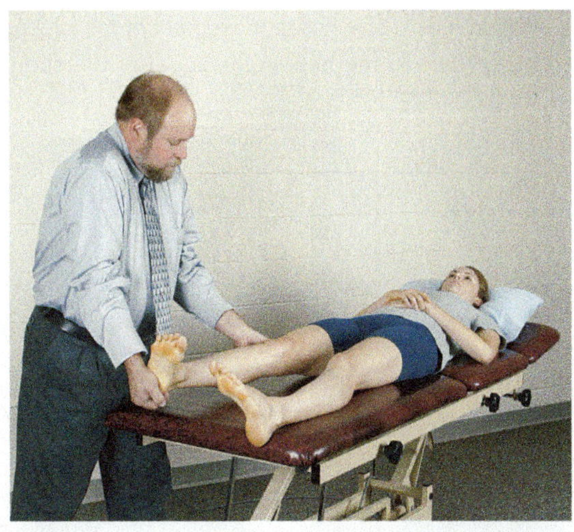

End position for hip medial rotation in supine with hip extended.

Joint(s):	Knee
Motion:	Flexion
Position:	Supine with hip flexed to 90 degrees
Hand placement:	Heel and distal femur

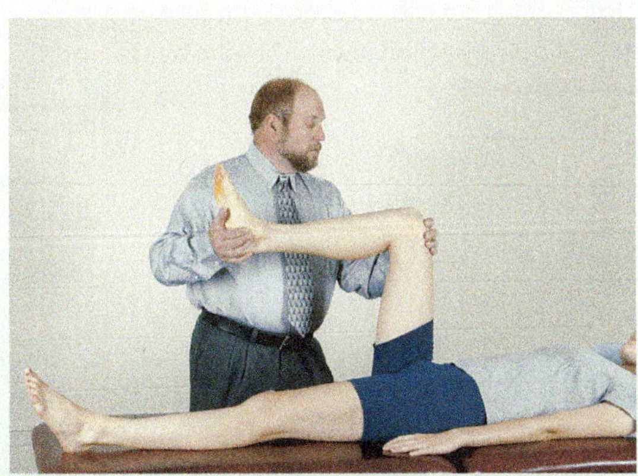

Midposition for knee flexion.

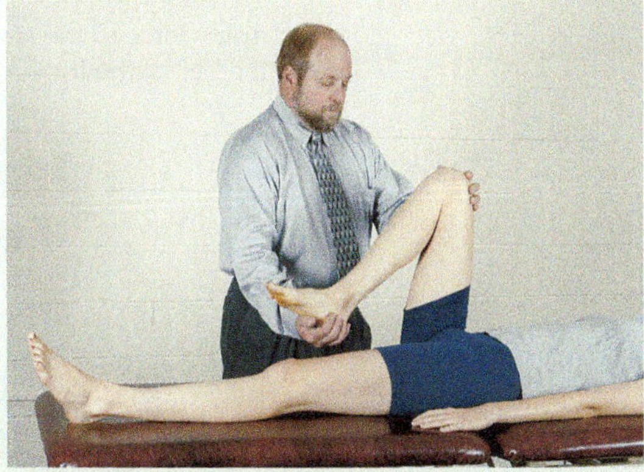

End position for knee flexion.

(continued)

PROCEDURE 8–1 Lower Extremity ROM Exercises: Anatomical Planes (*continued*)

Joint(s):	Ankle (talocrural)
Motion:	Plantar flexion
Position:	Supine
Hand placement:	Heel and dorsum of foot
Notes:	Motion should emphasize movement of the talocrural joint, not midfoot joints. Apply force to the heel in the superior direction (toward the head), not to the dorsum of the foot.

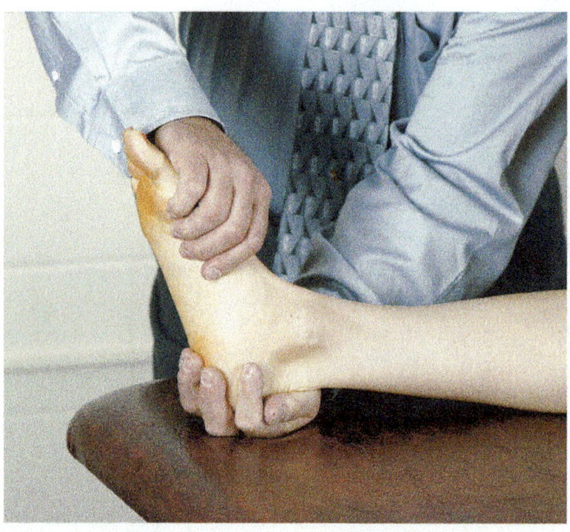

Starting position for ankle plantar flexion.

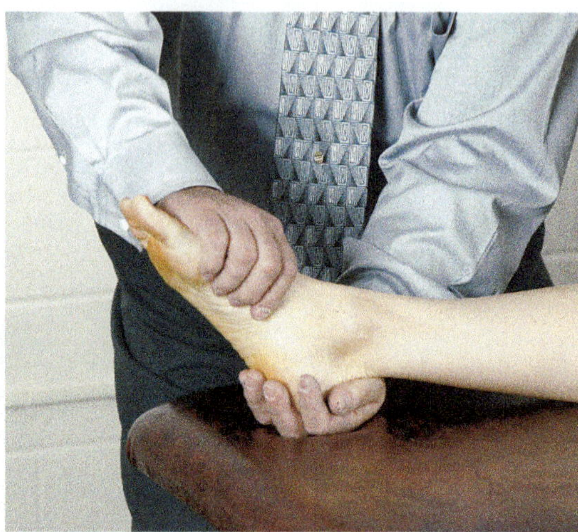

End position for ankle plantar flexion.

Joint(s):	Ankle (talocrural)
Motion:	Dorsiflexion
Position:	Supine with slight knee flexion
Hand placement:	Heel and posterior calf
Notes:	To move structures of the ankle joint and the one joint soleus muscle, flex the knee such that the gastrocnemius muscle does not limit motion. Apply force to the heel in the inferior direction (away from the head), not to the ball of the foot.

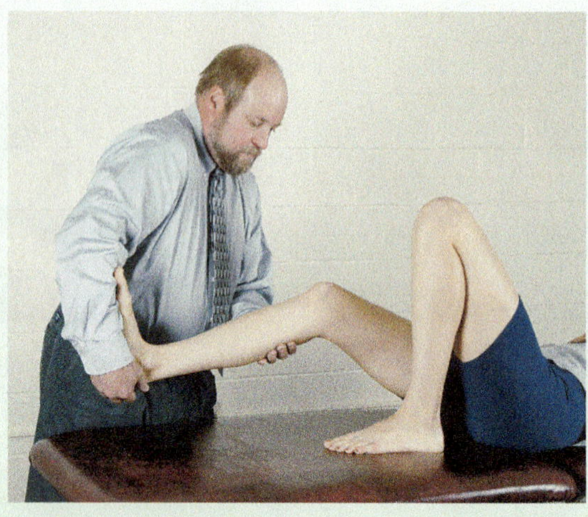

Position for ankle dorsiflexion.

Joint(s):	Foot (intertarsal)
Motions:	Inversion and eversion
Position:	Supine
Hand placement:	One hand grasps the heel to stabilize the leg. The other hand grasps the forefoot.

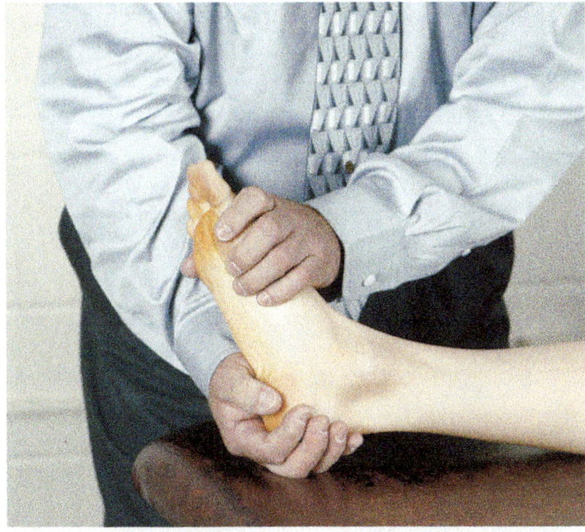
Starting position for foot inversion.

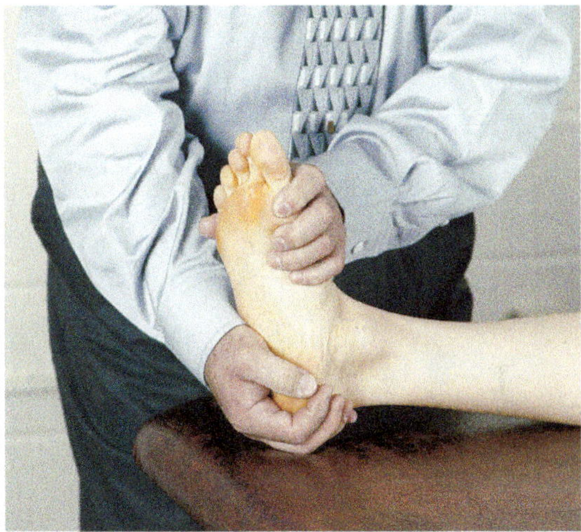
End position for foot inversion.

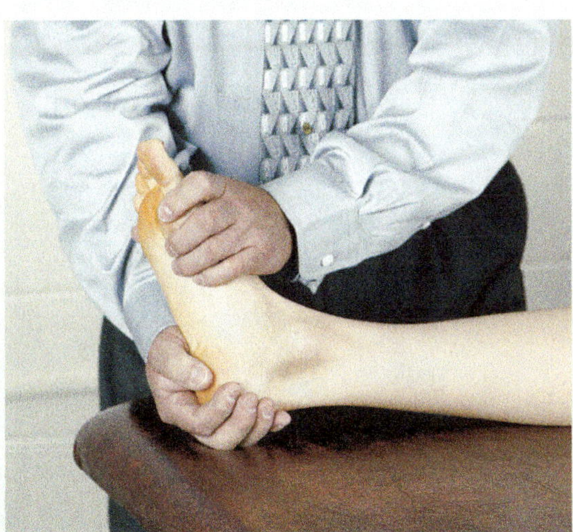
Starting position for foot eversion.

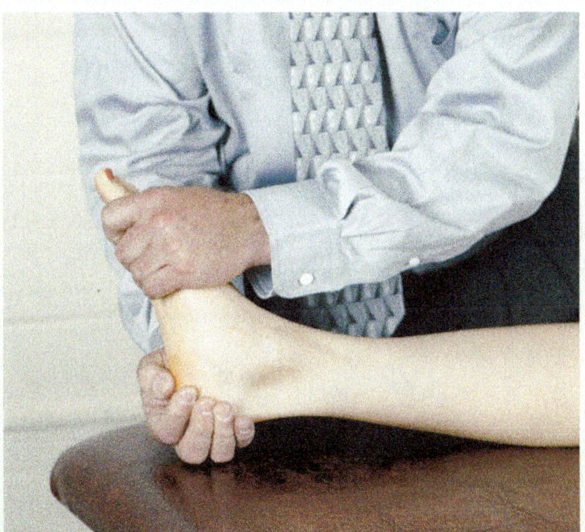
End position for foot eversion.

(continued)

PROCEDURE 8–1 Lower Extremity ROM Exercises: Anatomical Planes (*continued*)

Joint(s):	Toes (metatarsophalangeal and interphalangeal)
Motions:	Extension and flexion
Position:	Supine
Hand placement:	One hand stabilizes the foot and leg. The other hand moves the toes.

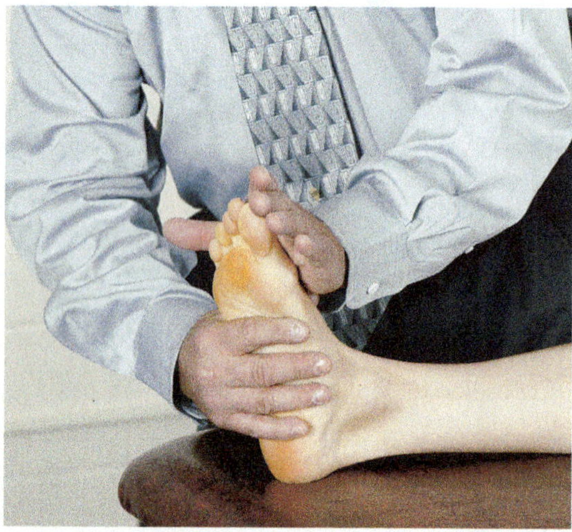

Starting position for toe flexion.

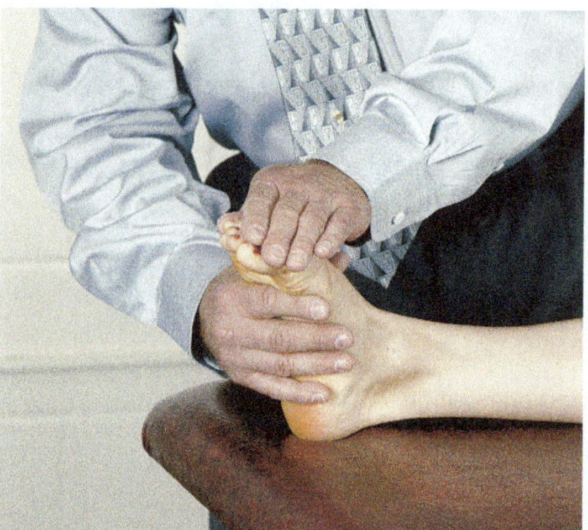

End position for toe flexion.

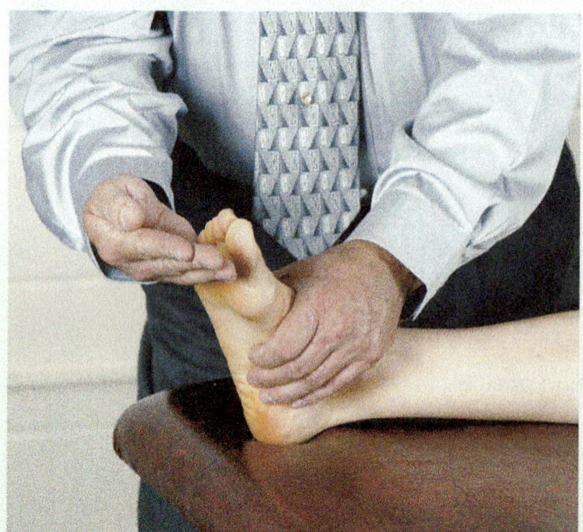

Starting position for toe extension.

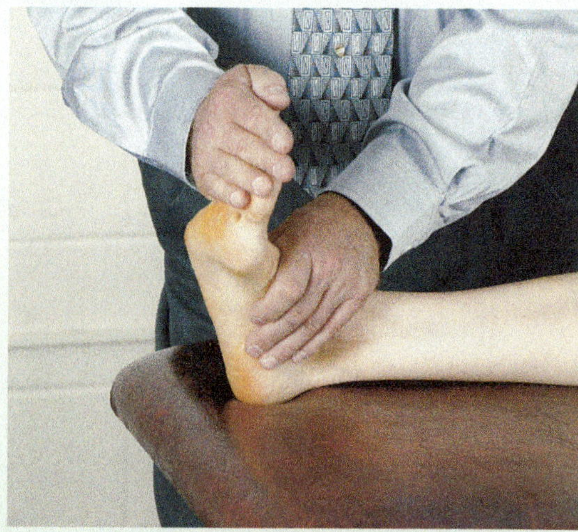

End position for toe extension.

Muscle Length

Joint(s):	Hip and knee
Muscles:	Semitendinosus, semimembranosus, biceps femoris
Motions:	Hip flexion with knee extension—straight leg raise (SLR)
Position:	Supine
Hand placement:	Heel and posterior knee
Notes:	This maneuver lengthens the multijoint muscles of the posterior thigh across both joints at which they act.
	Keep the knee extended.
	Do not allow the hip to rotate, adduct, or abduct. Do not allow the pelvis to rotate posteriorly.

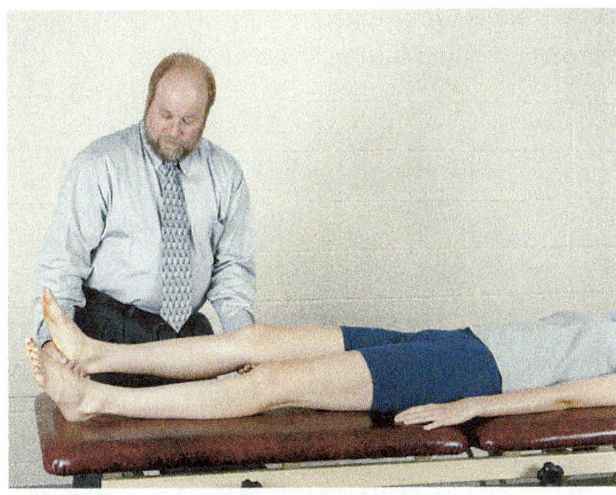

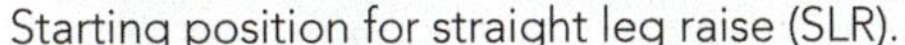
Starting position for straight leg raise (SLR).

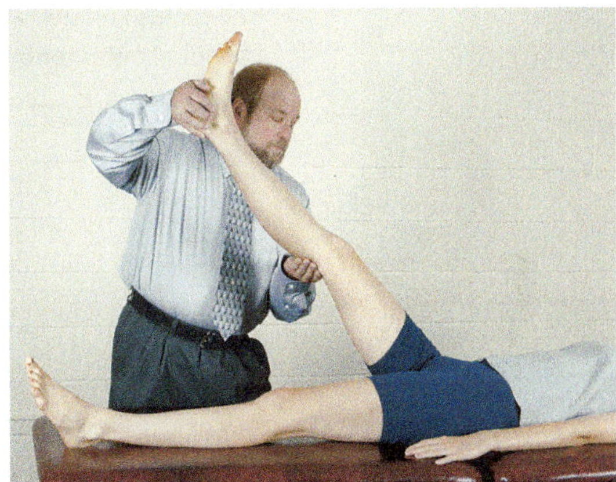

End position for hip flexion with knee extended (SLR).

Joint(s):	Hip
Muscle:	Tensor facia latae
Motions:	Extension and adduction
Position:	Sidelying
Hand placement:	One hand stabilizes the pelvis. The other hand and forearm support the leg.
Notes:	Do not substitute lateral pelvic motion for hip adduction motion.
	The tensor fascia latae flexes and abducts the hip and may assist in knee extension.
	Hip extension and adduction lengthen this muscle. There is controversy whether knee flexion lengthens this muscle.

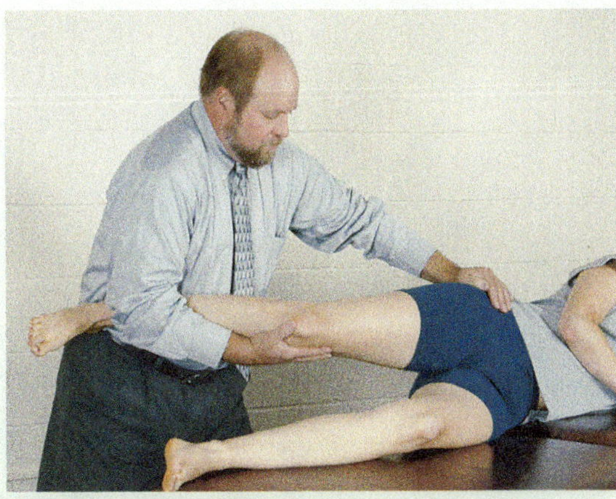

Starting position for tensor fascia latae lengthening.

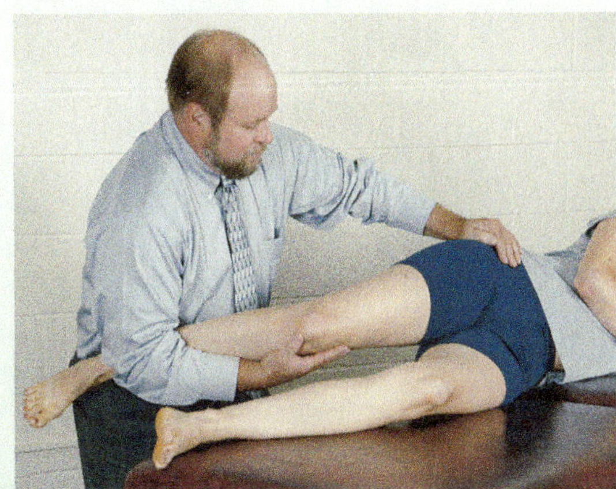

End position for tensor fascia latae lengthening.

(continued)

PROCEDURE 8–1 Lower Extremity ROM Exercises: Anatomical Planes (*continued*)

Joint(s):	Hip and knee
Muscle:	Rectus femoris
Motion:	Knee flexion with hip extended
Position:	Prone with hip extended
Alternative position:	Supine with knee at the end of the table
Hand placement:	One hand is on the posterior thigh or used to stabilize the pelvis. The other hand is on the distal tibia.
Notes:	The rectus femoris is a hip flexor and knee extensor. Do not allow anterior pelvic rotation or hip flexion to occur.

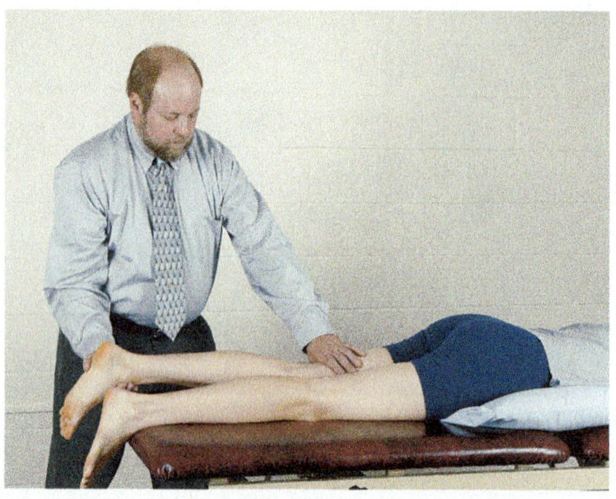

Starting position for rectus femoris range of motion.

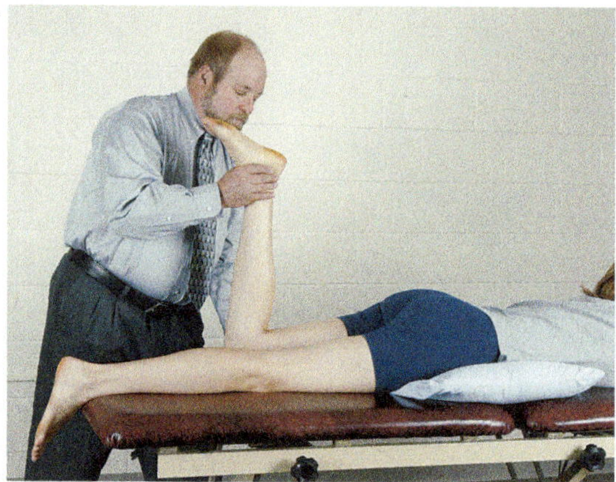

End position for rectus femoris range of motion.

Joint(s):	Ankle (talocrural)
Muscle:	Gastrocnemius
Position:	Supine with knee extended
Hand placement:	Heel and posterior leg
Notes:	To move the gastrocnemius muscle simultaneously across all joints over which it acts, keep the knee extended as the ankle is dorsiflexed. Apply force to the heel in an inferior direction (away from the head), not to the ball of the foot.

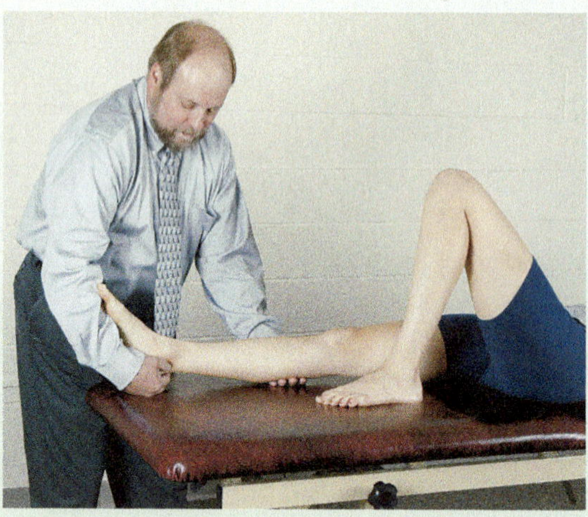

Starting position for gastrocnemius range of motion.

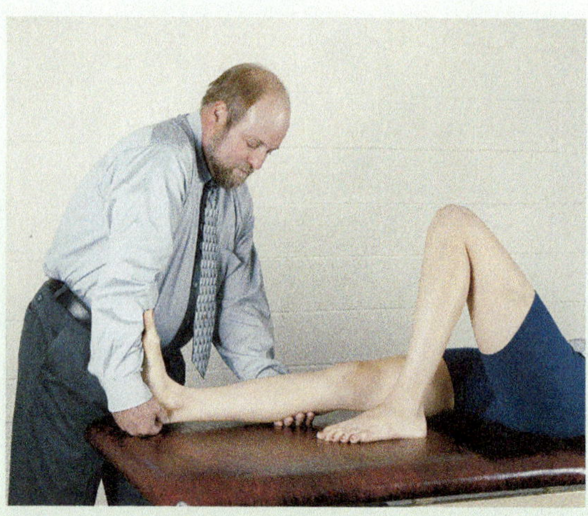

End position for gastrocnemius range of motion.

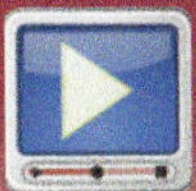

PROCEDURE 8–2 Lower Extremity ROM Exercises: PNF Diagonal Patterns

Pattern:
PNF diagonal 1 (D1) extension with knee extended
PNF diagonal 1 (D1) flexion with knee extended

Combining components of motion:

D1 extension with knee extended
- Hip: extension, abduction, medial rotation
- Knee: extended
- Ankle and foot: planar flexion, eversion

D1 flexion with knee extended
- Hip: flexion, adduction, lateral rotation
- Knee: extended
- Ankle and foot: dorsiflexion, inversion

Position: Supine

Hand placement: Heel and posterior thigh

Notes:
Knee extended (straight) indicates that the knee remains in complete extension throughout the movement of both patterns.

Not all motions of the foot and toes can be performed when the manual contact is on the patient's heel.

In PNF patterns, motion begins distally and progresses proximally, with the motions occurring more or less simultaneously.

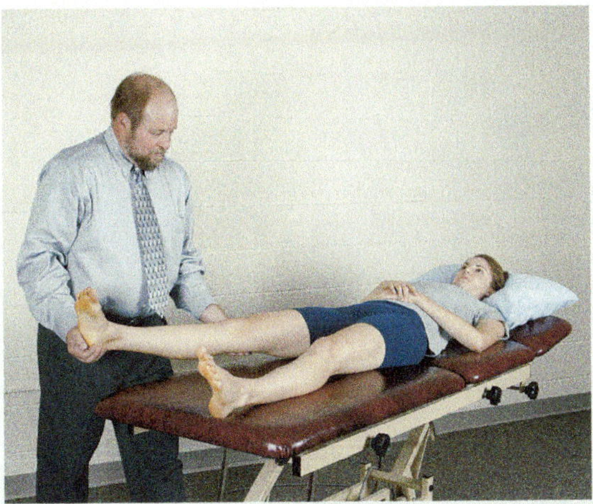

PNF D1 extension with knee extended.

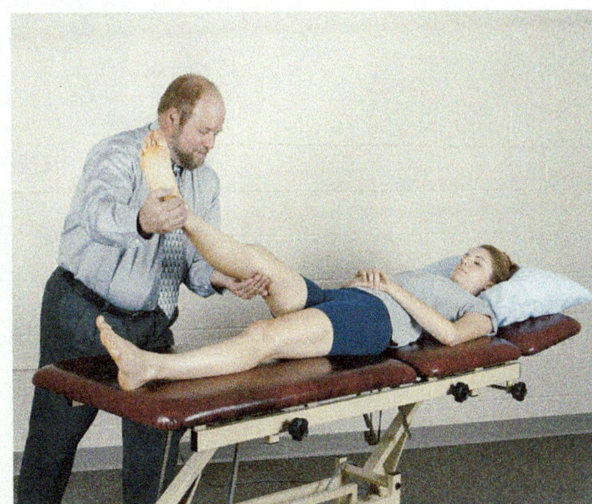

PNF D1 flexion with knee extended.

(continued)

PROCEDURE 8–2 Lower Extremity ROM Exercises: PNF Diagonal Patterns (*continued*)

Pattern:	PNF diagonal 1 (D1) extension with knee extension PNF diagonal 1 (D1) flexion with knee flexion
Combining components of motion:	D1 extension with knee extension Hip: extension, abduction, medial rotation Knee: extension Ankle and foot: plantar flexion, eversion D1 flexion with knee flexion Hip: flexion, adduction, lateral rotation Knee: flexion Ankle and foot: dorsiflexion, inversion
Position:	Supine
Hand placement:	Heel and posterior thigh
Notes:	Not all motions of the foot and toes can be performed when the manual contact is on the patient's heel. In PNF patterns, motion begins distally and progresses proximally, with the motions occurring more or less simultaneously.

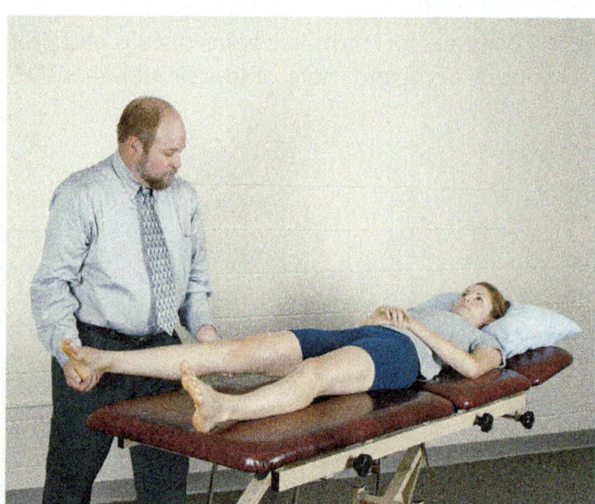

PNF D1 extension with knee extension.

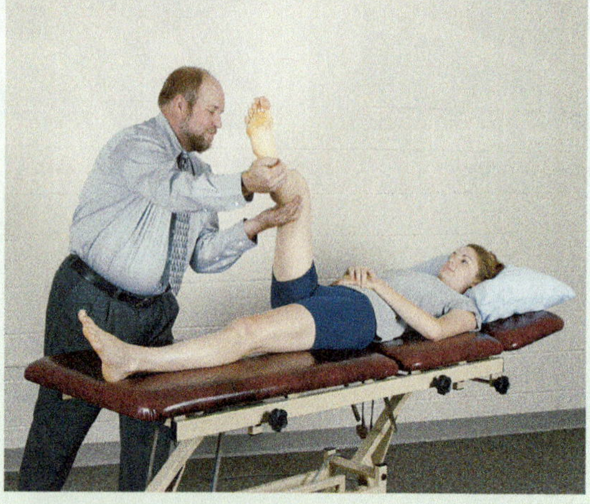

PNF D1 flexion with knee flexion.

Pattern:	PNF diagonal 1 (D1) extension with knee flexion PNF diagonal 1 (D1) flexion with knee extension
Combining components of motion:	D1 extension with knee flexion Hip: extension, abduction, medial rotation Knee: flexion Ankle and foot: plantar flexion, eversion D1 flexion with knee extension Hip: flexion, adduction, lateral rotation Knee: extension Ankle and foot: dorsiflexion, inversion
Position:	Supine
Hand placement:	Heel and posterior thigh
Notes:	Not all motions of the foot and toes can be performed when the manual contact is on the patient's heel. In PNF patterns, motion begins distally and progresses proximally, with the motions occurring more or less simultaneously.

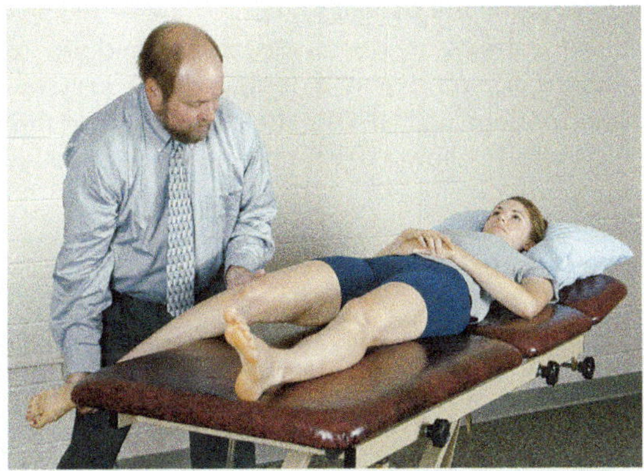

PNF D1 extension with knee flexion.

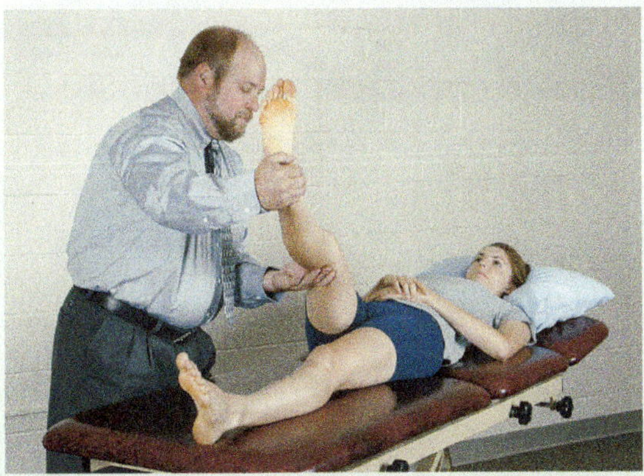

PNF D1 flexion with knee extension.

(continued)

PROCEDURE 8–2 Lower Extremity ROM Exercises: PNF Diagonal Patterns (*continued*)

Pattern:	PNF diagonal 2 (D2) extension with knee extended PNF diagonal 2 (D2) flexion with knee extended
Combining components of motion:	D2 extension with knee extended Hip: extension, adduction, lateral rotation Knee: extended Ankle and foot: plantar flexion, inversion D2 flexion with knee extended Hip: flexion, abduction, medial rotation Knee: extended Ankle and foot: dorsiflexion, eversion
Position:	Supine
Hand placement:	Heel and posterior thigh
Notes:	Knee extended indicates that the knee remains in complete extension throughout the movement of both patterns. Not all motions of the foot and toes can be performed when the manual contact is on the patient's heel. In PNF patterns, motion begins distally and progresses proximally, with the motions occurring more or less simultaneously. When performing PNF D2 patterns, the physical therapist/assistant must step and move to allow a patient's leg to move through the pattern completely and correctly.

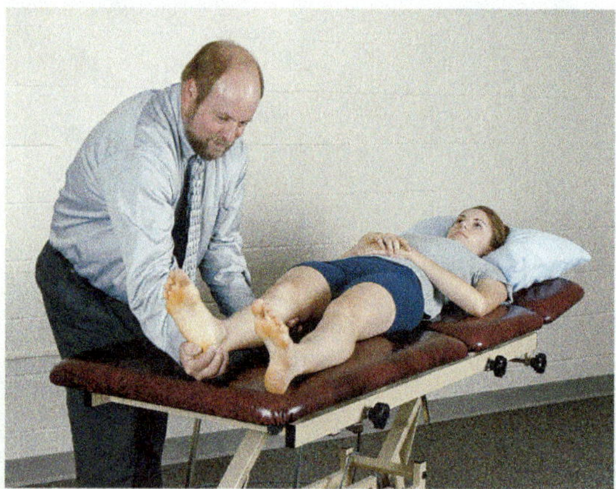

PNF D2 extension with knee extended.

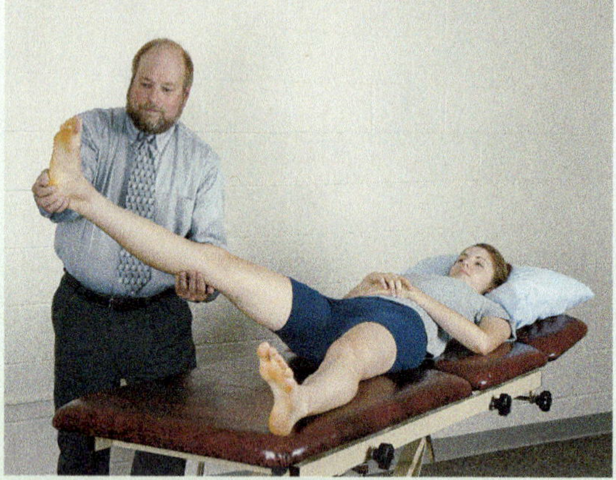

PNF D2 flexion with knee extended.

Pattern:	PNF diagonal 2 (D2) extension with knee extension PNF diagonal 2 (D2) flexion with knee flexion
Combining components of motion:	D2 extension with knee extension Hip: extension, adduction, lateral rotation Knee: extension Ankle and foot: plantar flexion, inversion D2 flexion with knee flexion Hip: flexion, abduction, medial rotation Knee: flexion Ankle and foot: dorsiflexion, eversion
Position:	Supine
Hand placement:	Heel and posterior thigh
Notes:	Not all motions of the foot and toes can be performed when the manual contact is on the patient's heel. In PNF patterns, motion begins distally and progresses proximally, with the motions occurring more or less simultaneously. When performing PNF D2 patterns, the physical therapist/assistant must step and move to allow a patient's leg to move through the pattern completely and correctly.

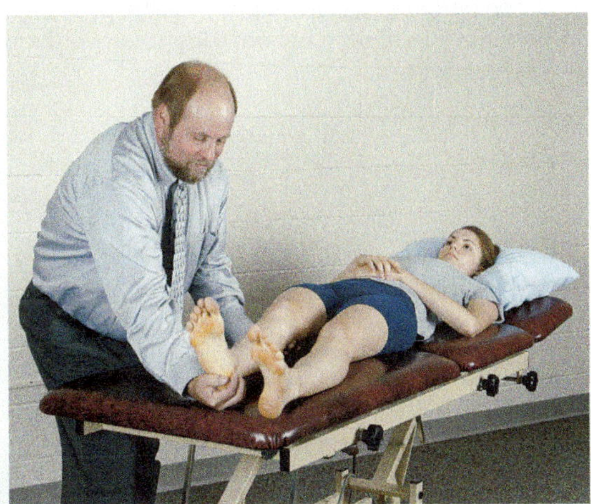

PNF D2 extension with knee extension.

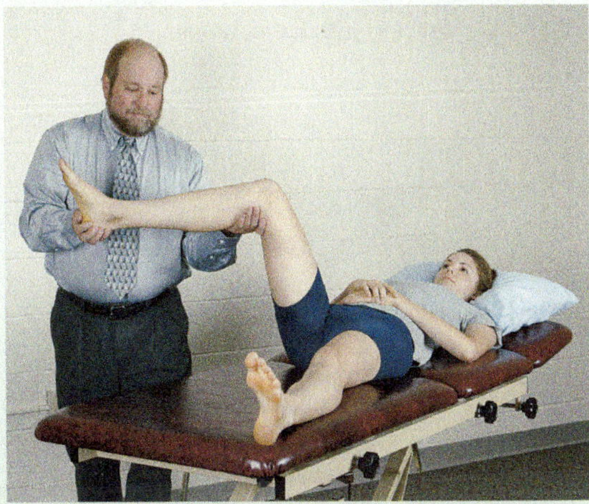

PNF D2 flexion with knee flexion.

(continued)

PROCEDURE 8–2 Lower Extremity ROM Exercises: PNF Diagonal Patterns (*continued*)

Pattern: PNF diagonal 2 (D2) extension with knee flexion
PNF diagonal 2 (D2) flexion with knee extension

Combining components of motion:

D2 extension with knee flexion
- Hip: extension, adduction, lateral rotation
- Knee: flexion
- Ankle and foot: plantar flexion, inversion

D2 flexion with knee extension
- Hip: flexion, abduction, medial rotation
- Knee: extension
- Ankle and foot: dorsiflexion, eversion

Position: Supine, knee flexed over end of the table

Hand placement: Heel and posterior thigh

Notes: Not all motions of the foot and toes can be performed when the manual contact is on the patient's heel.

In these patterns, motion begins distally and progresses proximally, with the motions occurring more or less simultaneously.

When performing PNF D2 patterns, the physical therapist/assistant must step and move to allow a patient's leg to move through the pattern completely and correctly.

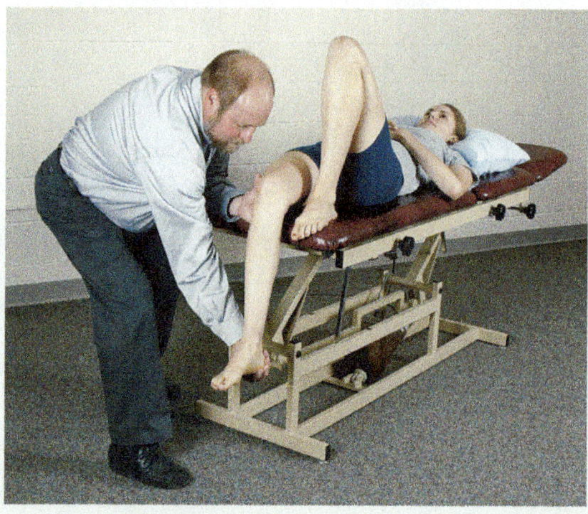

PNF D2 extension with knee flexion.

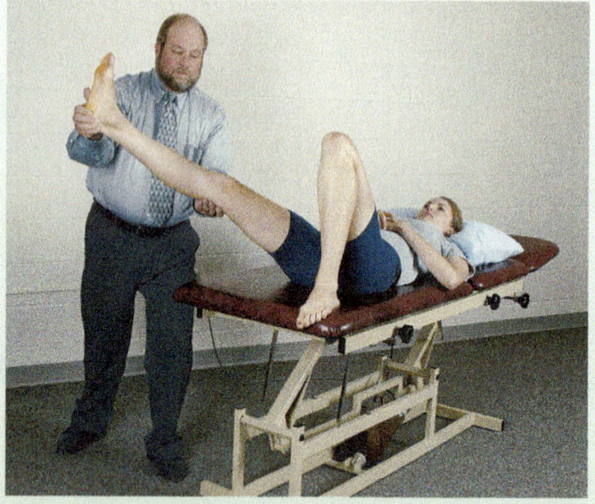

PNF D2 flexion with knee extension.

PROCEDURE 8–3 Upper Extremity ROM Exercises: Anatomical Planes

Joint(s):	Shoulder girdle (scapulothoracic)
Motions:	Protraction (abduction) and retraction (adduction) Elevation and depression Upward and downward rotation
Position:	Sidelying
Hand placement:	Place one hand over the acromion process and the other hand at the inferior angle of the scapula.
Notes:	The hand placement for each of the three pairs of motion is the same. There is a difference in the direction of force applied to the scapula.

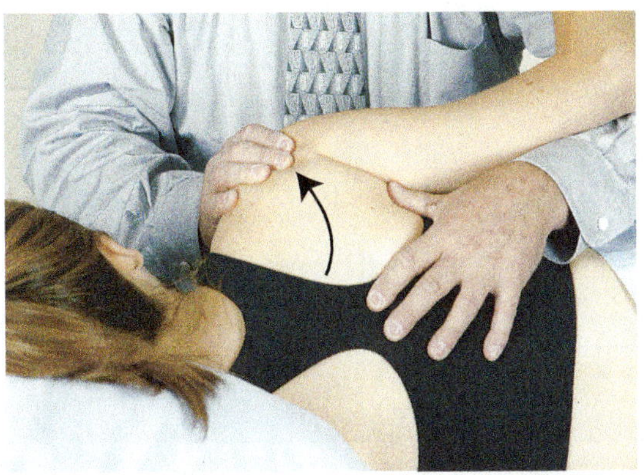

Scapular protraction (abduction).

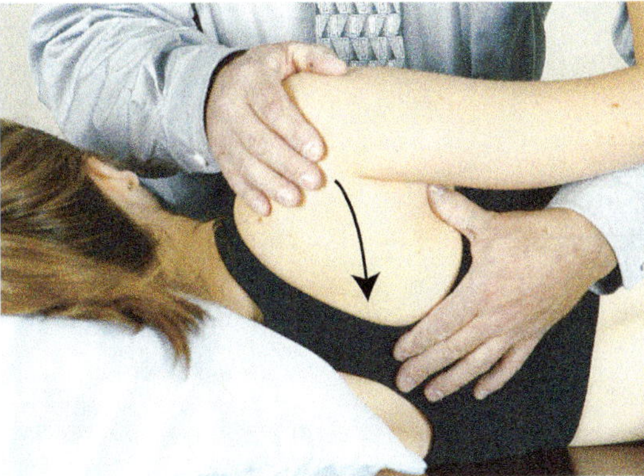

Scapular retraction (adduction).

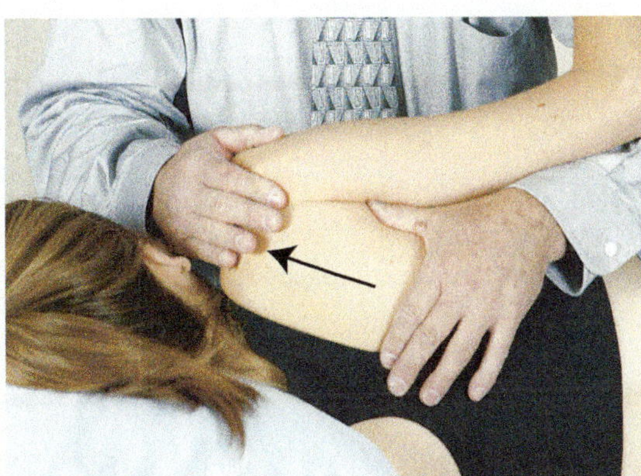

Scapular elevation.

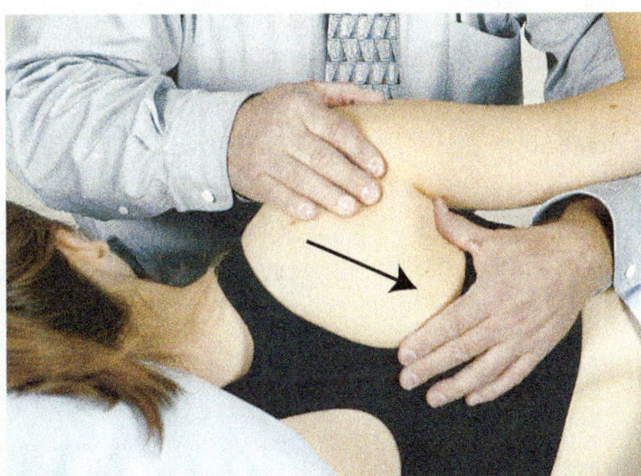

Scapular depression.

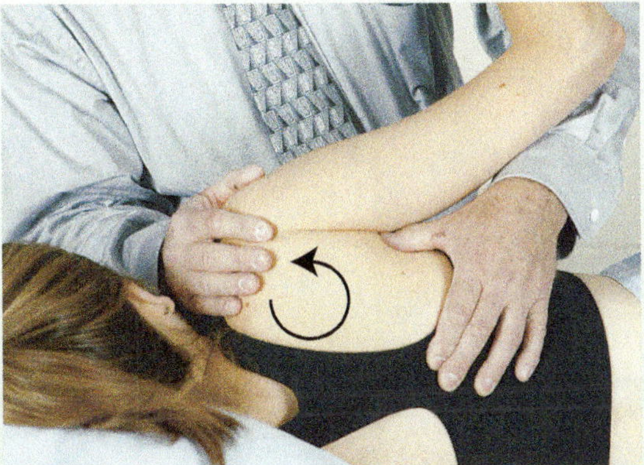

Scapular upward rotation.

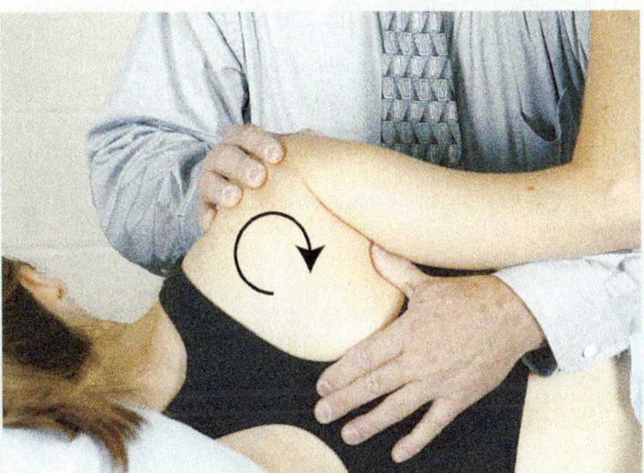

Scapular downward rotation.

(continued)

PROCEDURE 8–3 Upper Extremity ROM Exercises: Anatomical Planes (*continued*)

Joint(s):	Shoulder (glenohumeral)
Motion:	Flexion
Position:	Supine
Hand placement:	One hand supports the arm. The other hand grasps the wrist and hand. Hand placement may need to shift as movement occurs through full flexion.
Note:	Permit lateral rotation to avoid impingement.

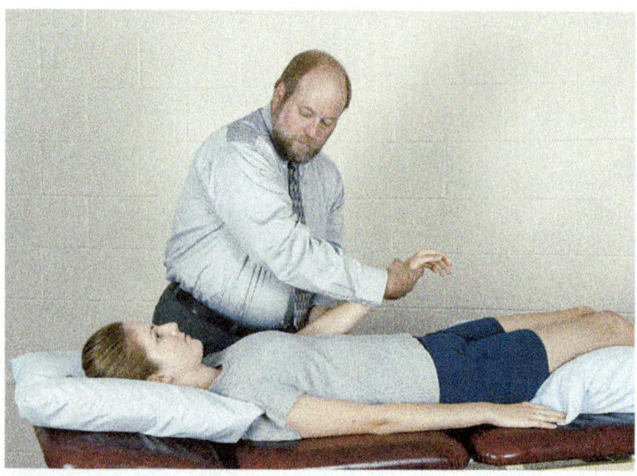

Beginning shoulder flexion.

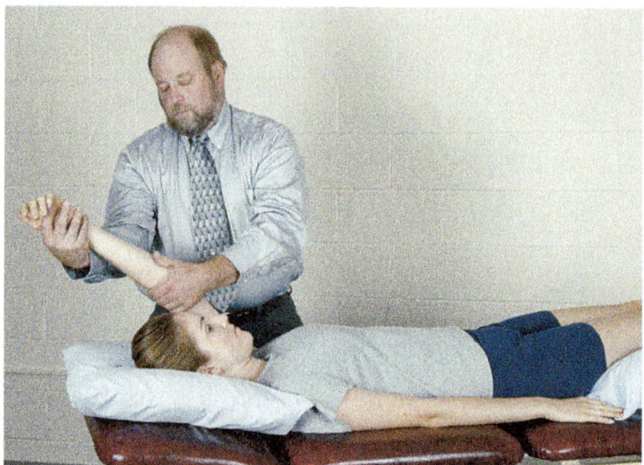

Ending shoulder flexion.

Joint(s):	Shoulder (glenohumeral)
Motion:	Extension
Position:	Sidelying
Alternative position:	Prone
Hand placement:	One hand supports the arm. The other hand supports the wrist and forearm.
Note:	When the end of the range of shoulder extension is reached, shoulder girdle motion will occur.

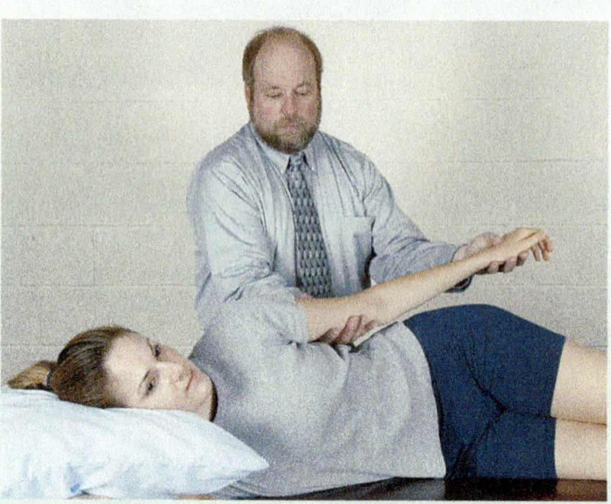

Beginning shoulder extension.

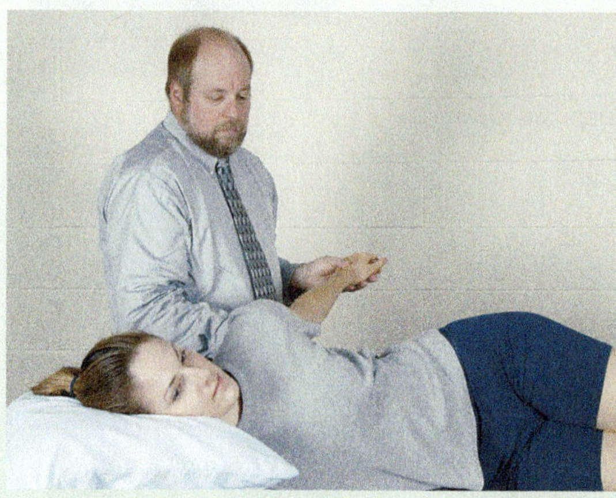

Ending shoulder extension.

Joint(s):	Shoulder (glenohumeral)
Motion:	Abduction
Position:	Supine
Hand placement:	One hand supports the arm. The other hand grasps the wrist and forearm.
Notes:	Avoid shoulder flexion and medial rotation during shoulder abduction. Permit lateral rotation to avoid impingement. The physical therapist/assistant must move to allow movement through complete range of motion.

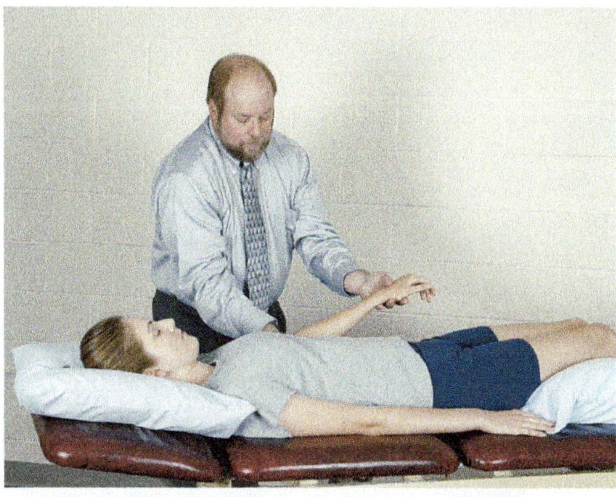

Beginning shoulder abduction.

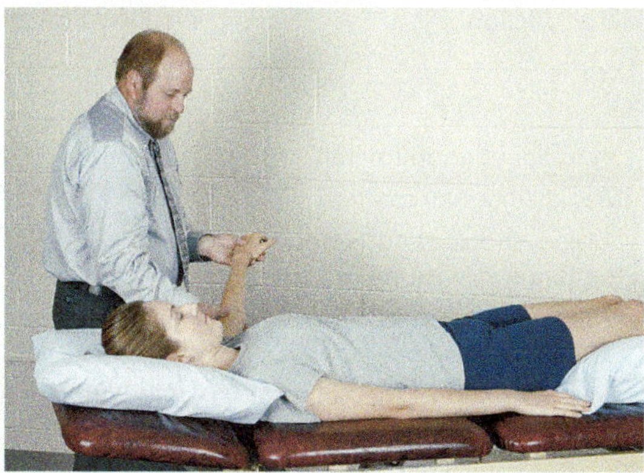

Midpoint of shoulder abduction.

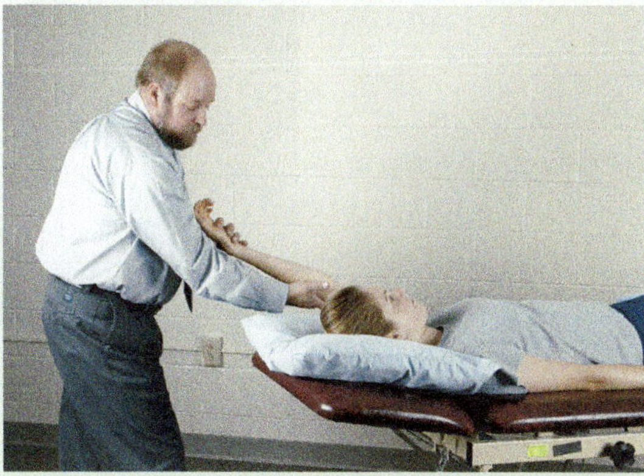

Ending shoulder abduction.

(continued)

PROCEDURE 8–3 Upper Extremity ROM Exercises: Anatomical Planes (*continued*)

Joint(s):	Shoulder (glenohumeral)
Motion:	Horizontal adduction
Position:	Supine, shoulder abducted to 90 degrees and elbow flexed to 90 degrees
Hand placement:	One hand supports the arm. The other hand grasps the wrist and hand.

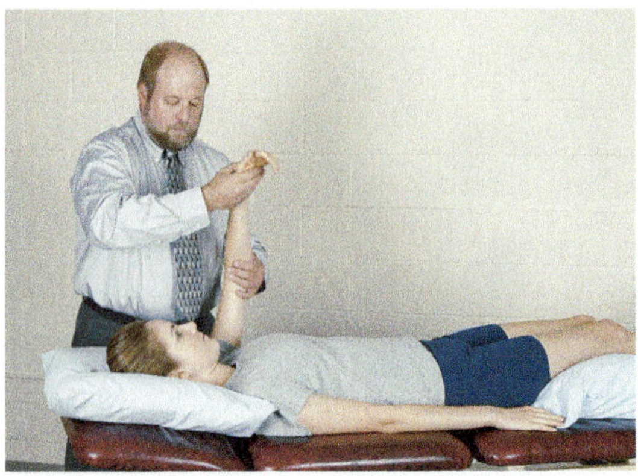
Midpoint of shoulder horizontal adduction.

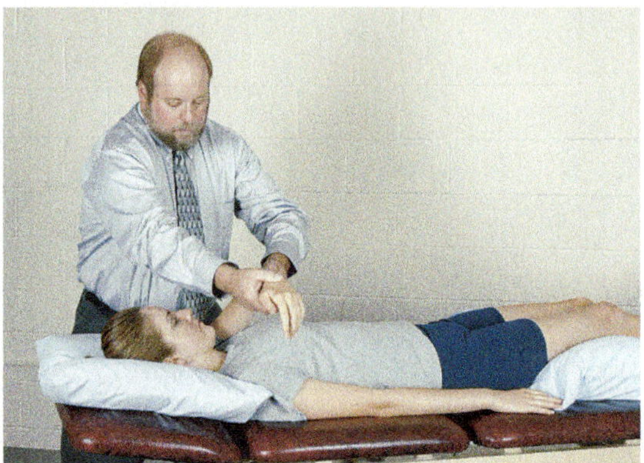
Ending shoulder horizontal adduction.

Joint(s):	Shoulder (glenohumeral)
Motion:	Medial (internal) rotation
Position:	Supine, shoulder abducted to 90 degrees, elbow flexed to 90 degrees, and the forearm in pronation
Hand placement:	One hand supports the arm. The other hand grasps the patient's wrist and forearm.
Note:	When the end of medial rotation ROM is reached, the shoulder girdle will start to move.

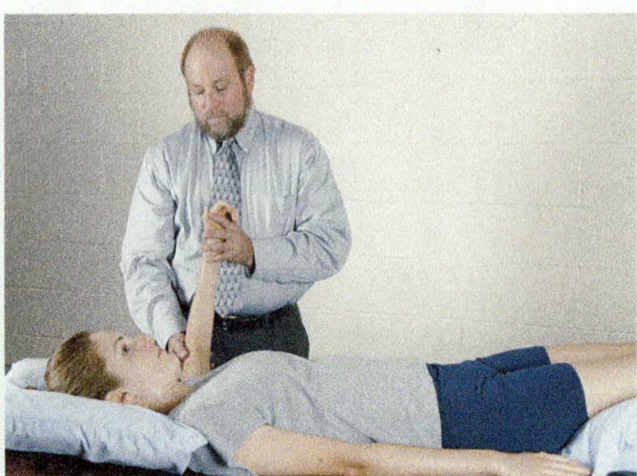
Starting position for shoulder medial rotation.

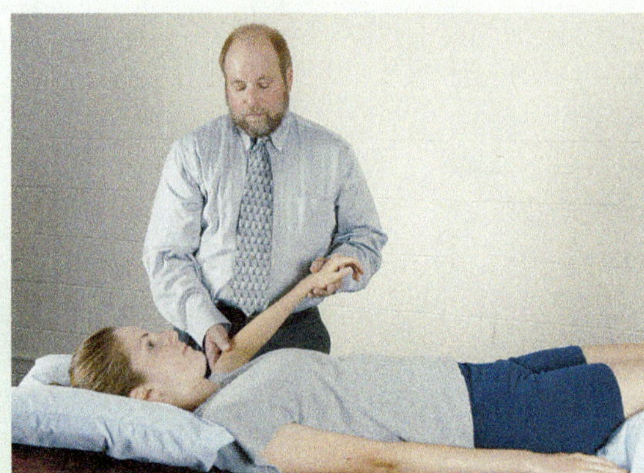
End position for shoulder medial rotation.

Joint(s):	Shoulder (glenohumeral)
Motion:	Lateral (external) rotation
Position:	Supine, shoulder abducted to 90 degrees, elbow flexed to 90 degrees, and forearm pronated
Hand placement:	One hand supports the arm. The other hand grasps the patient's wrist and hand.
Notes:	When the end of the range of lateral rotation is reached, the shoulder girdle will start to move into retraction. The patient may also extend the trunk when motion is limited.

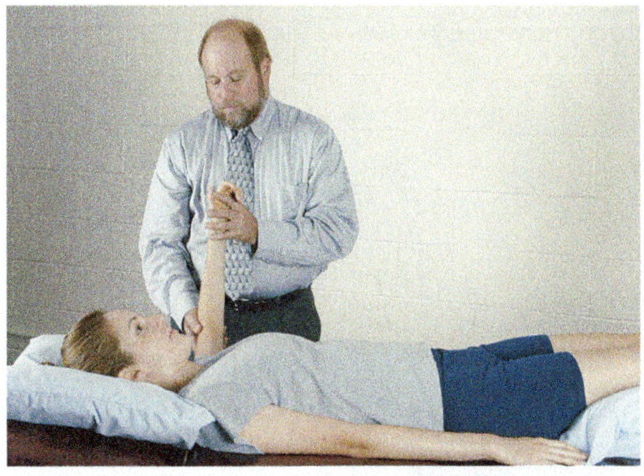

Starting position for shoulder lateral rotation.

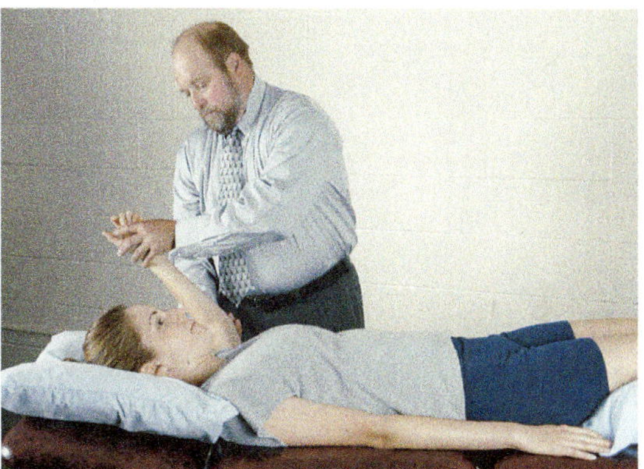

End position for shoulder lateral rotation.

Joint(s):	Elbow
Motions:	Flexion and extension
Position:	Supine, forearm supinated
Hand placement:	One hand supports the arm. The other hand grasps the patient's wrist and hand.
Note:	In this photograph, the shoulder is slightly flexed to allow visualization of the elbow.

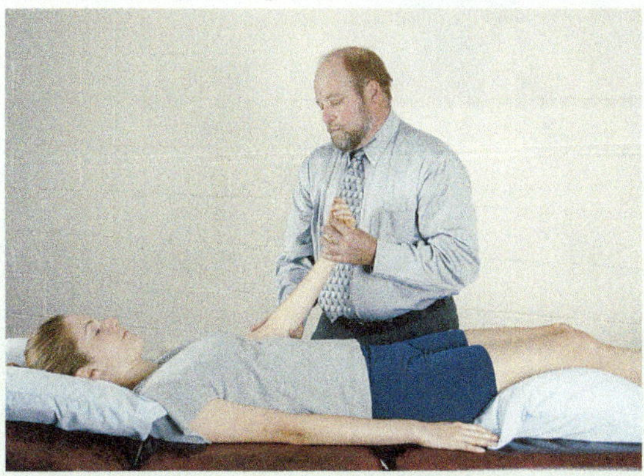

Elbow extension.

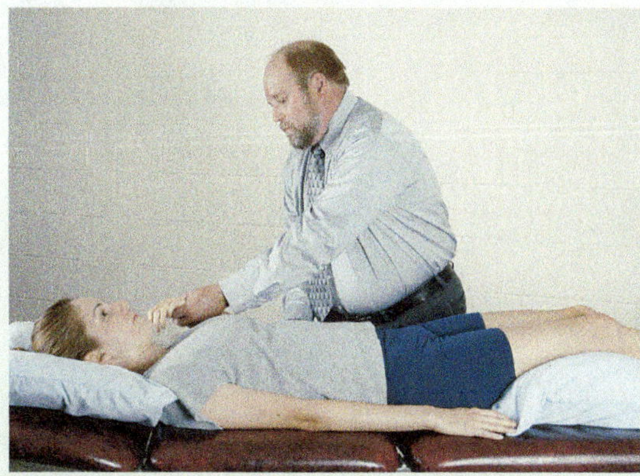

Elbow flexion.

(continued)

PROCEDURE 8–3 Upper Extremity ROM Exercises: Anatomical Planes (*continued*)

Joint(s):	Forearm (radioulnar)
Motions:	Pronation and supination
Position:	Supine, elbow flexed to 90 degrees
Alternative position:	Sitting
Hand placement:	One hand stabilizes the arm. The other hand grasps the distal forearm and supports the hand.
Notes:	This motion occurs in the forearm. Do not apply the force through the wrist by grasping the hand instead of the forearm.

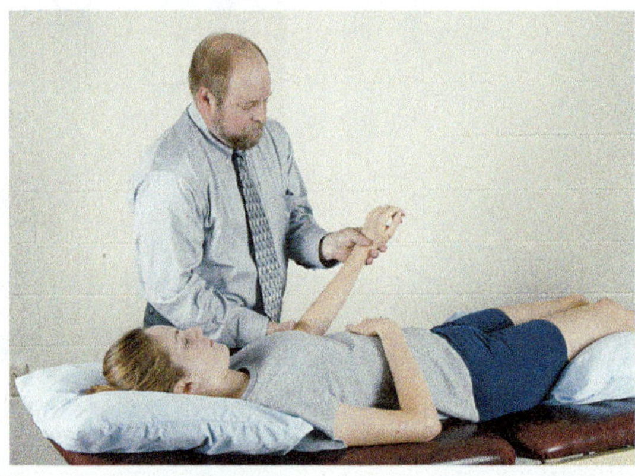

Forearm pronation.

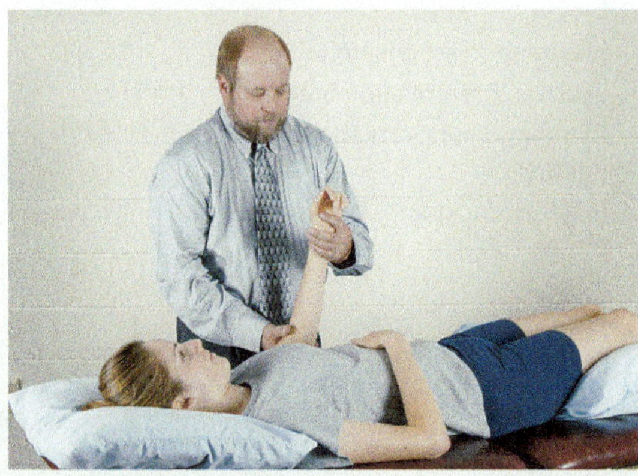

Midposition (neutral) of forearm.

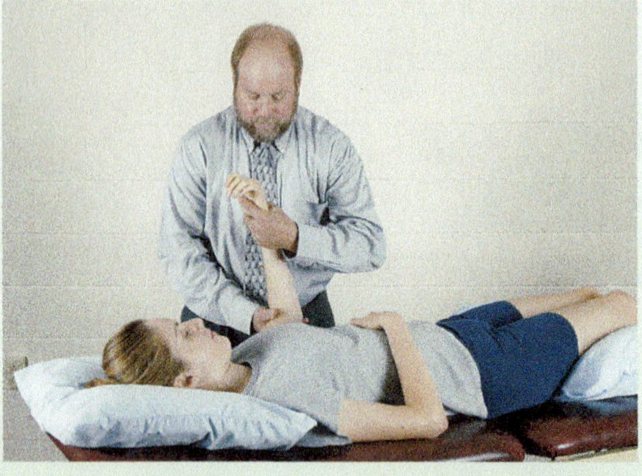

Forearm supination.

Joint(s):	Wrist (radiocarpal and intercarpal)
Motions:	Flexion and extension—finger motion is permitted
Position:	Supine, elbow flexed, and fingers free to move
Alternative position:	Sitting
Hand placement:	One hand stabilizes the arm and forearm. The other hand grasps the patient's hand.

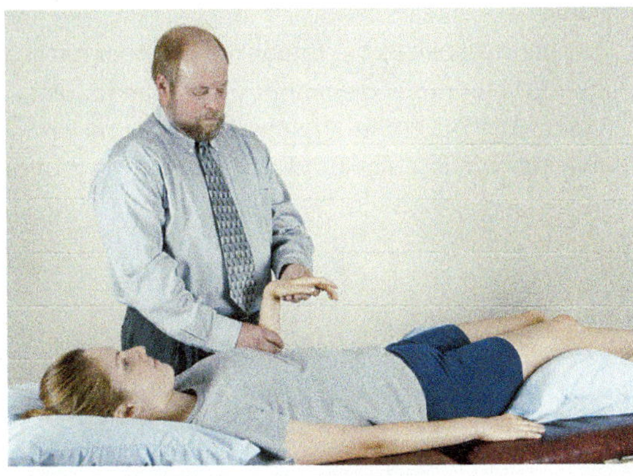

Wrist flexion fingers relaxed.

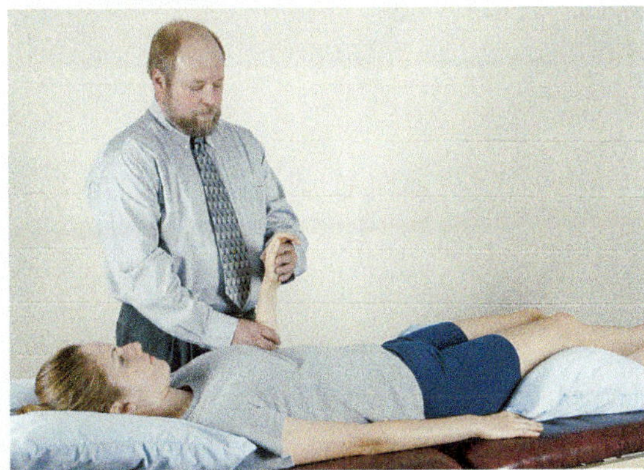

Midposition (neutral) of wrist.

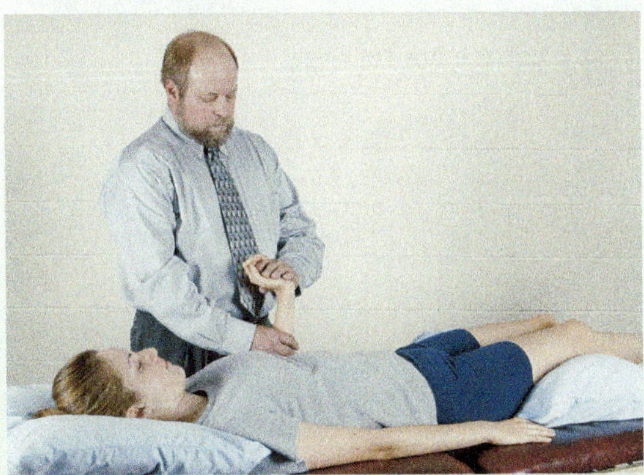

Wrist extension fingers relaxed.

(continued)

PROCEDURE 8–3 Upper Extremity ROM Exercises: Anatomical Planes (*continued*)

Joint(s):	Wrist (radiocarpal and intercarpal)
Motions:	Ulnar and radial deviation
Position:	Supine, elbow flexed, and forearm in midposition
Alternative position:	Sitting
Hand placement:	One hand stabilizes the forearm. The other hand grasps the patient's hand.
Notes:	The ROM for radial deviation is less than for ulnar deviation.
	Avoid wrist flexion and extension and forearm pronation and supination while performing ulnar and radial deviation motions.

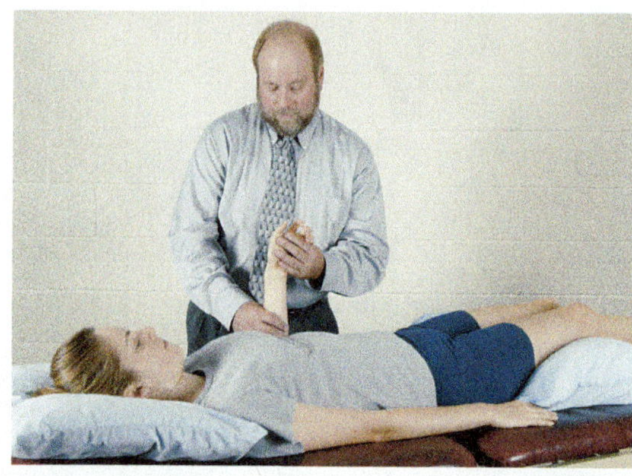

Ulnar deviation.

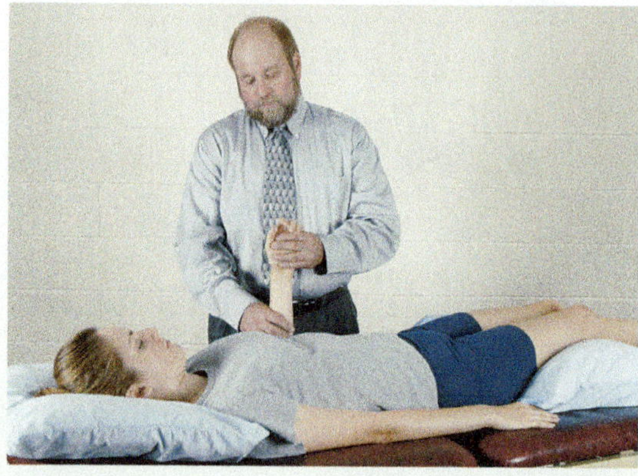

Midposition (neutral) of wrist.

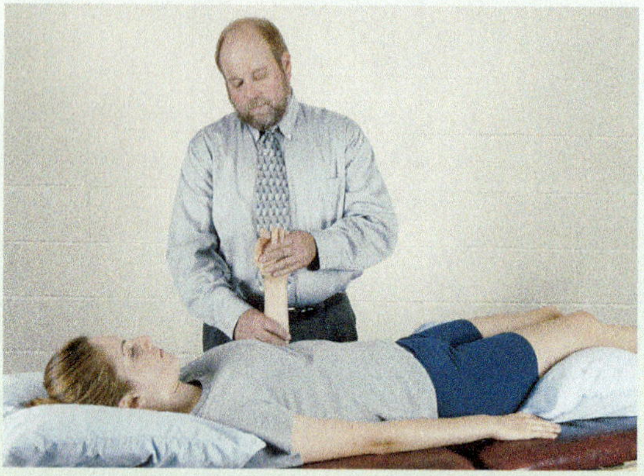

Radial deviation.

Joint(s):	Fingers (metacarpophalangeal and interphalangeal)
Motions:	Flexion and extension
Position:	Supine, elbow flexed to 90 degrees and wrist in neutral position
Alternative position:	Sitting
Hand placement:	One hand stabilizes the forearm and wrist. The other hand grasps the fingers or an individual digit.
Note:	Digits may be moved through the ROM at all joints and in all directions as a group or individually.

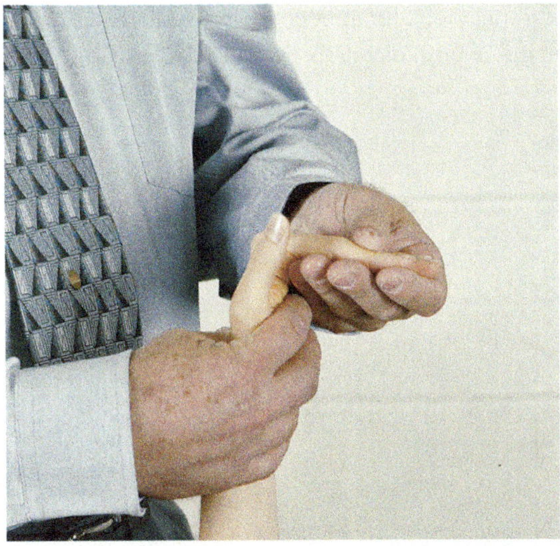

Finger flexion.

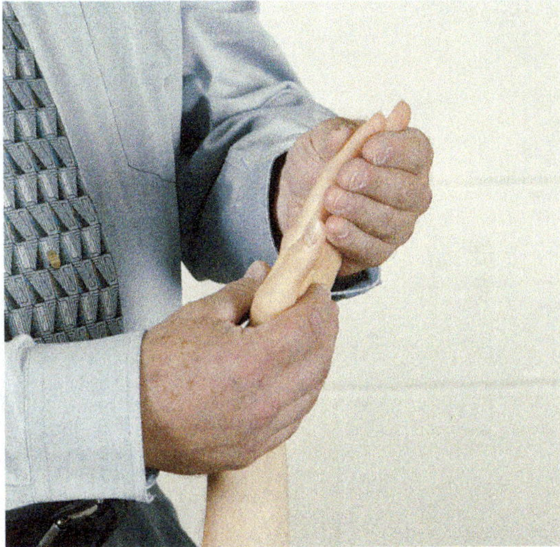

Neutral position of metacarpophalangeals with interphalangeal extension.

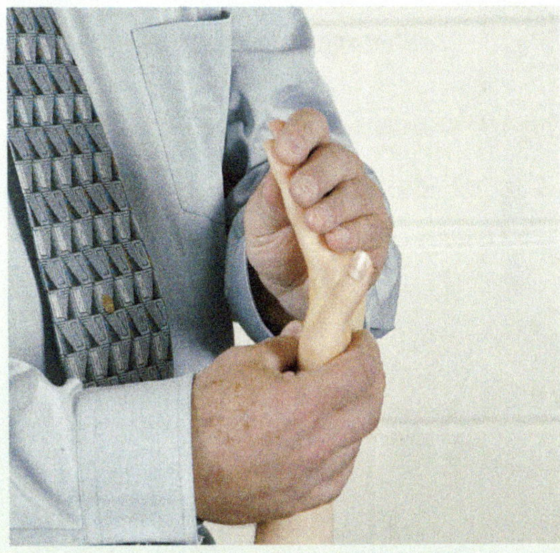

Finger extension.

(continued)

PROCEDURE 8–3 Upper Extremity ROM Exercises: Anatomical Planes (*continued*)

Joint(s):	Fingers (metacarpophalangeal)
Motions:	Abduction and adduction
Position:	Supine, elbow flexed to 90 degrees and wrist in neutral position
Alternative position:	Sitting
Hand placement:	One hand supports the hand and fingers, and the other hand grasps the finger to be moved through the ROM.
Notes:	The middle finger is the reference point for abduction and adduction. Movement of the middle finger in both directions is labeled abduction.

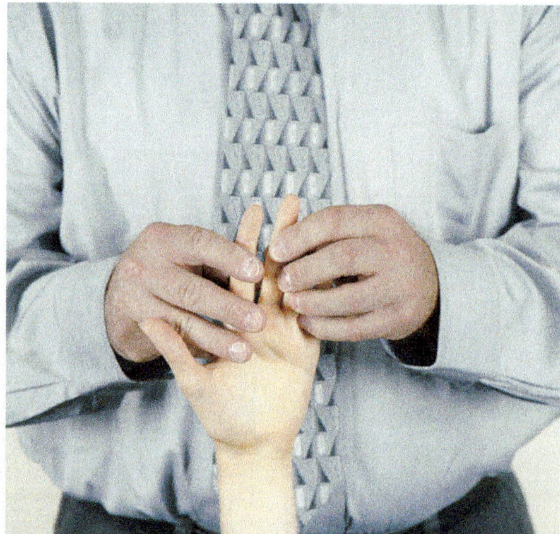

Starting position for finger abduction and adduction.

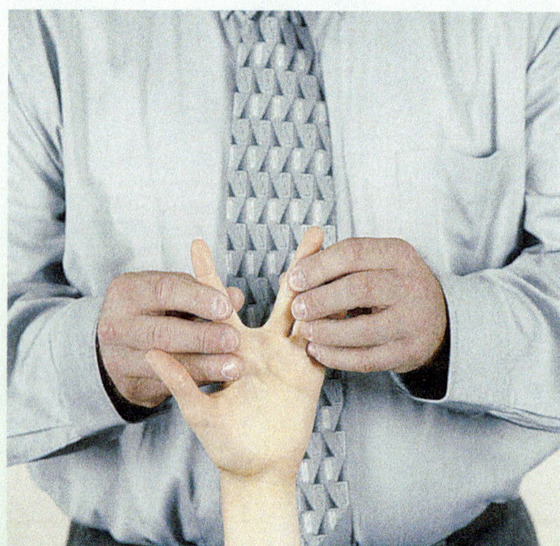

Finger abduction.

Joint(s):	Thumb (carpometacarpal) and fifth finger
Motion:	Opposition
Position:	Supine, elbow flexed to 90 degrees and wrist in anatomical position
Alternative position:	Sitting
Hand placement:	One hand grasps the thumb. The other hand grasps the fifth finger.
Notes:	To preserve function of the hand, maintain the arches of the hand. Opposition of the thumb and fifth finger can contribute to maintaining the arches of the hand.

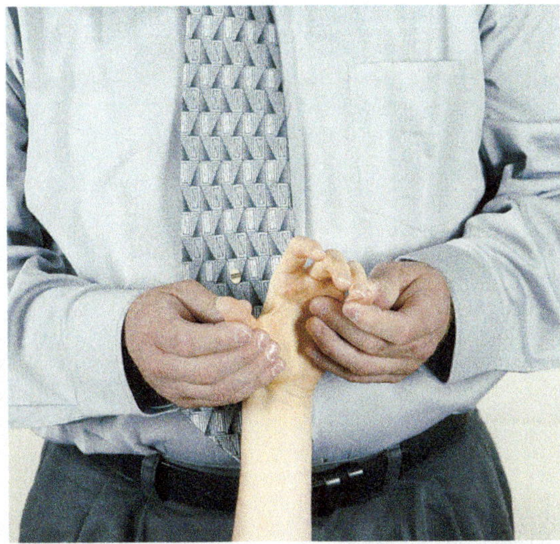

Beginning opposition.

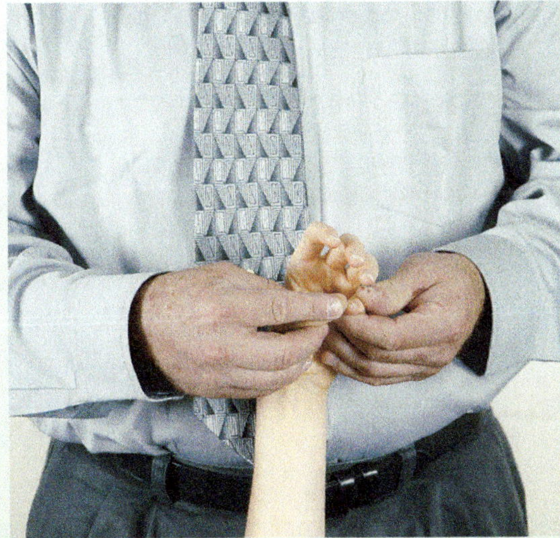

Opposition of thumb to fifth finger.

(continued)

PROCEDURE 8–3 Upper Extremity ROM Exercises: Anatomical Planes (*continued*)

Joint(s):	Thumb (carpometacarpal)
Motions:	Abduction and adduction
Position:	Supine, elbow flexed to 90 degrees, wrist in neutral position, and the thumb extended
Alternative position:	Sitting
Hand placement:	One hand grasps the thumb. The other hand grasps the patient's hand.
Note:	Maintaining the "web space" is vital for a functional hand.

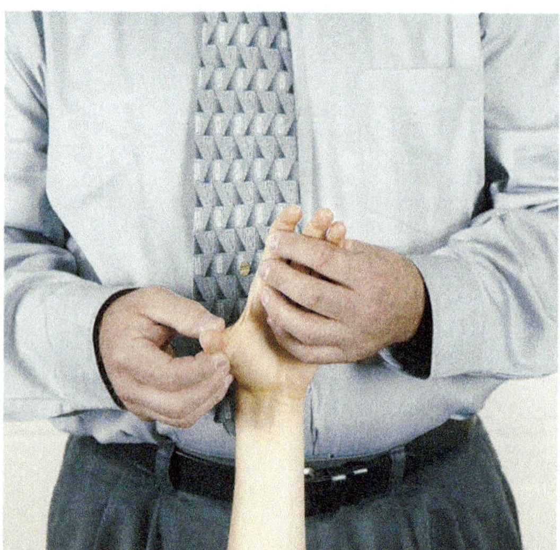

Thumb abduction.

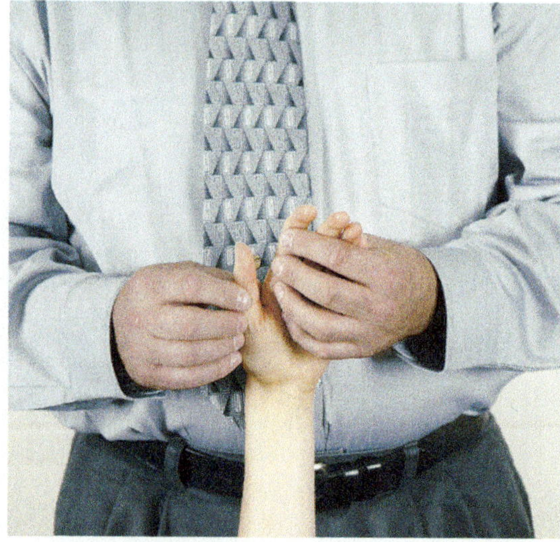

Thumb adduction.

Joint(s):	Thumb (carpometacarpal and metacarpophalangeal)
Motions:	Flexion and extension
Position:	Supine, wrist in neutral position
Alternative position:	Sitting
Hand placement:	One hand grasps the thumb. The other hand grasps the patient's hand.

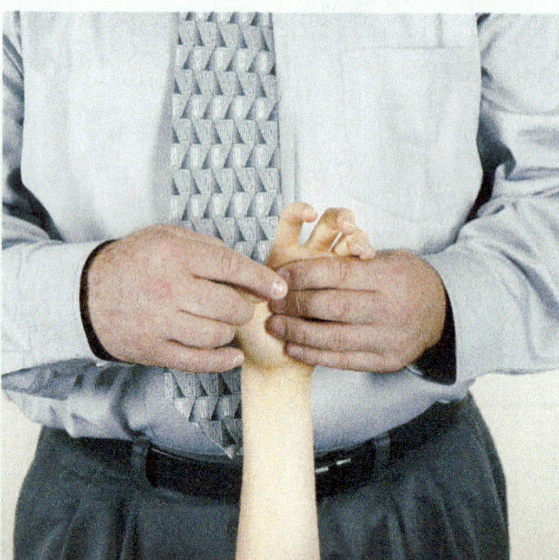

Thumb flexion.

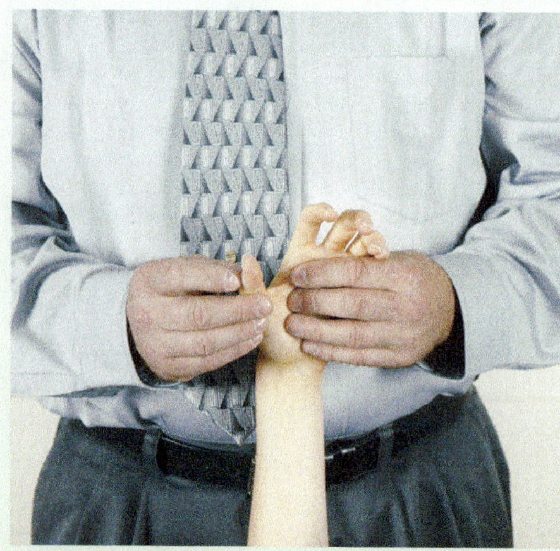

Thumb extension.

Muscle Length

Joint(s):	Shoulder (glenohumeral), elbow, and forearm
Muscle:	Biceps brachii
Motion:	Shoulder extension, elbow extension, and forearm pronation
Position:	Sidelying
Alternative position:	Sitting
Hand placement:	One hand supports the arm. The other hand grasps the patient's wrist and hand.
Notes:	To move the biceps muscle across both joints over which it acts requires elbow extension and forearm pronation with the shoulder in extension. This movement is achieved by first extending the shoulder and pronating the forearm through available ROM and then extending the elbow through its available ROM while maintaining shoulder extension and forearm pronation.

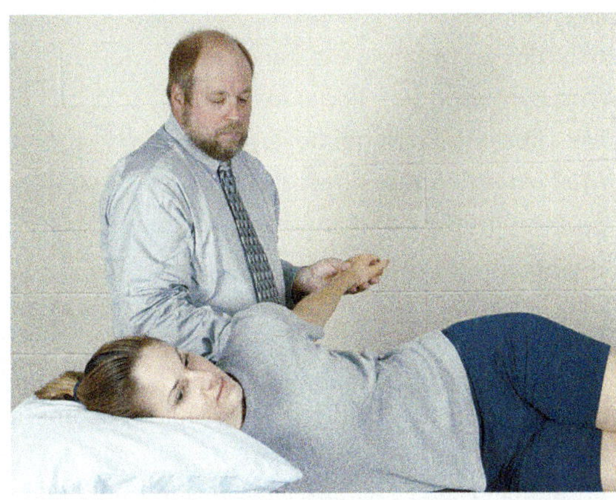

End position for biceps brachii muscle length.

Joint(s):	Shoulder (glenohumeral) and elbow
Muscle:	Triceps brachii
Motion:	Shoulder and elbow flexion
Position:	Supine
Hand placement:	One hand supports the arm. The other hand grasps the patient's wrist and hand.
Notes:	To move the triceps muscle across all joints over which it acts requires elbow flexion with the shoulder in flexion. This movement is achieved by first flexing the shoulder through its available ROM and then flexing the elbow through its available ROM while maintaining shoulder flexion.

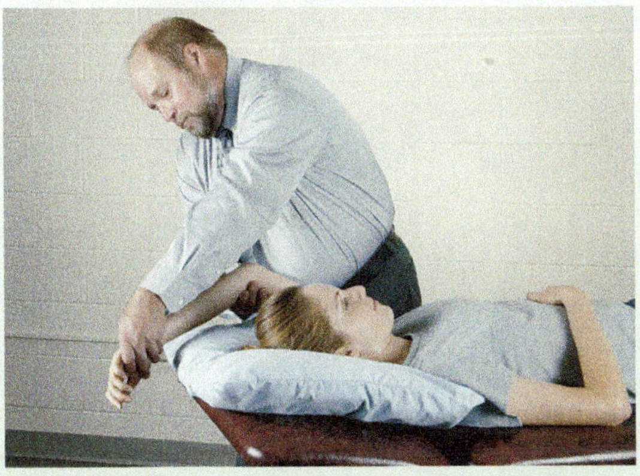

End position for muscle length of triceps brachii.

(continued)

PROCEDURE 8–3 Upper Extremity ROM Exercises: Anatomical Planes (*continued*)

Joint(s):	Elbow, wrist (radiocarpal and intercarpal), and fingers (metacarpophalangeal and interphalangeal)
Muscles:	Flexor digitorum superficialis Flexor digitorum profundus Palmaris longus Extensor digitorum Extensor digiti minimi Extensor indicis
Motions:	Wrist flexion with finger extension Wrist extension with finger extension Wrist flexion with finger flexion Wrist extension with finger flexion
Position:	Supine, elbow extended, forearm supinated
Alternative position:	Sitting
Hand placement:	One hand stabilizes the forearm. The other hand grasps the hand and fingers.
Notes:	These motions move (lengthen) multijoint muscles that cross the joints of the elbow, wrist, and fingers to the fullest extent possible. Although these muscles cross the elbow joint, the full effect of muscle lengthening can usually be achieved without regard for elbow joint position. Some patients should not have long finger flexors and extensors moved (lengthened) across all joints simultaneously, so they may develop tenodesis action.

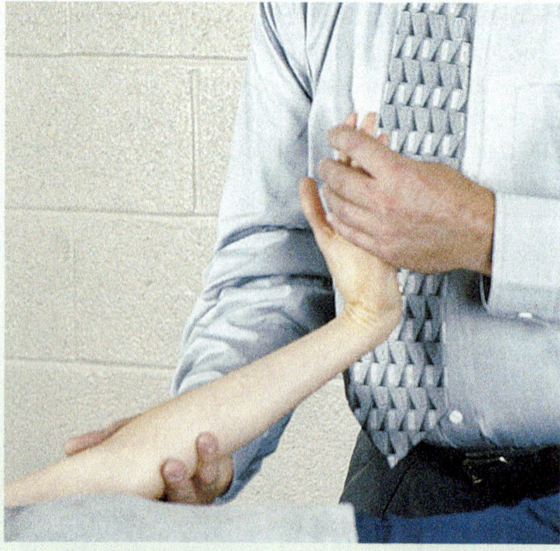

Wrist flexion with finger extension.

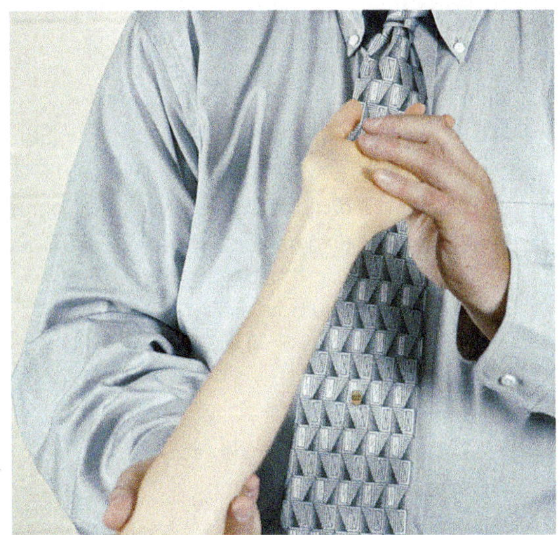

Wrist extension with finger extension.

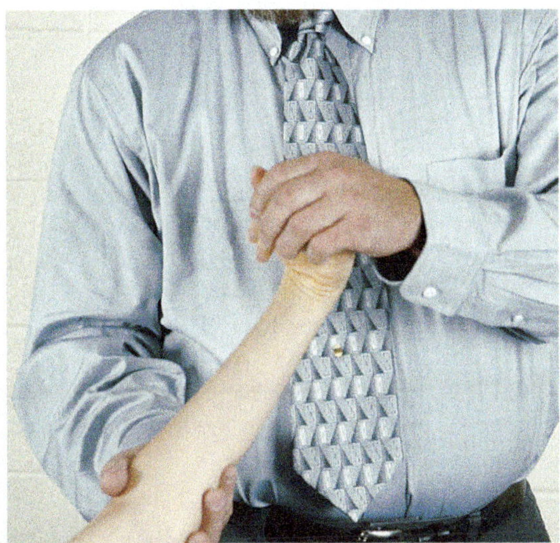

Wrist flexion with finger flexion.

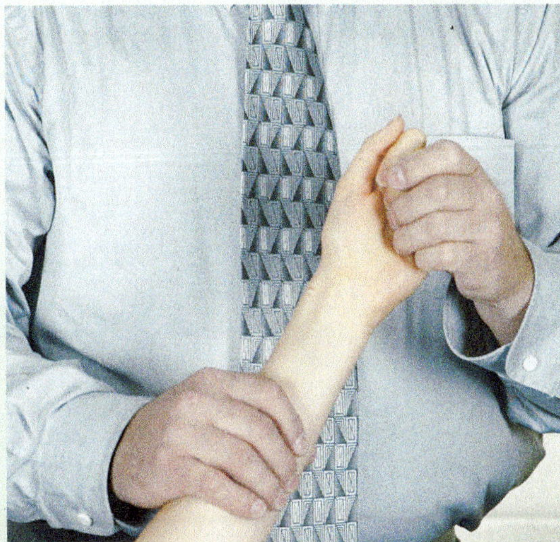

Wrist extension with finger flexion.

PROCEDURE 8–4 Upper Extremity ROM Exercises: PNF Diagonal Patterns

Pattern: PNF diagonal 1 (D1) extension with elbow extended
PNF diagonal 1 (D1) flexion with elbow extended

Combining Components of Motion:

D1 extension with elbow extended
- Shoulder: extension, abduction, medial rotation
- Elbow: extended
- Forearm: pronation
- Wrist: extension, ulnar deviation
- Digits: extension, abduction

D1 flexion with elbow extended
- Shoulder: flexion, adduction, lateral rotation
- Elbow: extended
- Forearm: supination
- Wrist: flexed, radial deviation
- Digits: flexion, adduction

Position: Supine

Hand placement: One hand supports the arm. The other hand grasps the patient's hand. When performing ROM of a patient's left upper extremity, the physical therapist/assistant's right hand controls the patient's left wrist and hand.

Notes: Elbow extended indicates that the elbow maintains extension throughout the movement of both patterns.

Not all motions of the hand and fingers occur when performed as passive range of motion.

In PNF patterns, motion begins distally and progresses proximally, with the motions occurring more or less simultaneously.

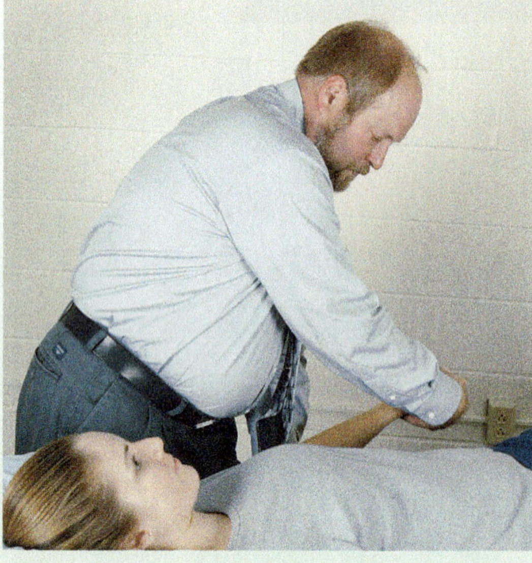

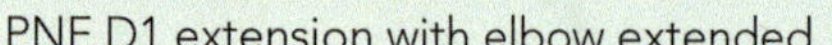

PNF D1 extension with elbow extended.

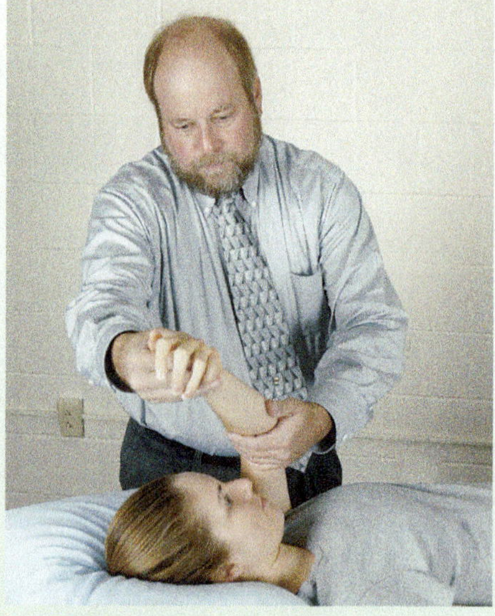

PNF D1 flexion with elbow extended.

Pattern:	PNF diagonal 1 (D1) extension with elbow extension PNF diagonal 1 (D1) flexion with elbow flexion
Combining components of motion:	D1 extension with elbow extension Shoulder: extension, abduction, medial rotation Elbow: extension Forearm: pronation Wrist: extension, ulnar deviation Digits: extension, abduction D1 flexion with elbow flexion Shoulder: flexion, adduction, lateral rotation Elbow: flexion Forearm: supination Wrist: flexion, radial deviation Digits: flexion, adduction
Position:	Supine
Hand placement:	One hand supports the arm. The other hand grasps the patient's hand. When performing range of motion of the patient's left upper extremity, the physical therapist/assistant's right hand controls the patient's left wrist and hand.
Notes:	Not all motions of the hand and fingers occur when performed as passive range of motion. In PNF patterns, motion begins distally and progresses proximally, with the motions occurring more or less simultaneously.

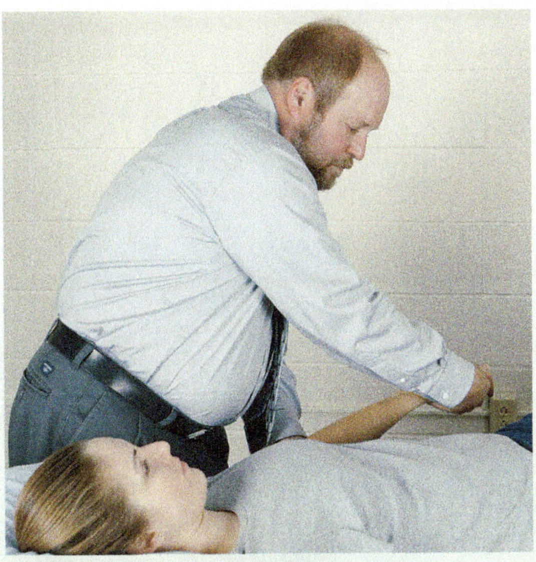

PNF D1 extension with elbow extension.

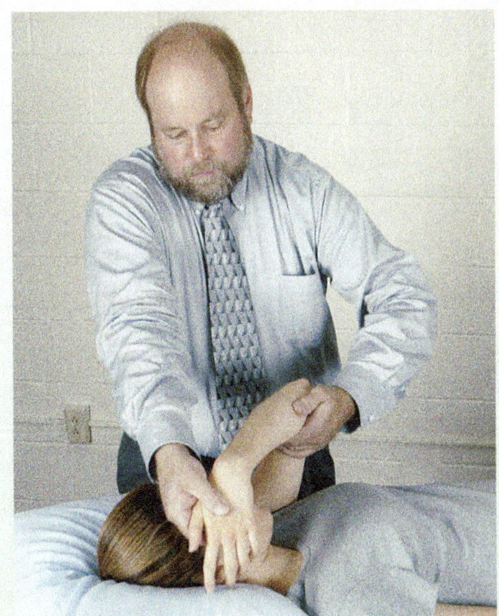

PNF D1 flexion with elbow flexion.

(continued)

PROCEDURE 8–4 Upper Extremity ROM Exercises: PNF Diagonal Patterns (*continued*)

Pattern: PNF diagonal 1 (D1) extension with elbow flexion
PNF diagonal 1 (D1) flexion with elbow extension

Combining components of motion:

D1 extension with elbow flexion
- Shoulder: extension, abduction, medial rotation
- Elbow: flexion
- Forearm: pronation
- Wrist: extension, ulnar deviation
- Digits: extension, abduction

D1 flexion with elbow extension
- Shoulder: flexion, adduction, lateral rotation
- Elbow: extension
- Forearm: supination
- Wrist: flexion, radial deviation
- Digits: flexion, adduction

Position: Supine

Hand placement: One hand supports the arm. The other hand grasps the hand. When performing ROM of a patient's left upper extremity, the physical therapist/assistant's right hand controls the patient's left wrist and hand.

Notes: Not all motions of the hand and fingers occur when performed as passive range of motion.

In PNF patterns, motion begins distally and progresses proximally, with the motions occuring more or less simultaneously.

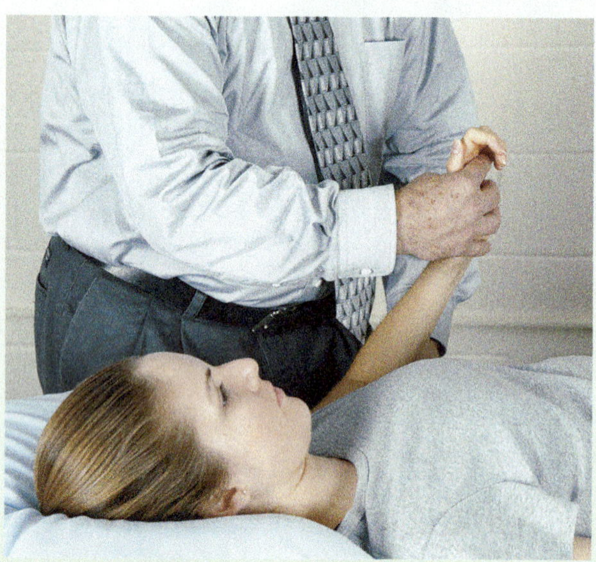
PNF D1 extension with elbow flexion.

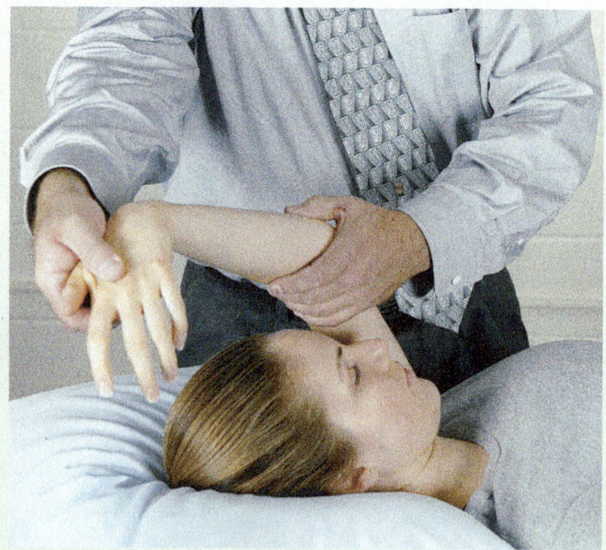
PNF D1 flexion with elbow extension.

Pattern:	PNF diagonal 1 (D1) extension—scapula PNF diagonal 1 (D1) flexion—scapula
Combining components of motion:	D1 extension: Scapula: depression, adduction, downward rotation D1 flexion: Scapula: elevation, abduction, upward rotation
Position:	Sidelying
Hand placement:	One hand is placed over the scapula. The other hand and forearm support the patient's upper extremity. When performing ROM of the patient's right scapula, the physical therapist/assistant's left hand is on the right scapula.
Note:	In PNF patterns, the motion occurs simultaneously.

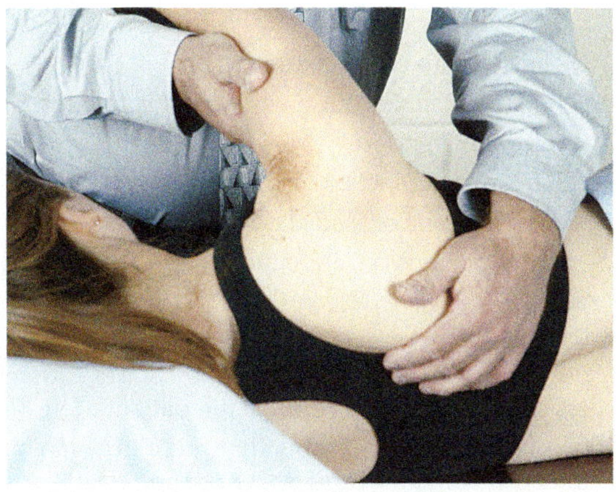

PNF D1 extension—scapula.

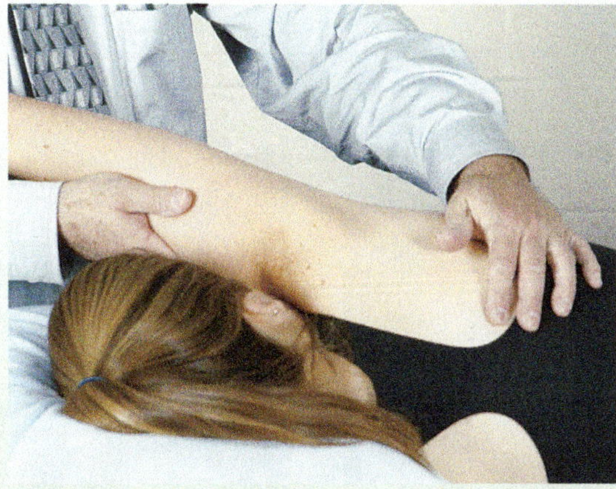

PNF D1 flexion—scapula.

(continued)

PROCEDURE 8–4 Upper Extremity ROM Exercises: PNF Diagonal Patterns (*continued*)

Pattern: PNF diagonal 2 (D2) extension with elbow extended
PNF diagonal 2 (D2) flexion with elbow extended

Combining components of motion: D2 extension with elbow extended
- Shoulder: extension, adduction, medial rotation
- Elbow: extended
- Forearm: pronation
- Wrist: flexion, ulnar deviation
- Digits: flexion, adduction
- Thumb: opposition

D2 flexion with elbow extended
- Shoulder: flexion, abduction, lateral rotation
- Elbow: extended
- Forearm: supination
- Wrist: extension, radial deviation
- Digits: extension, abduction

Position: Supine

Hand placement: One hand supports the arm. The other hand grasps the patient's hand. When performing ROM of the patient's left upper extremity, the physical therapist/assistant's right hand controls the patient's left wrist and hand.

Notes: Elbow extended indicates that the elbow maintains complete extension throughout the movement of both patterns.

Not all motions of the hand and fingers occur when performed as passive range of motion.

In PNF patterns, motion begins distally and progresses proximally, with the motions occurring more or less simultaneously.

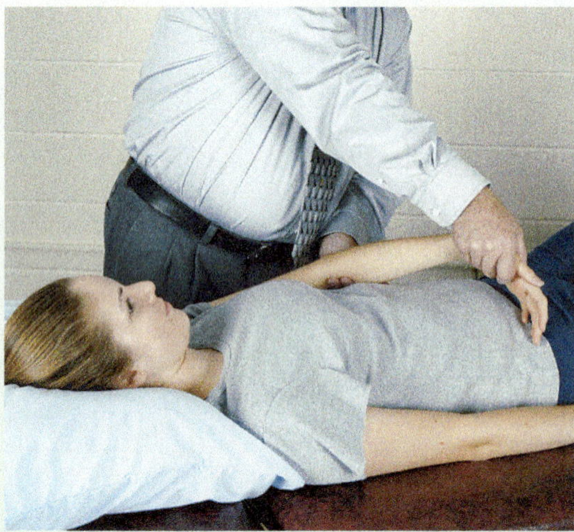
PNF D2 extension with elbow extended.

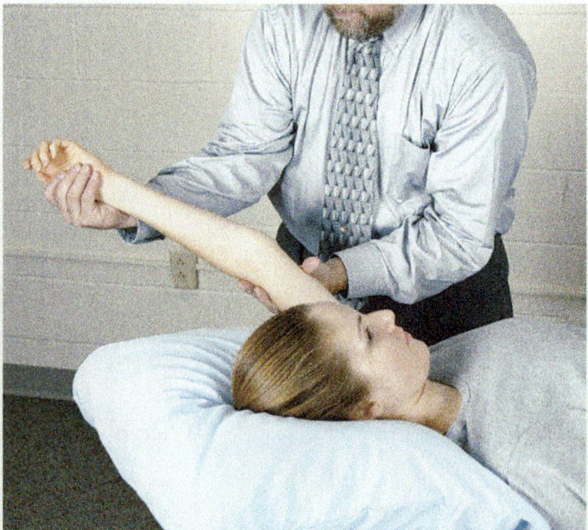
PNF D2 flexion with elbow extended.

Pattern: PNF diagonal 2 (D2) extension with elbow extension
PNF diagonal 2 (D2) flexion with elbow flexion

Combining components of motion:

D2 extension with elbow extension
- Shoulder: extension, adduction, medial rotation
- Elbow: extension
- Forearm: pronation
- Wrist: flexion, ulnar deviation
- Digits: flexion, adduction
- Thumb: opposition

D2 flexion with elbow flexion
- Shoulder: flexion, abduction, lateral rotation
- Elbow: flexion
- Forearm: supination
- Wrist: extension, radial deviation
- Digits: extension, abduction

Position: Supine

Hand placement: One hand supports the arm. The other hand grasps the patient's hand. When performing ROM of the patient's left upper extremity, the physical therapist/assistant's right hand controls the patient's left wrist and hand.

Notes: Not all motions of the hand and fingers occur when performed as passive range of motion.

In PNF patterns, motion begins distally and progresses proximally, with the motions occurring more or less simultaneously.

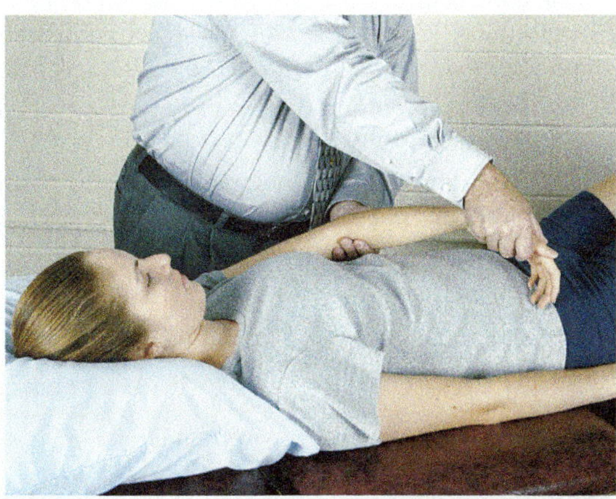

PNF D2 extension with elbow extension.

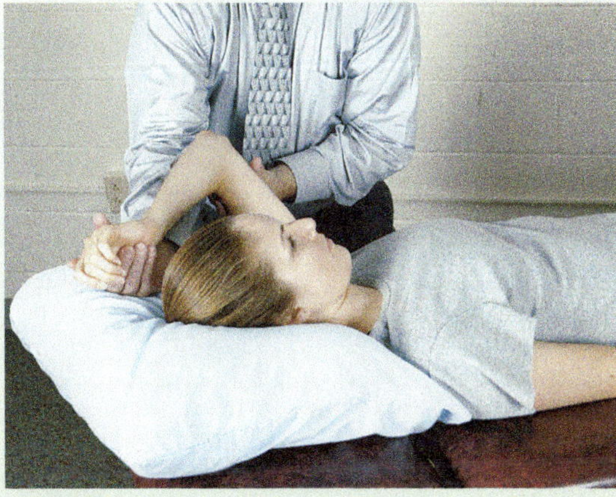

PNF D2 flexion with elbow flexion.

(continued)

PROCEDURE 8–4 Upper Extremity ROM Exercises: PNF Diagonal Patterns (*continued*)

Pattern:
PNF diagonal 2 (D2) extension with elbow flexion
PNF diagonal 2 (D2) flexion with elbow extension

Combining components of motion:
D2 extension with elbow flexion
- Shoulder: extension, adduction, medial rotation
- Elbow: flexion
- Forearm: pronation
- Wrist: flexion, ulnar deviation
- Digits: flexion, adduction
- Thumb: opposition

D2 flexion with elbow extension
- Shoulder: flexion, abduction, lateral rotation
- Elbow: extension
- Forearm: supination
- Wrist: extension, radial deviation
- Digits: extension, abduction

Position:
Supine

Hand placement:
One hand supports the arm. The other hand grasps the patient's hand. When performing ROM of the patient's left upper extremity, the physical therapist/assistant's right hand controls the patient's left wrist and hand.

Notes:
Not all motions of the hand and fingers occur when performed as passive range of motion.
In PNF patterns, motion begins distally and progresses proximally, with the motions occurring more or less simultaneously.

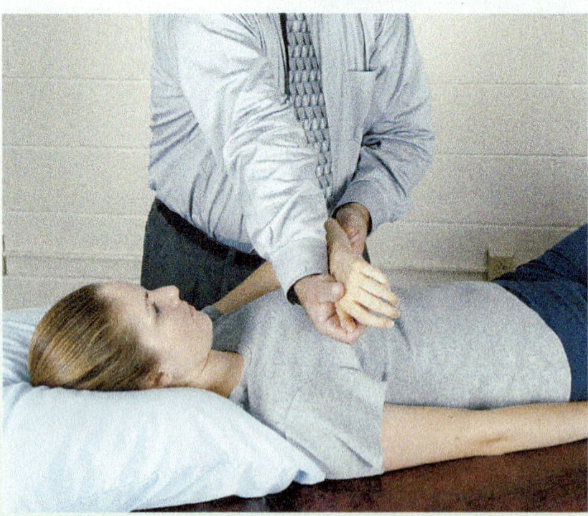
PNF D2 extension with elbow flexion.

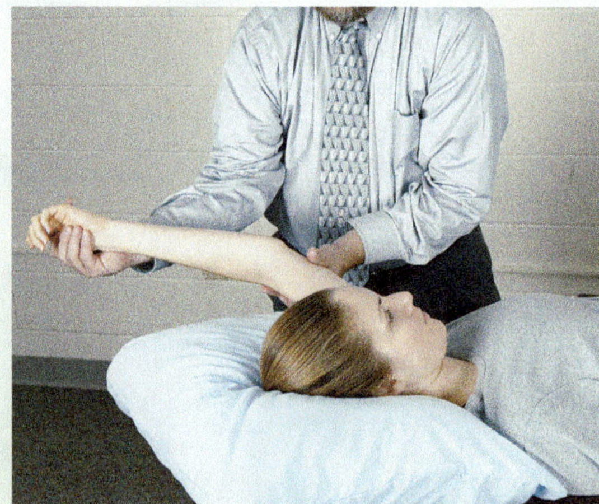
PNF D2 flexion with elbow extension.

Pattern:	PNF diagonal 2 (D2) extension—scapula PNF diagonal 2 (D2) flexion—scapula
Combining components of motion:	D2 extension Scapula: depression, abduction, downward rotation D2 flexion Scapula: elevation, adduction, upward rotation
Position:	Sidelying
Hand placement:	One hand is placed on the scapula. The other hand and forearm are used to support the patient's arm. When performing ROM of the patient's right scapula, the physical therapist/assistant's right hand grasps the right scapula.

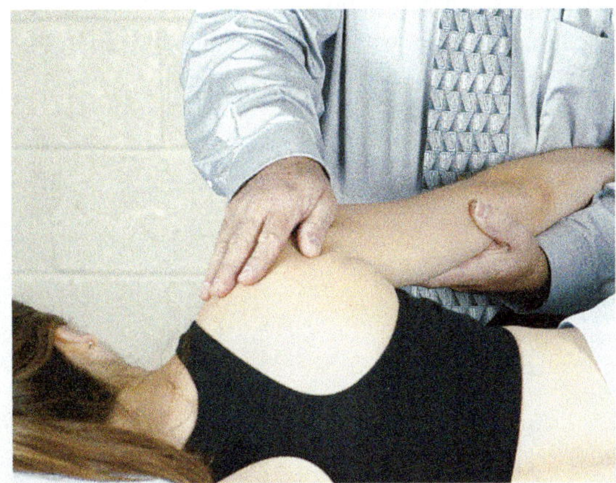

PNF D2 extension—scapula.

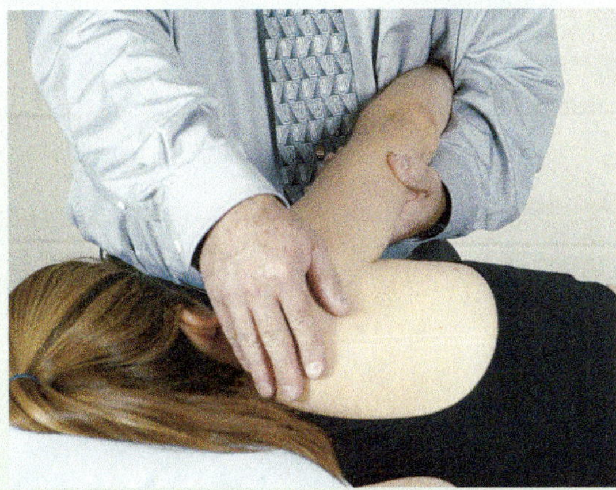

PNF D2 flexion—scapula.

PROCEDURE 8–5 Head, Neck, and Trunk ROM Exercises: Anatomical Planes

Joint(s):	Head and neck (atlantooccipital, atlantoaxial, and successive cervical spine joints)
Motions:	Flexion and extension
Position:	Supine
Hand placement:	One hand grasps each side of the head with the palms above the ears and the fingers spread over the occiput.
Notes:	When the treatment table does not have a head support that can be lowered, the patient must lie with his or her head over the end of the table. Carefully support the patient's head. Do not force movement. Movement begins with tucking of the chin rather than jutting the chin forward.

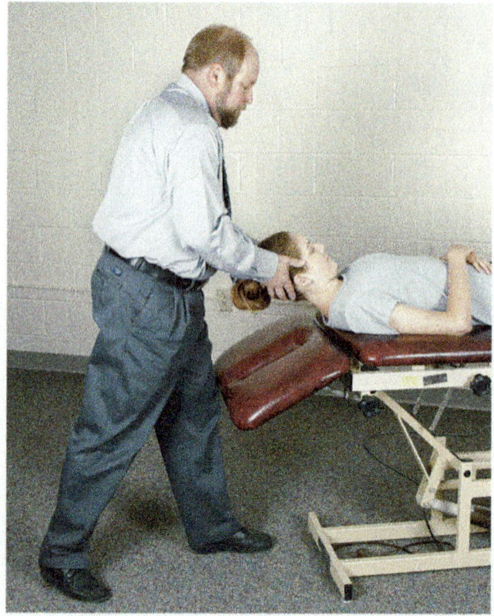

Head and neck (cervical spine) flexion.

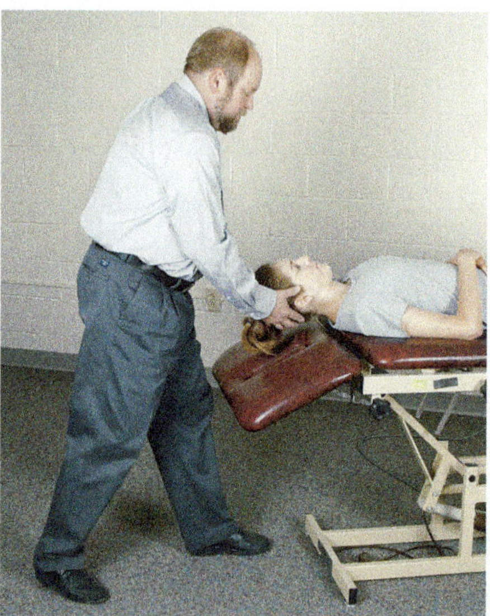

Neutral position of head and neck (cervical spine).

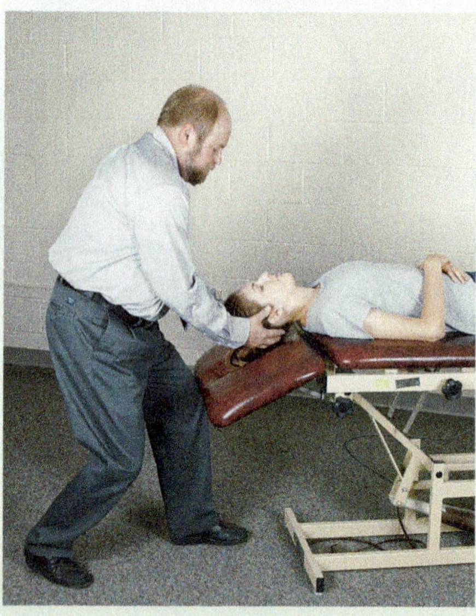

Head and neck (cervical spine) extension.

Joint(s):	Head and neck (atlantooccipital, atlantoaxial, and successive cervical spine joints)
Motions:	Lateral flexion
Position:	Supine
Hand placement:	One hand grasps each side of the head with the palms above the ears and the fingers spread over the occiput.
Notes:	Carefully support the patient's head. Do not force movement. Movement begins with tilting the ear to the shoulder rather than pushing the head laterally.

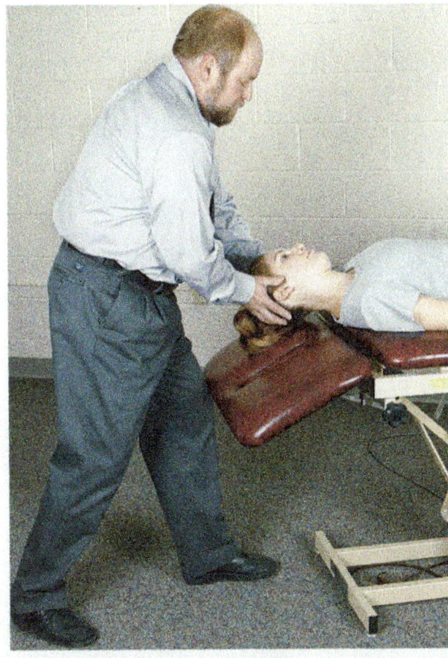

Lateral head and neck (cervical spine) flexion to the left.

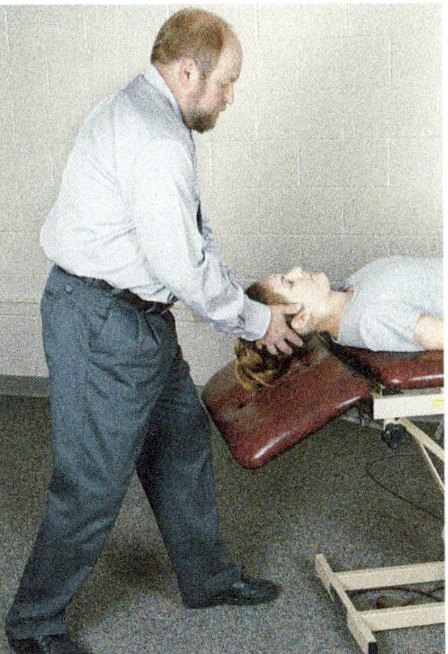

Neutral position of the head and neck (cervical spine).

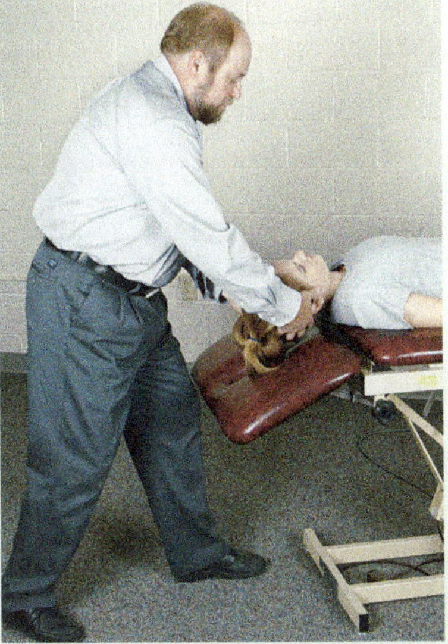

Lateral head and neck (cervical spine) flexion to the right.

(continued)

PROCEDURE 8–5 Head, Neck, and Trunk ROM Exercises: Anatomical Planes (*continued*)

Joint(s):	Head and neck (atlantooccipital, atlantoaxial, and successive cervical spine joints)
Motions:	Rotation
Position:	Supine
Hand placement:	One hand grasps each side of the head with the palms above the ears and the fingers spread over the occiput.
Notes:	Carefully support the patient's head. Do not force movement. Movement should not include flexion/extension or lateral flexion.

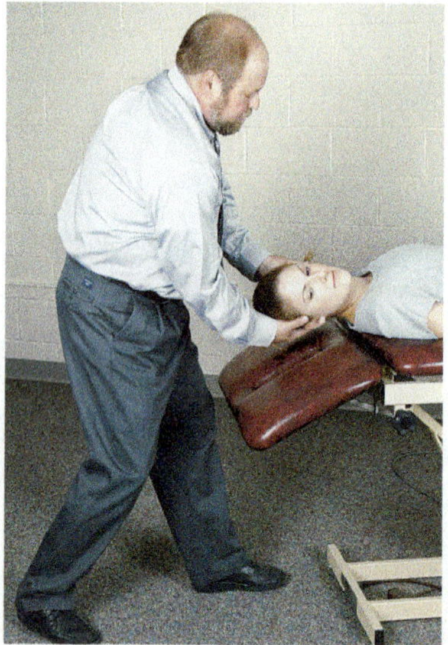

Head and neck (cervical spine) rotation to the right.

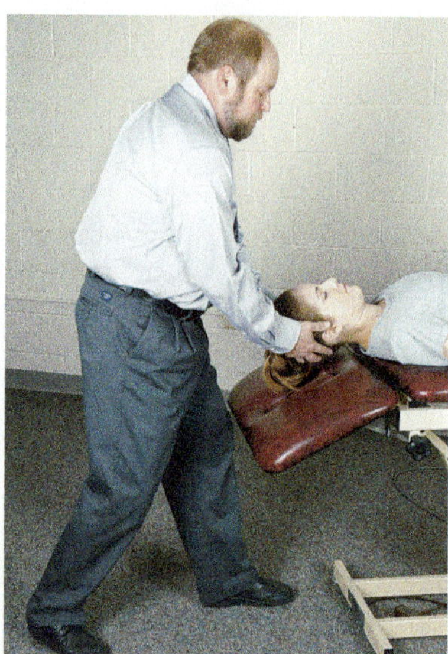

Neutral position of the head and neck (cervical spine).

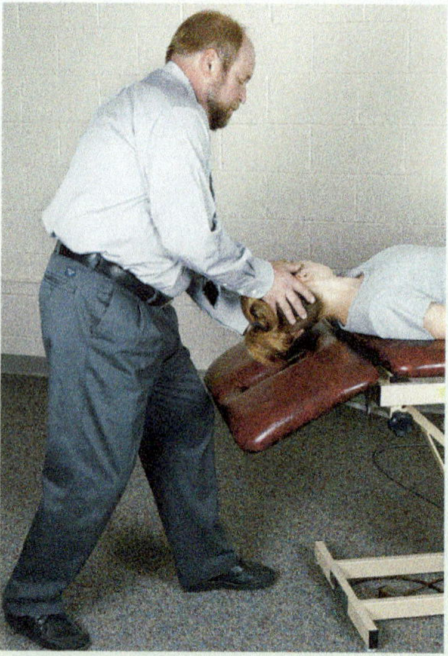

Head and neck (cervical spine) rotation to the left.

Joint(s):	Lower trunk (lumbar spine) and hip
Motion:	Lower trunk rotation
Position:	Supine, hips and knees flexed such that the patient's feet are resting flat on the supporting surface close to the buttocks
Hand placement:	One hand grasps the knees. The other hand stabilizes the pelvis.
Alternative placement:	Both hands are placed on the knees.
Notes:	The patient's shoulders remain on the supporting surface as the knees are moved from side to side. When a patient's upper trunk begins to roll, lower trunk rotation in that direction is completed.

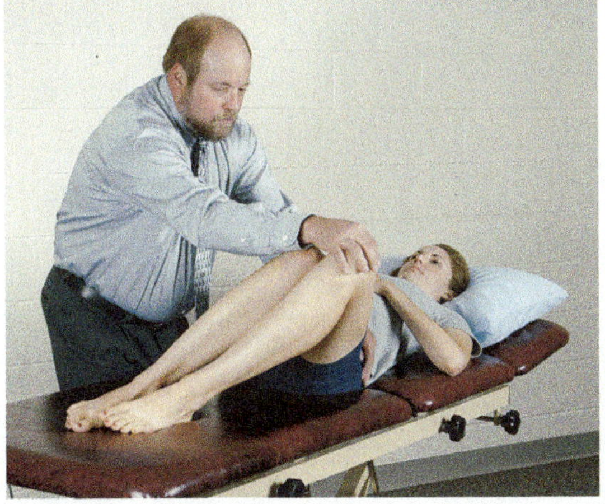

Lower trunk (lumbar spine) rotation to the left.

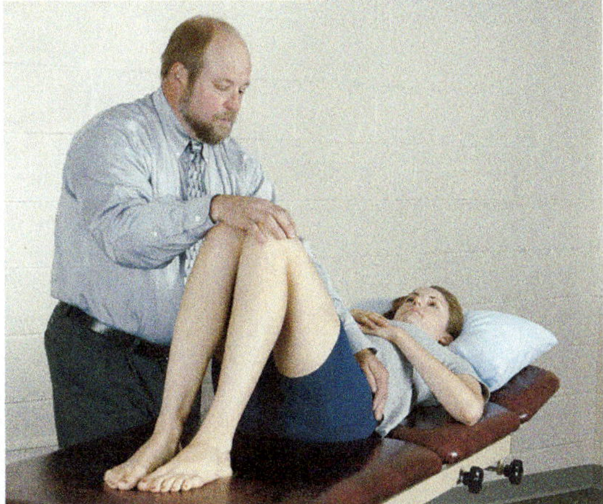

Neutral position of the lower trunk (lumbar spine).

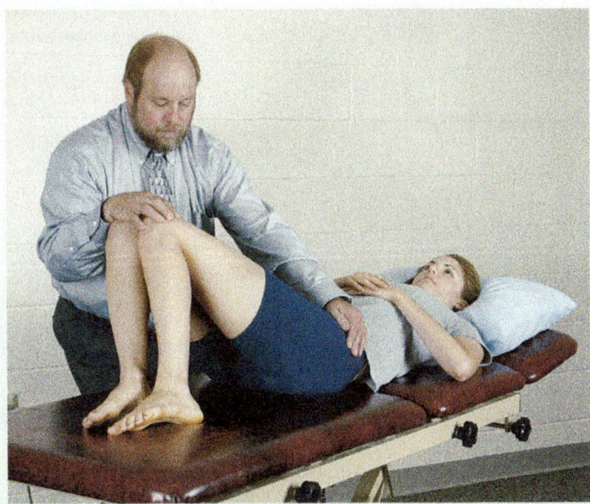

Lower trunk (lumbar spine) rotation to the right.

(continued)

PROCEDURE 8–5 Head, Neck, and Trunk ROM Exercises: Anatomical Planes (*continued*)

Joint(s):	Lower trunk (lumbar spine) and hip
Motion:	Lower trunk flexion
Position:	Supine, hips and knees flexed
Hand placement:	One arm supports the legs on the posterior aspect of the patient's thighs. The other hand supports the patient's feet as the lower trunk (lumbar spine) is flexed.

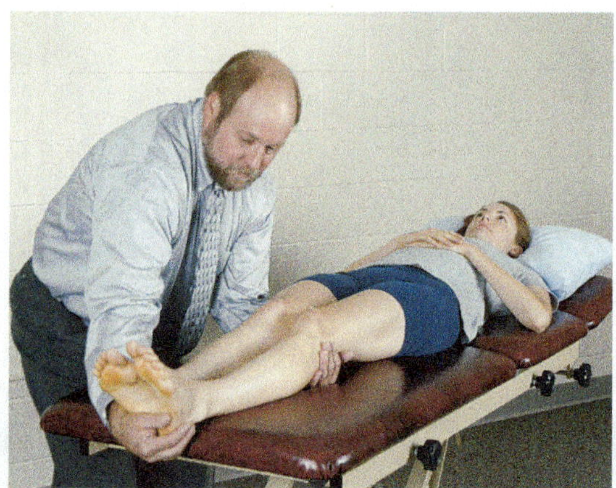

Starting position for lower trunk (lumbar spine) flexion.

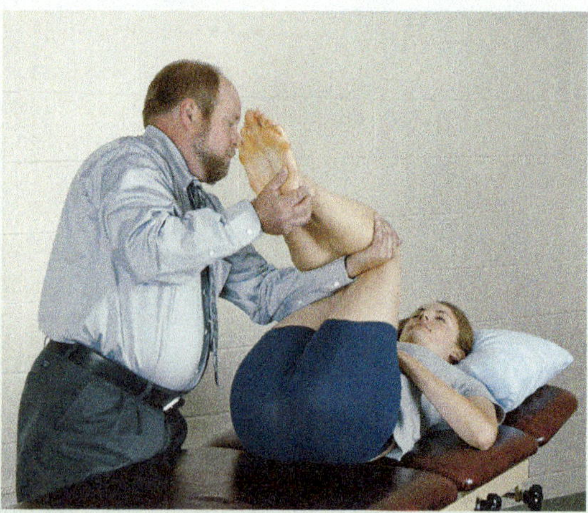

End position for lower trunk (lumbar spine) flexion.

Review Questions

1. What is the anatomical position, and what are the joint positions in the anatomical position?
2. What are the definitions of passive (PROM), active-assisted (AAROM), and active (AROM) range of motion?
3. When is it appropriate to use each type of ROM (PROM, AAROM, and AROM)?
4. How are body segments supported during performance of ROM exercises, including differences in support between PROM and AAROM.
5. What are the differences between joint ROM and muscle length?
6. How is muscle length ROM performed?
7. What are the different types of end feel, identifying joints that have each type of end feel caused by body structures, and identifying the body structures causing the end feel?
8. What are the differences in movement when a patient has normal muscle tone, spasticity, rigidity, and pain?
9. What are the definitions of the motions of flexion, extension, abduction, adduction, horizontal abduction, horizontal adduction, protraction, retraction, opposition, internal (medial) rotation, external (lateral) rotation, supination, pronation, inversion, and eversion?
10. What are the similarities and differences between anatomical plane motions and diagonal patterns of motion, including when each is most appropriate to use, the amount of motion that can be achieved in each, and the benefits of each?
11. What are the combining components of motion for each of the diagonal patterns?

Suggested Activities

1. Demonstrate selected procedures presented in this chapter, and then have students practice the procedures. Students perform the specific procedures on each other. Rotate partners periodically during practice sessions.
2. Students demonstrate procedures to classmates based on previous experience and pictures provided. Remaining students and faculty analyze performance. This assists students learning to analyze movement and to learn from printed material rather than demonstrations, which supports independent learning.
3. For most motions, identify type of end feel and the structures responsible. Use references from anatomy and kinesiology to confirm answers. Discuss how end feels may vary from expected as a result of age changes in ligaments, capsules, bone, skin, and internal joint structures.
4. Students prepare lists of motions that can be performed in prone, supine, sidelying, and sitting positions and on different surfaces such as mat on floor, treatment table, or bed. After practicing performing ROM in different positions and on different surfaces, discuss effect on clinician's body mechanics, ability to stabilize to ensure desired motion is achieved, and ability to move joint through full motion.
5. Practice performing PROM, AAROM, and AROM. Discuss when each is appropriate. Discuss how to explain to a patient your role in each.
6. Practice performing ROM exercises while a partner role-plays various diagnoses (see Case Studies for suggestions). The student role-playing the patient can add "character" to the role by being cooperative, uncooperative, in pain, hard of hearing, or lacking in ROM to enhance the activity. The "patient" must role-play the diagnoses and character consistently. Discuss what would be appropriate information to include in notes and what sections of notes where the information should be documented. Write a note documenting performing ROM for the patient your partner was role-playing.
7. Practice teaching "family and patients" and other healthcare providers how to perform ROM exercises. Discuss the important points about ROM to convey to others how to perform it and how to put information in terms others understand. Consider how to instruct others who do not understand and speak the same language as you.

Case Studies

Use these case studies to complete Suggested Activity 6. For each of the case studies that follow:

- Decide what type of ROM (PROM, AAROM, AROM) is appropriate.
- Decide which method, anatomical plane or diagonal pattern, is appropriate.
- Determine which multiarticular muscles must be included in the plan of care.
- Decide the frequency of providing ROM, the number of repetitions, and the number of sets.
- Discuss how to perform ROM when patients have abnormal tone.
- Discuss expected responses when performing ROM and the meaning if expected responses do or do not occur.
- Implement ROM intervention.
- Document intervention.

1. Patient is a 22-year-old status post-traumatic brain injury and is in a coma.
2. Patient is an 18-year-old with complete C6 spinal cord injury, presenting with moderate spasticity in the lower extremities.
3. Patient is a 59-year-old former executive with left hemiplegia, mild spasticity in the lower extremity, and moderate spasticity in the upper extremity.
4. Patient is a 44-year-old with multiple sclerosis, presenting with moderate spasticity in the lower extremities.
5. Patient is a 70-year-old with advanced Parkinson's disease, presenting with moderate to severe rigidity.
6. Patient is a 12-year-old with cerebral palsy, presenting with severe spastic quadriplegia.
7. Patient is a 70-year-old with right hemiplegia and flaccid extremities.

References

1. Knott, M, and Voss, D. E. (1968). *Proprioceptive neuromuscular facilitation* (2nd ed.). New York: Harper & Row.
2. Root, M. L., Orien, W. P., and Weed, J. H. (1977). *Normal and abnormal function of the foot: Clinical biomechanics—volume II.* Los Angeles: Clinical Biomechanics Corporation Publishers.
3. Warwick, R., and Williams, P. L. (1989). *Gray's anatomy* (37th ed.). Philadelphia: W. B. Saunders.
4. Sullivan, P. E., Markos, P. D., and Minor, M. A. D. (1982). *An integrated approach to therapeutic exercise: Theory and clinical application.* Reston, Virginia: Reston Publishing Company.

9

Transfer Activities

LEARNING OUTCOMES

Upon completion of this chapter, you will be able to:

1. List transfer activities, indicating those that are dependent, assisted, or independent.
2. Describe types and levels of assistance used when transferring patients.
3. Describe and demonstrate the use of teaching tips for transfer activities.
4. List the rules of, and demonstrate, proper body mechanics used during transfer activities.
5. Describe and demonstrate the proper use of gait belts during transfer activities.
6. Describe the purpose, and how, to prepare the environment in preparation for performing transfer activities.
7. Describe the purpose and proper use of counts and verbal cues.
8. Describe and perform correctly dependent, assisted, and independent transfer activities.

KEY TERMS

Assisted transfer activities
Close guarding
Contact guarding
Dependent transfer activities
Gait belts (transfer belts)
Generalizability
Independent transfer activities
Supervision

Introduction

The purpose of transfer activities is to move patients, or have patients move themselves, from one place (bed, chair, toilet, etc.) to another, permitting them to function in different environments or to use different pieces of equipment. Transfer activities may be performed independently by patients or with assistance of healthcare providers or family members. Each patient is examined, which may include, but not be limited to, strength, range of motion, pain, cognitive ability, and movement dysfunction. Others knowledgeable about a patient's functional capabilities may be interviewed, especially when a patient is not a reliable reporter. Physical therapists evaluate the results of the interview, systems review, and examination and then select an appropriate method of transfer that can be performed in a safe, effective, and efficient manner. Observation of performance and reevaluation of a patient's capabilities, within the physical therapist patient/client management process, may result in selection or modification of a different transfer activity.

Selection of a transfer activity includes determining the level of transfer activity and assistance necessary for the transfer. Levels of transfer activities are dependent, assisted, or independent. Description of assistance necessary for a transfer activity includes levels of assistance, amount of assistance, and type of assistance. Each of these factors is described in the following sections. Appropriate documentation requires inclusion of level of transfer, level of assistance, amount of assistance, and type of assistance.

A physical therapist sets the level of transfer activity as part of goal setting, both short- and long-term. The long-term goal is for the patient to achieve the maximum level of independent performance of a transfer activity that is consistently performed in a safe, effective, and efficient manner. Algorithms can be used to assist in decision making concerning the selection of the type of transfer activity, depending on a patient's abilities, as determined by the physical therapist's evaluation (see Figure 9–1 ■[1]).

■ Take Note
Safety of all person involved in transfer activities is of paramount importance. When in doubt about the safety of a transfer activity, seek assistance.

There is an interaction among levels and methods of transfer, levels of assistance, amount of assistance, and type of assistance. Each of these factors should be considered to ensure safe, effective, and efficient transfer activities. Documentation should include a clear description of these factors, so transfer activities are implemented consistently.

Safety must not be compromised by the selection, or during the performance, of a transfer activity.

Levels of Transfer Activities

Transfer activities may be independent, modified independent, assisted, or dependent. The level of transfer activity is based upon a patient's functional capabilities and safety of the patient and any assisting personnel. Transfer activities are usually named by the level and method of transfer, names of transfer activities, however, are not used consistently. As a patient improves, the level of transfer activity used by a patient may change (dependent → assisted → modified independent → independent).

Independent transfer activities: The patient performs all aspects of the transfer activity, including preparation, in a safe manner without transfer devices or assistance.

Modified independent transfer activities: The patient performs the transfer independently with transfer devices.

Assisted transfer activities: The patient participates actively, yet requires assistance.

Dependent transfer activities: The patient does not participate actively, or participates only minimally, and others perform all aspects of the transfer activity.

■ Take Note
Levels of transfer activities—independent, assisted, dependent.

Assistance

Levels of Guarding During Transfer Training Activities

Common terminology used to describe levels of guarding during transfer training activities is based, in part, on the scoring scale presented in the Functional Independence Measure (FIM).[2] When performing transfer training, the following terminology[3] describes

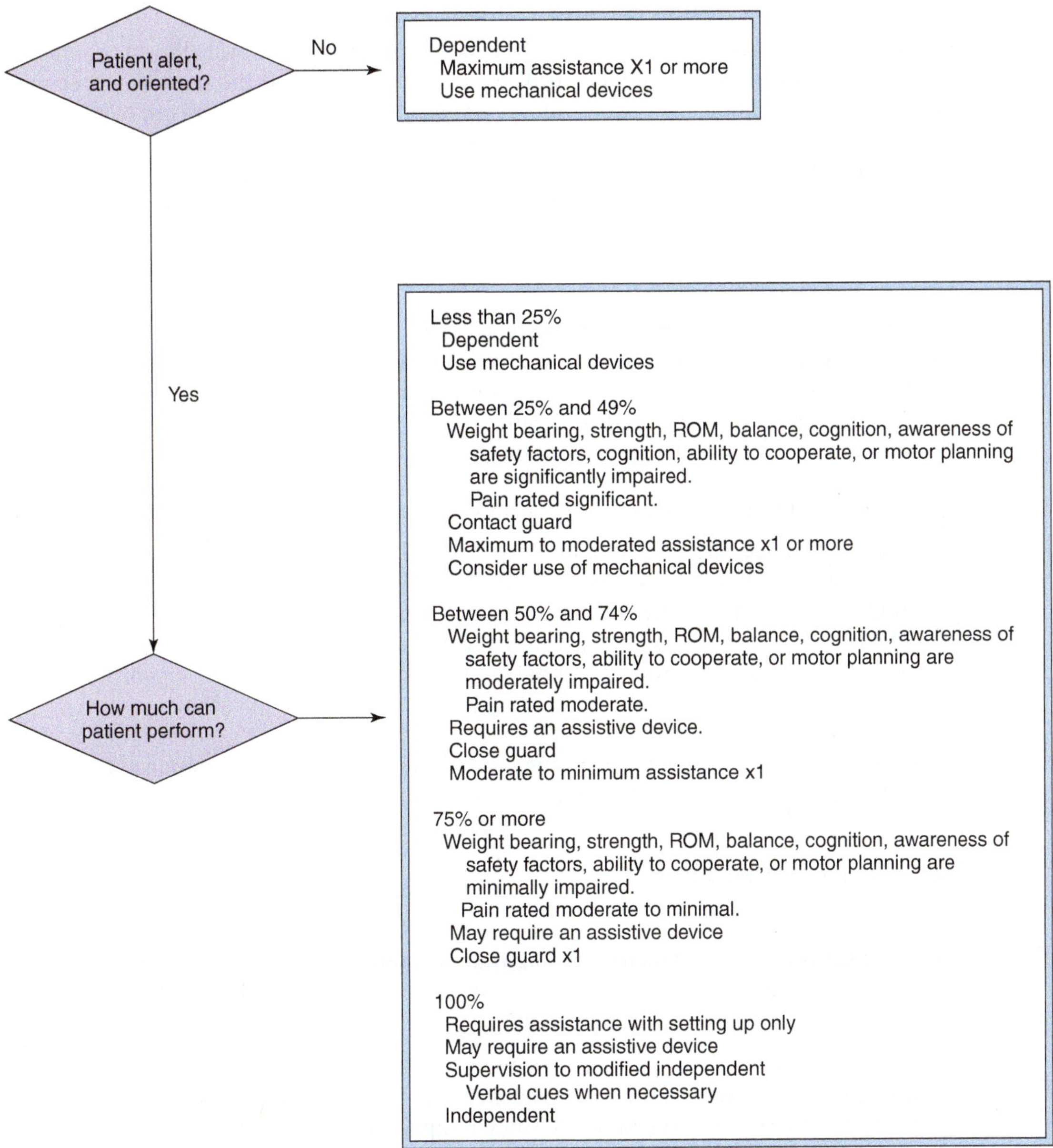

FIGURE 9–1 ■ Patient Transfer Assessment Flow Chart.

the level of guarding and the amount of assistance provided to a patient by the physical therapist/assistant.

1. **Supervision**: Physical therapist/assistant is near the patient and able to provide verbal or physical assistance as appropriate. It is unlikely that physical assistance will be required.
2. **Close guarding**: Physical therapist/assistant is positioned close to the patient, without contact with the patient. The likelihood of physical assistance being required is Fair.
3. **Contact guarding**: Physical therapist/assistant is positioned close to the patient, with hands on the patient/gait belt. The likelihood of physical assistance being required is High.
4. **Minimal (minimum) assistance**: A patient is able to perform 75% or more of an activity.
5. **Moderate assistance**: A patient is able to perform 50–74% of an activity.
6. **Maximal (maximum) assistance**: A patient is able to perform 0–49% of an activity.

Types of Guarding During Transfer Training Activities

■ **Take Note**

Types of assistance—verbal cuing, monitoring the environment, physical assistance.

Types of guarding include, but are not limited to, verbal cuing, monitoring the environment, and physical assistance. The goal of transfer training is to assist the patient to become independent or modified independent during transfer activities. This is achieved by reducing, as appropriate, the amount of assistance and guarding (maximal → moderate → minimal → contact guarding → close guarding → supervision → modified independent → independent). Included in this progression is the type of assistance (physical and verbal → verbal → independent).

Amounts of Assistance

When in doubt about the amount of assistance necessary for a patient to perform transfer training activities safely, obtain additional assistance. The number of persons needed to perform a transfer training activity safely is noted in your documentation. For example, when two people are required for a patient to perform the transfer training activity requiring moderate assistance, documentation should read "... moderate assistance X2 ..."

Types of Assistance

Types of assistance include, but are not limited to, verbal cuing, monitoring the environment, and physical assistance. The following are examples of types of assistance that might be needed by patients. A patient may require minimal physical assistance X1 for balance control. A second patient may require moderate physical assistance X2 for lifting. A third patient may require verbal cuing with supervision or close guarding. As a patient improves, the type of assistance may change (physical and verbal → verbal → no assistance).

Each of these factors, level of guarding, type of guarding, amount of assistance, and types of assistance needed to complete a transfer activity safely, is noted in your documentation.

General Guidelines

Teaching Tips

There are several components to teaching transfer activity techniques to patients, family, and other healthcare providers. Inclusion of these components leads to a safer, effective, and efficient transfer activity. These teaching tips are

1. Using demonstrations of the transfer activity assists patients and others in understanding what the transfer activity involves. One method of demonstration is for the patient and family to observe how a person with similar impairments performs the transfer activity. Another method is for you to demonstrate the transfer activity with the patient who is learning this activity.
2. The steps of a transfer activity can be practiced individually. This may make it easier for the patient with low endurance. For patients who do not initially recall all steps of a transfer activity, have the patient perform the steps they can remember, and guide them to complete the forgotten steps of the transfer activity.
3. Ensure that patients, or others assisting with transfer activities, know how to, and can, establish a safe environment in which the transfer activity can occur.
4. Some skills of transfer activities, such as locking a wheelchair and preparing the environment, are skills that can be used in other transfer activities once learned. In this way, transfer activities are generalized. **Generalizability** means that some skills learned for one transfer activity can be used when completing other transfer activities. Thus the skills of locking a wheelchair and preparing the environment are generalized when used for transferring from a wheelchair to a bed, transferring from a wheelchair to a couch, or transferring from a wheelchair to a toilet.
5. Learning of a transfer activity is enhanced by varying the context in which the transfer activity occurs. Start teaching in a closed environment, an environment in which there are few distractions. As the patient gains competence in performing the transfer

activity, practice can be performed in more open environments, one with distractions or increased complexities.

6. Learning of a transfer activity is promoted by practicing on different types of equipment, such as chairs/beds/couches of different heights, with soft or hard seats, or with and without armrests.
7. Mental practice, visualizing the steps of the transfer activity in sequence, assists learning the transfer activity. Ensuring that a patient understands the steps of a transfer activity requires that the patient be able to describe in sequence the steps of the transfer activity to you. Do not ask a patient the general question, "Do you understand?" Having a patient repeat the specific steps of a transfer activity serves as actual observation of the patient's mental practice. Actual physical performance of the transfer activity is necessary to attain competent performance of the activity, demonstrating that the patient can perform the transfer activity safely, effectively, and efficiently.

Body Mechanics

Proper attention to body mechanics and the relationship of the center of gravity and the base of support permit maintenance of the safest position while working with patients. Safe lifting and movement during transfer activities include

1. Maintaining the patient close to you
2. Maintaining an appropriately large base of support
3. Ensuring that your base of support can move with you as you move
4. Maintaining a static posture of the pelvis and spine to the greatest degree possible
5. Lifting using the large muscles of your legs
6. Not crossing your feet or legs as you move

Review the material on body mechanics presented in Chapter 3.

Manual Contacts

Positioning a patient close to you allows your hands to be placed on the appropriate aspect of a patient's anatomy to provide support or assistance (Figures 9–2 ■, 9–3 ■, and 9–4 ■). Support or assistance may be necessary under the buttocks or hips for lifting or assisting a patient to move. Manual contacts may be on a lateral aspect of a patient's trunk to indicate direction of movement or to provide assistance for balance.

■ **Take Note**

Manual contact can provide control and feedback.

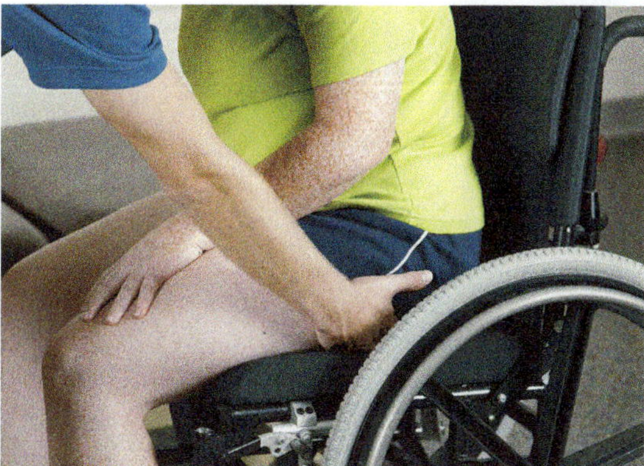

FIGURE 9–2 ■ By placing your hand under the patient's buttocks, a patient can be supported and assisted by lifting as the patient rises to standing.

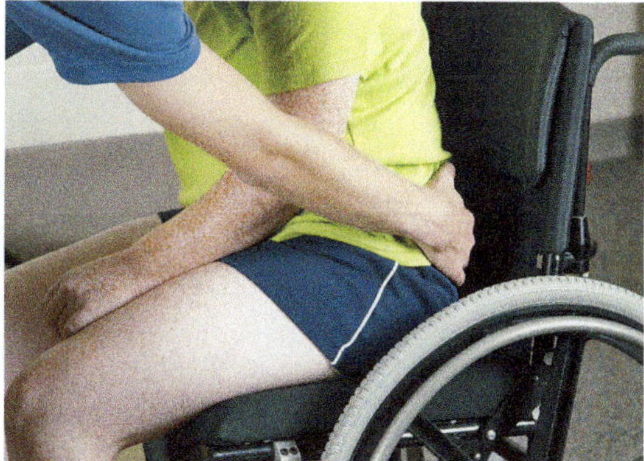

FIGURE 9–3 ■ By placing your hand on the posterolateral aspect of a patient's pelvis, the patient can be guided as she rises to standing. You are then in a position to control excessive lateral shift of the pelvis and can move your hand quickly to the posterior aspect of the pelvis to support or assist the patient when necessary.

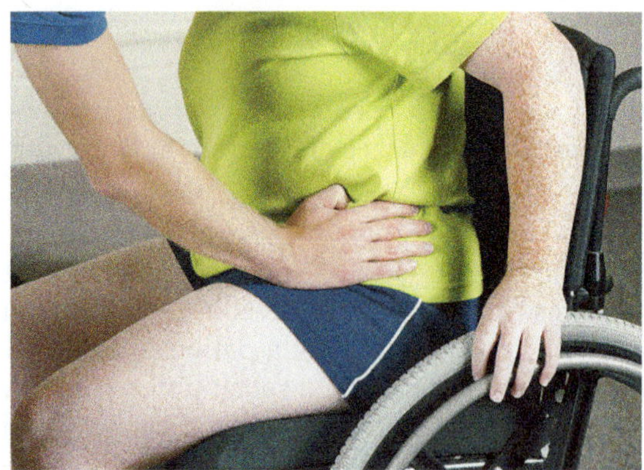

FIGURE 9–4 ■ By placing your hand on the anterolateral aspect of a patient's pelvis, you can guide or resist movement as the patient rises to standing. Resistance may provide facilitation, making the transfer activity easier, and teaches patients to bring the pelvis forward as they rise.

Gait Belts

Gait belts, sometimes called transfer belts, are straps with buckles or hook-and-loop closures for securing the belt around a patient's waist. A properly used gait belt provides a secure point of contact and control for whomever is assisting a patient during transfer activities. The straps are usually constructed of tightly woven material or leather and are available in different sizes. Some models of gait belts have handgrips at two or three points around the strap. When secured and used properly (Figure 9–5 ■), gait belts provide an additional method to support or assist during transfer activities. For large patients, or patients with lesions that limit options for manual contacts, gait belts provide a method of safely supporting or assisting a patient during transfer activities.

Improper use of gait belts reduces safety for both patients and those providing assistance. When a gait belt is not secured properly, it may become loose or move unexpectedly on a patient's body during transfer. Using a gait belt to hold a patient at arm's length keeps the patient farther from your base of support, making support and

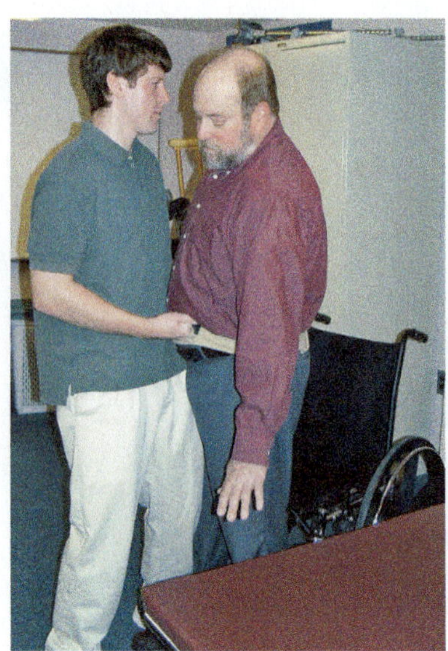

FIGURE 9–5 ■ Proper placement and use of gait belt for a transfer activity.

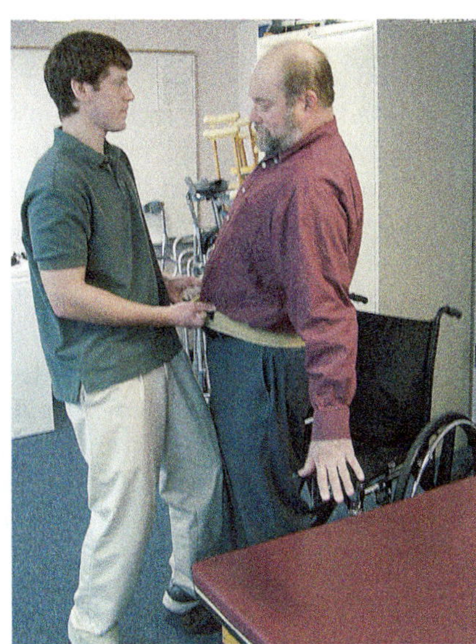

FIGURE 9–6 ■ Inappropriate use of gait belt to pull patient to standing, leading to lack of upper body control and excessive lumbar trunk extension.

assistance more difficult and placing more stress on your body. This will also become more uncomfortable for a patient because the gait belt is then more likely to be used for pushing or pulling, rather than support or assistance. Simply pushing, pulling, or lifting on gait or transfer belts alone may not provide specific support or assistance needed by patients during transfer activities and can injure a patient by placing significantly larger than usual stresses on body segments. As an example, when a patient is pulled to standing by incorrect use of a gait belt at the patient's waist, the patient generally assumes a position of excessive lumbar trunk extension, placing increased forces through the spine. In this instance, a physical therapist/assistant does not have control of the patient's upper body (Figure 9–6 ■). Use of gait belts by themselves does not provide the guidance that manual contacts do to help patients understand the direction movement. Use of a gait belt can be combined with manual contacts or use of your lower extremities to stabilize the patient's lower extremities (see Assisted Standing Pivot Transfer Activity, Procedure 9–12). Gait belts may be more useful for dependent transfer activities, especially when there is little prospect of the patient performing any or a significant amount of the transfer activity. Manual contacts may be more appropriate when a patient is able to participate significantly, such as when the goal is for a patient to be able to perform all or a majority of the transfer activity. Patient and personnel safety must be ensured whichever method is chosen.

In some settings or jurisdictions, gait belts may be required equipment. Each physical therapist is responsible for determining the administrative and legal requirements of practice in each specific setting or jurisdiction. Administrative or legal requirements for specific equipment exist in an effort to limit injury or liability. When specific equipment, such as gait belts, must be used, users must adhere to proper application and use of the equipment.

Preparing the Environment

When preparing the environment for transfer activities, consider the direction in which the patient will move—to the left or right. Ensure that movement will not be impeded by furniture or other equipment. Equipment that is needed should be within easy reach so you do not compromise patient safety. Specific considerations for preparing the environment for each transfer activity are covered as each transfer activity procedure is presented in this chapter. When performing transfer activities, avoid wearing jewelry that can become entangled with or scratch patients. Additional considerations for preparing an environment can be found in Chapter 3.

Instructions and Verbal Cues

Patients should always be informed about a transfer activity by the person in charge prior to initiating performance of the transfer activity. Included in the information provided is the patient's role and actions to be performed during the transfer activity. Explanations must be provided in a manner that is understood by patients, using nontechnical terms and using the assistance of a language interpreter when appropriate. When more than one person is involved in assisting with the transfer activity, the person in charge is also responsible for indicating the responsibilities of each participant.

■ **Take Note**
Verbal cues are action words.

Counts and verbal cues are used to synchronize actions of all participants in the transfer activity. When assistance of more than one person is required to assist in the performance of a transfer activity, the person at the head of the patient is usually responsible for providing the counts and verbal cues. Counting is used to synchronize all participants in preparation for the verbal cue that initiates the ensuing action. A verbal cue, such as "lift," is the word that indicates the specific action to be performed when the action word is spoken. An appropriate set of a count and verbal cue to initiate a transfer activity is presented in the following sequence.

1. "I will count to three and then give the verbal cue to lift."
2. "When I say 'lift,' we will lift."
3. The person providing the count and verbal cue checks visually and verbally to ensure that all assistants and the patient are ready before the transfer activity is initiated.
4. The person providing the count and verbal cue then says "One, two, three, lift."

Completing the Transfer Activity

A transfer activity is not complete until (1) the patient is securely in the new position, (2) manual contacts, and thus control, are removed, (3) appropriate positioning and draping is completed, (4) necessary equipment is placed within usable reach, and (5) you have confirmed that the patient feels secure and comfortable. When these five actions have been performed satisfactorily, the transfer activity is complete.

Modifications of Procedures

Examples of methods for performing transfer activities, or positioning of patients and those assisting with transfer activities, are presented in this text, but clinical decision making must be applied in all situations.

Sizes and abilities of patients, and those assisting in transfer activities, and the environment in which transfer activities occur will vary. Therefore specific steps within a transfer activity, or certain positions used for a transfer activity, may need to be modified for safe, effective, and efficient performance of transfer activities. The clinical decision as to the selection of the transfer activity and assistance is vital to the safety of patients and personnel, as well as to the ultimate ability of patients to achieve their optimal outcomes.

Sliding Transfer Activity

A sliding transfer can be used to transfer a patient between two treatment tables, a treatment table and cart, or a cart and bed. As a dependent transfer, three people are needed to transfer an average-size adult. For a patient who can independently perform this transfer with supervision or minimal assistance, the assistance of one person to stabilize the cart or provide minimal verbal or physical assistance may be necessary.

Position the cart parallel to, and against, the treatment table, and secure it with the patient's head at the head of the treatment table or cart.

NOTE: In the following illustrations, two treatment tables are used. The first treatment table represents a cart or gurney and will be referred to as a cart. The second treatment table represents a treatment table or bed and will be referred to as a treatment table.

PROCEDURE 9–1 Sliding Transfer Activity: Cart to Treatment Table

1. A "draw" sheet may be used to move ("draw") the patient from cart to treatment table. Cloth sheets are most often used as draw sheets. "Slippery" sheets may be used when available to decrease friction. A draw sheet is placed under the patient. The strongest and safest way to grasp a "draw" sheet is with the forearms supinated. The portions of the sheet to each side of the patient are rolled and grasped close to the patient.

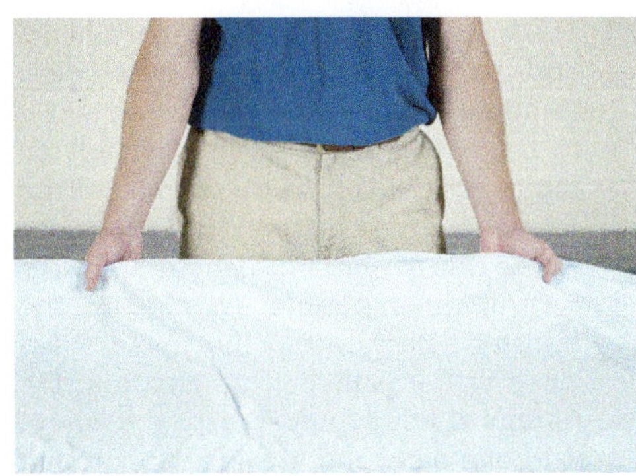

2. When patients are unable to control the head and neck, the person standing at the patient's head supports the patient's head by placing one arm under the patient's shoulders while cradling the patient's head.

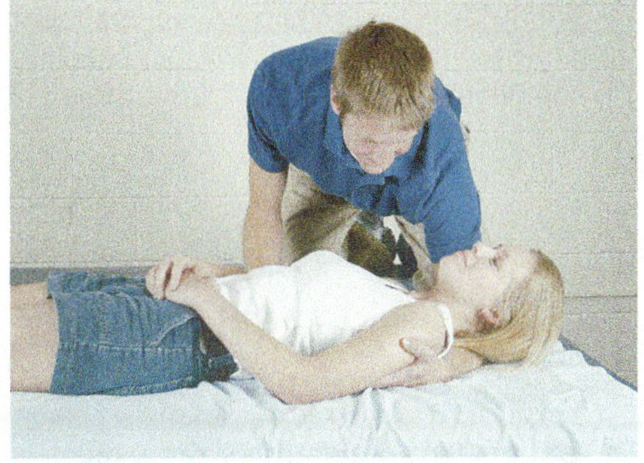

3. When a patient's extraneous movements cannot be controlled during a transfer activity, or if a patient is agitated, a sheet wrapped around the patient can be used to provide control of the patient's extremities.

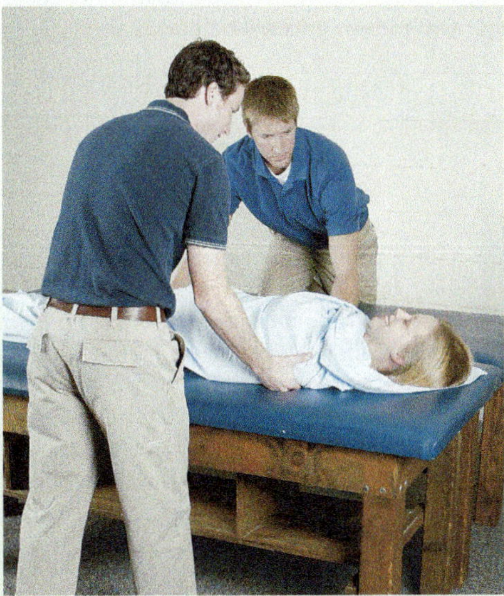

(continued)

PROCEDURE 9–1 Sliding Transfer Activity: Cart to Treatment Table (*continued*)

4. Two people, one at the patient's head, and the other at the lower extremities, stand on the side to which the patient is to be moved. A third person stands on the opposite side. The person who will be supporting the patient's head should be on the side to which the patient is moving.

   All three people assisting in the transfer activity grasp the rolled sheet close to the patient. The person at the patient's head may grasp the sheet with one hand and provide support and control of the patient's head by encircling the patient's head and shoulders with the other arm. When the two people on the side to which the patient is to be moved are not able to reach across the treatment table to lift the patient, they may kneel on the treatment table to which the patient is to be transferred.

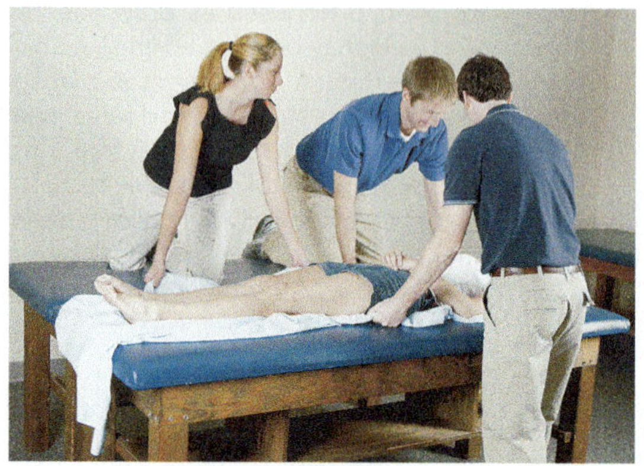

5. On the counts and verbal cues of the person coordinating the transfer, the patient is lifted and moved from the cart toward the treatment table. In some cases a patient will be able to be transferred from the cart to the table in one movement. In other cases, two movements will be necessary.

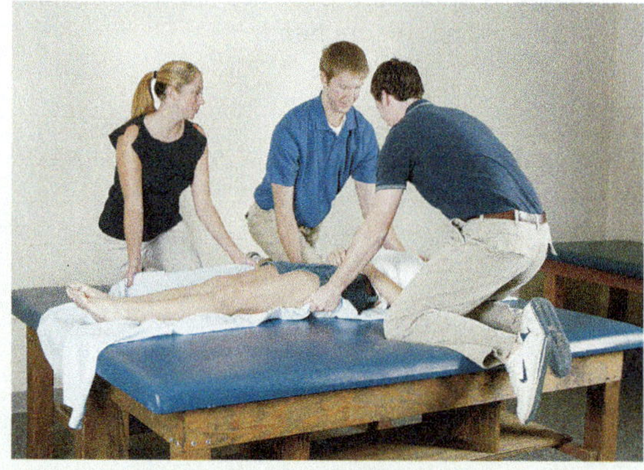

6. If the patient cannot be moved all the way from the cart to the table in one motion, the patient is rested after part of the transfer activity is performed. While the patient is rested in this position, the people on the side to which the patient is being moved start to remove themselves from the treatment table, and the person on the side from which the patient is being moved may kneel on the cart to complete the transfer. The transfer is completed by finishing movement of the patient to the treatment table and ensuring that the patient is safe in the new position.

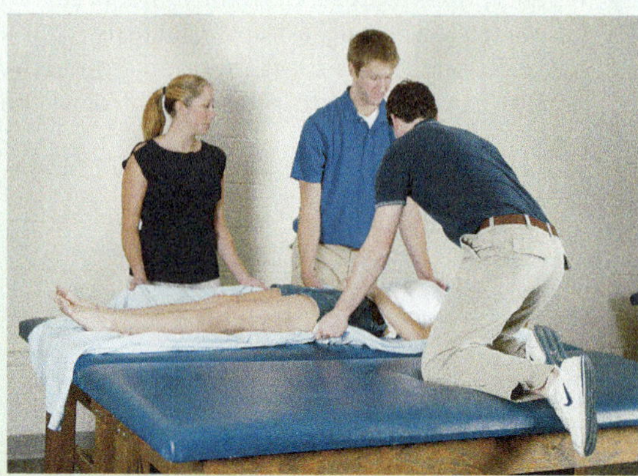

Three-Person Carry Transfer Activity

When two surfaces cannot be arranged parallel to each other, or a sliding transfer is deemed unsafe, a three-person carry is used. A three-person carry, a dependent transfer, is another method to transfer a patient between two treatment tables, a treatment table and cart, or a cart and bed. As the name of the transfer implies, three people are required to transfer an average-size adult.

NOTE: In the following photos, two treatment tables are used. The first treatment table represents a cart or gurney and will be referred to as a cart. The second treatment table represents a treatment table or bed and will be referred to as a treatment table.

PROCEDURE 9–2 Three-Person Carry Transfer Activity

1. A cart is positioned and secured at a right angle to a treatment table, with the head of the cart at the foot of the table or the foot of the cart at the head of the table.

   All three people assisting with the transfer stand with their feet in stride, slightly apart, and knees flexed, on the same side of the cart. The three people are positioned so one person supports the patient's head and upper trunk, one person supports the patient's midsection, and one person supports the lower extremities. The strongest person should be at the patient's head or middle position, depending on distribution of the patient's weight.

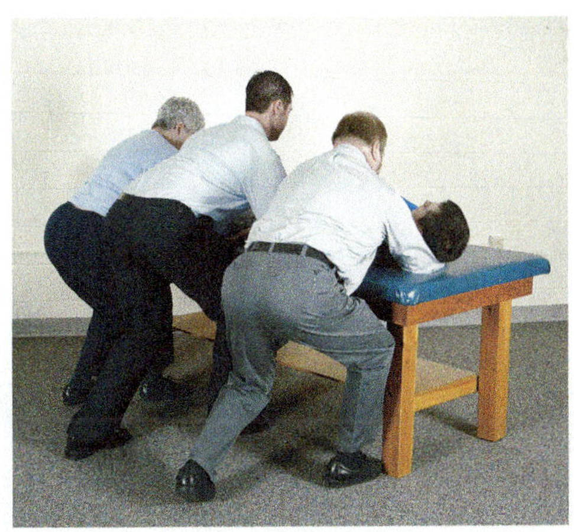

2. All three people assisting with the transfer slide their arms under the patient such that their elbows are on the cart, and the patient is cradled from head to foot.

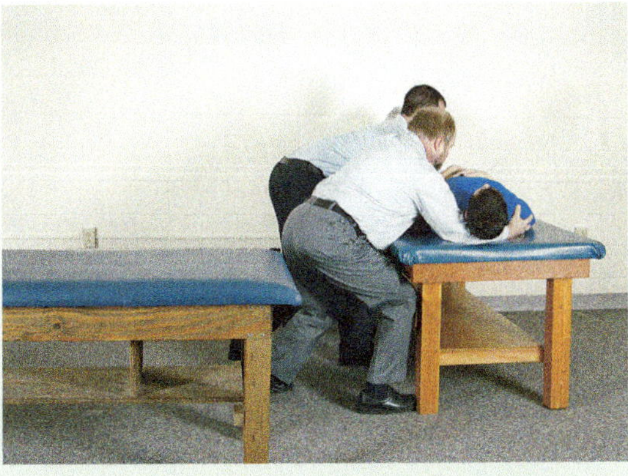

(continued)

PROCEDURE 9–2 Three-Person Carry Transfer Activity (*continued*)

3. Using proper body mechanics, move the patient to the edge of the cart when the verbal cue "move" is given.

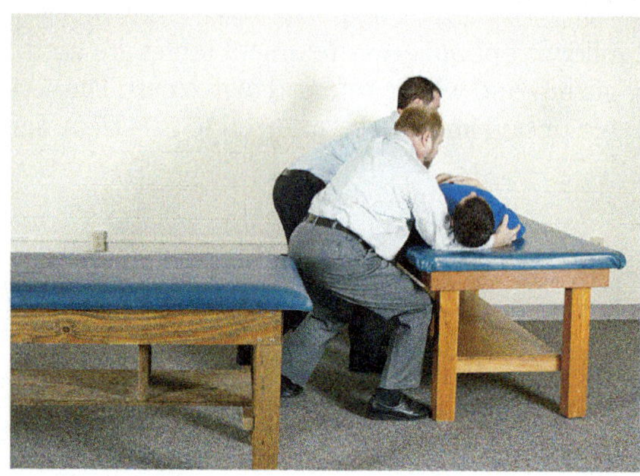

4. Flex your elbows to logroll the patient toward you when the verbal cue "roll" is given. The patient is now cradled in the bend of everyone's elbows, bringing the patient's weight closer to the base of support of the people assisting in the transfer.

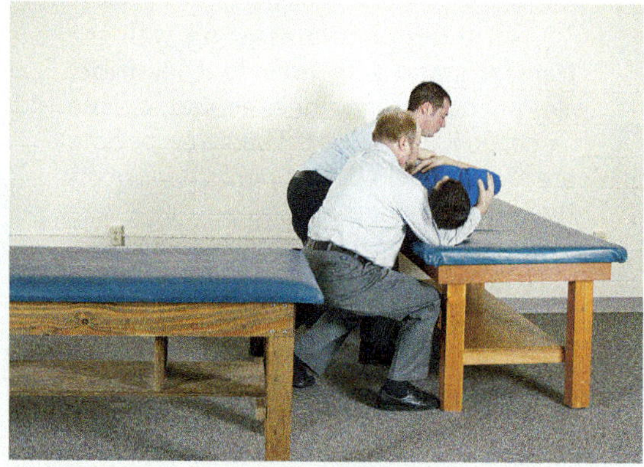

5. Using proper body mechanics, on the verbal cue "lift," stand and lift the patient from the cart.

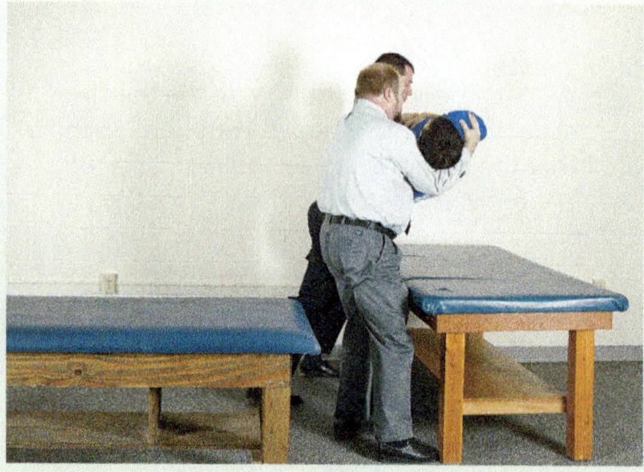

6 On the verbal cue "pivot," walk backward while pivoting the patient 90 degrees. On completion of the 90-degree pivot, the patient is aligned parallel to the treatment table, and the persons performing the transfer activity are in line facing the treatment table.

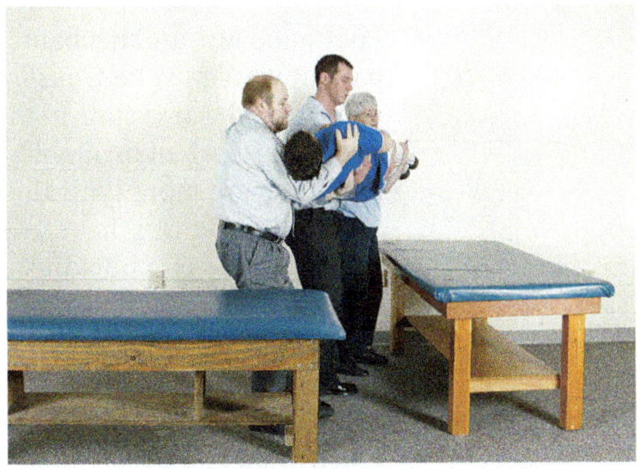

7 On the verbal cue "forward," move forward in unison to the treatment table. When at the edge of the treatment table, stand in stride with the feet slightly apart.

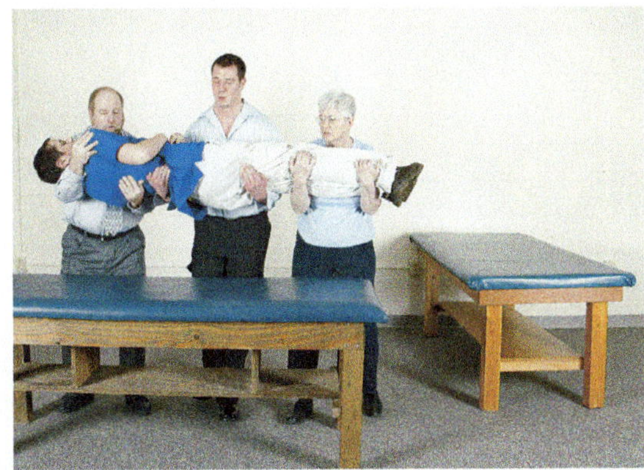

8 On the verbal cue "lower," flex your lower extremities, lowering the patient to the treatment table. Rest your elbows on the edge of the treatment table.

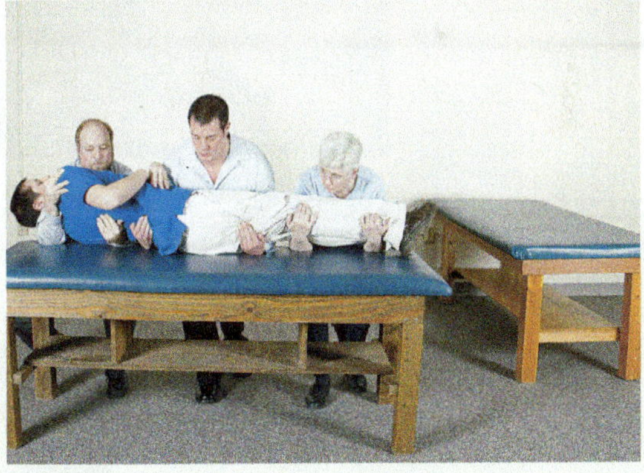

9 On the verbal cue "unroll," uncradle the patient onto the treatment table. Move the patient to the center of the treatment table, and position in proper alignment. Remove your arms carefully.

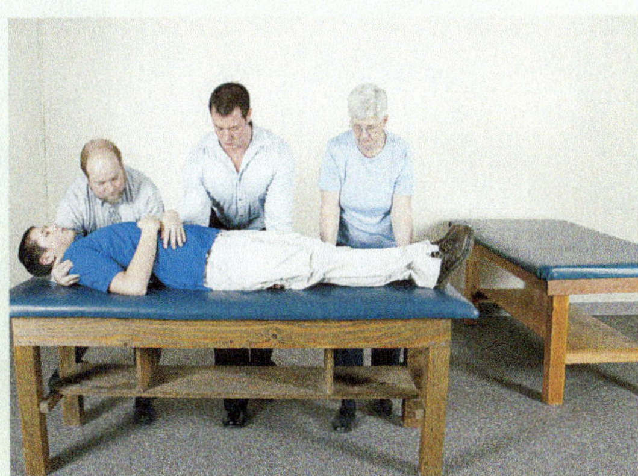

Hydraulic Lift Transfer Activity

Hydraulic lifts are mechanical devices that provide a method for one person to transfer a patient who must be transferred dependently. The term *hydraulic* is derived from the use of fluid under pressure to move the arm of a lift. Facilities use power-operated hydraulic patient lifts when available, particularly for bariatric patients. Patient hydraulic lifts for home use are more typically manually operated.

Hydraulic lifts have caster wheels for positioning and maneuvering. The base of hydraulic lifts can be adjusted to a widened position to fit around a wheelchair or other equipment. The base is placed in the narrow position when the patient is being moved to make maneuvering easier. To change the width of the base, the long lever attached to the base is moved from one side to the other (**Figures 9–7** ■ and **9–8** ■). This lever is locked by either a slotted mechanism at the bottom of the lever, or by a cam locking mechanism that is activated and deactivated by twisting the lever.

A hydraulic release valve (**Figure 9–9** ■) on the front of the lift's upright is closed to allow the arm of the hydraulic lift to be raised and opened slowly to allow lowering of the

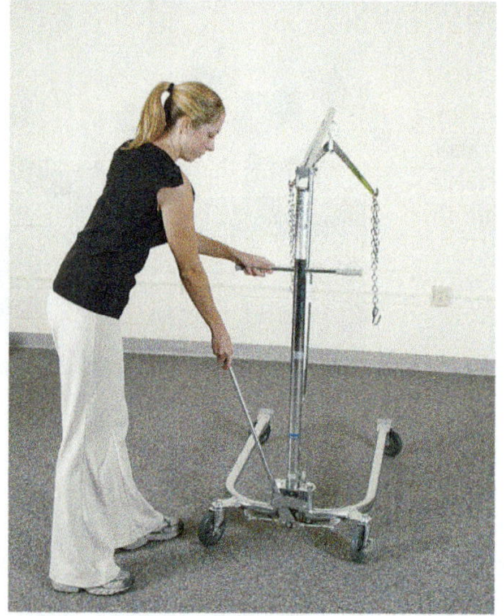

FIGURE 9–7 ■ Narrowing the base of a hydraulic lift.

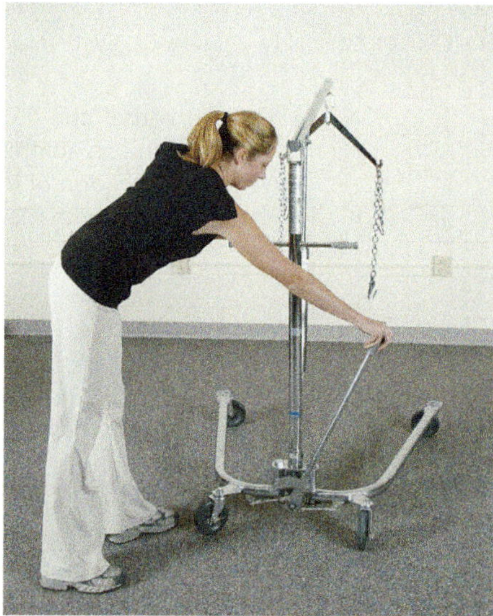

FIGURE 9–8 ■ Widening the base of a hydraulic lift.

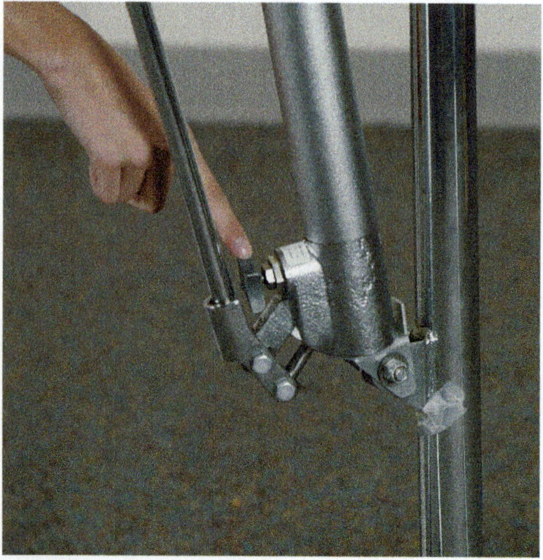

FIGURE 9–9 ■ Hydraulic release valve knob for lift arm.

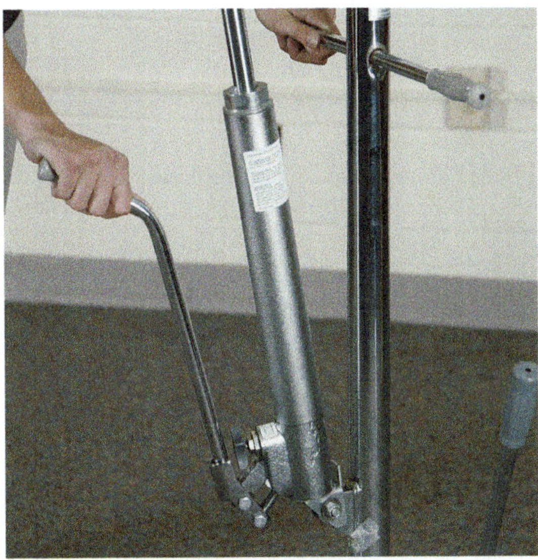
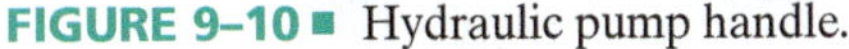

FIGURE 9–10 ■ Hydraulic pump handle.

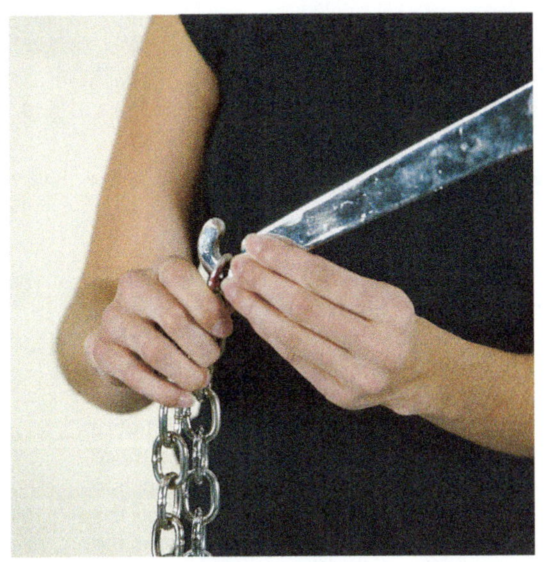

FIGURE 9–11 ■ Attaching chains to spreader bar.

lift arm. After checking that the hydraulic release valve is closed, pump the handle to raise the arm of the hydraulic lift (Figure 9–10 ■).

Patients are supported by a sling, which is attached to a spreader bar on the lift arm by two chains with hooks (Figure 9–11 ■). Slings are made of a variety of fabrics. Some slings are one piece, others are two pieces, and some slings also provide head support. Position slings so seams are on the outside, away from the patient, to avoid pressure areas.

Chain lengths may be adjusted to accommodate the height of individual patients. The chains are attached to each side of the spreader bar such that each chain is divided into two unequal segments, approximately one-third and two-thirds, respectively. The shorter segment will be attached to the upper part of the sling, supporting the patient's back. The longer segment will be attached to the lower part of the sling, supporting the patient's lower extremities. In this way, when a patient is lifted, he or she is in a sitting position. Chain hooks are attached from the inside of the sling to the outside (Figure 9–12 ■). This reduces the likelihood of patients being injured by the hook.

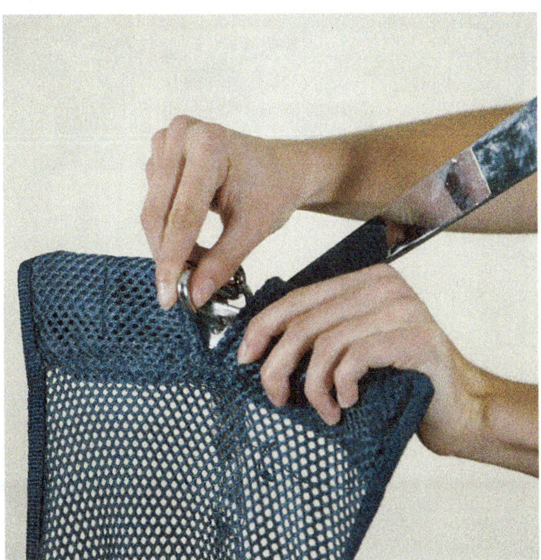

FIGURE 9–12 ■ Attaching chain hooks to sling.

PROCEDURE 9–3 Hydraulic Lift Transfer Activity

The wheelchair for this transfer activity is positioned with wheels locked before patient/sling positioning is initiated.

1. Position a sling under the patient by rolling the patient onto one side and properly positioning the sling on the treatment table. Proper positioning of the sling depends on the type of sling (one- or two-piece and with or without head support), proportions of the patient's height, and size of the sling. With a one-piece sling without head support, the upper section of the sling is positioned at approximately the upper thoracic area, and the distal edge of the lower section of the sling should not extend into the popliteal fossa.

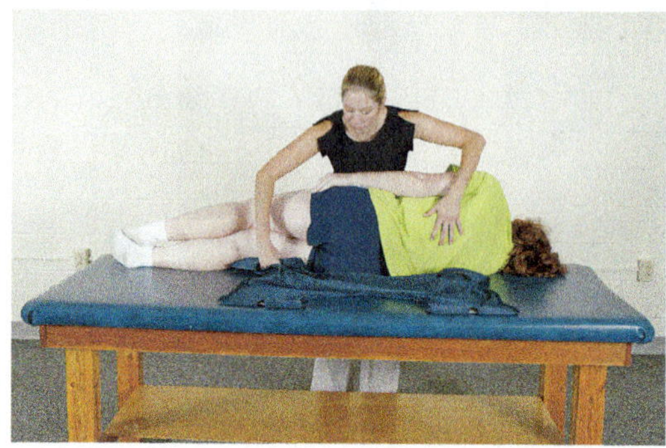

2. Roll the patient onto the patient's other side, smoothing the fabric of the sling to allow proper positioning of the sling. Roll the patient to a supine position on the sling.

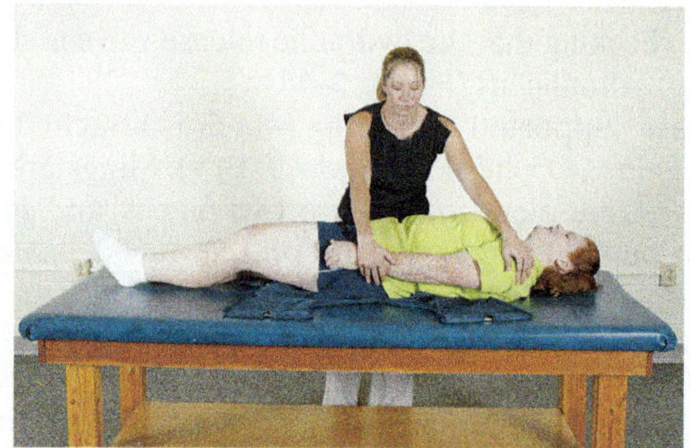

3. Once the patient is positioned on the sling, move the hydraulic lift into position with the spreader bar and chains suspended across the patient, being careful not to strike the patient with either the spreader bar or chains. Both ends of each chain are attached to their respective sides of the sling.

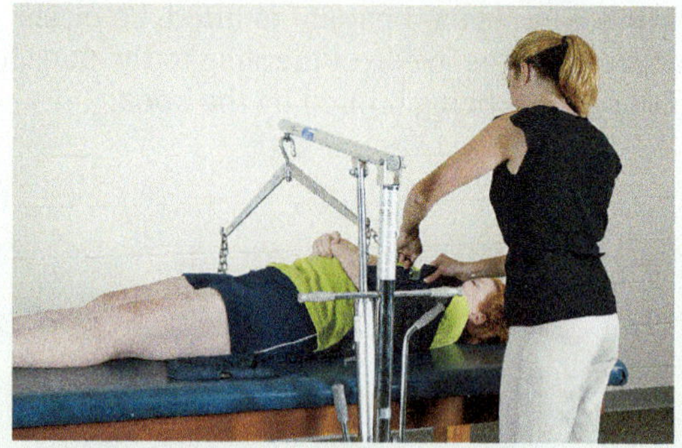

4. With the hydraulic release valve closed, pump the handle to lift the patient to a safe sitting position.

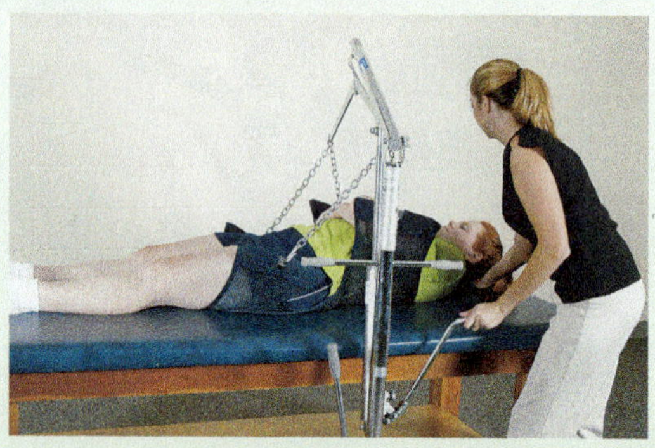

5 As the patient' torso is lifted above the treatment table, place an arm under the patient's lower extremities to lift the legs from the treatment table.

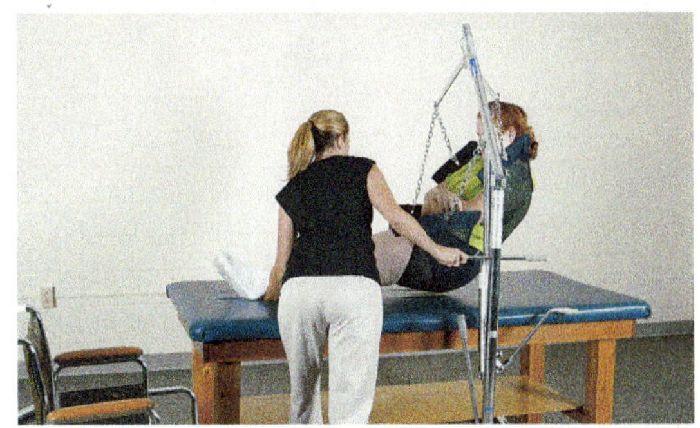

6 Cradling the patient's lower extremities, rotate the lower extremities so they are over the side, and clear, of the treatment table.

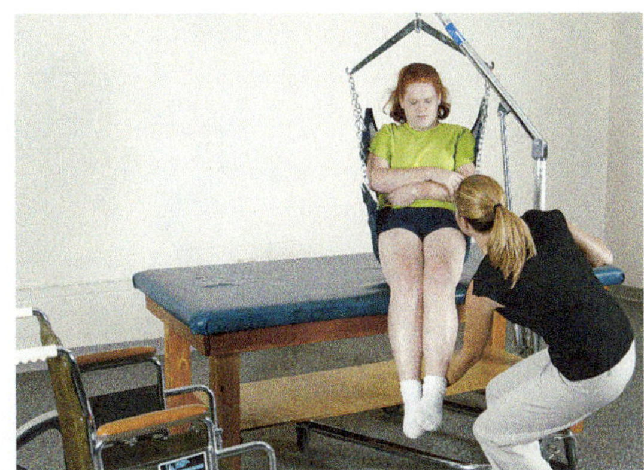

7 You may need to steady the patient to prevent excessive sway as the hydraulic lift, with patient, is maneuvered. Move the patient to a locked wheelchair, and place the base of the hydraulic lift in the wide position to fit around the perimeter of the wheelchair.

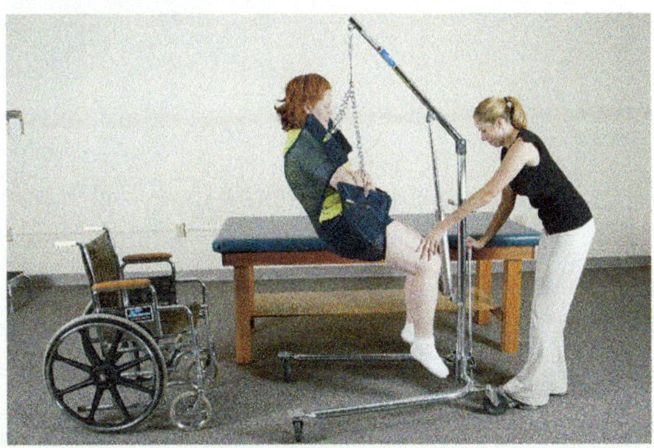

8 Maneuver the hydraulic lift to position the patient directly over the seat of a locked wheelchair, with the patient facing in the proper orientation before starting to lower the patient.

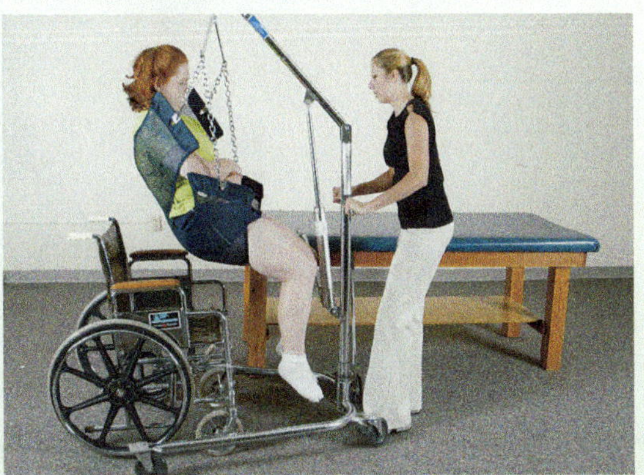

(continued)

PROCEDURE 9–3 Hydraulic Lift Transfer Activity (*continued*)

9. Slowly open the hydraulic release valve to lower the patient into the wheelchair. Seating a patient properly in a wheelchair requires the application of slight pressure at the knees or thighs toward the back of the wheelchair. This positions the patient into the wheelchair such that the patient is positioned fully into the wheelchair.

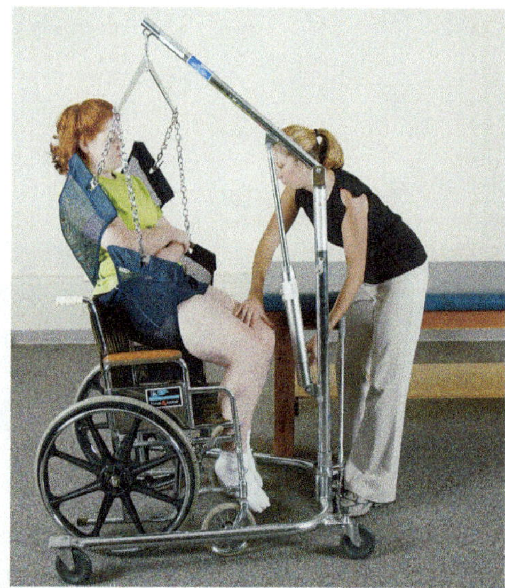

10. Once the patient is seated in the wheelchair, close the hydraulic release valve to avoid the potential of the hydraulic lift arm lowering further and striking the patient.

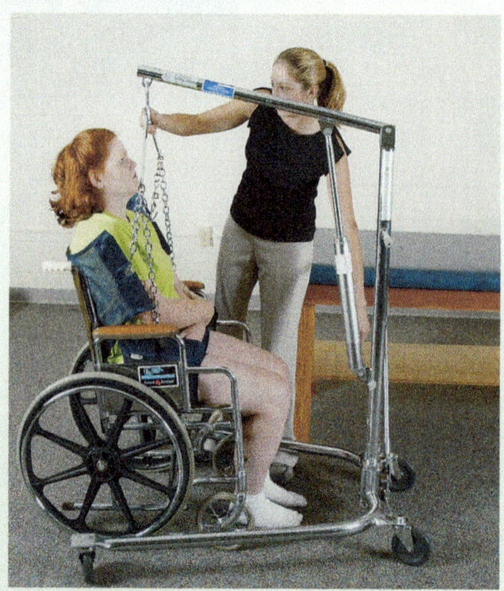

11 After determining that a patient can maintain sitting without assistance, remove the chains from the sling and move the hydraulic lift away from the patient. Hold the chains and spreader bar to reduce the potential that they might swing and strike the patient as the hydraulic lift is removed.

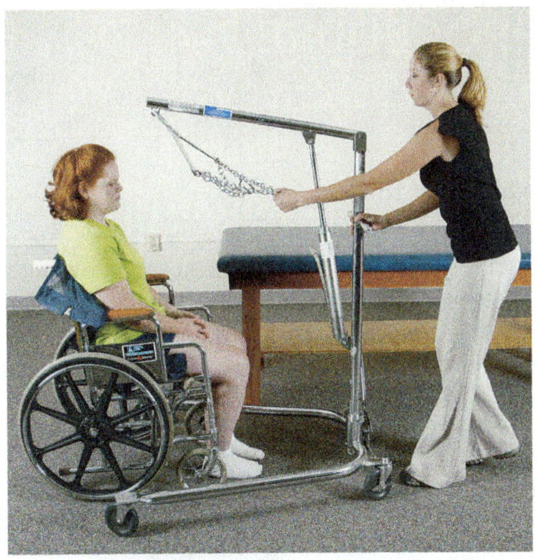

12 A one-piece sling is left in place under the patient, hence the initial need to position a sling appropriately to avoid pressure from the seams. When a two-piece sling is used, the upper portion of the sling, which is behind the patient's back, may be removed, whereas the portion under the patient's thighs remains in place.

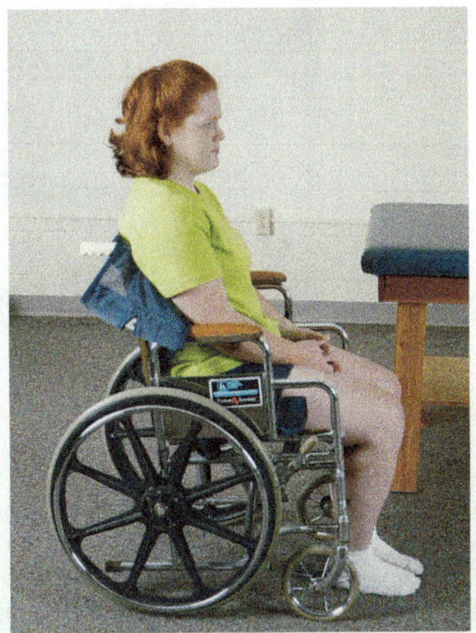

13 Secure the wheelchair's pelvic stabilizer, and properly place the patient's feet on the wheelchair footrests.

Two-Person Lift Transfer Activity

A two-person lift, a dependent transfer requiring maximum assistance of two persons, can be used to move a patient between two surfaces that are significantly different in height. When the height difference between surfaces is minimal, other transfer activities may be more appropriate.

A patient participates in this transfer by crossing the upper extremities in front of the trunk. Patients must be able to maintain an upper extremity position of shoulder girdle depression, shoulder extension, adduction, internal rotation, and elbow flexion at approximately 90 degrees to assist in successful completion of the transfer.

PROCEDURE 9–4 Two-Person Lift Transfer Activity

Wheelchair to Floor

1. Position the wheelchair close, and parallel, to the surface to which the patient will be transferred. Engage the wheel locks. Remove the patient's feet from the footrests, raise the footplates, and remove the footrests or swing the footrests out of the way. Remove the armrest from the side of the wheelchair to which the patient will be transferred.
2. The person at the head of the patient, standing behind the patient, reaches under the patient's upper extremities and grasps the opposite wrists of the patient (left on right and right on left). This prevents the patient from abducting the upper extremities during the transfer activity.

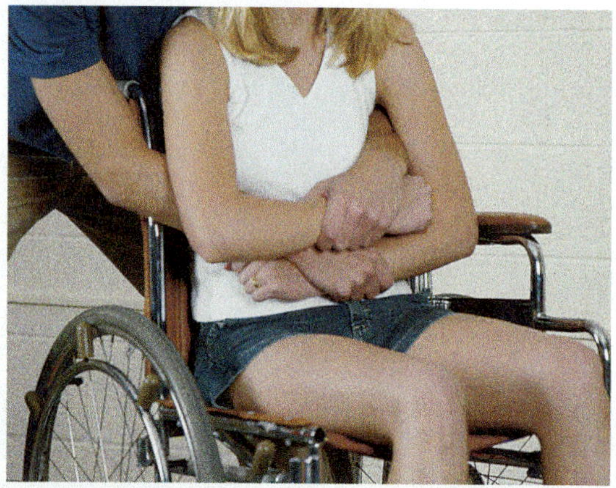

3. The person at the head of the patient places one foot on either side of the drive wheel and leans around the push handle on the side to which the transfer will occur.

   A second person faces in the direction of the intended transfer activity and squats with feet in stride. Although starting in a half-kneeling position may seem easier for the second person, starting in a half-kneeling position necessitates movement into a squatting position, increasing the risk of injury to all participants. This person places one arm under the patient's thighs and the other arm under the patient's legs.

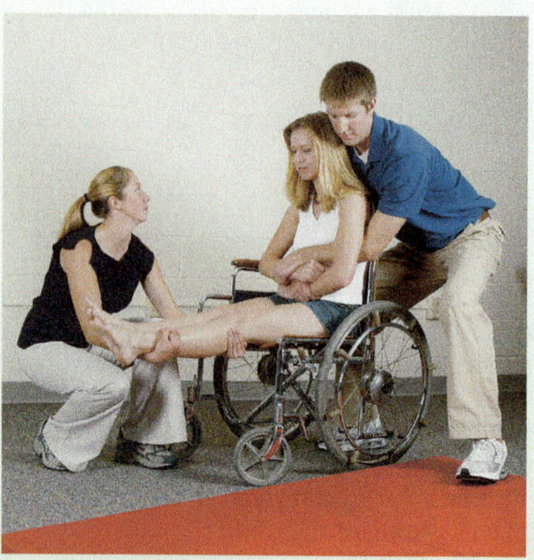

4. On the verbal cue "lift," using proper body mechanics, both people simultaneously rise and lift the patient to a height that ensures clearance of all parts of the wheelchair.

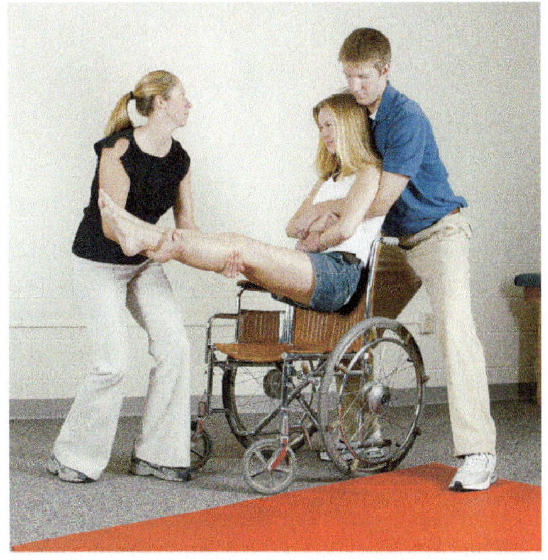

5. On the verbal cue "move," both people move in unison. The person at the patient's head steps to the side, and the person supporting the patient's lower extremities steps forward to position the patient over the floor mat. While lifting and moving, the person supporting the patient's lower extremity may also pull the patient's lower extremities away from the wheelchair to assist in clearing the patient's torso from the wheelchair.

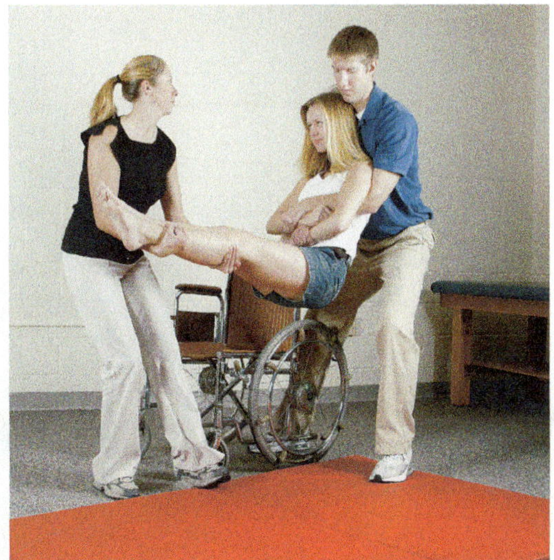

6. On the verbal cue "lower," using proper body mechanics squat and lower the patient to the floor.

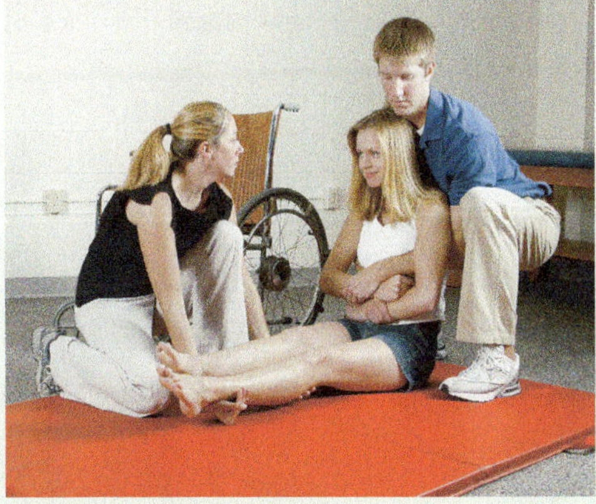

7. Continue contact with the patient for support until the patient is able to maintain a safe and comfortable position.

(continued)

PROCEDURE 9–4 Two-Person Lift Transfer Activity (*continued*)

Floor to Wheelchair

1. Position the wheelchair close, and parallel, to the surface to which the patient will be transferred. Engage the wheel locks. Raise the footplates, and remove the footrests or swing the footrests out of the way. Remove the armrest from the side of the wheelchair to which the patient will be transferred.
2. Squatting behind the patient with feet in stride and slightly apart, the person at the patient's head reaches under the patient's upper extremities and grasps the opposite wrists of the patient (left on right and right on left). This prevents the patient from abducting the upper extremities during the transfer activity.
3. A second person faces in the direction of the intended transfer activity, squatting with feet in stride. Although starting in a half-kneeling position may seem easier for the second person, starting in a half-kneeling position necessitates movement into a squatting position, increasing the risk of injury to all participants. The second person places one arm under the patient's thighs and the other arm under the patient's legs.

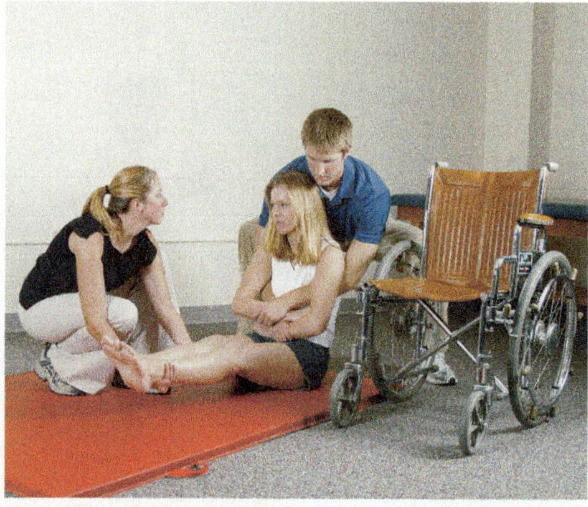

4. On the verbal cue "lift," using proper body mechanics, both people rise simultaneously and lift the patient to a height that ensures clearance of all parts of the wheelchair.

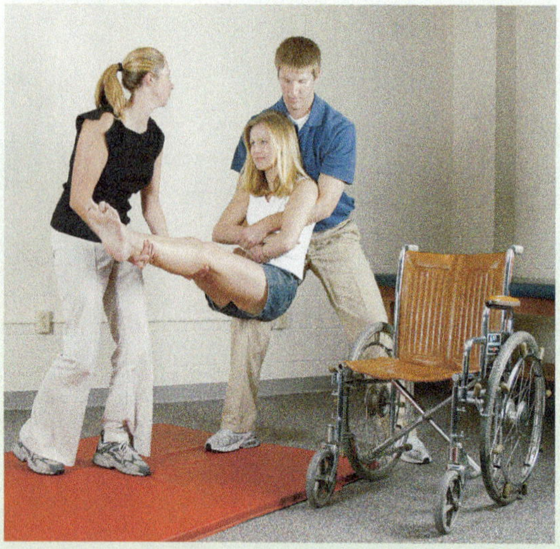

5 On the verbal cue "move," both people move in unison. The person at the patient's head steps to the side, and the person supporting the patient's lower extremities steps forward to position the patient over the wheelchair seat. While moving and lifting, the person supporting the patient's lower extremities may also pull the patient's lower extremities away from the wheelchair to assist in clearing the patient's torso from the wheelchair.

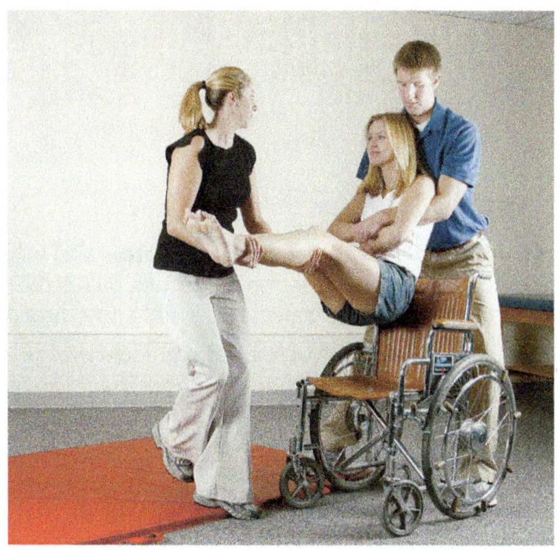

6 On the verbal cue "lower," use proper body mechanics to lower the patient into the wheelchair. While lowering the patient, the person supporting the patient's lower extremities may also push the patient's lower extremities toward the back of the wheelchair so the patient is appropriately seated on the wheelchair seat.

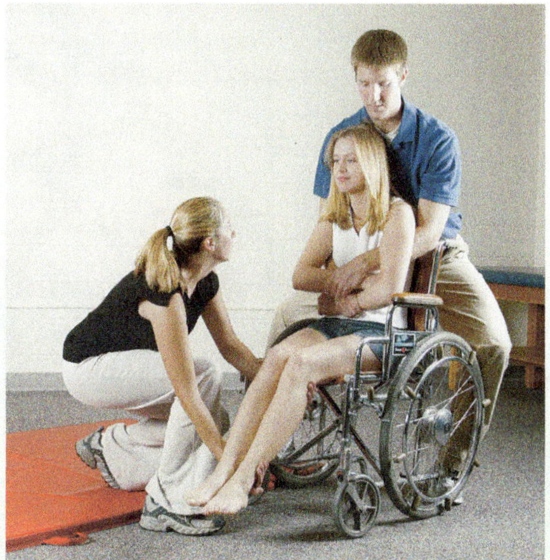

7 Continue contact with the patient for support until the patient is able to maintain a safe and comfortable position.

Assist to Front of Seat Transfer Activity

A patient must be able to maneuver to the front of any seat, including a wheelchair seat, couch, bed, or treatment table, prior to standing or performing transfer activities. Sitting on the front of a seat allows patients to move their center of gravity over their base of support, placing their force directly downward, rather than backward or to the side, as they perform the transfer activity. Being positioned on the front of a wheelchair seat also provides better clearance of a wheelchair's drive wheels when performing transfer activities to the side.

When patients are unable to maneuver forward on a seat independently, several methods can be used to assist. As a patient's ability improves, assistance is reduced until the patient is performing the transfer activity independently.

PROCEDURE 9–5 Assist to Front of Seat Transfer Activity

Side-to-Side Weight Shifting

1. Position the wheelchair appropriately, and engage the wheel locks. Remove the patient's feet from the footplates, raise the footplates, place the patient's feet on the floor, and remove the footrests from the wheelchair when possible, or swing them out of the way.
2. Standing in front of the patient and in stride, place one arm around the patient's shoulders from one side and the other arm under the thigh of the opposite lower extremity.
3. Shift the patient's weight away from the supported lower extremity.

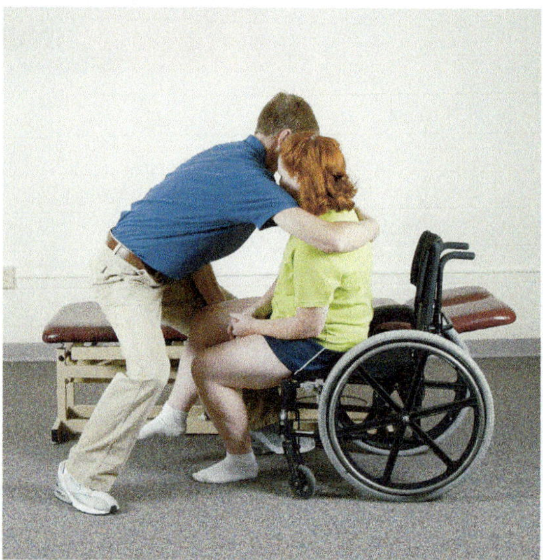

4. While the thigh and buttock are unloaded, assist the patient to move the unloaded thigh and buttock forward.

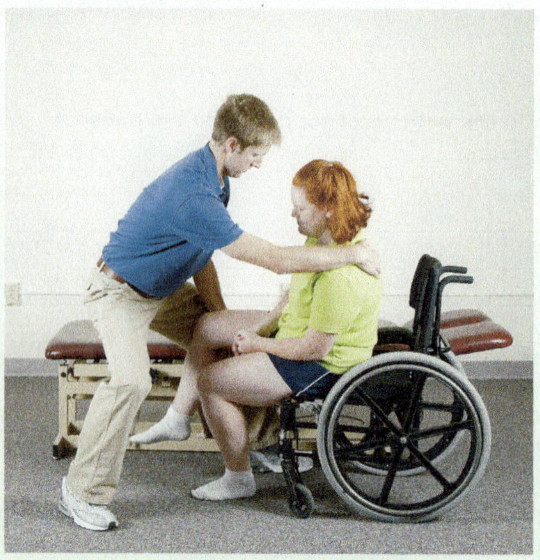

5. Return the supported lower extremity to the wheelchair seat as the patient returns to an erect sitting position.

6. Reverse your arm positions. Repeat steps 2–6, alternating sides, until the patient is properly positioned at the front of the wheelchair seat. You must continue contact for support until a patient is able to maintain a safe and comfortable position.

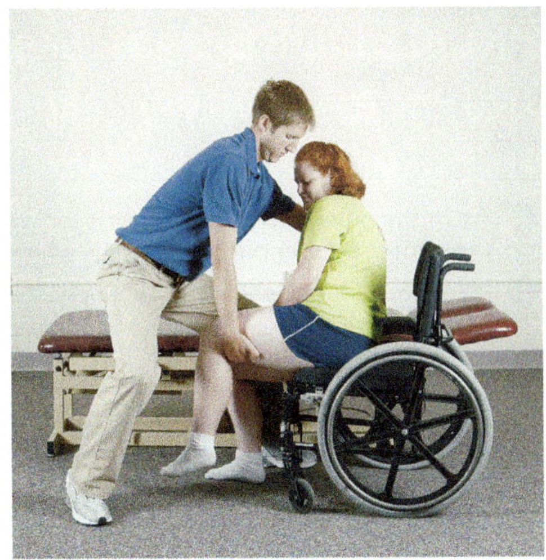

Pelvic Slide

1. Position the wheelchair appropriately, and engage the wheel locks. Remove the patient's feet from the footplates, raise the footplates, place the patient's feet on the floor, and remove the footrests from the wheelchair or swing them out of the way.

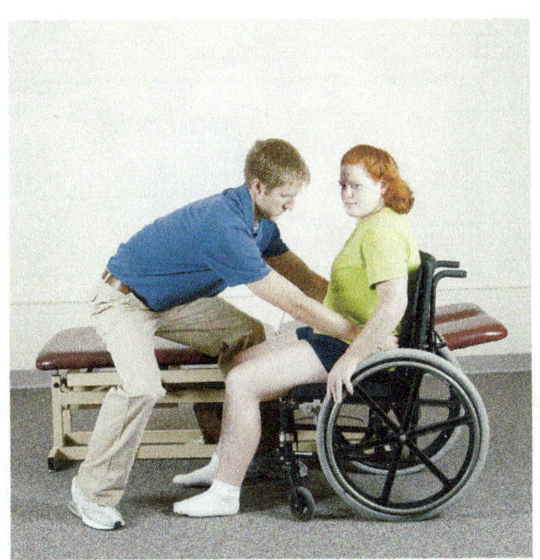

2. Standing in front of the patient and in stride, squat to place both hands behind the patient's pelvis to assist the patient in moving the pelvis forward.

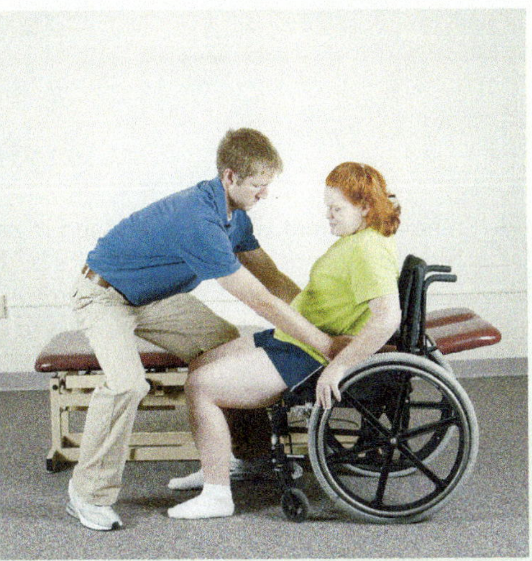

(continued)

PROCEDURE 9–5 Assist to Front of Seat Transfer Activity (*continued*)

3. Assist the patient to slide the pelvis forward toward the front of the wheelchair seat while keeping the patient's upper back against the wheelchair back.
4. Place your hands behind the patient's shoulders to assist the patient in moving the trunk and head forward so the patient can assume an erect sitting position.

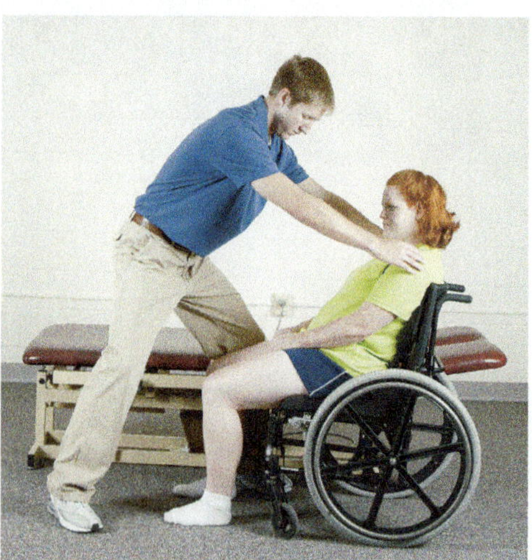

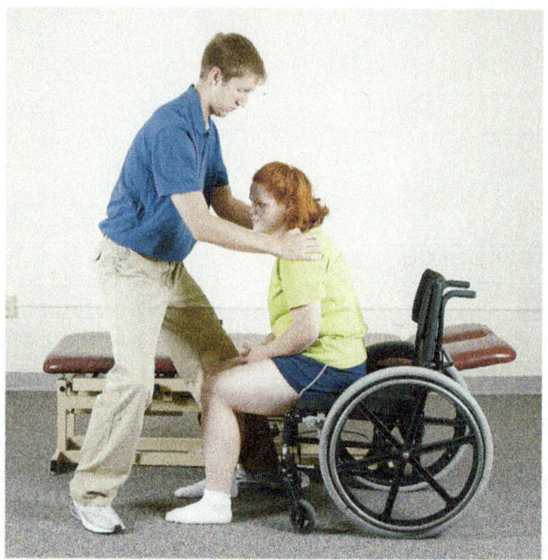

5. Continue contact for support until the patient is able to maintain a safe and comfortable position.

Sitting Push-Up

1. Position the wheelchair appropriately, and engage the wheel locks. Remove the patient's feet from the footplates, raise the footplates, place the patient's feet on the floor, and remove the footrests from the wheelchair when possible, or swing them out of the way.
2. Standing in front of the patient and in stride, place both hands under the patient's buttocks to assist the lift as the patient performs a push-up, or behind the patient's pelvis to assist the patient in moving the pelvis forward.

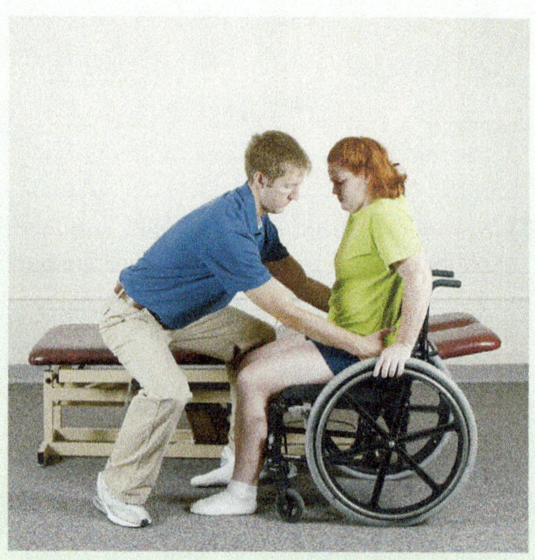

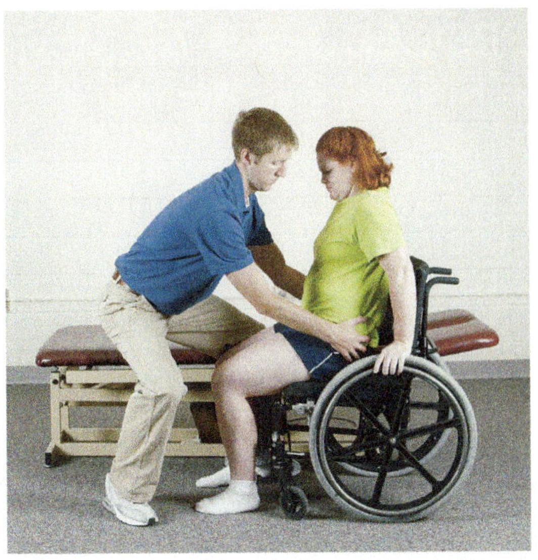

3 As the patient performs the push-up, provide the assistance the patient needs in moving the pelvis forward toward the front of the wheelchair seat.

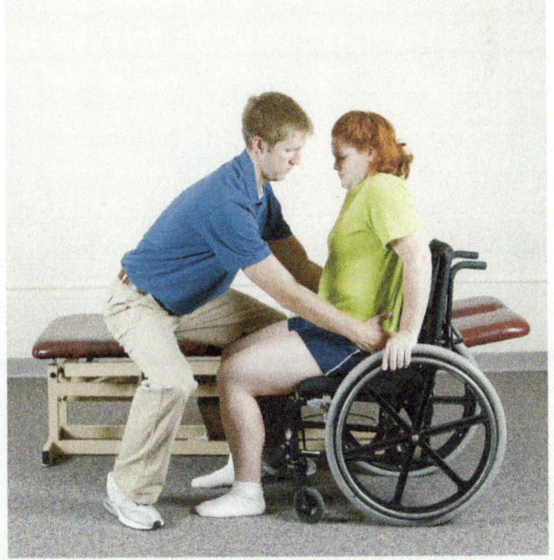

4 Each time the patient lowers to the wheelchair seat, it is closer to the front of the wheelchair seat.

5 Repeat steps 2–4 until the patient is properly positioned at the front of the wheelchair seat.

6 Continue contact to maintain support until the patient is able to maintain a safe and comfortable position.

Moving from Front of Seat Transfer Activity

When patients sit on the front of a seat, including wheelchair, couch, bed, or treatment table and are unable to move more completely onto the seating surface, you can assist by using a reversal of the side-to-side weight shifting or push-up maneuvers used to move a patient forward on a seat. Guard against a patient sliding off the front of the seat as the patient's weight is shifted.

PROCEDURE 9–6 Moving from Front of Treatment Table Transfer Activity

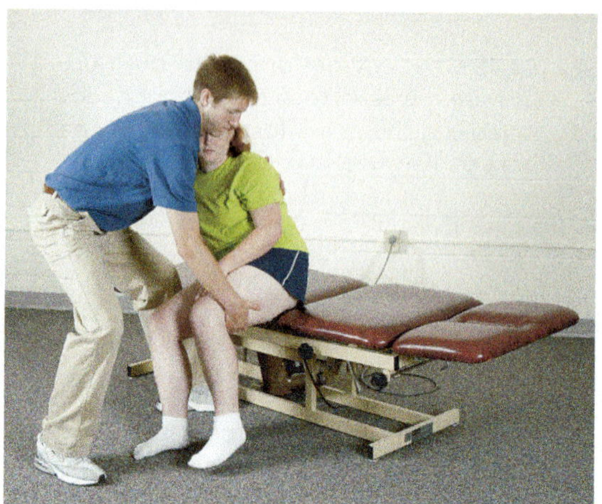

1. Standing in front of the patient and in stride, place one arm around the patient's shoulders from one side and the other arm under the thigh of the opposite lower extremity.
2. Shift the patient's weight away from the supported lower extremity.

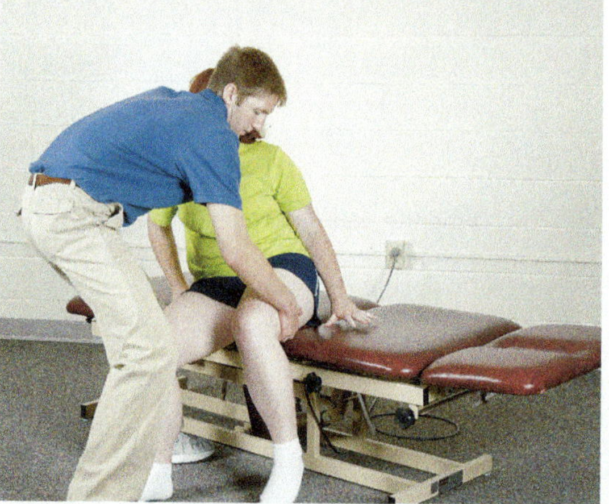

3. While the thigh and buttock are unloaded, assist the patient to move the unloaded thigh and buttock backward.
4. Return the supported lower extremity to the treatment table as the patient returns to an erect sitting position.

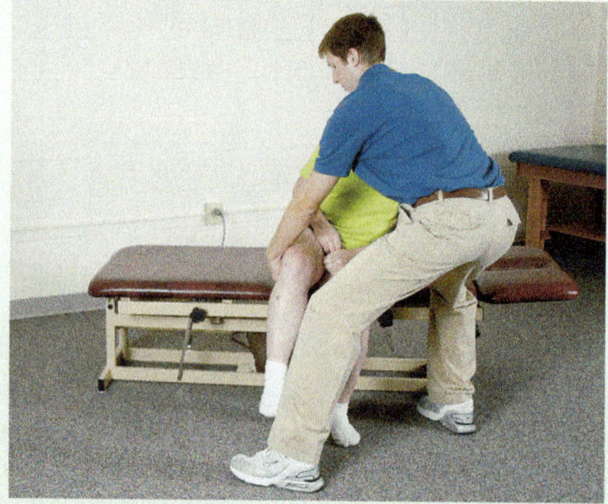

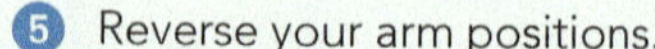

5. Reverse your arm positions.
6. Repeat steps 1–5, alternating sides, until the patient is properly positioned on the treatment table, or at the back of the wheelchair seat.
7. Continue contact for support until the patient is able to maintain a safe and comfortable position.

Dependent Standing Pivot Transfer Activity

The dependent standing pivot transfer activity is an assisted transfer requiring the maximum assistance of one person. The dependent standing pivot transfer can be used to move patients unable to stand independently, but who can bear some weight through their lower extremities, including patients with weakness, paresis, or paralysis. This transfer activity can be used with patients whose weight, stature, and impairments, and the size and strength of the person assisting in the transfer activity, allow safe, effective, and efficient movement.

PROCEDURE 9–7 Dependent Standing Pivot Transfer Activity

1. Place the wheelchair adjacent and parallel to a treatment table or bed, and engage the wheel locks. Remove the patient's feet from the footplates, raise the footplates, place the patient's feet on the floor, and remove the footrests from the wheelchair when possible, or swing them out of the way. Remove the armrest nearest the treatment table.
2. Move the patient to the front of the wheelchair seat to facilitate clearing the wheel.
3. Provide stability for the patient's lower extremities during the transfer activity by "blocking" the patient's lower extremities. Blocking the lower extremities is performed in different ways for different transfer activities. In this transfer activity, block the patient's knees by placing your feet and knees outside the patient's feet and knees. Thus the patient's knees are held between your knees by squeezing your knees together. When transferring from a wheelchair to treatment table, place your foot that is closest to the treatment table a little behind your other foot, which places you in stride.
4. Patients may rest their head on your shoulder. The patient's head may be rested on either shoulder. When the patient's head is placed on the side toward which the transfer activity will occur, the patient will be able to see the space/surface to which she is moving. When the patient's head is placed on the side away from which the transfer activity will occur, the physical therapist/assistant will be able to see the space/surface to which he is moving. The choice of head placement is part of clinical decision making.

    Alternatively, patients may place their upper extremities around your upper back, but *not* around your neck. The purpose of the placement of the patient's arms in this method is to provide control for the patient's upper trunk, and not for the patient to "pull" on you.

    After blocking the patient's lower extremities, place your hands under the patient's buttocks.

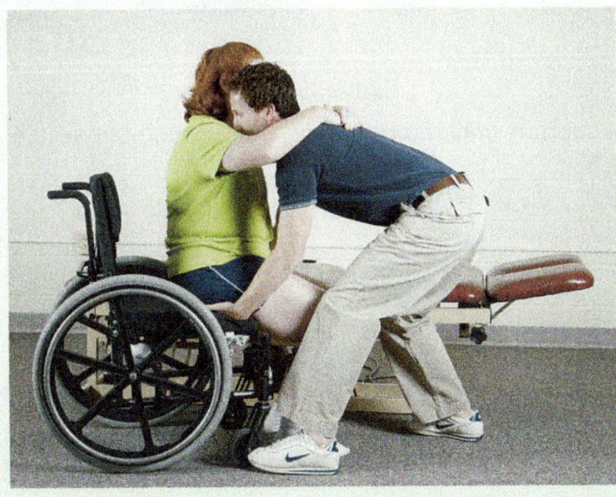

(continued)

PROCEDURE 9–7 Dependent Standing Pivot Transfer Activity (*continued*)

5 Initiate a rocking motion to develop momentum on the count "one, two, three."

6 On the verbal cue "up," use proper body mechanics to lift the patient from the wheelchair. The lift should only be high enough to clear the wheelchair and the height of the treatment table.

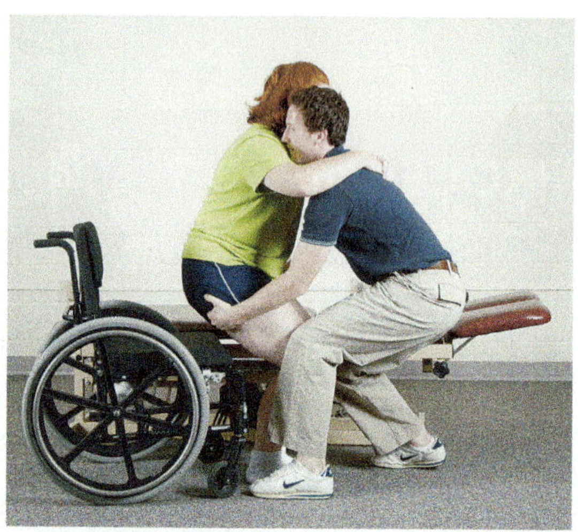

7 On the verbal cue "pivot," pivot toward the treatment table, rotating the patient. As the patient reaches a position over the treatment table, lower the patient to a sitting position.

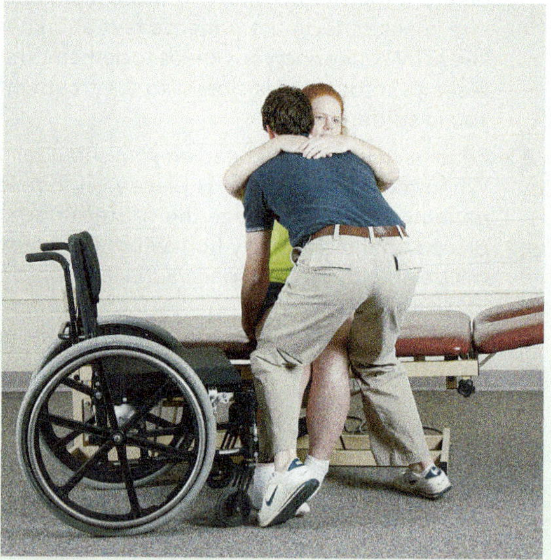

8 Continue contact for support until the patient is able to maintain a safe and comfortable position.

Dependent Sitting Pivot Transfer Activity

The dependent sitting pivot transfer activity is a variation of the dependent standing pivot transfer activity. The dependent sitting pivot transfer activity is used for patients who are unable to stand independently, but can bear some weight on their lower extremities. This includes patients with weakness, paresis, or paralysis. Patients must have sufficient range of motion that permits full flexion of the trunk on the thighs.

PROCEDURE 9–8 Dependent Sitting Pivot Transfer Activity

1. Position the wheelchair close, and parallel, to the surface to which the patient will be transferred. Engage the wheel locks. When moving out of a wheelchair, remove the patient's feet from the footrests, raise the footplates, and remove the footrests or swing the footrests out of the way. When moving into a wheelchair, raise the footplates and remove the footrests or swing the footrests out of the way. Remove the armrest from the side of the wheelchair to which the patient will be transferred.
2. To facilitate clearing the wheelchair drive wheel, move the patient to the front of the wheelchair seat.
3. Stand in front of the patient and in stride. When transferring from a wheelchair to a treatment table, place your foot closest to the treatment table a little behind your other foot, and one foot on either side of the patient's lower extremities.
4. To provide stability for the patient's lower extremities during the dependent sitting pivot transfer activity, "block" the patient's lower extremities. Blocking the lower extremities is performed in different ways for different transfer activities. Block the patient's lower extremities by placing your feet and knees outside the patient's feet and knees, squeezing the patient's knees between your knees.
5. Have the patient flex forward, resting the head and upper body on the legs, or on your thigh on the side opposite the direction in which the pivot will occur.

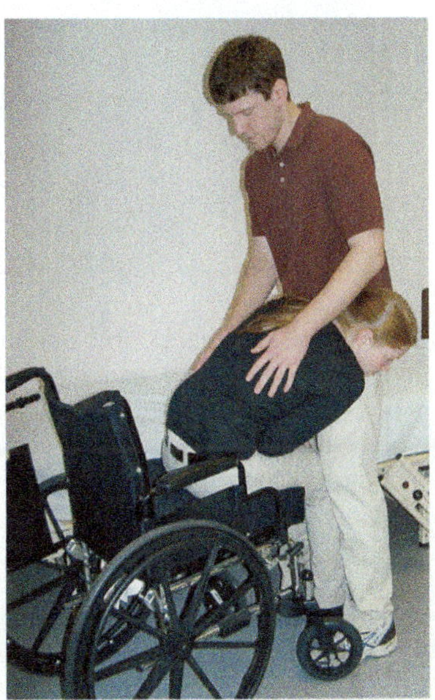

6. Place your hands under the patient's buttocks.

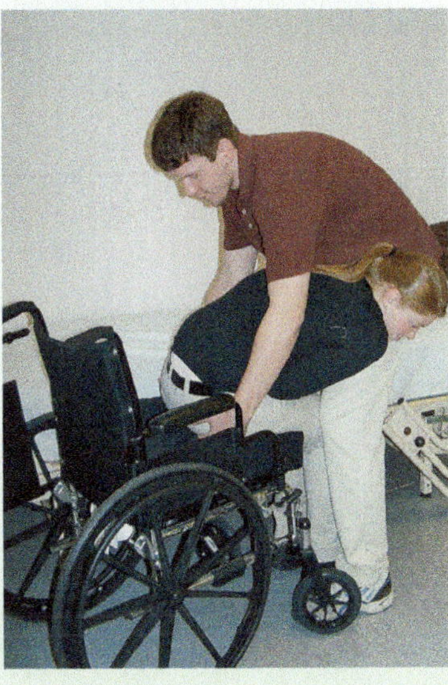

(continued)

PROCEDURE 9–8 Dependent Sitting Pivot Transfer Activity (*continued*)

7. Initiate a rocking motion to develop momentum on the count "one, two, three."

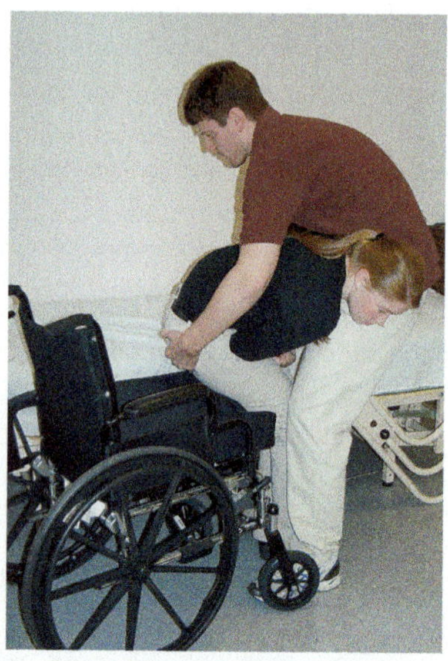

8. On the verbal cue "up," use proper body mechanics to lift the patient from the wheelchair. The lift should only be high enough to clear the wheelchair and the height of the treatment table.

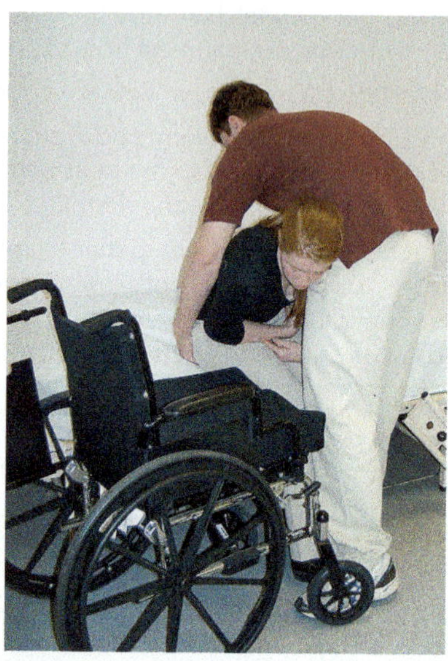

9. On the verbal cue "pivot," pivot toward the treatment table, rotating the patient. As the patient reaches a position over the treatment table, lower the patient to a sitting position.

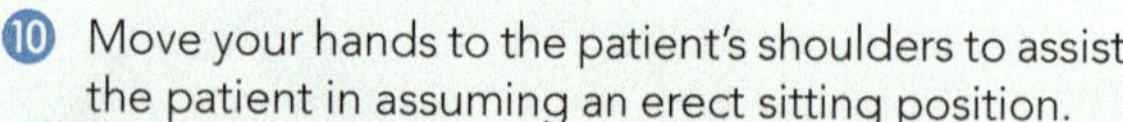

10. Move your hands to the patient's shoulders to assist the patient in assuming an erect sitting position.

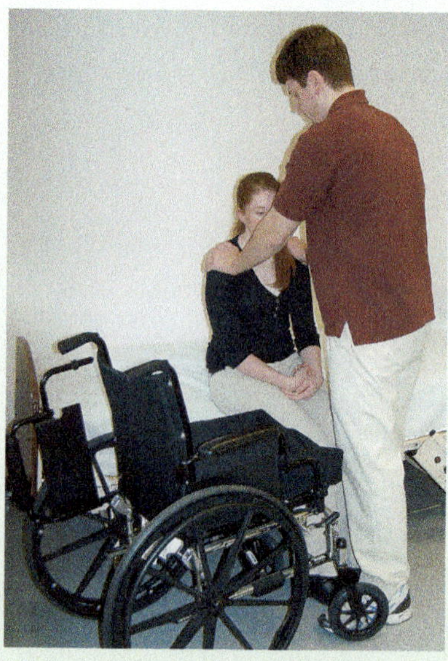

11. Continue contact for support until the patient is able to maintain a safe and comfortable position.

Squat Pivot Transfer Activity

The squat pivot transfer activity is an assisted transfer activity that requires minimal assistance of one person. The squat pivot transfer activity is used when patients can sit, stand, pivot, and bear weight on the lower extremities, but need physical assistance and verbal cues to perform the transfer activity safely.

When transferring between two adjacent surfaces, attaining a fully erect standing position is not always necessary.

PROCEDURE 9–9 Squat Pivot Transfer Activity

1. Place a wheelchair parallel, or at a slight angle, to the treatment table or bed, and engage the wheel locks. Raise the footplates, and remove the footrests from the wheelchair or swing them out of the way. Remove the armrest on the side of the wheelchair to which the patient will transfer.

2. With the patient seated toward the front of the treatment table, seat yourself on a stool in front of the patient. Block both of the patient's thighs by squeezing them between your knees. Place both of your hands on the posterolateral lower thoracic region.

   Assist the patient to perform an anterior pelvic tilt and extension of the upper back while the patient shifts weight forward onto her feet. This results in the patient being in proper position to rise from the treatment table.

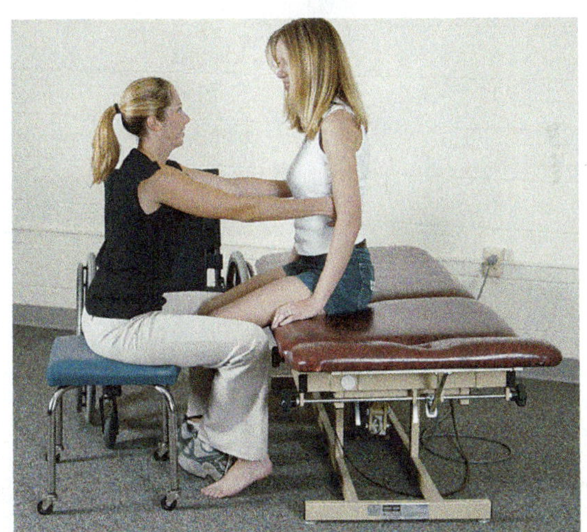

3. Without coming to a complete standing position, the patient rises and pivots toward the wheelchair. When not able to move directly to the wheelchair, the patient can perform an intermediate movement to a new position on the treatment table.

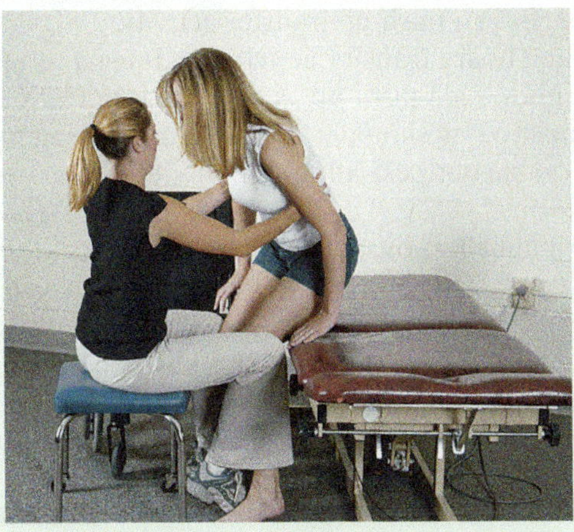

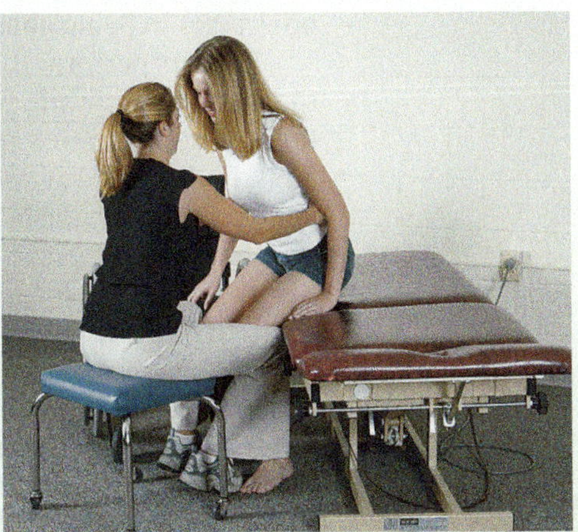

(continued)

PROCEDURE 9–9 Squat Pivot Transfer Activity (*continued*)

4. The patient repeats the sequence until seated in the wheelchair. As a patient's capabilities progress, the patient may be able to complete the transfer activity in one pivot movement.

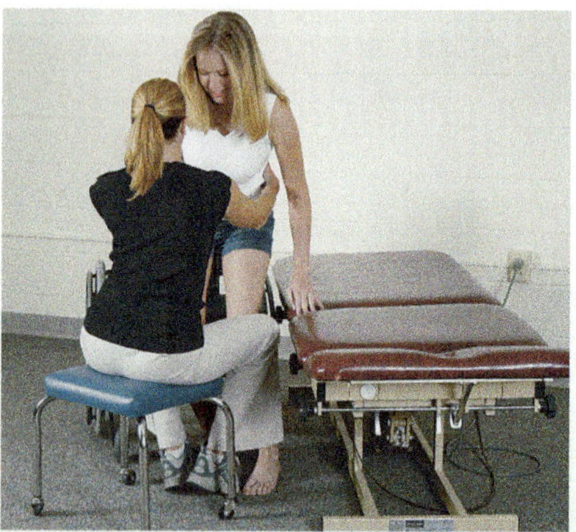

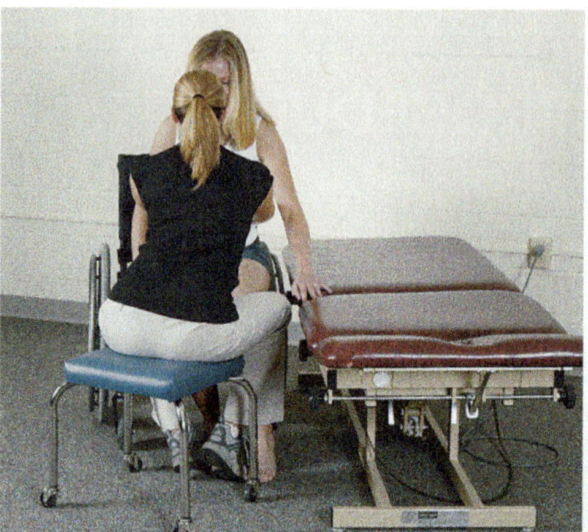

5. Continue contact to support the patient until the patient is able to maintain a safe and comfortable position.

Sliding Board Transfer Activity

The sliding board transfer activity is an assisted or independent transfer activity that may require moderate or no assistance. The sliding board transfer activity is used when patients have enough strength to lift most of the weight off the buttocks and sufficient sitting balance to move in a sitting position, but are not able to perform a push-up transfer activity. The sliding board transfer activity can be used as an intermediate activity as the patient progresses to being able to perform a push-up transfer activity.

Patients perform the sliding board transfer activity by doing a series of push-ups, and sliding sideways while performing each push-up. A push-up is performed by extension of the upper extremities accompanied by shoulder depression, allowing patients to lift their body. Reducing body weight on the buttocks allows a patient to slide toward the treatment table during each push-up.

Patients may place their palms flat on the sliding board, grasp the armrest or drive wheel of the wheelchair, or make a fist and place the outside of their fist on the sliding board to achieve higher lift during push-ups. Patients must not grasp the edge of the sliding board, which places the distal ends of fingers under the sliding board, causing fingers to be pinched as push-ups are performed. The upper extremity on the side to which the patient will transfer must be placed slightly away from the patient's body. In this way the patient can move along the sliding board without this upper extremity limiting sideways movement on the sliding board.

NOTE: In the illustrations presenting the sliding board transfer activity, assistance is being provided for balance.

PROCEDURE 9–10 Sliding Board Transfer Activity

Wheelchair to Treatment Table

1. Position a wheelchair parallel, or at a slight angle, to a treatment table or bed, and engage the wheel locks. Remove the patient's feet from the footrests, raise the footplates, and remove the footrests or swing the footrests out of the way. Remove the armrest from the side of the wheelchair to which the patient will transfer.

   Have the patient move to the front of the wheelchair seat.

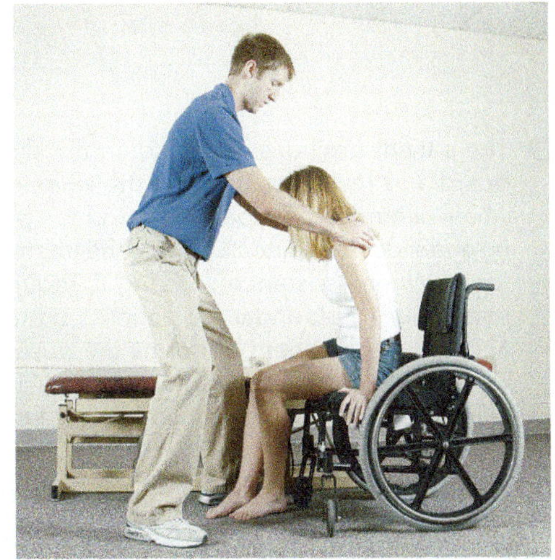

2. Assist the patient, when necessary, in placing a sliding board well under the buttocks. To place the sliding board, the patient leans to the side away from the treatment table. When leaning in this direction, the buttock on the side of the treatment table rises, making it possible to place the sliding board under the buttock. Ensure that the patient is not pinched between the sliding board and the wheelchair seat.

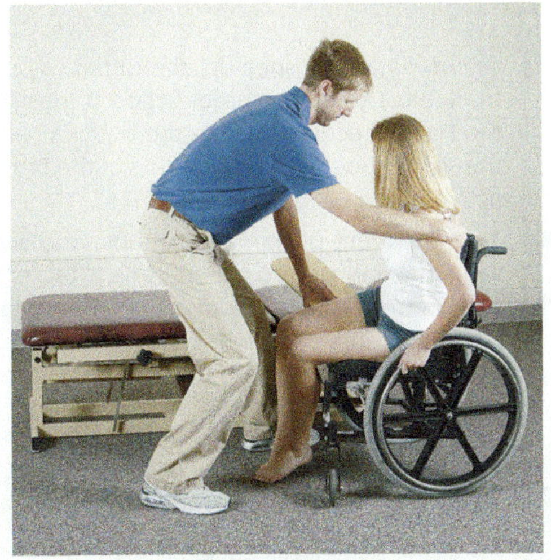

3. The patient returns to an upright sitting position, with the buttock nearest the treatment table resting on the sliding board. Guard the patient by standing in front of the patient and blocking the patient's knees if necessary to prevent the patient from sliding off the sliding board.

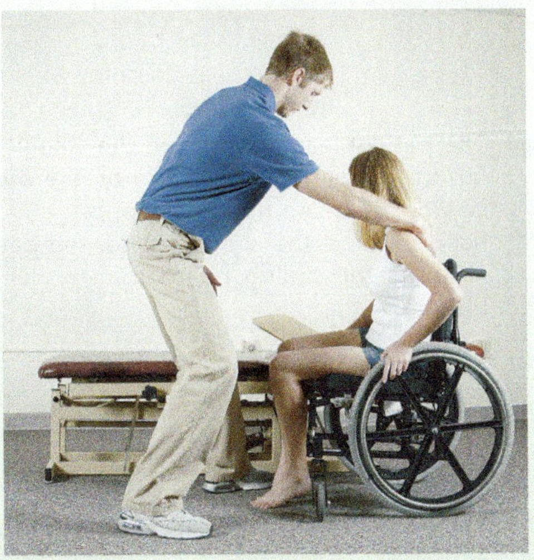

(continued)

PROCEDURE 9–10 Sliding Board Transfer Activity *(continued)*

4. The patient positions one hand on the sliding board and the other hand on the wheelchair wheel or armrest. The patient performs a push-up and slides the buttocks toward the treatment table. When assistance in lifting is required, place your hands under the patient's buttocks and lift as the patient performs the push-up. When a patient needs assistance for balance, place your hands on the patient's shoulders.

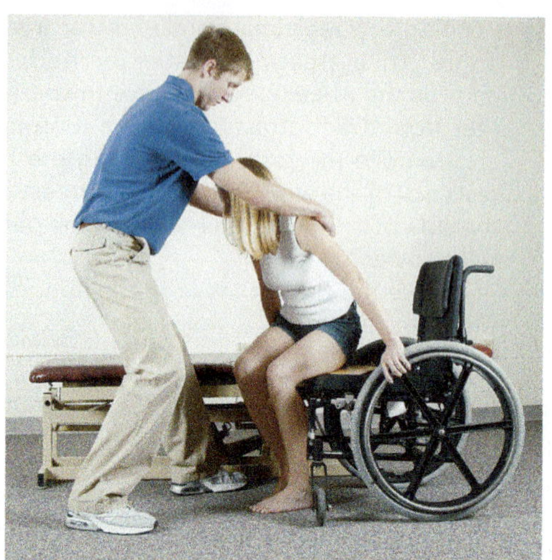

5. As the patient pushes up, the patient's upper trunk must rotate in the direction opposite to the transfer activity to slide the buttocks along the sliding board in the direction of the transfer activity.
6. As the patient performs push-ups, and slides while moving toward the treatment table, the arm on the side away from the treatment table pushes on the wheelchair wheel or armrest, the wheelchair seat, and eventually the sliding board. This sequence is repeated until the patient is on the treatment table and only one buttock remains on the sliding board.

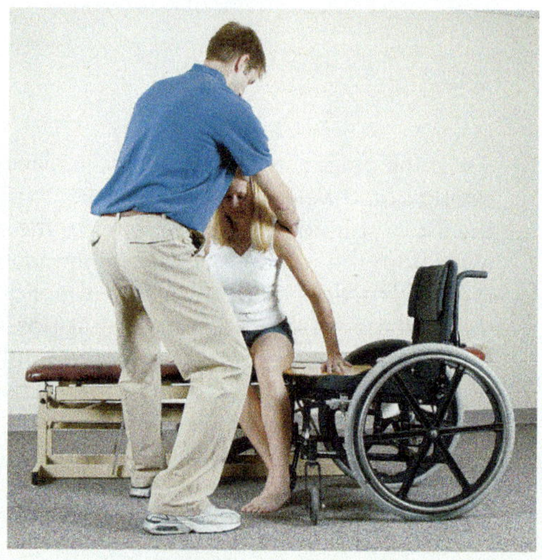

7. The patient leans away from the wheelchair, raising the buttock remaining on the sliding board. Using one hand for support, and one hand to move the sliding board, the patient removes the sliding board from under the buttock.

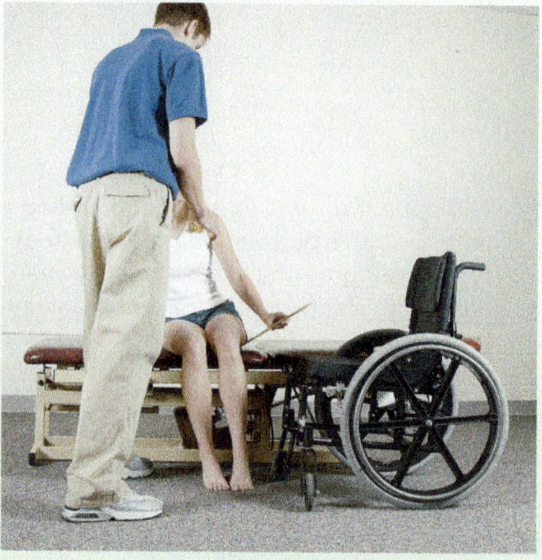

8. Continue contact to support the patient until the patient is able to maintain a safe and comfortable position.

Treatment Table to Wheelchair

The sliding board transfer activity from treatment table to the wheelchair using a sliding board is essentially the same as the wheelchair to treatment table sliding board transfer activity.

1. Position a wheelchair parallel, or at a slight angle, to a treatment table or bed, and engage the wheel locks. Raise the footplates, and remove the footrests or swing the footrests out of the way. Remove the armrest from the side of the wheelchair to which the patient will be transferred.
   Have the patient move to the front of the treatment table.

2. The patient leans away from the wheelchair, causing the buttock on the side of the wheelchair to rise. The patient then places the sliding board under the raised buttock and returns to an upright sitting position. Ensure that the patient is not pinched between the sliding board and the treatment table.

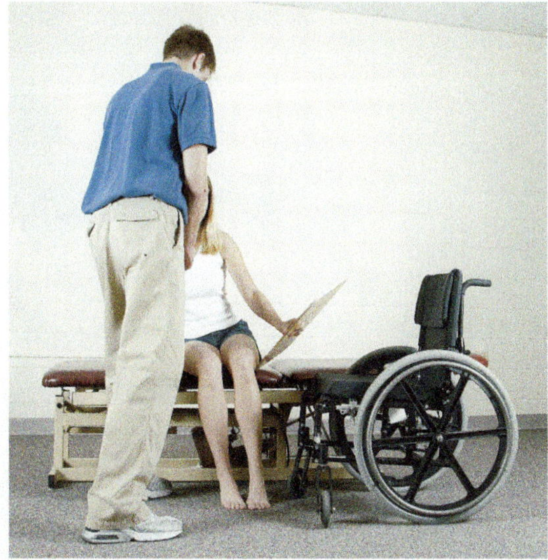

3. The patient positions one hand on the treatment table, and the other hand on the wheelchair wheel, or armrest, or sliding board. The patient performs a push-up and slides the buttocks toward the wheelchair. When assistance in lifting is required, place your hands under the patient's buttocks and lift as the patient performs the push-up. When a patient needs assistance for balance, place your hands on the patient's shoulders.

4. Using push-ups, the patient slides toward the wheelchair. As the patient reaches the wheelchair, the arm closest to the wheelchair pushes down on the wheelchair seat and then on the wheelchair drive wheel or armrest. As the patient pushes up, the patient's upper trunk must rotate in the direction opposite to the transfer activity to slide the buttocks along the sliding board in the direction of the transfer activity.

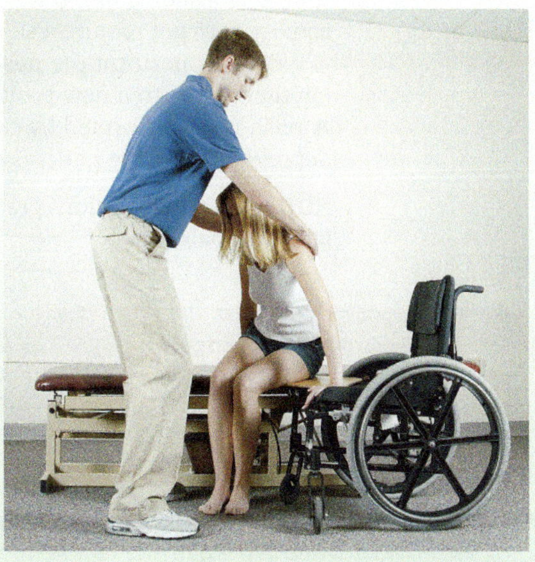

(continued)

PROCEDURE 9–10 Sliding Board Transfer Activity (*continued*)

5 Once the patient is seated over the chair, the sliding board is removed by having the patient lean away from the treatment table, which causes the buttock remaining on the sliding board to rise. Using one arm to maintain stability and one arm to move the sliding board, the patient removes the sliding board and returns to an erect seated position on the wheelchair seat.

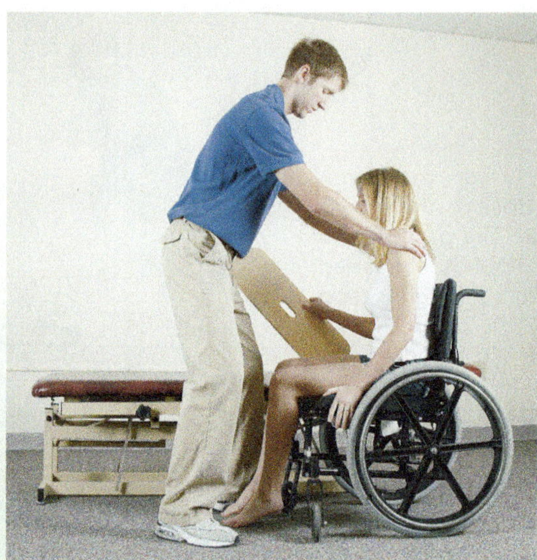

Push-Up Transfer Activity

The push-up transfer activity is an assisted or independent transfer activity that may require moderate assistance to no assistance. The push-up transfer activity is used when patients have enough strength to lift themselves from the supporting surface and sufficient sitting balance to move in a sitting position. A push-up transfer activity is performed in a manner similar to a sliding board transfer activity, except that performance of a push-up transfer activity does not require a sliding board.

Patients perform the push-up transfer activity by using a series of push-ups, lowering themselves to a new position in the direction of the transfer following each push-up. A push-up is performed by extension of the upper extremities accompanied by shoulder depression, allowing patients to lift their body from the supporting surface.

NOTE: In the illustrations presenting the push-up transfer activity, assistance is being provided for balance.

PROCEDURE 9–11 Push-Up Transfer Activity

Wheelchair to Treatment Table

1 Position a wheelchair parallel, or at a slight angle, to a treatment table or bed, and engage the wheel locks. Remove the patient's feet from the footrests, raise the footplates, and remove the footrests or swing the footrests out of the way. Remove the armrest from the side of the wheelchair to which the patient will be transferred. The patient moves to the front of the wheelchair seat.

2. Patients may place their palms flat on the supporting surface, grasp the armrest or drive wheel of the wheelchair, or make a fist and place the outside of their fists on the supporting surface to achieve the necessary lift height during push-ups. The upper extremity on the side to which the patient will transfer must be placed slightly away from the patient's body. In this way the patient moves toward the transfer destination without this upper extremity limiting sideways movement.
3. Guard the patient by standing in front of the patient. Block the patient's knees, if necessary, to prevent the patient from sliding forward. When assistance in lifting is required, place your hands under the patient's buttocks and lift as the patient performs the push-up. When a patient needs assistance for balance, place your hands on the patient's shoulders.
4. The patient performs push-ups and moves sideways to lower closer to, or on, the treatment table. As the patient pushes up, the patient's upper trunk must rotate in the direction opposite to the transfer activity to move the body in the direction of the transfer activity. As a patient's capabilities progress, a push-up transfer may be completed using only one push-up.

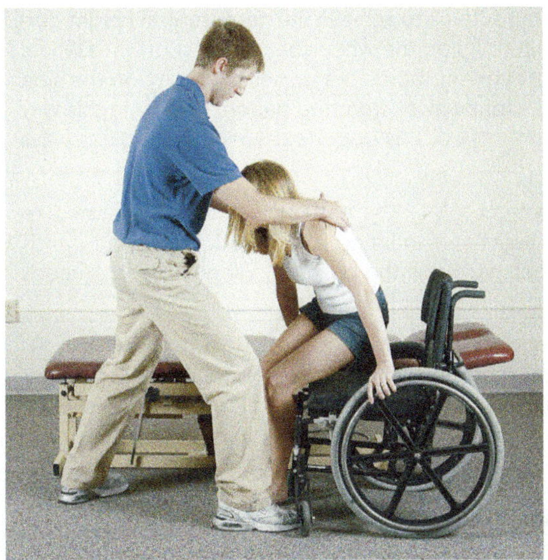

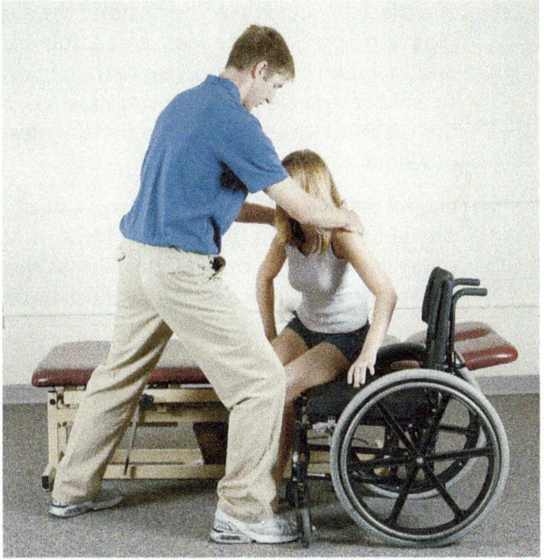

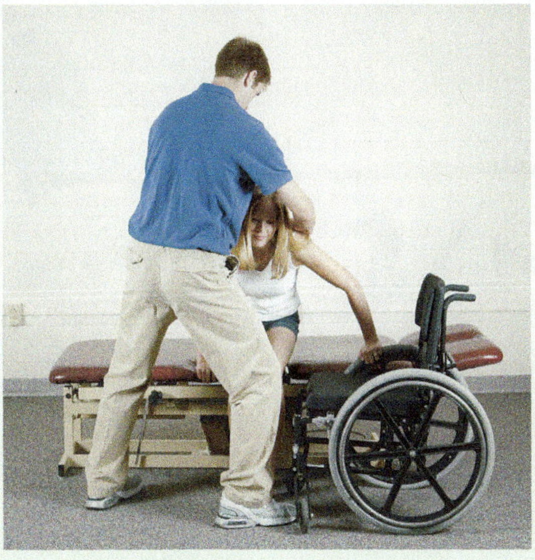

5. Continue contact to support the patient until the patient is able to maintain a safe and comfortable position.

(continued)

PROCEDURE 9–11 Push-Up Transfer Activity (*continued*)

Treatment Table to Wheelchair

A push-up transfer activity from treatment table to the wheelchair is essentially the same as the wheelchair to treatment table transfer activity.

1. Position a wheelchair parallel, or at a slight angle, to a treatment table or bed, and engage the wheel locks. Raise the footplates and remove the footrests or swing the footrests out of the way. Remove the armrest from the side of the wheelchair to which the patient will be transferred. The patient moves to the edge of the treatment table.
2. Patients may place their palms flat on the supporting surface of the treatment table, or make a fist and place the outside of their fists on the supporting surface to achieve the necessary lift height during push-ups. Some patients place one upper extremity on the wheelchair armrest or drive wheel and maintain the other upper extremity on the treatment table. The upper extremity on the side to which the patient will transfer must be placed slightly away from the patient's body. In this way the patient moves toward the transfer destination without this upper extremity limiting sideways movement.
3. Guard the patient by standing in front of the patient. Block the patient's knees, if necessary, to prevent the patient from sliding forward. When assistance in lifting is required, place your hands under the patient's buttocks and lift as the patient performs the push-up. When a patient needs assistance for balance, place your hands on the patient's shoulders.
4. The patient performs push-ups and moves sideways to lower closer to, or onto, the wheelchair. As the patient pushes up, the patient's upper trunk must rotate in the direction opposite to the transfer activity to move the body in the direction of the transfer activity. As a patient's capabilities progress, a push-up transfer may be completed using only one push-up.

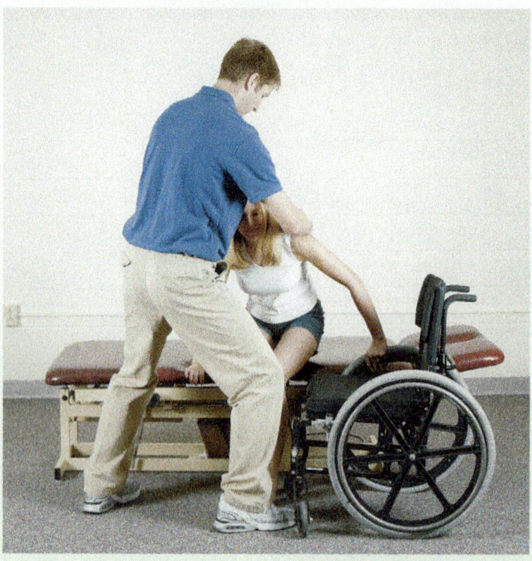

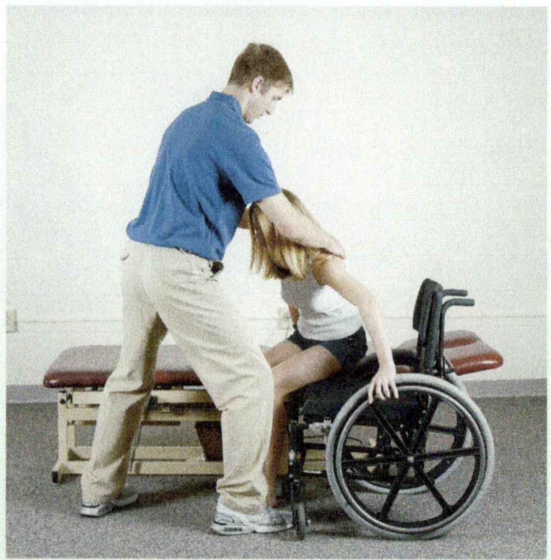

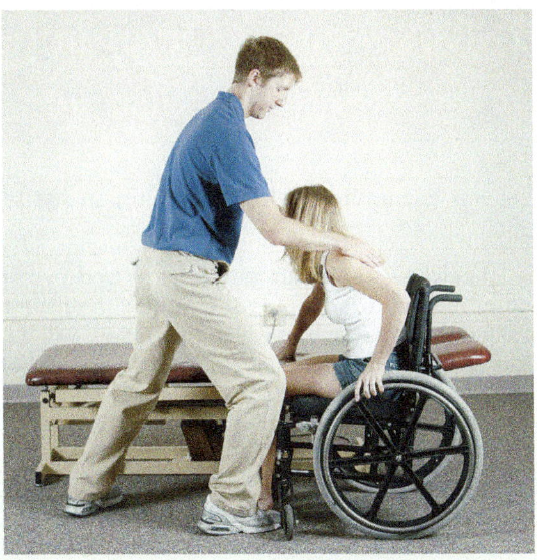

5 Continue contact to support the patient until the patient is able to maintain a safe and comfortable position.

Assisted Standing Pivot Transfer Activity

The assisted standing pivot transfer activity is an assisted transfer that may require moderate to minimal assistance of one person. The assisted standing pivot transfer activity is used when patients can sit, stand, pivot, and bear full weight on at least one lower extremity, but have some weakness, paresis, paralysis, or loss of balance or sensation, which necessitates assistance to transfer safely. This transfer is also used to teach patients to transfer independently. As a patient progresses, the amount of assistance provided to a patient is reduced until the highest possible level of independence is achieved.

■ **Take Note**
Practice transfers to both sides.

Generally, when patients have more involvement on one side than the other, transferring toward the stronger side is easier. This direction can be used during initial transfer activities to ensure success and bolster a patient's confidence. When first teaching patients to transfer, moving toward the uninvolved side is easier and safer for many patients because they are moving toward the side in which the lower extremity can provide support. Patients, however, need to be able to transfer to both sides, and transfer activities should be practiced to both sides. Teaching patients to transfer toward the involved side reinforces a patient's awareness and use of the involved side.

When unsure of a patient's capability, guard the patient's uninvolved lower extremity to ensure support on at least one side during the transfer activity. Always guard the hip and knee on the same side, whether guarding the uninvolved or involved side, by having a knee in contact with the anterolateral aspect of the patient's knee, and a hand in contact with the patient's pelvis. This permits you to prevent the hip and knee from flexing, and thus maintaining an extended lower extremity during the standing portion of the transfer activity.

■ **Take Note**
Guard the hip and knee on the same side of the patient.

PROCEDURE 9–12 Assisted Standing Pivot Transfer Activity

Guarding a Patient's Right Lower Extremity While Performing an Assisted Standing Pivot Transfer Activity to the Right

1. When transferring from a wheelchair to a treatment table or bed by pivoting to the right, a patient is positioned so the treatment table is to the right during the transfer. Position the wheelchair close, and parallel, to the surface to which the patient will be transferred. Engage the wheel locks. When moving out of a wheelchair, remove the patient's feet from the footrests, raise the footplates, and remove the footrests or swing the footrests out of the way. When moving into a wheelchair, raise the footplates, and remove the footrests or swing the footrests out of the way.
2. Move the patient to the front of the wheelchair seat, and position the patient's feet below the front of the wheelchair seat.
3. Stand in stride with your right foot medial to the patient's right foot. This position provides a base of support in the direction of the transfer activity and permits both you and the patient to move without tangling feet once the patient is standing. This position also allows you to move the patient's foot with your foot if the patient does not pivot as the transfer proceeds.

   Guard the patient's right knee with your right knee and the right side of the patient's pelvis with your left hand. This position prevents the patient from collapsing at these joints. Your right hand is on the patient's left shoulder to prevent the patient from falling to the left.

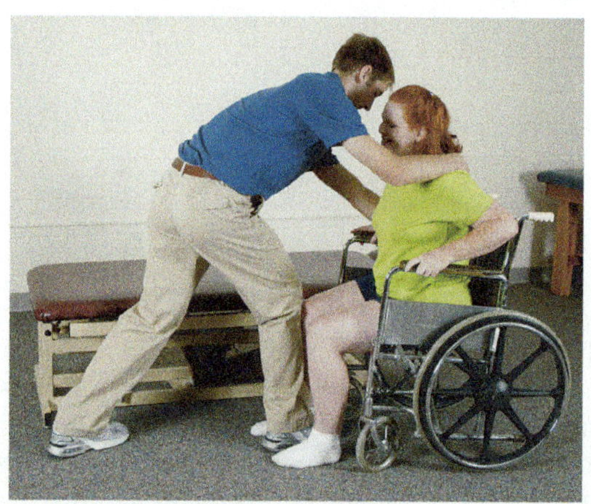

4. The patient initiates standing by leaning forward and pushing to standing using the armrest of the wheelchair.

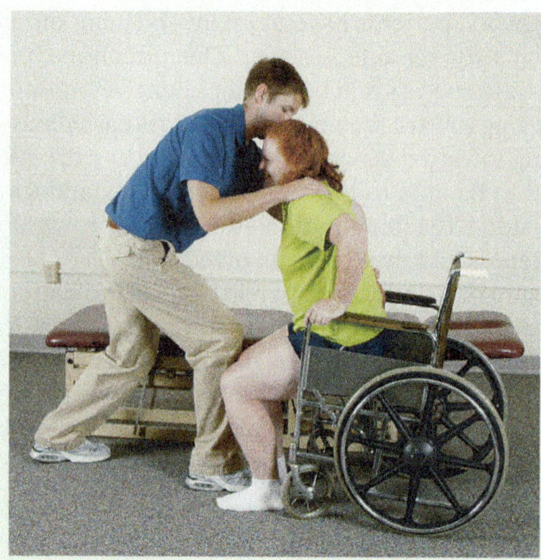

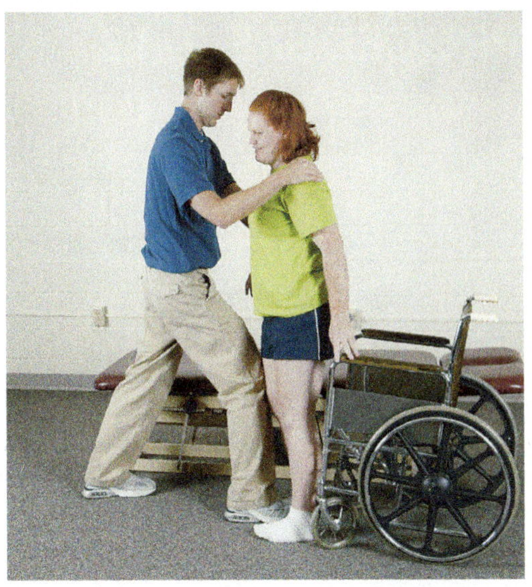

5 The patient attains a standing position and pauses to adjust to the upright position. As the patient progresses, the duration of the pause can be shortened, or the pause can be deleted.

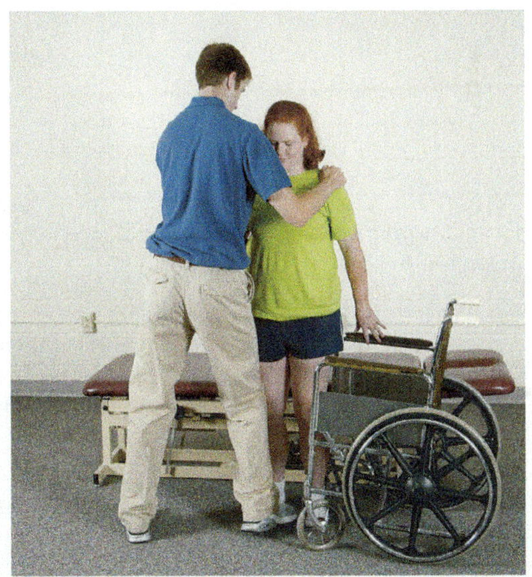

6 The patient pivots to the right, toward the treatment table. Pivot with the patient, maintaining guarding.

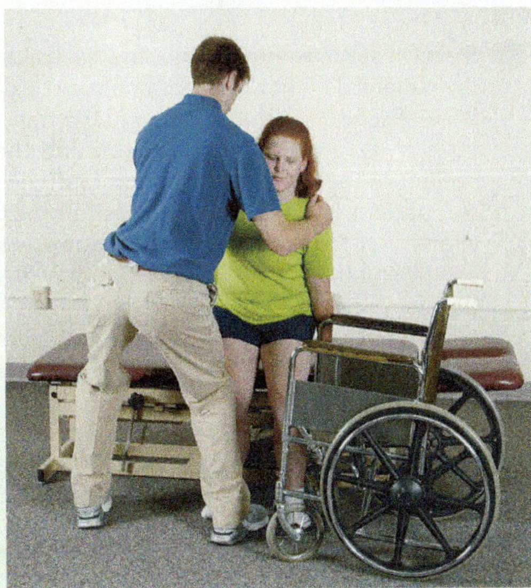

7 The patient lowers to the treatment table.

(continued)

PROCEDURE 9–12 Assisted Standing Pivot Transfer Activity (*continued*)

8 Continue contact for support until the patient is able to maintain a safe and comfortable position.

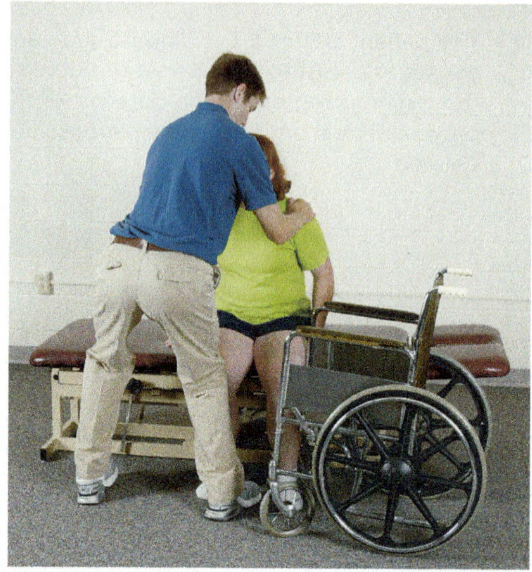

Guarding a Patient's Left Lower Extremity While Performing an Assisted Standing Pivot Transfer Activity to the Right

1 When transferring from a wheelchair to a treatment table or bed by pivoting to the right, a patient is positioned so the treatment table is to the right during the transfer. Position the wheelchair close, and parallel, to the surface to which the patient will be transferred. Engage the wheel locks. When moving out of a wheelchair, remove the patient's feet from the footrests, raise the footplates, and remove the footrests or swing the footrests out of the way. When moving into a wheelchair, raise the footplates, and remove the footrests or swing the footrests out of the way.

2 Move the patient to the front of the wheelchair seat, and position the patient's feet below the front of the wheelchair seat.

3 Stand in stride with your right foot lateral to the patient's left foot. This position provides a base of support in the direction of the transfer activity, and permits both you and the patient to move without tangling feet once the patient is standing. This position also allows you to move the patient's foot with your foot if the patient does not pivot as the transfer proceeds.

Guard the patient's left knee with your right knee and the left side of the patient's pelvis with your right hand. This position prevents the patient from collapsing at these joints. Your left hand is on the patient's right shoulder to prevent the patient from falling to the right.

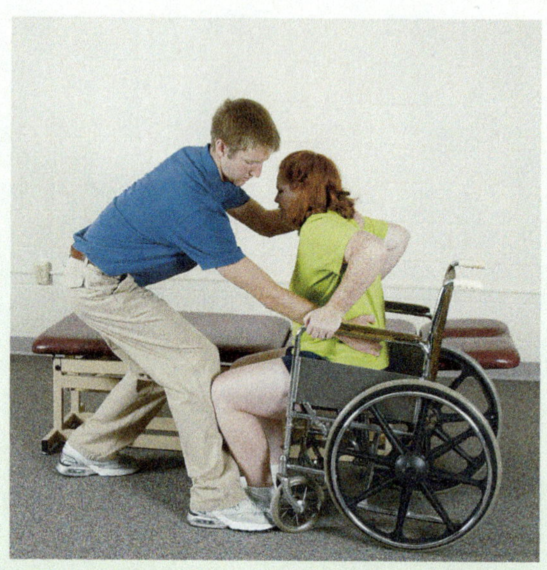

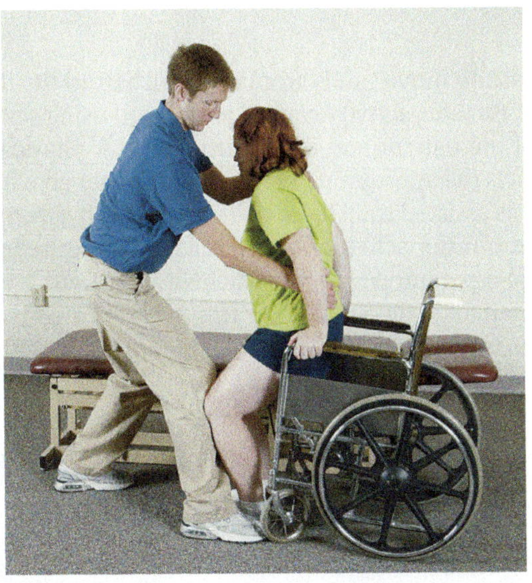

4 The patient initiates standing by leaning forward and pushing to standing using the armrest of the wheelchair.

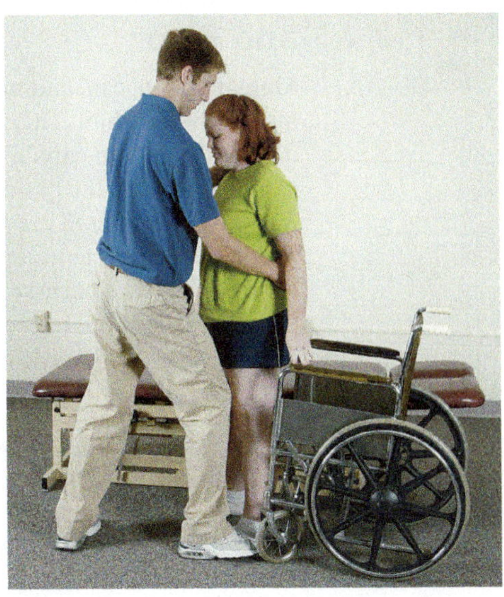

5 The patient attains a standing position and pauses to adjust to the upright position. As the patient progresses, the duration of the pause can be shortened, or the pause can be deleted.

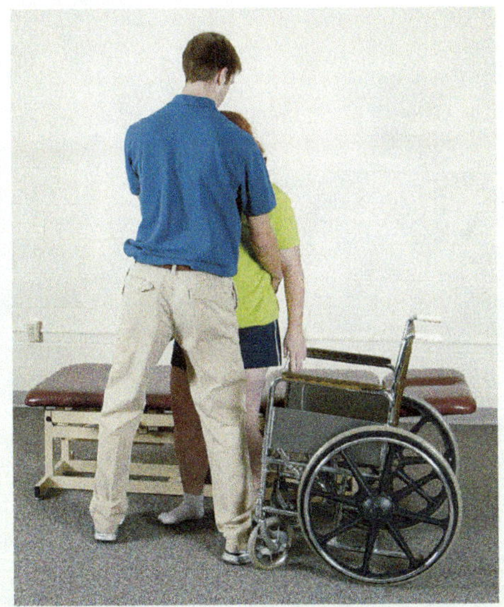

6 The patient pivots to the right, toward the treatment table. You pivot with the patient, maintaining guarding.

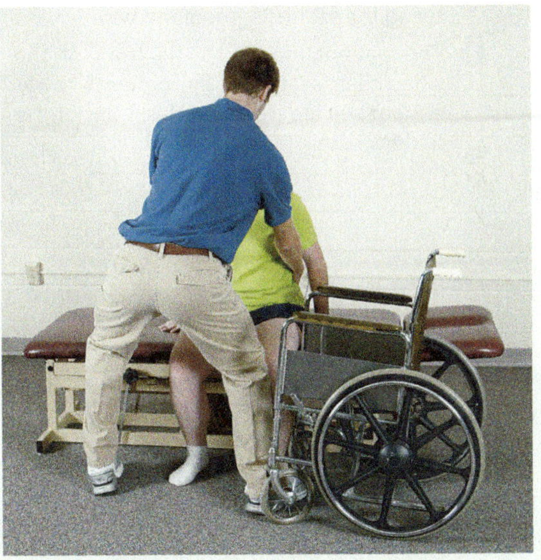

7 The patient lowers to the treatment table.

8 Continue contact for support until the patient is able to maintain a safe and comfortable position.

Independent Transfer Activities Between Wheelchair and Floor

Many patients can, and must, learn to move safely from a wheelchair to the floor and back into the wheelchair. This type of transfer activity can be performed using several methods, depending on the capabilities of the patient and the environment. A physical therapist, in conjunction with the patient, selects the appropriate methods of transfer activities. The transfer activities selected may begin as assisted transfer activities (physical or verbal assistance) and then progress to independent transfer activities. Transfer activities between a wheelchair and the floor are necessary when a patient wants to participate in activities on the floor, if the patient falls out of a wheelchair, or if the wheelchair tips over.

In the following illustrations transfer activities are being performed with supervision.

PROCEDURE 9–13 Independent Transfer Activities Between Wheelchair and Floor

Forward Lowering: Wheelchair to Floor Transfer Activity

1. Position the wheelchair with the caster wheels forward to increase the base of support of the wheelchair.
2. Engage the wheel locks. Remove the patient's feet from the footrests, raise the footplates, and remove the footrests or swing the footrests out of the way.
3. The patient moves to the front of the wheelchair seat, and the patient's lower extremities are positioned in front of the patient, with knees extended.

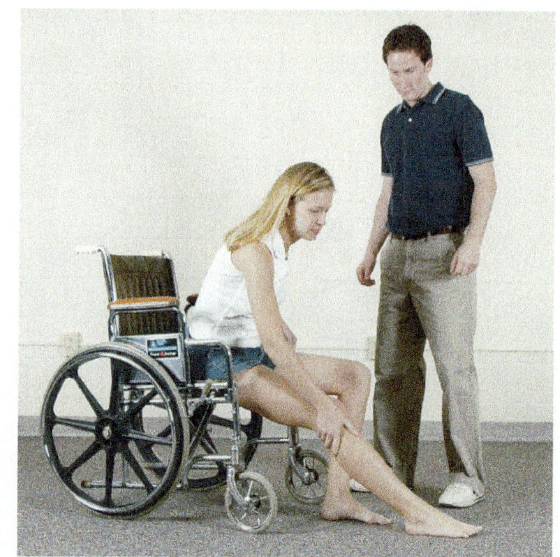

4. The patient positions one hand on the side, and toward the front, of the wheelchair seat or the lower portion of a desk armrest, and the other hand on a caster wheel or floor. Hand placements depend on the patient's size, strength, and range of motion (ROM).

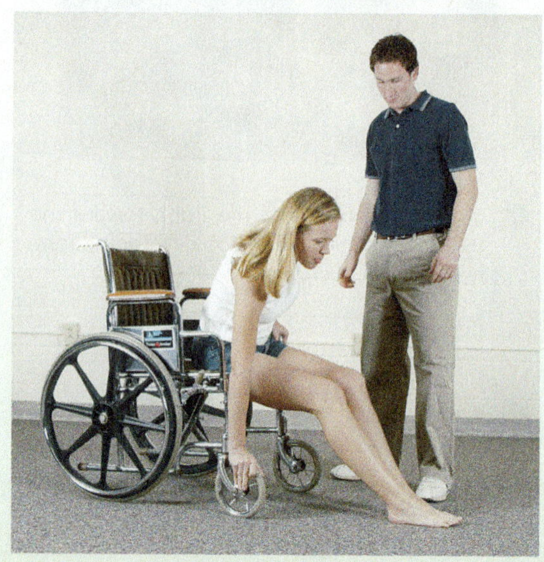

5. The patient initially extends the upper extremities to lift the body from the wheelchair seat, moves the body forward, and then lowers to the floor by flexing the upper extremities.

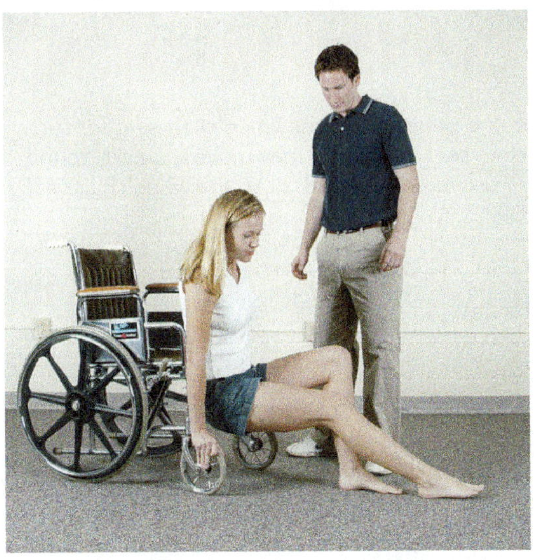

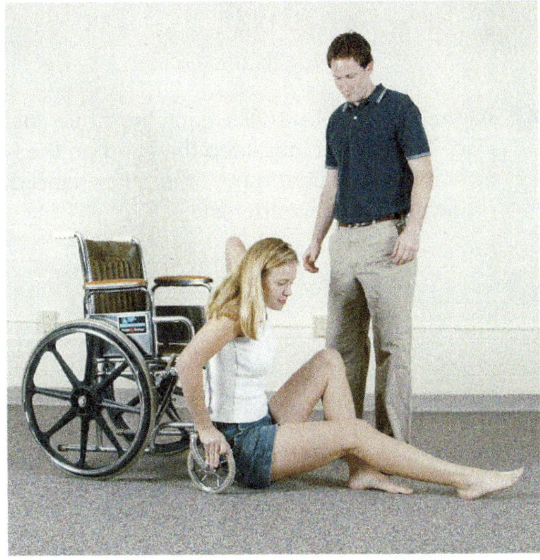

Backward Lift: Floor to Wheelchair Transfer Activity

1. Position the wheelchair with the caster wheels forward to increase the base of support of the wheelchair.
2. Engage the wheel locks. Raise the footplates, and remove the footrests or swing the footrests out of the way.
3. The patient assumes a long-sitting position with knees extended, and back toward, and close to, the front of the wheelchair.
4. The patient places one hand on the side, and toward the front, of the wheelchair seat, and places the other hand on a caster wheel or floor. Hand placements depend on the patient's size, strength, and ROM.

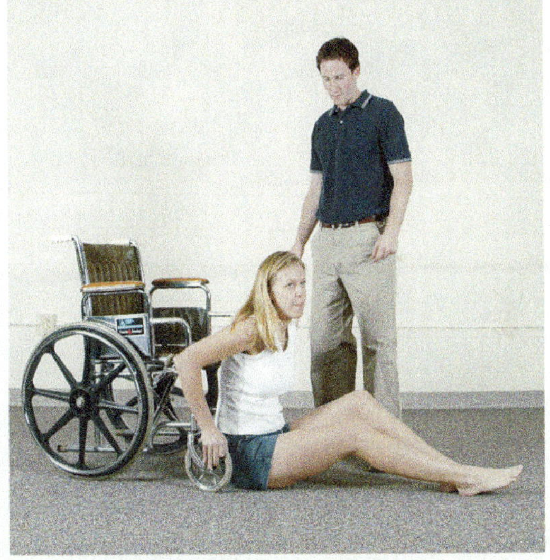

5. The patient pushes up by extending the upper extremities, depressing the shoulder girdles, and flexing the head and neck.

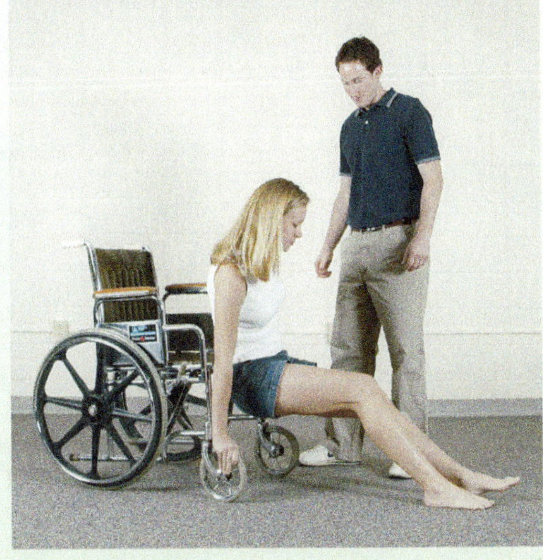

(continued)

PROCEDURE 9–13 Independent Transfer Activities Between Wheelchair and Floor (*continued*)

6 As the patient's buttocks reach the wheelchair seat, the patient uses the wheelchair seat for support. The patient may keep the hand on the wheelchair seat in place or may move it quickly to the armrest. The patient moves the other hand quickly from the caster or floor to the wheelchair seat or lower part of the armrest.

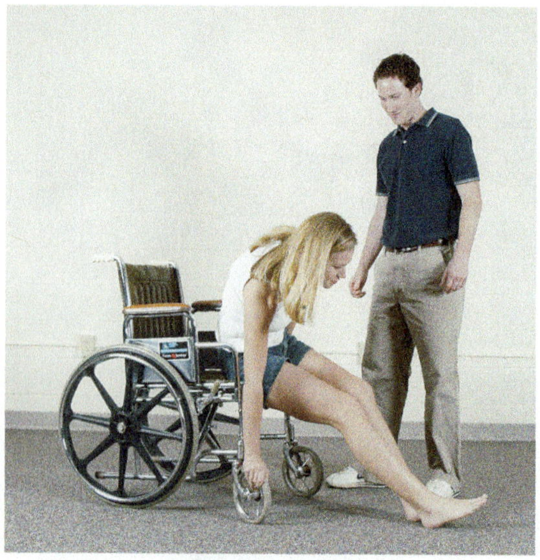

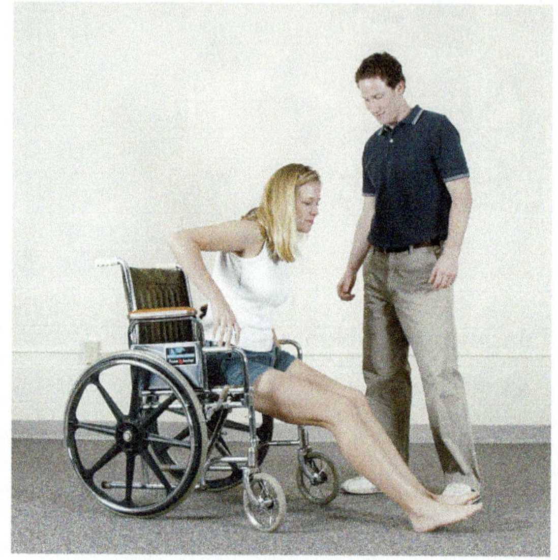

7 Using both upper extremities, the patient moves well back onto the wheelchair seat.

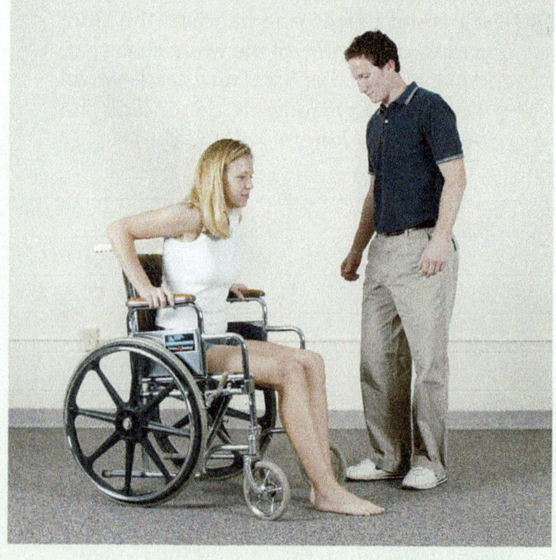

8 The transfer is complete once the footrests are reattached and repositioned and the patient's feet are placed appropriately on the footplates.

Backward Lift Using a Step Stool: Floor to Wheelchair Transfer Activity

When a patient is unable to perform an independent floor-to-wheelchair transfer, a step stool may be used.

1. Position the wheelchair with the caster wheels forward to increase the base of support of the wheelchair.
2. Engage the wheel locks. Raise the footplates, and remove the footrests or swing the footrests out of the way. Place a step stool close to, and in front of, the wheelchair.
3. The patient assumes a long-sitting position with knees extended and back toward, and close to, the stool.
4. The patient places both hands on the sides of the step stool.

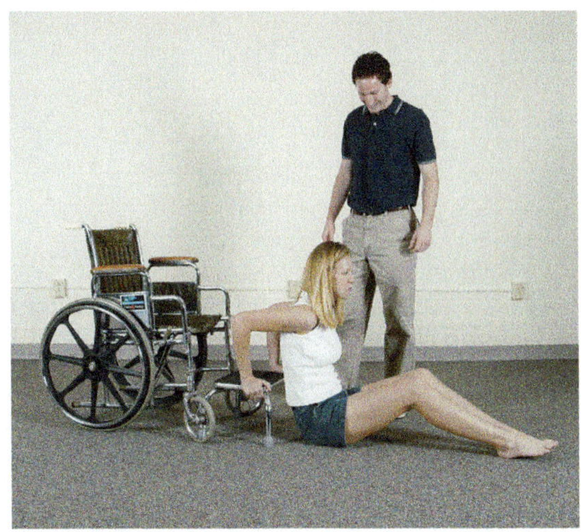

5. The patient pushes up by extending the upper extremities, depressing the shoulder girdles, and flexing the head and neck to lift and assume a sitting position on the step stool.

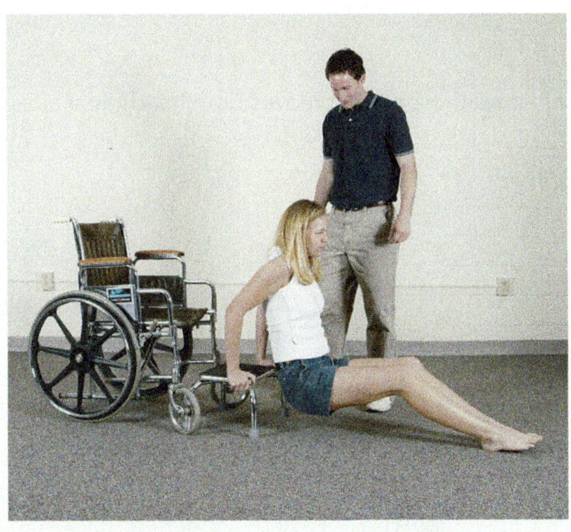

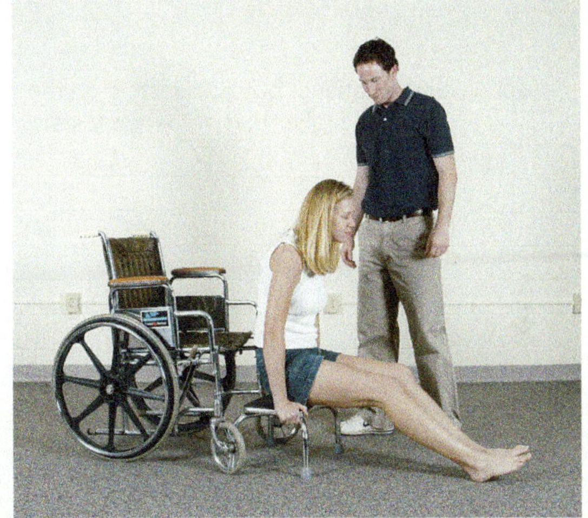

6. Sitting on the step stool, the patient places both hands on the sides and toward the front of the wheelchair seat or the lower part of desk armrests when available. Hand placements depend on the patient's size, strength, and ROM.

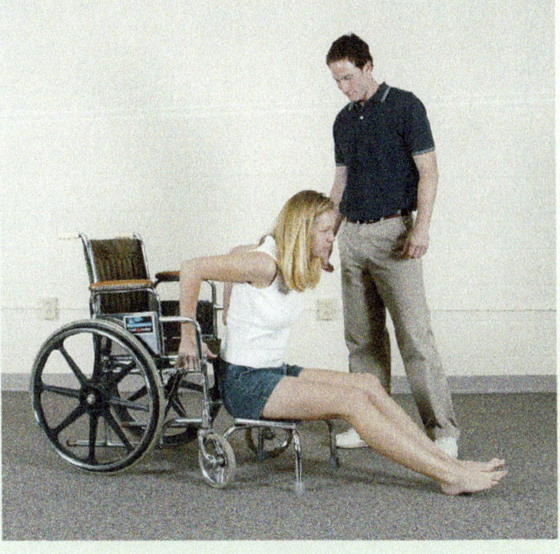

(continued)

PROCEDURE 9–13 Independent Transfer Activities Between Wheelchair and Floor (*continued*)

7. The patient pushes up by extending the upper extremities, depressing the shoulder girdles, and flexing the head and neck to raise the buttocks above the level of the wheelchair seat.

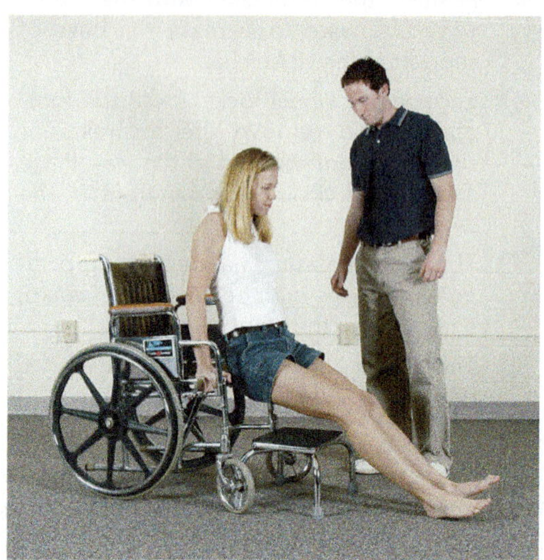

8. With the patient's buttocks resting on the wheelchair seat, the patient moves both hands, one at a time, to the higher part of the armrests.

9. Using both upper extremities, the patient moves well back onto the wheelchair seat.

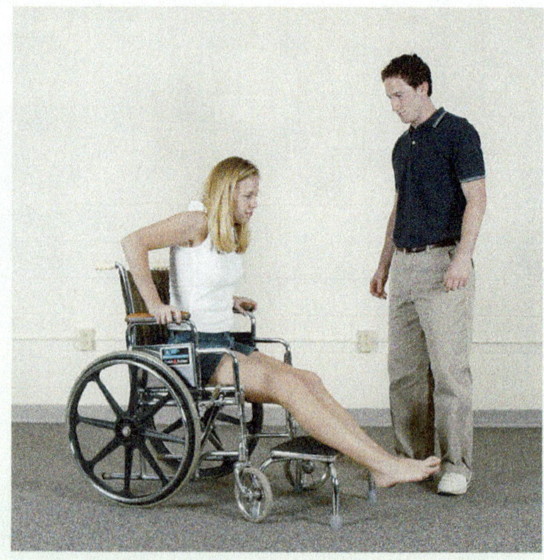

10. Remove the step stool from its position in front of the wheelchair, attach and re-position the footrests, and place the patient's feet appropriately on the footplates.

Turn Around: Wheelchair to Floor Transfer Activity

1. Position the wheelchair with the caster wheels forward to increase the base of support of the wheelchair.
2. Engage the wheel locks. Remove the patient's feet from the footrests, raise the footplates, and remove the footrests or swing the footrests out of the way.
3. The patient moves to the front of the wheelchair seat and turns partially onto one hip.

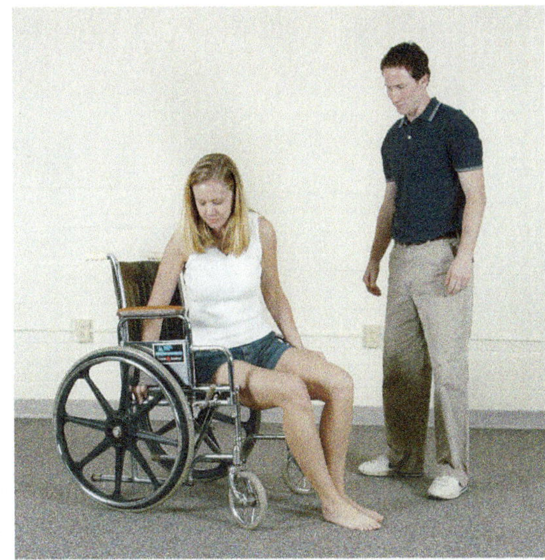

4. The patient moves the right hand behind to grasp the left side of the seat and moves the left hand across the front of the body to grasp the right side of the seat.

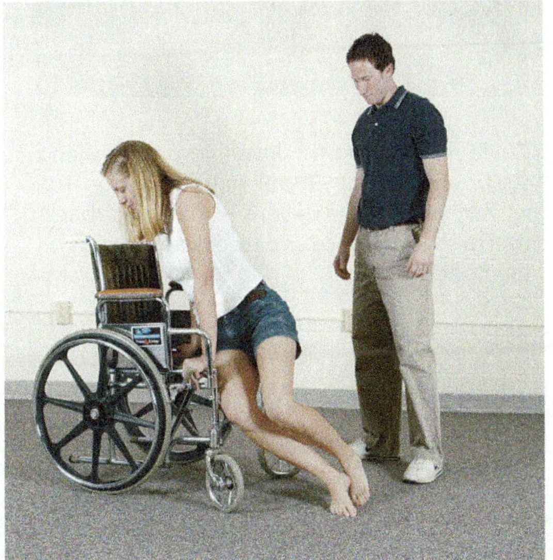

5. Extending the upper extremities while depressing the shoulder girdles, the patient lifts and turns to face the back of the wheelchair and then lowers to a kneeling position on the floor in front of the wheelchair.

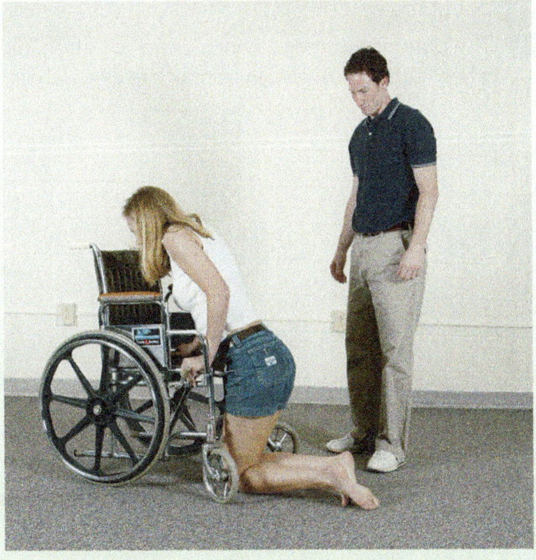

(continued)

PROCEDURE 9–13 Independent Transfer Activities Between Wheelchair and Floor (*continued*)

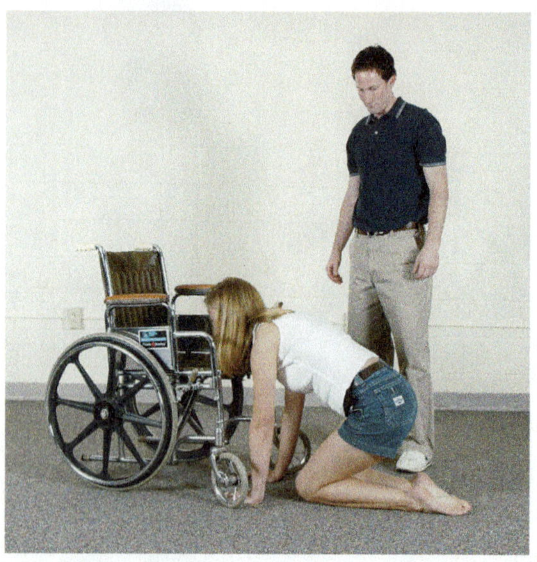

6. While maintaining the kneeling position, and supported by the upper extremities on the wheelchair seat, the patient "knee-walks" backward a short distance and places both hands on the floor.

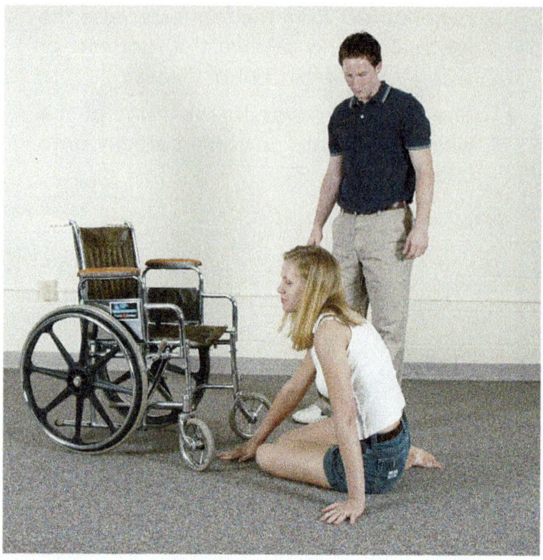

7. The patient assumes a side-sitting position.

Turn Around: Floor to Wheelchair Transfer Activity

1. Position the wheelchair with the caster wheels forward to increase the base of support of the wheelchair.
2. Engage the wheel locks. Raise the footplates, and remove the footrests or swing the footrests out of the way.
3. The patient assumes a hands-knees position, or a heel-sitting position, in front of the wheelchair.

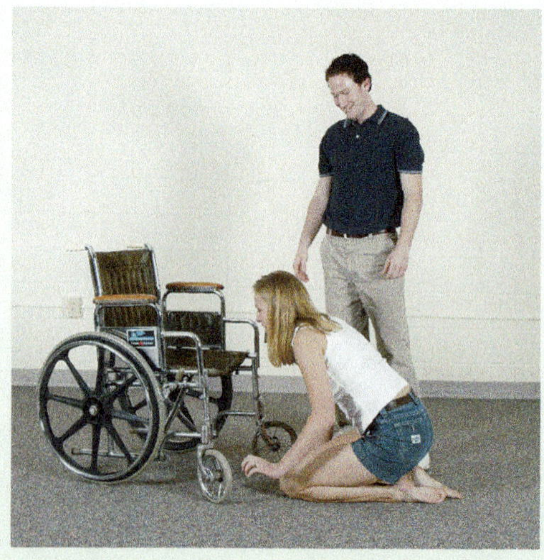

4 The patient places one hand on the side, and toward the front of, the wheelchair seat and the other hand on the caster wheel or floor, and pushes into a kneeling position. The hand on the caster wheel or floor is then moved to the wheelchair seat.

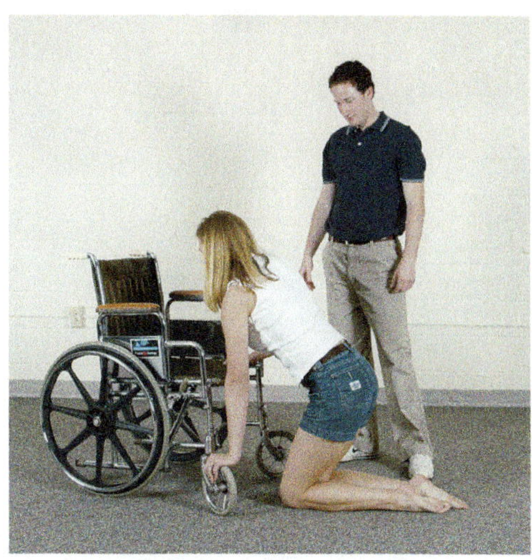

5 Some patients have the capability to push to the kneeling position with both hands on the sides of the wheelchair seat.

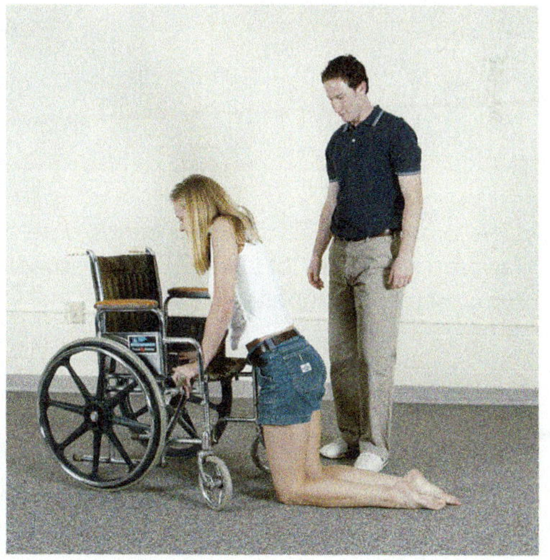

6 The patient pushes up by extending the upper extremities and depressing the shoulder girdles, lifting and starting to turn, and then lowers to rest one hip on the wheelchair seat.

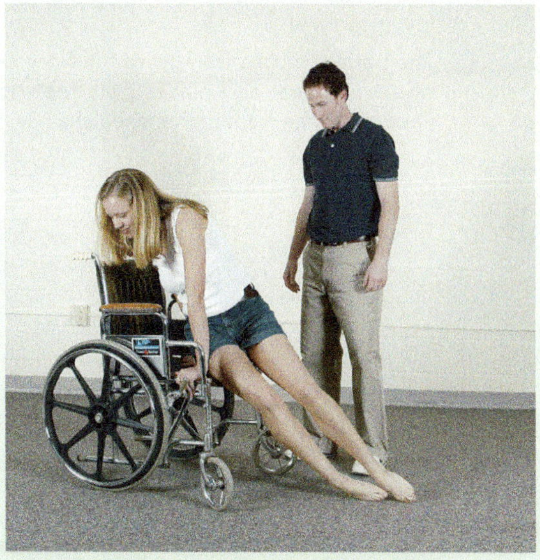

(continued)

PROCEDURE 9–13 Independent Transfer Activities Between Wheelchair and Floor (*continued*)

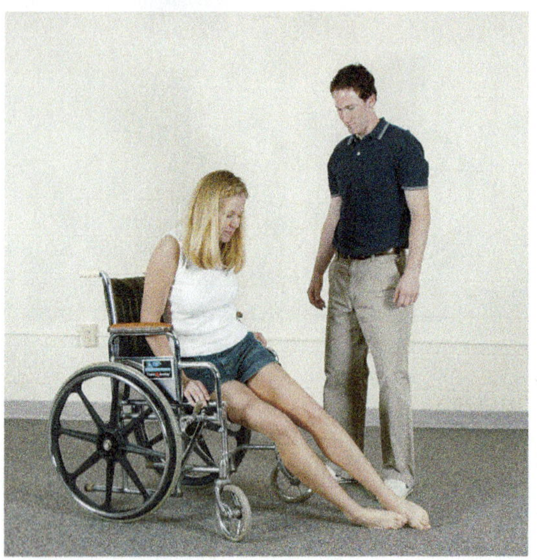

7 The patient repositions both hands onto the appropriate sides of the wheelchair seat, or armrests, and completes the turn.

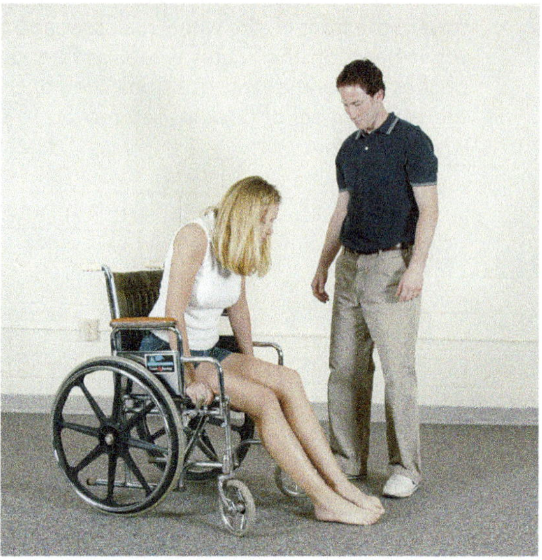

8 The patient can then position properly in the wheelchair.

Forward to Hands-Knees via Kneeling: Wheelchair to Floor Transfer Activity

1. Position the wheelchair with the caster wheels forward to increase the base of support of the wheelchair.
2. Engage the wheel locks. Raise the footplates, and remove the footrests or swing the footrests out of the way.
3. The patient moves forward to the front of the wheelchair seat and places both feet on the floor under the front of the wheelchair seat.

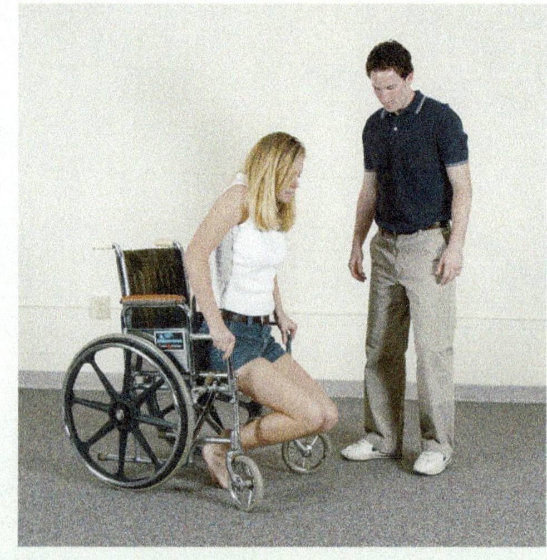

4 Grasping the lower portion of the desk armrests or the sides of the wheelchair seat, the patient lowers to a kneeling position.

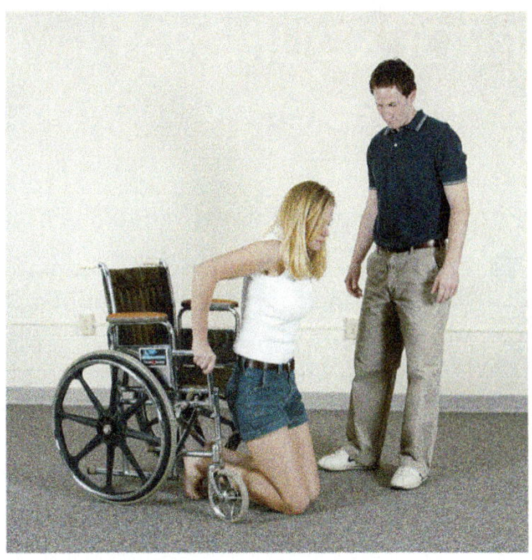

5 Holding the lower portion of a desk armrest or the wheelchair seat with one hand, the patient reaches forward to the floor with the other hand.

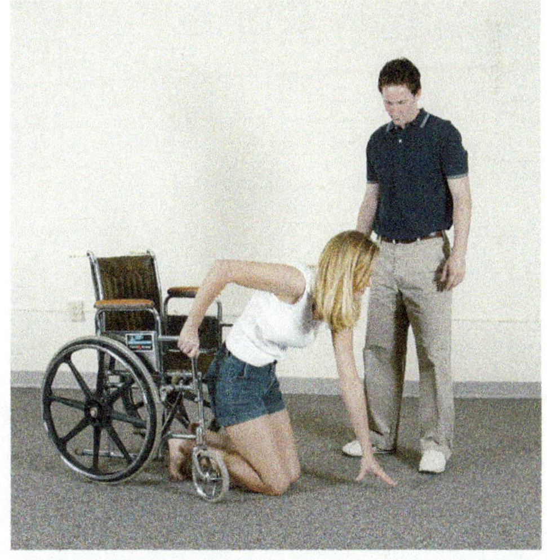

6 When supported with both knees and one upper extremity on the floor, the patient moves the other upper extremity to the floor, assuming a hands-knees position.

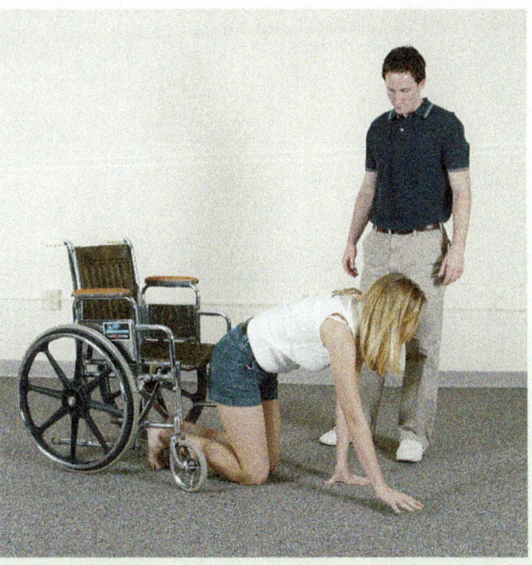

(continued)

PROCEDURE 9–13 Independent Transfer Activities Between Wheelchair and Floor (*continued*)

Forward to Hands-Knees: Wheelchair to Floor Transfer Activity

1. Position the wheelchair with the caster wheels forward to increase the base of support of the wheelchair.
2. Engage the wheel locks. Raise the footplates, and remove the footrests or swing the footrests out of the way.
3. The patient moves forward to the front of the wheelchair seat and places both feet on the floor under the front of the wheelchair seat.

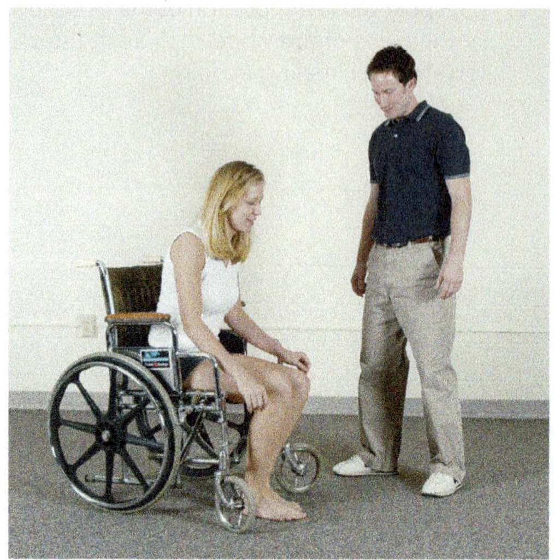

4. The patient reaches toward the floor with both upper extremities, creating forward momentum to move from the wheelchair seat.

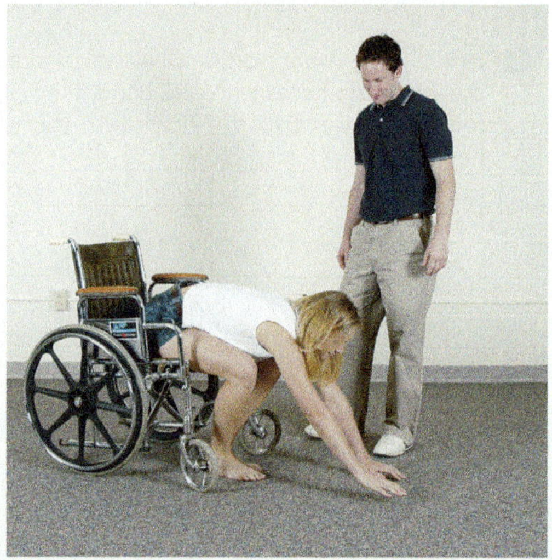

5. With support through the upper extremities, the patient shifts weight onto the upper extremities. Momentum brings the lower portion of the body forward so the patient assumes a hands-knees position on the floor.

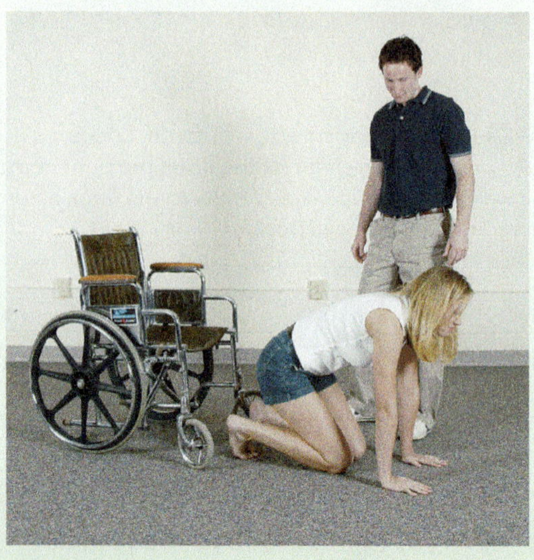

Review Questions

1. What are the differences and similarities between dependent, assisted, modified independent, and independent transfer activities?
2. What are the purposes of counts and verbal cues during transfer activities?
3. What are the sequences for performing the following transfer activities?
   Sliding transfer: cart to treatment table
   Three-person carry
   Hydraulic lift
   Two-person lift
   Assist to front of seat (three methods)
   Moving from front edge of seat
   Dependent standing pivot
   Dependent sitting pivot
   Squat pivot
   Sliding board
   Push-up
   Assisted standing pivot (two methods)
   Independent transfer activities between wheelchair to floor and return
4. What are the rules of proper body mechanics to use during transfer activities?
5. What are the levels of guarding and types and amount of assistance used and documented during transfer activities?
6. What is the proper use of gait belts during transfer activities?
7. Which transfer activities are considered dependent, assisted, and independent?
8. What is purpose of preparing the environment before initiating transfer activities?
9. What are the teaching tips used when teaching transfer activities?

Suggested Activities

1. Demonstrate transfer activity procedures shown in this chapter.
2. Practice transfer activities working in groups of 2 to 4 people, with each student participating in each role required in the transfer activity.
3. Practice transfer activities with partners role-playing the patient. Students should role-play patients with different diagnoses such as CVA (right or left hemiplegia), spinal cord injury (quadriplegia or paraplegia), multiple sclerosis, cerebral palsy, or Parkinson's disease. Students role-playing patients can add "character" to enhance the activity by being cooperative or noncooperative, in pain, hard of hearing, apprehensive, faint, flaccid, or spastic. Students playing the role of a patient must role-play the diagnosis and character consistently.
4. Practice teaching transfer activities to students role-playing patients, families, and other healthcare providers.
5. Document patient/client management actions of transfer activities using the note format indicated by your instructor.

Case Studies

For the following case studies, develop a progression of transfer activities appropriate for progressing a patient from dependent to independent (as much as feasible) transfer status. Note transfer activity methods, amount, and type of assistance.

1. The patient is a 23-year-old female with a diagnosis of multiple sclerosis. She was independent in all ADLs and ambulated with a cane for balance until 2 weeks ago. At that time, she experienced an exacerbation that has left her totally dependent in all transfer activities and unable to ambulate. She becomes faint when moved from supine to sitting, or sitting to standing, too quickly. She is expected to recover most of her prior level of independence.
2. The patient is a 63-year-old male with left CVA onset 20 hours ago, presenting with right hemiplegia and global aphasia (both receptive and expressive aphasia). The cause was a blood clot. Because he received immediate medical treatment, recovery is anticipated to be nearly complete. At present, he is dependent in all ADLs, including transfer activities and ambulation.

3. The patient is an 18-year-old male who sustained a complete T12–L1 spinal cord lesion in a motorcycle accident 2 weeks ago. Following surgery, he is wearing a thoraco-lumbar-sacral orthosis (TLSO). He has medical clearance to begin transfer activity training while wearing his TLSO.
4. The patient is a 23-year-old female with cerebral palsy presenting with spastic quadriplegia. While living with her parents, her father lifted her for all transfer activities. Following her recent college graduation, she is living in a group home for the first time. She ambulates by using a power wheelchair. The staff of the group home requests assistance in selecting appropriate transfer activities. The staff would like a program to assist her in becoming an active participant in her transfer activities. Would the transfer activity method selected be different if she was 5 feet tall weighing 250 pounds, versus 5 feet tall weighing 96 pounds?
5. The patient is a 49-year-old female with severe rheumatoid arthritis. She is 5 feet 3 inches tall and weighs 175 pounds. Transfer activities are currently accomplished using a hydraulic lift. She ambulates by using a power wheelchair. Because her arthritis is in remission at this time, she would like to learn to transfer without the hydraulic lift so she can get out in the community more.

Reference

1. Occupational Health and Safety Agency for Healthcare (OHSAH) in British Columbia. (2002). *Safe patient & resident handling—acute and long term care sectors handbook*. Vancouver, BC: Author, p. 8.

10

Gait Training with Ambulatory Assistive Devices

LEARNING OUTCOMES

Upon completion of this chapter, you will be able to:

1. List indications for use of ambulatory assistive devices for gait.
2. Describe and discuss the uses of parallel bars during gait training.
3. Describe and discuss the use of the tilt table during gait training.
4. List and discuss the causes of fatigue during gait training and methods to reduce the effects of fatigue.
5. Discuss the effect of patient concentration on gait training.
6. Describe the use of a scale to teach weight-bearing limits.
7. Describe methods of instruction appropriate for gait training.
8. List activities that a patient must master to be independent in gait training with an assistive device.
9. List assistive-device selection in sequence from those providing most stability to least stability.
10. List assistive-device selection in sequence from those requiring the most coordination to least coordination.
11. List evaluations used to determine appropriate ambulatory assistive devices for different patients and pathologies.
12. List contraindications to the use of ambulatory assistive devices.
13. Adjust the height of ambulatory assistive devices properly.
14. Describe various styles of walkers, crutches, and canes.
15. Describe and demonstrate common gait patterns used with ambulatory assistive devices.
16. Describe and demonstrate how to guard a patient properly when using ambulatory assistive devices during gait training on level surfaces, stairs, and curbs; the assumption of sitting from standing and standing from sitting; moving through doorways; falling without injury; and resumption of standing after falling.
17. Instruct a patient in the proper method of using various ambulatory assistive devices to perform different gait patterns on level surfaces, stairs, and curbs; moving through doorways; the assumption of sitting from standing and standing from sitting; falling without injury; and resumption of gait standing after falling.

KEY TERMS

- Ambulation
- Ambulatory assistive devices
- Close guarding
- Contact guarding
- Folding walkers
- Full weight bearing (FWB)
- Gait pattern
- Gait training
- Hemi-walkers
- Knee walkers
- Maximal (maximum) assistance
- Minimal (minimum) assistance
- Moderate assistance
- Non–weight bearing (NWB)
- Partial weight bearing (PWB)
- Reverse walkers
- Ring walkers
- Stair-climbing walkers
- Supervision
- Toe touch weight bearing (TTWB)
- Weight bearing
- Weight bearing as tolerated (WBAT)
- Wheeled walkers

Introduction

Ambulatory assistive devices provide external support during gait training in an upright posture. Ambulatory assistive devices permit safe gait training for patients with impairments who could not otherwise ambulate. Three major indications for using ambulatory assistive devices during gait are

1. Structural deformity, amputation, injury, or disease resulting in decreased ability to bear weight through the lower extremities
2. Muscle weakness or paralysis of the trunk or lower extremities
3. Inadequate balance

Ambulatory assistive devices increase a patient's base of support. Base of support is defined as the area within the boundaries created by the ambulatory assistive devices and patients' feet. Increasing a patient's base of support creates a larger area within which the patient's center of gravity can shift without loss of balance. Ambulatory assistive devices provide a method of redistributing weight normally borne by the lower extremities to the upper extremity(ies).

A large variety of ambulatory assistive devices, and variations, exists. Ambulatory assistive devices come in several sizes—tall, standard, junior, and child. Most ambulatory assistive devices are adjustable within a given range, and there is usually some overlap of adjustment between sizes. Included in this chapter are common ambulatory assistive devices, including parallel bars, crutches, canes, and walkers, but not orthotic or prosthetic devices, wheelchairs, or scooters.

The terms *ambulation* and *gait training* refer to different activities. **Ambulation** is a mobility activity. **Gait training** is the process of teaching a patient to ambulate. Gait training is terminology used by the Centers for Medicare and Medicaid Services (CMS) to mean the provision of services by an appropriate professional.

Ambulatory Assistive Devices

Walkers

Walkers provide a relatively large degree of stability and are generally easy to use. The base of support provided by a walker is the area within the four legs of the walker, or between the front legs of the walker and the patient's foot or feet in contact with the floor when the lower extremities are behind the walker. Walkers are chosen for patients with generalized weakness, debilitating conditions, a need to reduce weight bearing on one or both lower extremities, relatively poor balance and coordination, or an inability to use crutches. Walkers are often chosen for use by elderly patients.

Walkers are U-shaped in a horizontal plane, with four legs to which wheels may be attached when appropriate. During use a patient stands within the U, facing the crossbar, and grasps the handgrips on the sides of the upper portion of the walker (Figure 10–1 ▪).

Walkers are made of aluminum and are adjustable in height. To adjust the height of a walker, the walker is inverted (Figure 10–2 ▪). Each leg has a push-button lock with a telescoping leg (Figure 10–3 ▪). Adjust all legs to the same height.

Most walkers are **folding walkers**, making it possible to decrease their size and making them easier to place in a car or out of the way in public spaces (Figure 10–4 ▪). Various mechanisms exist by which walkers can be folded.

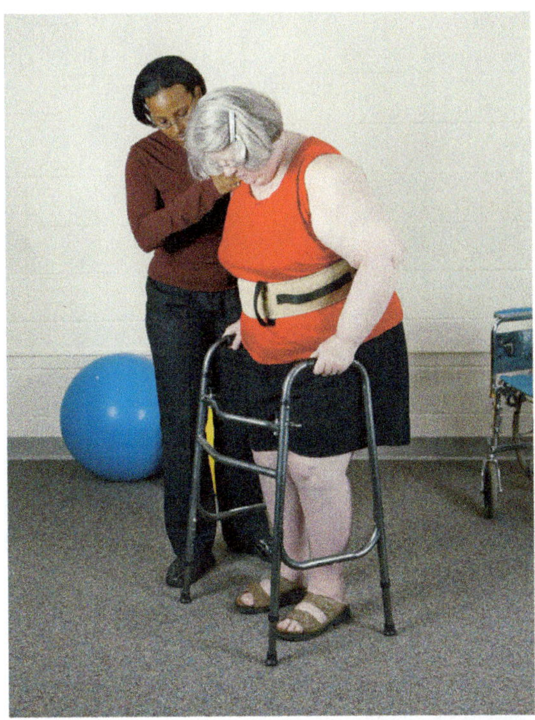

FIGURE 10–1 ■ Patient supporting self with walker.

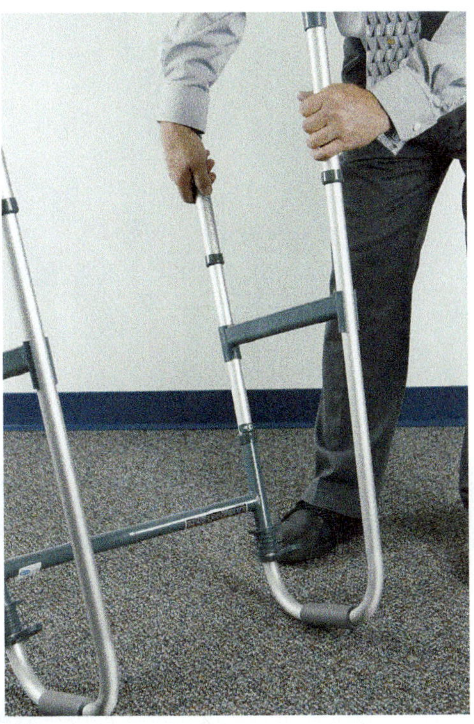

FIGURE 10–2 ■ Walker inverted to adjust height.

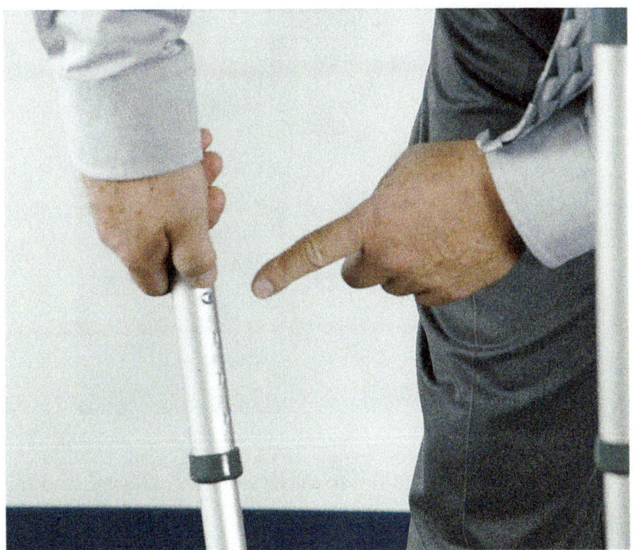

FIGURE 10–3 ■ Push button for height adjustment on walker.

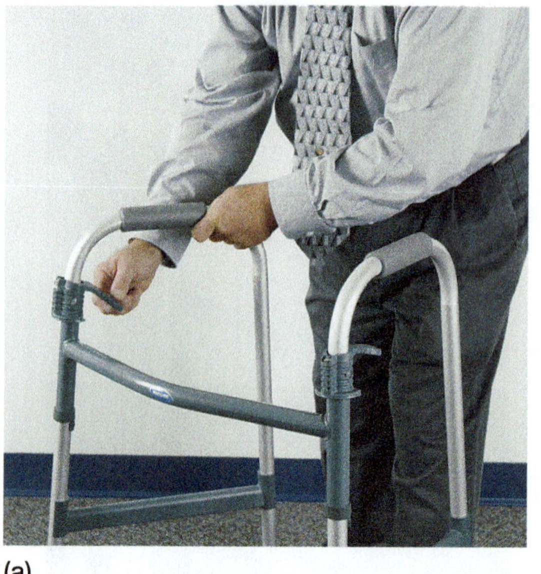
(a)

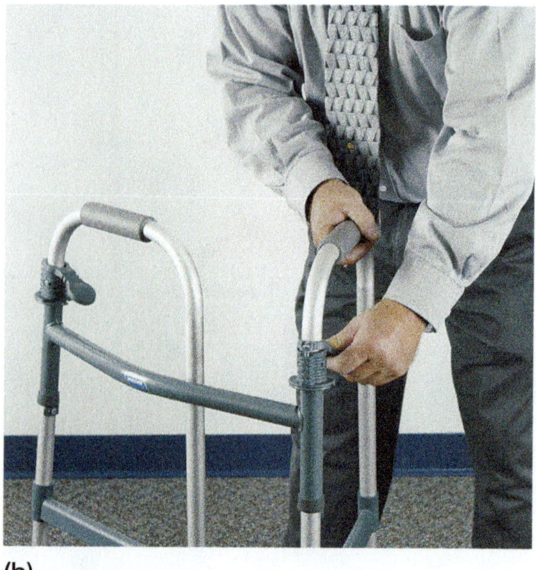
(b)

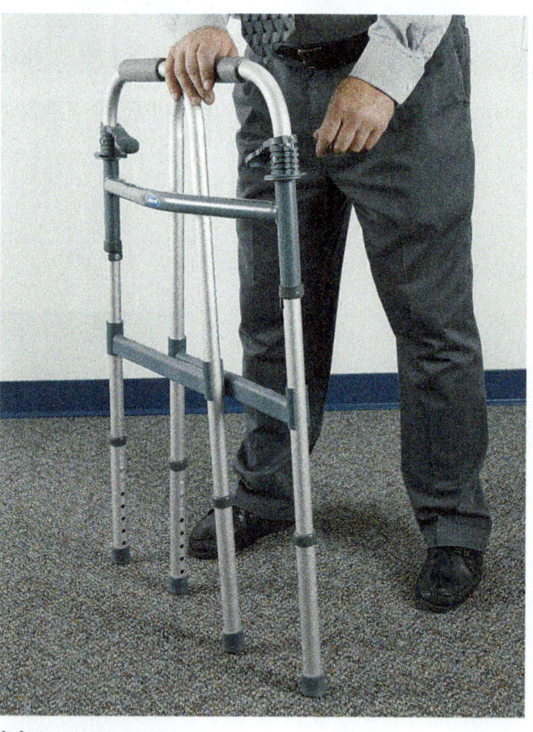
(c)

FIGURE 10–4 ■ The sides of a folding walker fold flat to allow for easier storage and transport.

A number of the variations of walkers are described next. On most walkers, a platform for the forearm can be attached for patients who are unable to bear weight through their hand, wrist, or forearm, or who have poor grasp (Figure 10–5 ■). Other accessories such as baskets are available, making walkers more functional for users.

Wheeled walkers are available with either two or four wheels (Figure 10–6 ■). Walkers with four wheels should have a brake that is activated during weight bearing on the walker to ensure stability. Wheeled walkers may also have seats that can be folded out of the way during ambulation.

Stair-climbing walkers are available for patients who must use stairs frequently because ascending and descending stairs using a regular walker is a challenge. This walker has an additional pair of handgrips on the rear legs to be used when the patient is on the stairs

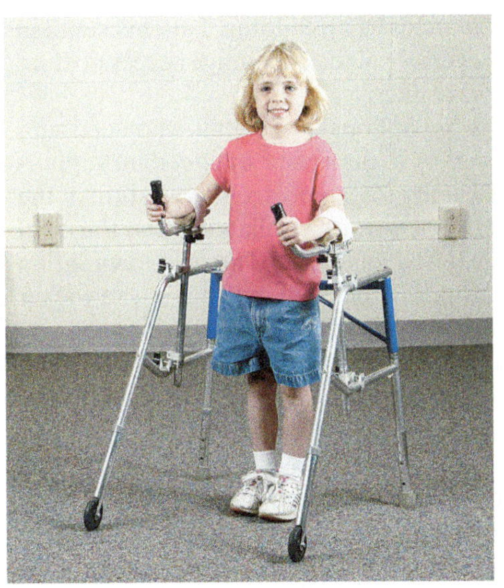

FIGURE 10–5 ■ Reverse walker with forearm platform attachments.

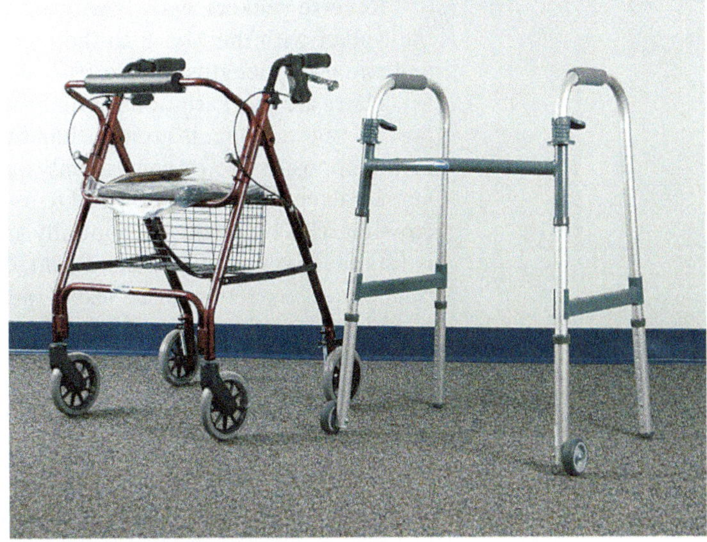

FIGURE 10–6 ■ Four-wheeled walker with brake (left) and two-wheeled walker (right).

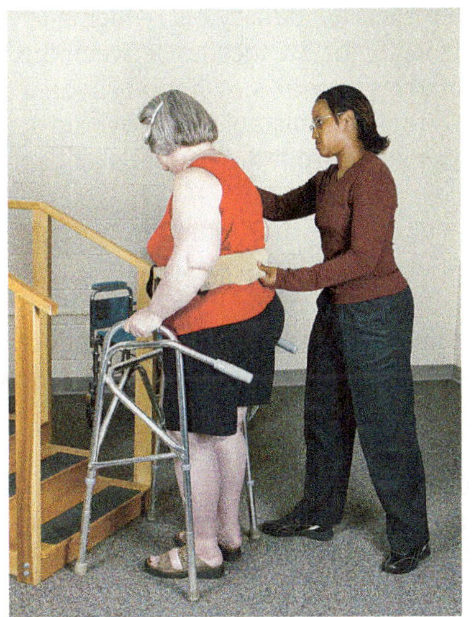

FIGURE 10–7 ■ Stair-climbing walker.

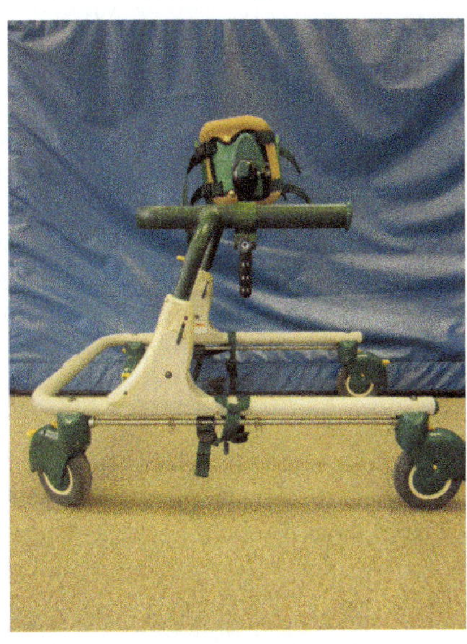

FIGURE 10–8 ■ Ring walker.

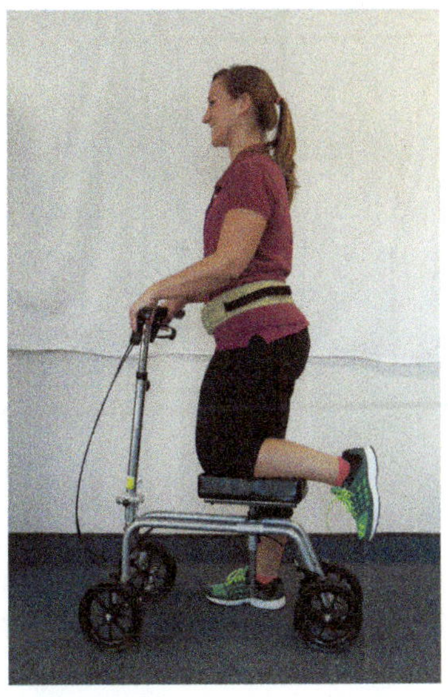

FIGURE 10–9 ■ Knee walker.

(Figure 10–7 ■). These handgrips increase the anterior/posterior dimension of the walker, increasing difficulty of maneuvering in small areas.

Ring walkers are walkers with trunk support and are indicated for patients with adequate reciprocal lower extremity movements, but lacking adequate trunk support. Ring walkers are larger than standard walkers in all three dimensions, have four wheels, and do not fold (Figure 10–8 ■). An *adduction board* may be added to a ring walker. Adduction boards are suspended from the frame of the walker to prevent a patient's lower extremities from adducting during the swing phase of gait.

Reciprocal walkers are designed with joints that permit each side of the walker to be advanced independently. A reciprocal walker is used when patients lack strength or balance to lift a walker completely to advance the walker during gait.

Knee walkers are ambulatory assistive devices for patients with transtibial amputations or who are unable to bear weight through the lower leg and foot for other reasons (Figure 10–9 ■). Patients place their involved lower leg on the cushioned leg support, bearing weight through the knee, and grasp the steering handlebar. The lower extremity that is on the floor propels the patient.

Reverse walkers, with or without wheels, often are used by children. Patients stand in the walker with their back to the cross bar. The reverse walker encourages erect posture and equal step lengths. Figure 10–5 shows a reverse walker.

There are two variations of **hemi-walkers**. Both are options for patients who need support on one side that is greater than can be provided by a quad cane, but need no support on the opposite side, or can use only one upper extremity for support. One variation of the hemi-walker, sometimes referred to as a walkcane, is one side of a walker without the front crossbar. This variation is essentially an extra-large based quad cane. The second variation is a standard walker with a handle attached to the center of the front crossbar so the walker can be maneuvered with the use of only one upper extremity. This second variation is also considered an adaptation of a standard walker, and not a separate type of walker. As with standard walkers, ambulation on stairs is a problem because of the large base of support.

Axillary Crutches

Axillary crutches provide a moderate degree of stability and are more challenging to use than walkers. The base of support for a person using two axillary crutches is the area within the patient's one or two feet on the floor, and the two crutch tips. Axillary crutches are generally chosen for patients with weakness of one or both lower extremities, a need to reduce weight bearing on one or both lower extremities, balance, impairment, or a need for some trunk support.

Typically, each axillary crutch has two parallel upper supports, which join to a single lower support. At the top of the two parallel upper supports is an axillary bar, which may be covered with a soft axillary pad. Handgrips, adjustable in height, are located between the upper and lower ends of the two parallel supports. Handgrips may or may not be covered with a soft handgrip. The single leg at the bottom of the crutch is adjustable and covered at its bottom with a crutch tip. During use, axillary crutches extend from the patient's axillae to the floor.

Axillary crutches were traditionally made of wood, but now are more commonly made of aluminum (Figure 10–10 ■). Wing nuts and bolts are used to adjust crutch length and handgrip height of wooden crutches. Push-button locks and telescoping legs are used on most aluminum crutches, although handgrips on aluminum crutches may still use wing nuts and bolts for adjustment.

Forearm (Lofstrand) Crutches

Forearm (Lofstrand) crutches (Figure 10–11 ■) provide more ease of movement but less trunk support than axillary crutches. The base of support for a person using forearm crutches is the area bounded by the patient's foot or feet on the floor and the two crutch

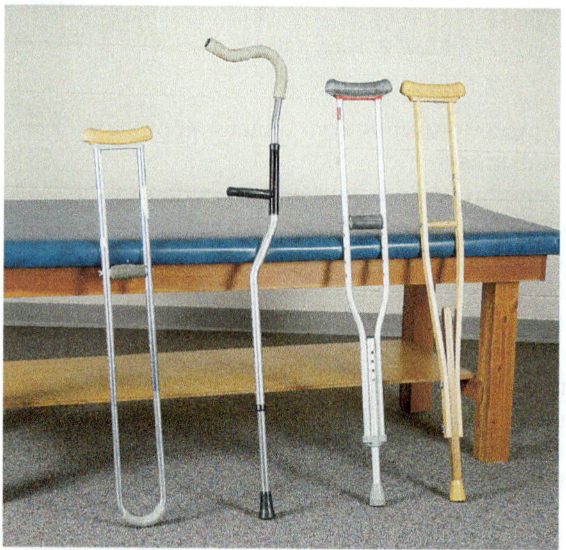

FIGURE 10–10 ■ A variety of aluminum and wooden axillary crutches.

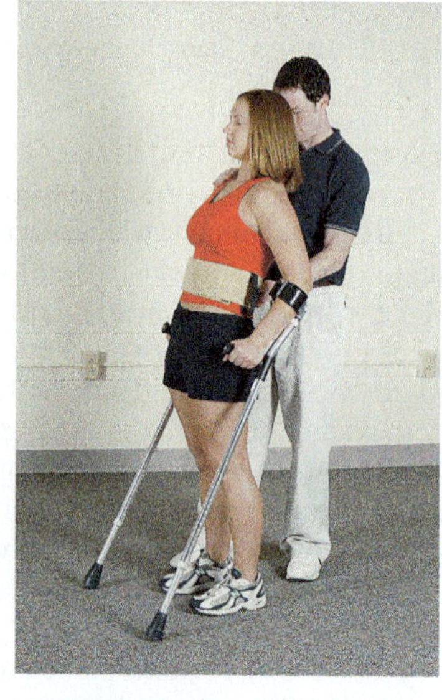

FIGURE 10–11 ■ Patient using forearm (Lofstrand) crutches.

tips. The cuff around the forearm permits patients to use their hands without dropping the crutch. Forearm crutches are recommended for patients with the same problems as would require axillary crutches, with the exception of decreased trunk stability. Patients who will need crutches permanently or for long periods of time may find forearm crutches more desirable because they are less cumbersome and more maneuverable than axillary crutches.

Forearm crutches have a single adjustable support leg with an adjustable cuff at the top to surround the forearm and an adjustable handgrip. Adjustments to the cuff allow the cuff to be raised or lowered and for the cuff to be narrowed or widened to accommodate a patient's forearm size. During use, forearm crutches extend from the floor to the forearms.

Canes

Standard canes (**Figure 10–12** ■) are generally chosen for patients with minimal weakness of the lower extremity(ies), who require slight weight-bearing reduction, or who need assistance with balance. The base of support for a patient using one cane is the area bounded by the patient's feet and the single cane tip. When using two canes, the base of support is the area bounded by the patient's feet and the two cane tips.

The most common styles of single-point standard canes are "J" canes and offset canes. Both of these standard canes have a handgrip and shaft, with a tip at the bottom end of the shaft. A J cane's handgrip extends in a smooth curve directly onto the shaft, so forces applied to the handgrip are not directly over the tip. The offset cane's shaft is offset under the handgrip, allowing forces applied to the handgrip to be directly over the tip. During use a patient holds a cane vertically in one hand, and the cane extends from the floor to the hand. Standard canes provide limited stability and weight-bearing capability.

■ Take Note

The variety of cane handgrips allows for a selection that can accommodate a patient's hand size and impairments.

Both styles of standard canes are constructed of aluminum or wood. Aluminum canes are adjustable using push-button locks and telescoping legs. Some aluminum canes have a ring around the lower end of the shaft that is part of the adjustment system. Wooden canes can be cut to adjust length, meaning they can only be shortened.

A variation of the standard cane is a quad cane, so named because it has four feet. Quad canes are available in two base sizes, large and small (**Figure 10–13** ■). The design of a quad cane makes it stable during ambulation. The four feet also allow the quad cane to remain upright and readily available for use when a patient is not holding the cane. Because of these benefits, quad canes are commonly used by patients with

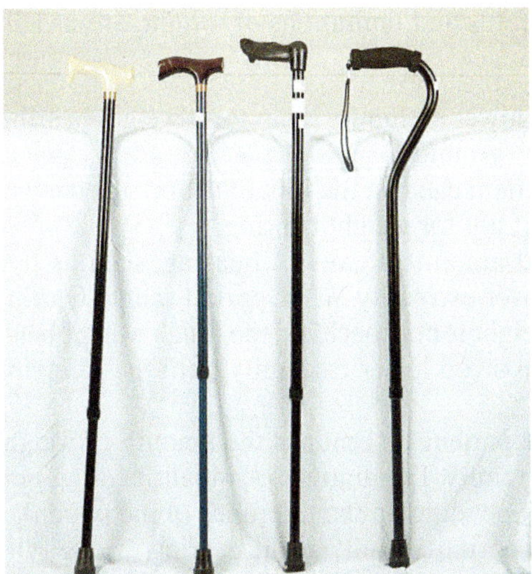

FIGURE 10–12 ■ A variety of standard canes.

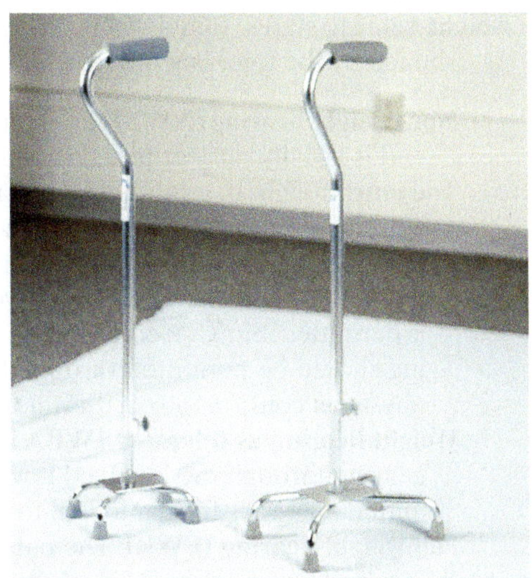

FIGURE 10–13 ■ Small-base quad cane (left) and large-base quad cane (right).

limited or no use of one upper extremity. A disadvantage of large base quad canes is that the larger base does not permit it to be placed on a standard stair tread unless turned sideways.

Quad canes are chosen for patients with impairments that are similar to, but greater than, patients who use standard canes. The base of support for a patient using one quad cane is the area bounded by the patient's feet and the base of the quad cane. When using two quad canes, the base of support is the area bounded by the patient's feet and the bases of the two quad canes. Patients may initially use a quad cane and transition to a standard cane as their abilities increase.

Quad canes are constructed of aluminum, using a telescoping upper shaft for height adjustment. The offset handgrip style is used for quad canes. The outer legs of quad cane bases are angled outward from the base to a greater degree than the inner legs to increase the base of support provided. During use the wider angled legs are placed away from the patient to avoid interference with a patient's feet during gait. Bases on quad canes can be rotated so the same cane can be used on either the right or left side, maintaining appropriate outward orientation of the larger legs with respect to handgrip orientation. Handgrips for all types of canes are available in varied shapes and textures to make grasp easier.

Ambulating with Assistive Devices

A **gait pattern** is defined as a selected sequence of movements for the ambulatory assistive device(s) and lower extremities. Important considerations for selecting a gait pattern include, but are not limited to, weight-bearing status, strength, range of motion, balance, stability, coordination, general condition, and living environment. The referring physician provides weight-bearing status. The specific gait pattern is determined by the physical therapist.

Weight-Bearing Status

Weight bearing is the amount of weight that can be borne on a lower extremity during standing or ambulation. The amount of weight bearing permitted is dependent on the patient's pathology, impairment, and medical management. When ambulating with ambulatory assistive devices, lifting of the body to decrease weight bearing on the lower extremities is achieved by shoulder girdle depression and elbow extension.

The amount of weight bearing through a lower extremity can vary from full weight bearing to non–weight bearing. During gait training, weight bearing through the lower extremities is reduced by shifting the transmission of forces to the upper extremities and thus through the ambulatory assistive device(s). Five commonly used terms describe weight-bearing status. Initial weight-bearing status and limitations of weight, are usually determined by the referring physician.

Non–weight bearing (NWB): The involved lower extremity is not to be weight bearing, and is usually not permitted to touch the ground.

Toe touch weight bearing (TTWB): The patient can rest the foot of the involved lower extremity on the ground for balance, but not for weight bearing.

Partial weight bearing (PWB): A limited amount of weight bearing, such as five pounds, is permitted for the involved lower extremity. When partial weight bearing is permitted, but a specific amount of weight is not specified, toe touch weight bearing should be permitted through the involved lower extremity until the referring physician confirms a specific amount.

Weight bearing as tolerated (WBAT): The patient determines the amount of weight bearing through the involved lower extremity. The amount of weight bearing permitted may vary from minimal to full, depending on the tolerance of the patient.

Full weight bearing (FWB): The patient is permitted full weight bearing through the involved lower extremity. Ambulatory assistive devices are not required to decrease weight bearing but may be used for assistance with balance.

Gait Patterns

The gait patterns described in the following sections are for forward progression. These patterns, however, are also used for turning and backward progression.

THREE-POINT GAIT PATTERN A three-point gait pattern is used when a walker or two ambulatory assistive devices, crutches or canes, are required. A three-point gait pattern has two variations, step-to and step-through. The three-point step-to gait pattern has the patient move the trailing lower extremity only up to the ambulatory assistive device(s). The three-point step-through gait pattern has the patient move the trailing lower extremity beyond the ambulatory assistive devices and involved lower extremity. When the ambulatory assistive device is a walker, using a three-point step-through gait pattern results in the patient taking small steps so as to not step beyond the cross bar. A modification of the three-point step-through gait pattern occurs when patients ambulating with crutches become proficient and advance both lower extremities simultaneously beyond the crutches.

The walker or both ambulatory assistive devices are considered "one point," and each lower extremity is considered "one point." Thus the name three-point gait pattern.

A three-point gait pattern permits weight bearing to be varied from non–weight bearing to partial weight bearing to full weight bearing as appropriate and possible, given the ambulatory assistive device used. A three-point gait pattern is used by patients with impairments that include, but are not limited to, weight-bearing status, strength, pain, decreased balance or stability, or injury/surgery.

Usually, the three-point step-to gait pattern is a precursor to the three-point step-through gait pattern, as patients use the step-to variation while learning to ambulate with the ambulatory assistive device(s). There may, however, be patients with significant impairments who may only be able to ambulate by using the step-to variation. When appropriate, encourage patients to use the step-through gait pattern to achieve a faster and more normal step length pattern.

The examples that follow demonstrate the use of two crutches. The use of two canes follows the same pattern, but requires that both lower extremities are almost full weight bearing. When a walker is used, the walker is advanced as a unit, mimicking the simultaneous advancement of two crutches or two canes.

Three-Point Step-to Gait Pattern Both ambulatory assistive devices are advanced forward and placed on the floor approximately one step length. The patient advances the involved lower extremity forward between the two ambulatory assistive devices so that the ball of the foot is placed at a point in line with the tip of ambulatory assistive devices (**Figure 10–14 ■**).

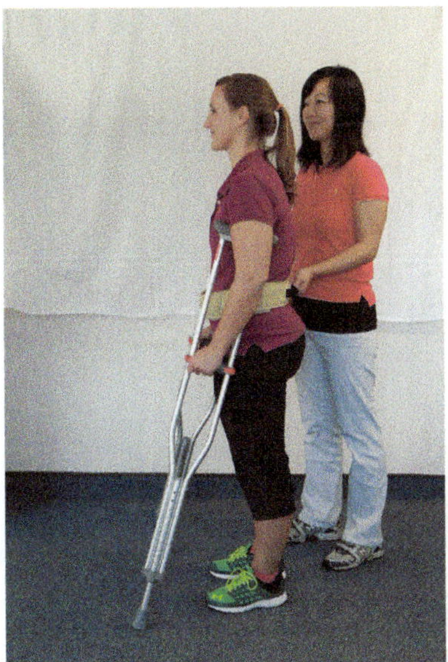

FIGURE 10–14 ■ Three-point step-to gait pattern—part 1.

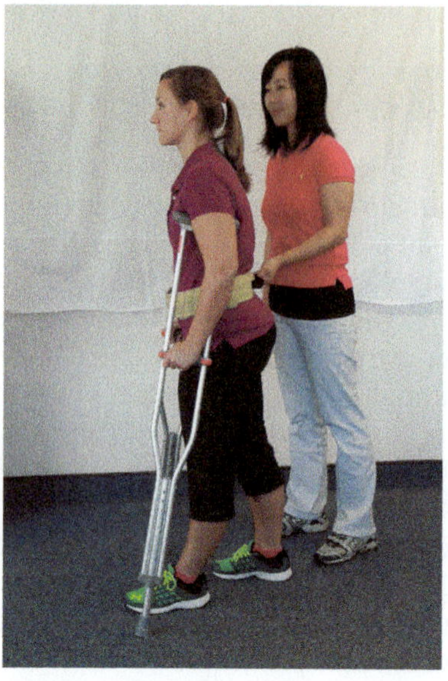

FIGURE 10–15 ■ Three-point step-to gait pattern—part 2.

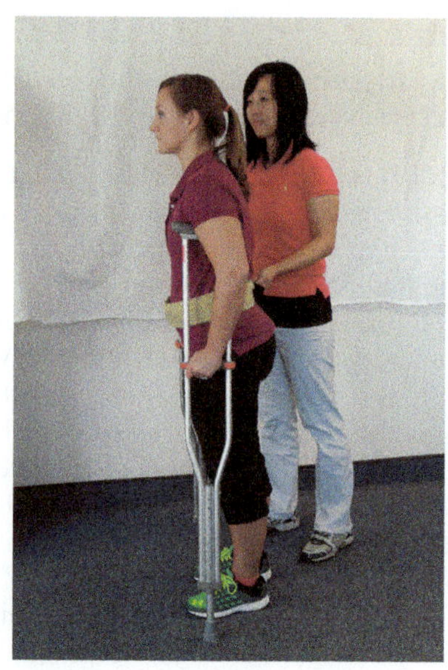

FIGURE 10–16 ■ Three-point step-to gait pattern—part 3.

The patient shifts weight-bearing to the upper extremities and involved lower extremity if permitted by weight-bearing status. The patient then advances the uninvolved lower extremity forward to a point in line with the tip of the ambulatory assistive devices and involved lower extremity (Figure 10–15 ■). The patient shifts weight bearing to the uninvolved lower extremity in preparation for the next forward movement of the ambulatory assistive devices and involved lower extremity (Figure 10–16 ■). This three-part sequence is repeated as the patient continues to ambulate.

As patients become more confident, they move the ambulatory assistive devices and involved lower extremity forward simultaneously, increasing the speed of ambulation.

Three-point step-through gait pattern Both ambulatory assistive devices are advanced forward and placed on the floor approximately one step length (Figure 10–17 ■).

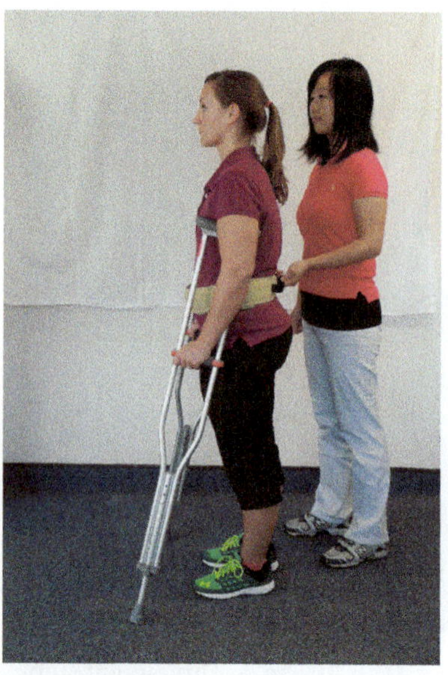

FIGURE 10–17 ■ Three-point step-through gait pattern—part 1.

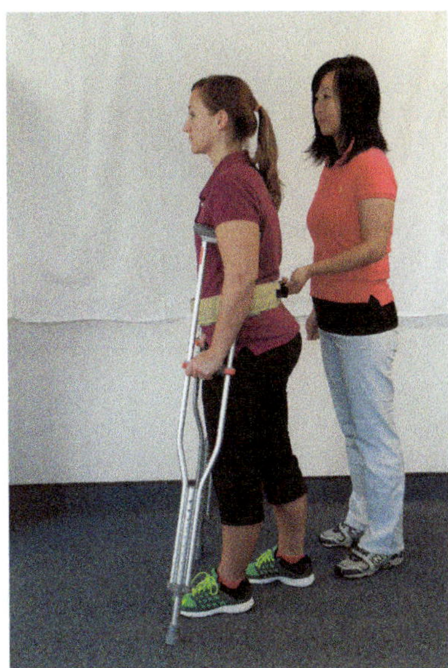

FIGURE 10–18 ■ Three-point step-through gait pattern—part 2.

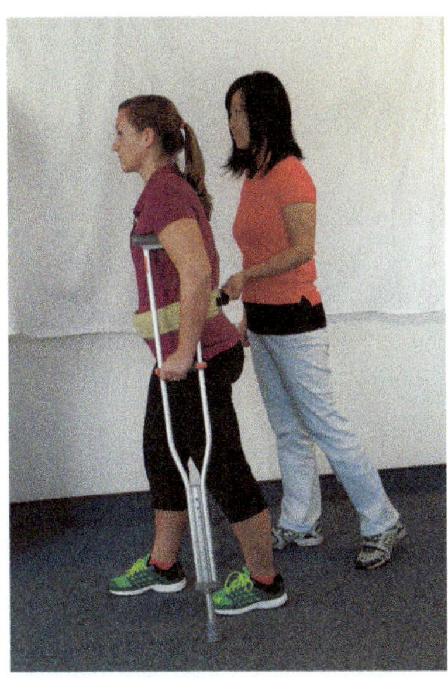

FIGURE 10–19 ■ Three-point step-through gait pattern—part 3.

The patient advances the involved lower extremity forward between the two ambulatory assistive devices so that the ball of the foot is placed at a point in line with the tip ambulatory assistive devices (Figure 10–18 ■).

The patient shifts weight bearing to the upper extremities and involved lower extremity if permitted by weight-bearing status. The patient then advances the uninvolved lower extremity forward past the ambulatory assistive devices. The patient shifts weight-bearing to the uninvolved lower extremity in preparation for the next forward movement of the ambulatory assistive devices and involved lower extremity. This three-part sequence is repeated as the patient continues to ambulate (Figure 10–19 ■).

As patients become more confident, they move the ambulatory assistive devices and involved lower extremity forward simultaneously, increasing the speed of ambulation.

FOUR-POINT GAIT PATTERN A four-point gait pattern is often described as a deliberate two-point gait pattern. This gait pattern is used when two ambulatory assistive devices, such as two canes or two crutches, are required. When using a four-point gait pattern, each ambulatory assistive device and each lower extremity is advanced independently, and each is considered "one point." A complete cycle includes "four points," thus the name four-point gait pattern.

A four-point gait pattern requires weight bearing status to be nearly full or full weight bearing. The four-point gait pattern is used by patients with impairments of, but may not be limited to, weight-bearing, strength, pain, balance, stability, coordination, or deconditioning. A four-point gait pattern may be used as a starting point to teach patients the pairing of the opposite upper and lower extremities before using the two-point gait pattern.

The patient advances one crutch forward approximately one step length (Figure 10–20 ■).

The opposite lower extremity is advanced so the ball of the foot is placed at a point in line with the crutch tip on the opposite side (Figure 10–21 ■).

The patient moves the other crutch forward approximately one step length beyond the first crutch and lower extremity (Figure 10–22 ■).

The opposite lower extremity is advanced so the ball of the foot is at a point in line with the crutch tip on the opposite side. This four-part sequence is repeated as the patient continues to ambulate (Figure 10–23 ■).

TWO-POINT GAIT PATTERN A two-point gait pattern is used when two ambulatory assistive devices, such as two canes or two crutches, are required. Each combination of one

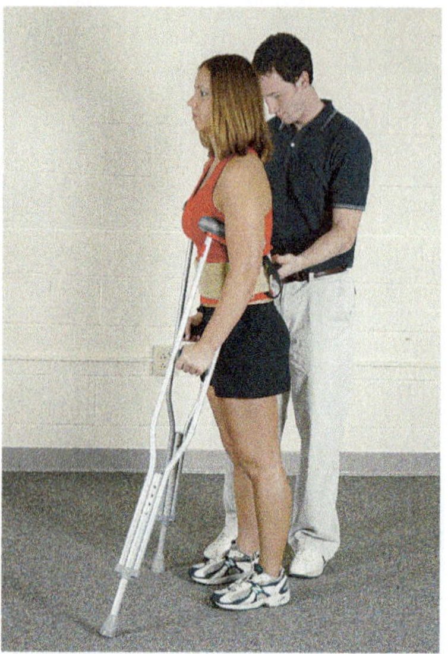

FIGURE 10–20 ■ Four-point gait pattern—part 1.

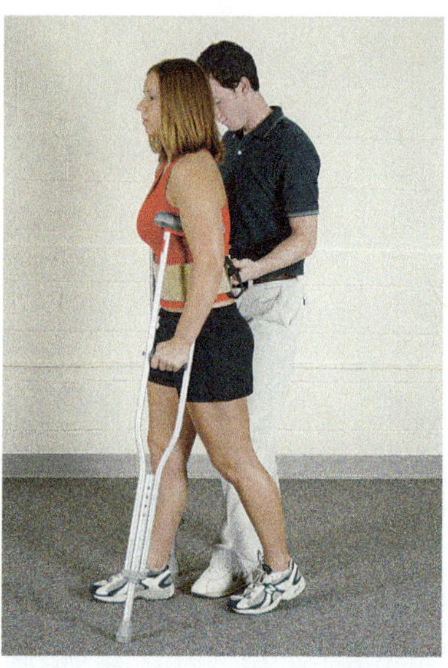

FIGURE 10–21 ■ Four-point gait pattern—part 2.

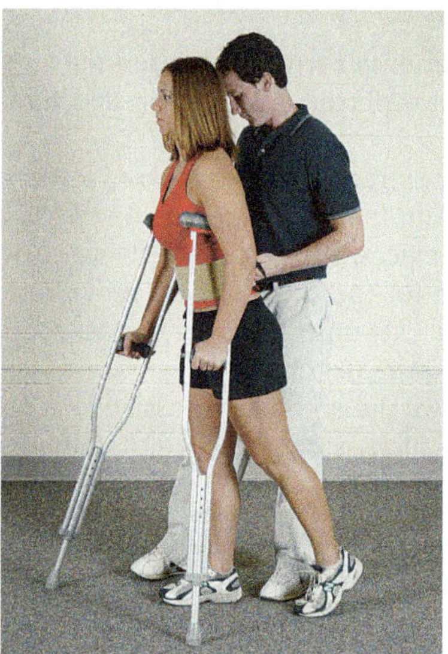

FIGURE 10–22 ■ Four-point gait pattern—part 3.

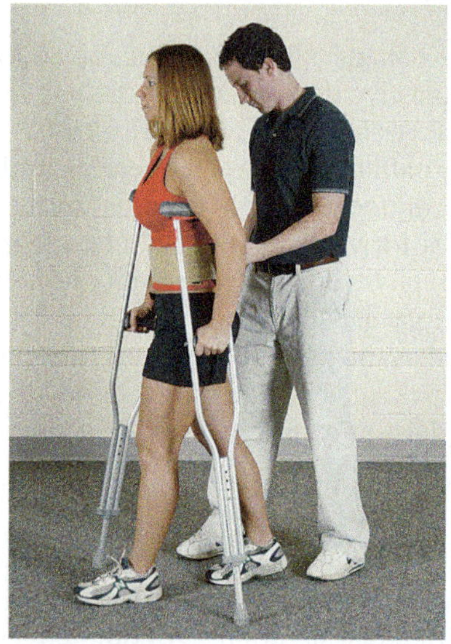

FIGURE 10–23 ■ Four-point gait pattern—part 4.

ambulatory assistive device and the opposite lower extremity is advanced simultaneously and is considered "one point." A complete cycle includes "two points," thus the name two-point gait pattern.

A two-point gait pattern requires weight bearing to be nearly full or full weight bearing. This gait pattern is used by patients with impairments of, but may not be limited to, weight-bearing, strength, pain, balance, stability, coordination, or general deconditioning.

The patient lifts and moves one cane and the opposite lower extremity forward approximately one step length simultaneously (**Figure 10–24** ■).

When the cane and lower extremity have been placed on the ground, the patient shifts weight to these supports. The patient then steps forward with the other cane and its opposite lower extremity beyond the other cane and lower extremity. This two-part sequence is repeated as the patient continues to ambulate (**Figure 10–25** ■).

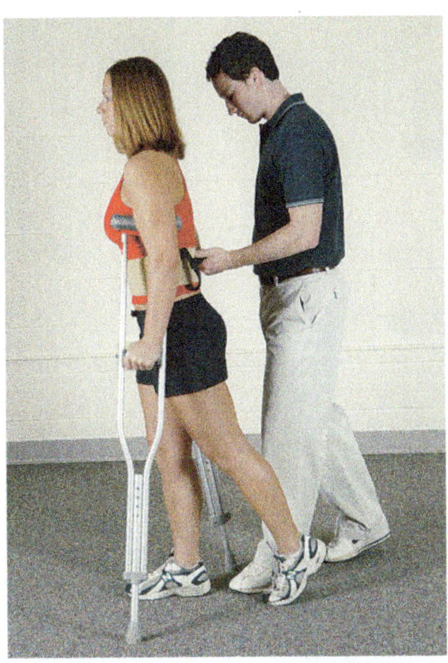

FIGURE 10–24 ■ Two-point gait pattern—part 1.

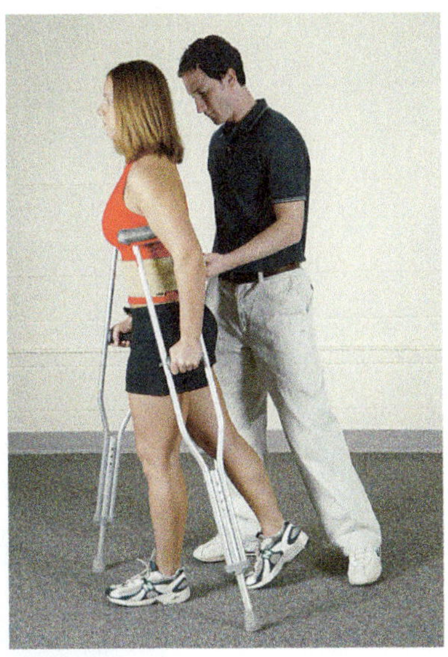

FIGURE 10–25 ■ Two-point gait pattern—part 2.

SWING-TO GAIT PATTERN A swing-to gait pattern requires the use of two crutches or a walker. The ambulatory assistive device(s) are advanced simultaneously, and then both lower extremities are advanced to a point in line with the ambulatory assistive device(s). The lower extremities "swing-to" the ambulatory assistive device(s), thus the name of the gait pattern.

This gait pattern is used by patients with paresis or paralysis of the lower extremities and lower trunk. Because the lower extremities are paretic or paralyzed, upper trunk movements and lower extremity orthotic devices are necessary.

Usually, the swing-to gait pattern is a precursor to the swing-through gait pattern, using the swing-to pattern to learn to ambulate. When appropriate, encourage patients to use the swing-through gait pattern to achieve faster and more efficient ambulation.

While weight bearing through the lower extremities, the patient moves both crutches forward simultaneously (Figure 10–26 ■).

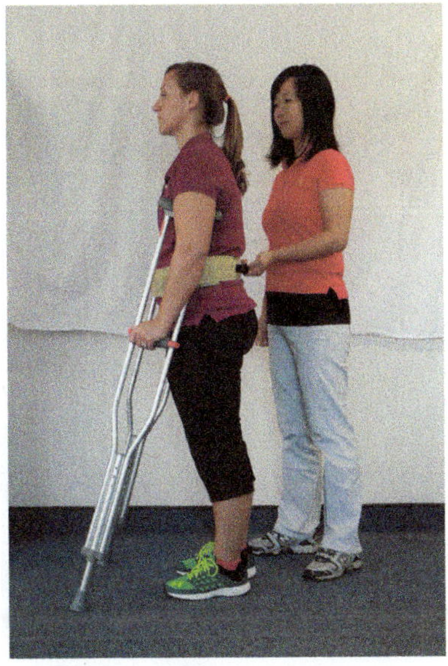

FIGURE 10–26 ■ Swing-to gait pattern—part 1.

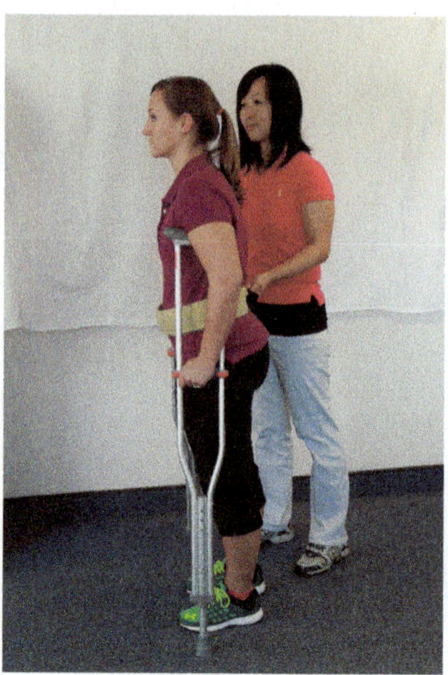

FIGURE 10–27 ■ Swing-to gait pattern—part 2.

The patient shifts weight bearing onto the crutches. Using head and upper trunk movement and shoulder girdle depression with elbow extension, the patient lifts and advances both lower extremities forward simultaneously. The lower extremities are placed on the floor so the balls of the feet are approximately at a point in line with the crutch tips (Figure 10–27 ■). This two-part sequence is repeated as the patient continues to ambulate.

SWING-THROUGH GAIT PATTERN A swing-through gait pattern requires the use of two crutches. The crutches are advanced simultaneously, and then both lower extremities are advanced to a point beyond the crutches. The lower extremities "swing-through" the crutches, thus the name of the gait pattern.

This gait pattern is used by patients with paresis or paralysis of the lower extremities and trunk. Because the lower extremities are paretic or paralyzed, upper trunk movements and lower extremity orthotic devices are necessary.

While weight bearing through the lower extremities, the patient moves both crutches forward simultaneously (Figure 10–28 ■).

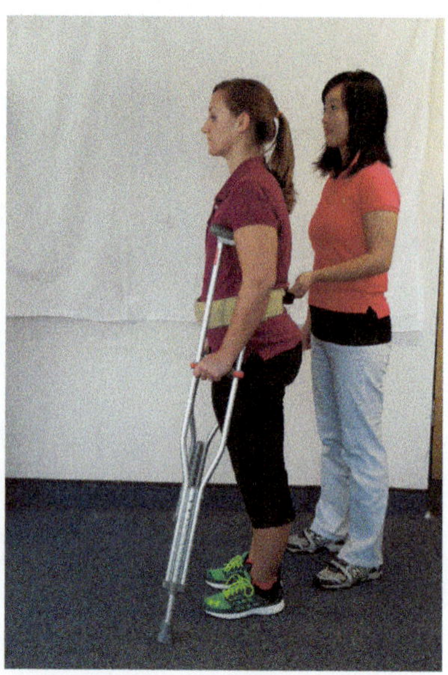

FIGURE 10–28 ■ Swing-through gait pattern—part 1.

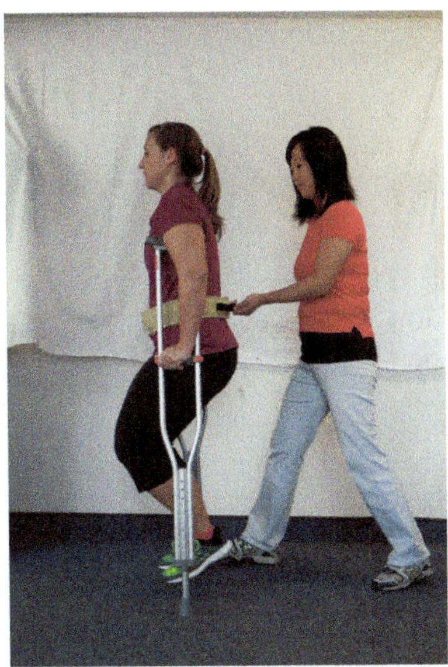

FIGURE 10–29 ■ Swing-through gait pattern—part 2.

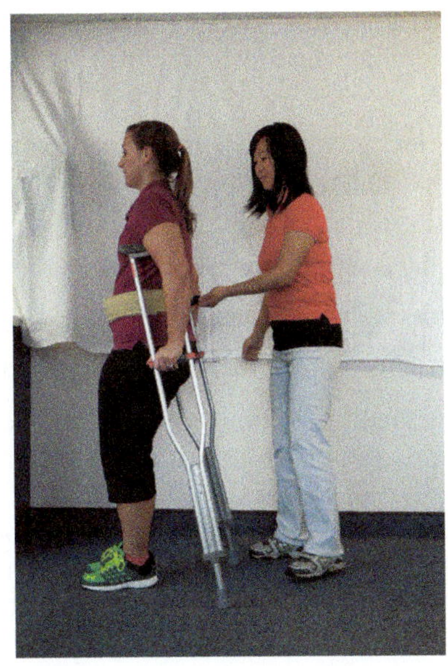

FIGURE 10–30 ■ Swing-through gait pattern—part 3.

The patient shifts weight bearing onto the crutches and using head and upper trunk movement and shoulder girdle depression with elbow extension, lifts and advances both lower extremities forward simultaneously (Figure 10–29 ■).

The lower extremities are placed on the floor so the feet are beyond the crutch tips. This two-part sequence is repeated as the patient continues to ambulate (Figure 10–30 ■).

Guarding During Gait Training Activities

The purpose of guarding during gait training activities is to protect the patient from excessive weight bearing, loss of balance, or falling. Safety must not be compromised by the selection, or during the performance, of gait training activities. Those assisting the patient must provide appropriate guarding during gait training activities. The level and type of guarding during gait training activities is determined by the physical therapist. As a patient improves, the level and type of guarding decreases to the minimum amount possible without compromising patient safety.

■ **Take Note**

Proper guarding techniques provide safety for patients and physical therapists/assistants.

Gait Belts

Proper guarding requires use of a gait belt. Guarding by holding onto the patient's belt may be uncomfortable for the patient because the narrow belt or belt buckle can bind or pinch the patient. Holding clothing is not appropriate because clothing does not fit firmly enough to provide control during guarding or may tear and provide no support. A gait belt should fit snugly around the patient's waist. There may or may not be handles for grasping the gait belt. Hold the gait belt with the forearm in supination for a stronger grip. Initially, grasp the gait belt with one hand and place the other hand on the patient's trunk over the shoulder girdle on the side to which you are standing.

Levels of Guarding During Gait Training Activities

Common terminology describing levels of guarding is based on the scoring scale presented in the Functional Independence Measure (FIM).[1] When performing gait training, the following terminology[2] describes the amount of assistance provided to a patient by the physical therapist/assistant. When no assistance is required, the patient is described as being independent. When the only assistance a patient requires is an ambulatory assistive device, the patient is described as having modified independence.

1. **Supervision**: Physical therapist/assistant is near the patient and able to provide verbal or physical assistance as appropriate. It is unlikely that physical assistance will be required.

2. **Close guarding**: Physical therapist/assistant is positioned close to the patient, without contact with the patient. The likelihood of physical assistance being required is Fair.
3. **Contact guarding**: Physical therapist/assistant is positioned close to the patient, with hands on the patient/gait belt. The likelihood of physical assistance being required is High.
4. **Minimal (minimum) assistance**: A patient is able to perform 75% or more of an activity.
5. **Moderate assistance**: A patient is able to perform 50–74% of an activity.
6. **Maximal (maximum) assistance**: A patient is able to perform 25–49% of an activity.

When in doubt about whether one person can provide the amount of assistance necessary for a patient to perform gait training activities safely, obtain additional assistance. The number of persons needed to perform a gait training activity safely is noted in your documentation. For example, when two people are required for a patient to perform the gait training activity requiring moderate assistance, documentation should read ". . . moderate assistance X 2. . . ."

Types of Guarding

■ **Take Note**

Type of assistance—verbal cuing, monitoring the environment, physical assistance.

Types of guarding include, but are not limited to, verbal cuing, monitoring the environment, and physical assistance. The following are examples of types of guarding that might be needed by patients. A patient may require minimal physical assistance X 1 for balance control. A second patient may require moderate physical assistance X 2 for assistance with assuming a standing position with appropriate ambulatory assistive devices. A third patient may require only verbal cuing.

The goal of gait training is to assist the patient to become independent or modified independent during ambulation. This is achieved by reducing, as appropriate, the amount of assistance (maximal → moderate → minimal → contact guarding → close guarding → supervision → modified independent → independent). Included in this progression is the type of assistance (physical and verbal → verbal → independent).

Guarding During Gait Training Activities

■ **Take Note**

Caution—Be alert to patient balance and movement. Be prepared to prevent or control a fall.

In all situations, persons guarding patients during gait training activities must be positioned in a way that permits those guarding the patient to move with the patient and to avoid interference with the patient's movements. Safe guarding of patients during gait training activities requires being alert to a patient's associated conditions such as orthostatic hypotension, mentation and alertness, position, movements, and fatigue, as well as obstacles in the environment.

During early stages of gait training, a patient usually leans away from weight bearing on the involved lower extremity because they fear pain or further injury if too much weight is placed on the involved lower extremity. By guarding on a patient's uninvolved side, you are in the best position to pull a patient into your base of support, reducing the risk of increased weight bearing on an involved lower extremity. Pulling the patient into your base of support is the safer method for preventing a fall for both the patient and yourself. When a patient starts to fall, you are better able to provide support and protection of an involved lower extremity by shifting the patient's weight onto the uninvolved lower extremity. For these reasons, initial gait training usually begins by guarding patients on the uninvolved side. As a patient's capabilities improve, you may switch to guarding from the patient's involved side, thereby encouraging upright posture and appropriate use of the involved lower extremity.

■ **Take Note**

For safety, initial guarding should be from the side of the patient's uninvolved lower extremity.

In and Out of a Wheelchair

When a patient arises from or sits in a chair, stand in stride to one side and slightly behind the patient (Figure 10–31 ■). In some instances, you may stand in front of the patient, as for an assisted standing pivot transfer. Standing in front of the patient permits the provision of physical assistance and moves the patient into your base of support.

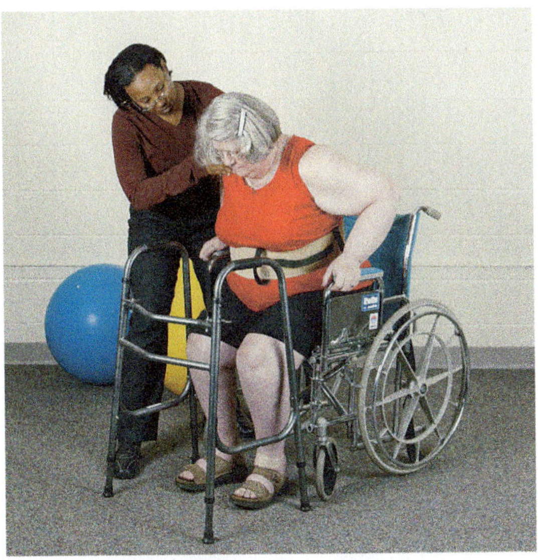

FIGURE 10–31 ■ Position for guarding during assumption of standing.

Level Surfaces

When patients ambulate with *contact guarding,* stand in stride directly behind the patient and the assistive device on the side on which you are guarding. Grasp the gait belt with your forearm in supination, and place your other hand over the patient's shoulder girdle, not on the upper extremity. When a hand is placed on the patient's upper extremity, it may interfere with the patient's freedom of motion needed to control ambulatory assistive devices. When the patient improves significantly, remove your hand from the patient's shoulder girdle if doing so will not compromise patient safety.

As the patient ambulates, move your "outside" (the one most lateral to the patient) foot as the patient moves the ambulatory assistive device on the side on which you are guarding. Move your "inside" foot (the one directly behind the patient) as the patient moves the lower extremity on the side on which you are guarding.

When the patient progresses, stand in stride behind and to the side of the patient on the side on which you are guarding. Grasp the gait belt with your forearm in supination. Your other hand may or may not be in contact with the patient's shoulder girdle (Figure 10–32 ■).

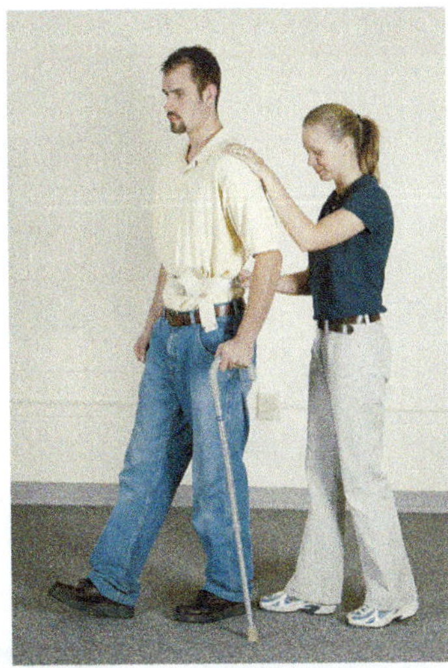

FIGURE 10–32 ■ Starting position for close guarding during ambulation.

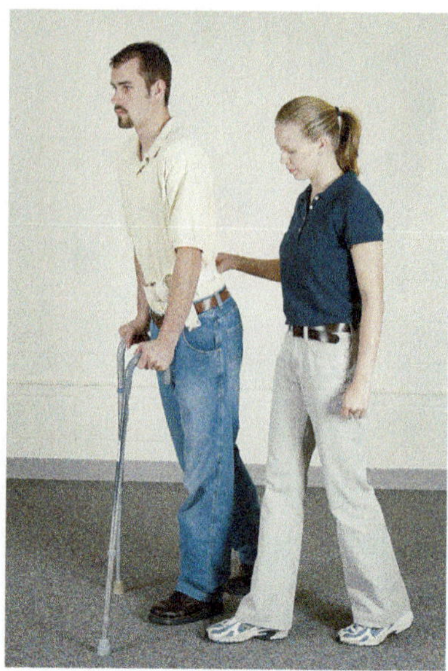

FIGURE 10–33 ■ Moving with patient for close guarding during ambulation.

As the patient ambulates, move your "outside" foot as the patient moves the ambulatory assistive device on the side on which you are guarding. Move your "inside" foot as the patient moves the lower extremity on the side on which you are guarding (**Figure 10–33** ■).

Eventually, *supervision guarding,* walking near the patient without contact or holding the gait belt, may be the only guarding that is needed.

Falling

When a patient starts to fall, you must decide whether to maintain the patient in an upright position or to permit a controlled lowering to the floor in a manner that will prevent injury to the patient or yourself. By guarding on a patient's uninvolved side, you are in the best position to pull a patient into your base of support and away from their involved lower extremity to prevent falls (**Figure 10–34** ■). When lowering a patient to the floor in a controlled manner, enlarge your base of support by moving your lower extremity(ies),

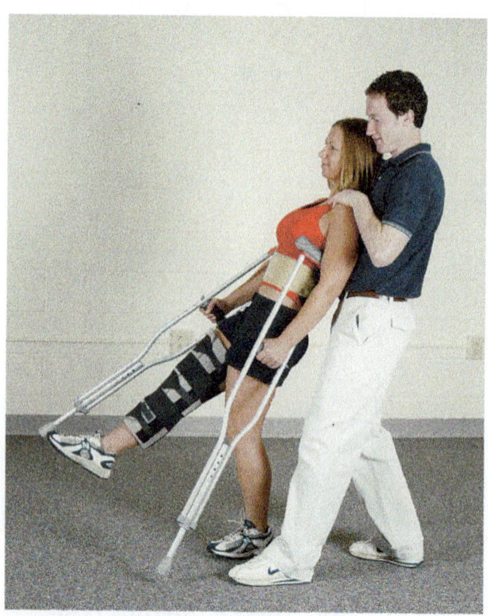

FIGURE 10–34 ■ Guarding to prevent falling.

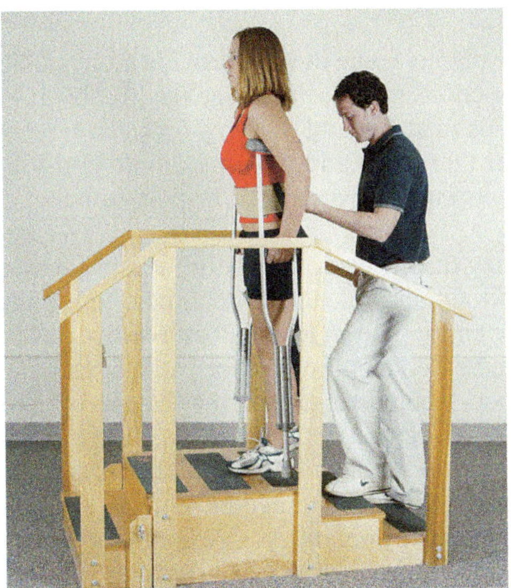

FIGURE 10–35 ■ Position for guarding patient ascending stairs.

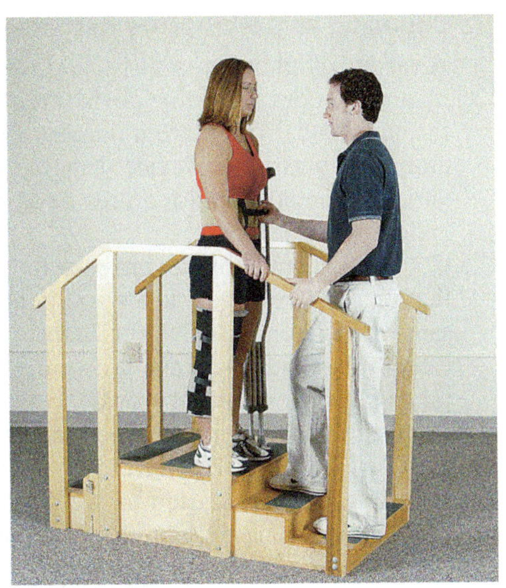

FIGURE 10–36 ■ Position for guarding patient descending stairs.

keeping the patient within your base of support. Avoid becoming entangled with the patient and the ambulatory assistive devices as you move to control lowering the patient to the floor.

Be alert at all times to a patient's movements, balance, and alertness and react quickly to prevent or control a fall. You must also be alert to your position and movements with respect to the patient.

Ascending/Descending Stairs

Position yourself below the patient when guarding as the patient ascends and descends stairs (**Figures 10–35** ■ and **10–36** ■). Grasp the patient's gait belt with one hand and a handrail with the other hand. Holding a handrail provides a point of stability to halt a fall. Stand in stride on the stairs, placing one foot on the first step below the patient, and your other foot on the second step below the patient, thus standing on different stair treads. A stride position provides a larger base of support within which you can shift your weight and position as the patient moves, placing you in position to move the patient into your base of support should the patient begin to fall. Being close to the patient enables you to use your body, as well as your arms, to control a patient.

■ **Take Note**

When guarding a patient ascending/descending stairs, hold the handrail with one hand for stability to prevent a fall.

Occasionally a second person is needed to guard a patient learning to ascend and descend stairs. The second person stands in stride on the stairs above the patient and also holds the gait belt and handrail.

Physical Therapy Patient/Client Management Process

The physical therapy patient/client management process is used to select ambulatory assistive device, gait pattern, and level of guarding to be employed. Documentation of a patient's abilities must support these selections. Subsequent changes in patient abilities must be documented to support decisions to change ambulatory assistive devices, gait patterns, and level of guarding.

Interventions that develop and increase each patient's capabilities, such as strength, balance, and coordination, may be needed to ensure proficiency in selected ambulatory activities. For many reasons, such as health insurance coverage or distance to a clinic, time available to improve a patient's capabilities is often not available. Patients must become as proficient as possible in all necessary skills prior to discharge.

Once a physical therapist has chosen the ambulatory assistive device, a physical therapist assistant can implement gait training as directed by the physical therapist.

Choosing an Ambulatory Assistive Device

A variety of ambulatory assistive devices are available. Some devices provide more stability and support, and some devices require more coordination during use (see Tables 10–1 through 10–5). There are a number of variations in styles and features for each type of ambulatory assistive device. Together, physical therapists and patients should consider variations in style and features of ambulatory assistive devices with respect to benefits and drawbacks for use.

As a patient's abilities increase, the patient may change to an ambulatory assistive device that provides relatively less stability and support. Other patients may continue to use the same ambulatory assistive device throughout the entire time an ambulatory assistive device is required. When progressive disorders create increased impairments for patients, ambulatory assistive devices that provide relatively greater stability and support may be appropriate.

Decisions concerning selection of ambulatory assistive devices are based on a patient's impairments as determined during the examination and evaluation of a number of aspects, including, but not limited to, weight-bearing status, strength, range of motion, balance, stability, coordination, general condition, and living environment. As an example, a patient with a fractured lower extremity who must be non–weight bearing may use either crutches or a walker. When a patient has sufficient strength, balance, and coordination, crutches may be the ambulatory assistive device of choice. When a patient has poor stability, coordination, or a medically debilitating condition, a walker may be the ambulatory assistive device of choice. Thus a patient's weight-bearing status, strength, and balance, among other aspects, are matched to the ambulatory assistive device.

Information needed to make an appropriate choice of ambulatory assistive devices includes the stability provided by the device (**Table 10–1** ▪), amount of patient coordination required to use the device (**Table 10–2** ▪), amount of weight-bearing permitted (**Table 10–3** ▪), amount of patient strength (**Table 10–4** ▪), and degree of balance impairment (**Table 10–5** ▪).

Table 10–1 ▪ Stability provided by device, from most to least stable

1	Parallel bars
2	Walker
3	Axillary crutches
4	Forearm (Lofstrand) crutches
5	Two canes
6	One cane

Table 10–2 ▪ Patient coordination required to use device, from least to most coordination

1	Parallel bars
2	Walker
3	One cane
4	Two canes
5	Axillary crutches
6	Forearm (Lofstrand) crutches

Table 10–3 ▪ As the amount of weight bearing permitted is reduced and the number of involved limbs increases, the more external support is needed

Amount of WB	Unilateral LE WB Restriction	Bilateral LE WB Restriction
PWB almost full WB	1 standard cane	2 standard canes
↓PWB	1 crutch	Lofstrand crutches
↓↓PWB	2 canes	2 crutches or walker
↓↓↓PWB	2 crutches	2 crutches or walker
TT	2 crutches or walker	Unable to walk
NWB	2 crutches or walker	Unable to walk

Table 10–4 ▪ As strength decreases and the number of limbs involved increases, the more external support is needed

Amount of Strength	Unilateral LE Weakness	Bilateral LE Weakness
Minimal weakness	1 standard cane	2 standard canes
↓Strength	1 quad cane	2 quad canes
↓↓Strength	1 crutch	Lofstrand crutches
Significant weakness	2 crutches or walker	2 crutches or walker

Table 10–5 ▪ As balance impairment increases, the more external support is needed

Degree of Balance Impairment	Ambulatory Assistive Device Appropriate
Minimal	1 cane or 1 forearm crutch
Moderate	2 canes, 2 crutches, or walker
Severe	2 crutches or walker and guarding

Choosing a Gait Pattern

A physical therapist selects a gait pattern based on weight-bearing status permitted and number of limbs involved (Table 10–6 ▪), strength and number of limbs involved (Table 10–7 ▪), and severity of balance impairment (Table 10–8 ▪). Environments in which a patient will be ambulating, such as stairs, ramps, uneven ground, and types of doorways, may require adaptations or modifications of the chosen gait pattern.

As patients improve and gain confidence in use of the ambulatory assistive device, the gait pattern may change. As an example, a patient may move from a three-point step-to gait pattern to a three-point step-through gait pattern. This type of change requires increased control of the ambulatory assistive devices and improved balance and strength. Changes in gait pattern will also change as weight-bearing status changes. As an example, as a lower extremity fracture heals, a patient may move from a non–weight-bearing status to a partial weight-bearing status.

Table 10–6 ▪ Choosing a gait pattern considering weight-bearing status and number of limbs involved

Type of WB	Unilateral LE WB Restriction	Bilateral LE WB Restriction
PWB	3 point	2 or 4 point
TTWB	3 point or swing through	Unable to walk
NWB	3 point or swing through	Unable to walk

Table 10–7 ▪ Choosing a gait pattern considering strength impairment and number of limbs involved

Amount of Strength	Unilateral LE Weakness	Bilateral LE Weakness
Minimal weakness	3 point	2 or 4 point
Moderate weakness	3 point	Swing through (may need orthoses)
Significant weakness	3 point or swing through (may need orthoses)	Swing through (probably will need orthoses)

Table 10–8 ▪ Choosing a gait pattern considering severity of balance impairment

Balance Impairment	Gait Pattern
Minimal impairment	3 point
Moderate impairment	2, 3, or 4 point
Significant impairment	3 or 4 point and guarding

The choice of ambulatory assistive device may affect the gait pattern selected. As an example, a patient with generalized weakness or poor balance may use a walker because it provides more stability. When using a walker, patients might use a three-point step-to, but not a three-point step-through gait pattern. As another example, a patient with minimal balance problems using two canes may begin ambulating with a four-point gait pattern and then move to a two-point gait pattern as coordination when using the ambulatory assistive devices improves, or balance improves.

Choosing Guarding Level

The level of guarding to ensure safety is chosen by a physical therapist during development of a plan of care and before a patient arises from a bed or a chair. A level of guarding is chosen based on data from the examination. Although the evaluation may indicate that a low level of guarding, such as close guarding, may be appropriate, contact guarding is used during initial gait training activities to ensure safety. When it is determined that a patient expected to be able to perform gait training activities with close guarding can do so, initial contact guarding can change to close guarding, as planned. The level of guarding can decrease as patients improve performance of gait training activities. When a patient has a progressive condition, the level of guarding must be adjusted as the patient's abilities decline.

Teaching Tips

Methods of Instruction

Before a patient begins an ambulatory activity, describe and demonstrate proper performance of the ambulatory activity. Demonstration is the primary method of instruction. Verbal descriptions reinforce demonstration and must be simple. Having a patient observe other patients performing the ambulatory activity *correctly* is another useful method of instruction.

■ Take Note
Teaching techniques—demonstration and verbal description.

Select specific ambulatory activities to be mastered in order of difficulty. As an example, gait training on level surfaces should be well advanced before beginning gait training on stairs. A patient's learning capabilities must be balanced with imposed time constraints of treatment sessions or hospital discharge, without compromising patient health and safety.

As you will not always be available to instruct patients in how to perform tasks outside a rehabilitation setting, patients must learn how to solve problems on their own when performing ambulatory activities. Present novel situations and ask patients how they might proceed in the new situation, prior to a patient attempting the actual maneuver.

■ Take Note
Caution—Ensure patient's orientation, alertness, and ability to follow directions.

Training Environment

Initial ambulatory activity training should occur in an environment that is as free of distractions as possible. Select and monitor the environment to ensure patient safety. When patients improve, more complex environments are used to simulate a more natural environment.

■ Take Note
Motor learning principle—simple to complex environment.

Effect of Patient Fatigue and Concentration on Performance of Gait Training Activities

Fatigue may occur during ambulatory activity training, as a result of:

1. Performing an activity that has not been performed recently
2. Using ambulatory assistive devices during gait training activities
3. Greater levels of concentration required to perform gait training activities
4. Physiological responses to the stresses of injury or illness

These factors can cause the patient to fatigue rapidly. Fatigue, both physical and mental, may interfere with learning and performing ambulatory activities. Frequent rest periods or several shorter training sessions may decrease the effects of fatigue during initial ambulatory training sessions.

■ Take Note
To monitor fatigue, use vital signs and perceived exertion scales.

A patient's need to concentrate is very high when initially learning to use an ambulatory assistive device and gait pattern properly. Patients often look at their feet and ambulatory assistive devices because visual input of foot and assistive device location with respect to their body is necessary for coordination and safety. Because patients are paying attention to foot and assistive device position, you must ensure safety by reducing distraction from other objects and activities in the immediate area.

High levels of concentration exhibited by patients during ambulatory activity training may interfere with ability to respond to other inputs, such as conversation and objects in the environment. Patients may stop ambulation to answer questions. Initially, conversation not directly related to gait training activity should be avoided. Later, however, such additional inputs can be used to test the degree to which patients have mastered ambulatory activities. When ambulatory activities have again become an automatic activity, patients will be able to respond to questions and attend to the environment. As gait becomes automatic, patients usually start to look around as they ambulate. At this time patients can take over the responsibility of monitoring the environment for themselves, and more complex and distracting environments can be used for gait training activity.

■ Take Note
Motor learning principle—single task to multitask.

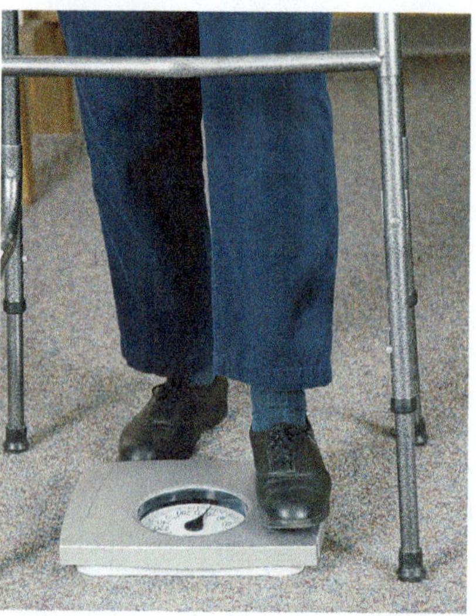

FIGURE 10–37 ■ Using one scale to measure weight bearing.

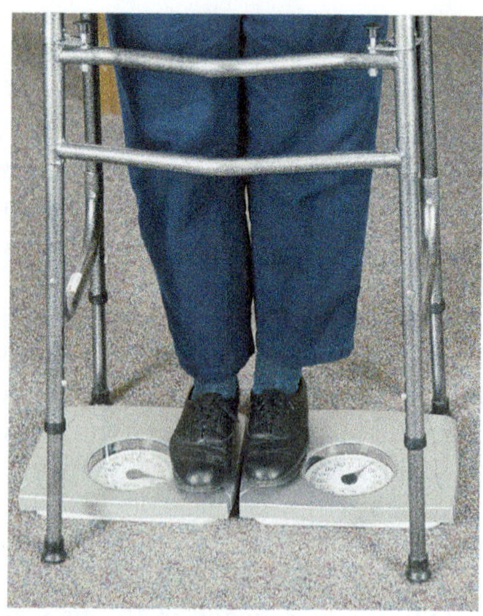

FIGURE 10–38 ■ Using two scales to measure weight bearing.

Demonstrating Levels of Weight Bearing

When a patient has a weight-bearing restriction, bathroom scales can be used to demonstrate different levels of weight bearing and the accompanying sensation. When using this method, the lower extremity not placed on the scale must be placed on a solid surface. The amount of weight bearing on the involved lower extremity is increased slowly until weight bearing reaches the level permitted (Figure 10–37 ■). Two scales may be used, with one lower extremity placed on each scale, to encourage equal weight bearing when full weight bearing is permitted (Figure 10–38 ■).

Use of Parallel Bars

Gait training activities with ambulatory assistive devices often begin at the parallel bars, either within the parallel bars or alongside one of the parallel bars. Parallel bars provide maximum stability while requiring the least amount of coordination from patients. Patients can become accustomed to upright posture while learning a gait pattern in the relative safety of parallel bars. Ambulatory assistive devices can be adjusted while a patient stands in parallel bars (Figure 10–39 ■). Patients may, however, become too dependent on parallel bars. Patients should progress to ambulation with ambulatory assistive devices other than parallel bars as rapidly as is safely possible.

When parallel bars are not available, other stable objects should be used. These objects may include, but are not limited to, handrails in hallways or stable pieces of furniture.

■ **Take Note**
Motor learning principle—practice in a variety of environments.

■ **Take Note**
Selection of ambulation skills to be taught is based on determination of environment(s) in which patient will be ambulating.

Sequence of Gait Training Activities

To be independent, patients using ambulatory assistive devices must learn to (1) move from sitting to standing and standing to sitting positions, (2) ambulate on level or uneven surfaces, (3) move through doorways, and (4) ascend and descend stairs. Patient education must be provided for as many, if not all, combinations of environments in which gait training may occur.

An important task is to teach patients to check that ambulatory assistive devices are in safe working condition. Rubber tips will not grip the floor properly if they become worn excessively or if dirt fills the grooves. Wing nuts on crutches often loosen with use and should be checked regularly to ensure they are tightened appropriately. Push buttons used for adjustment do not always seat completely and may become disengaged.

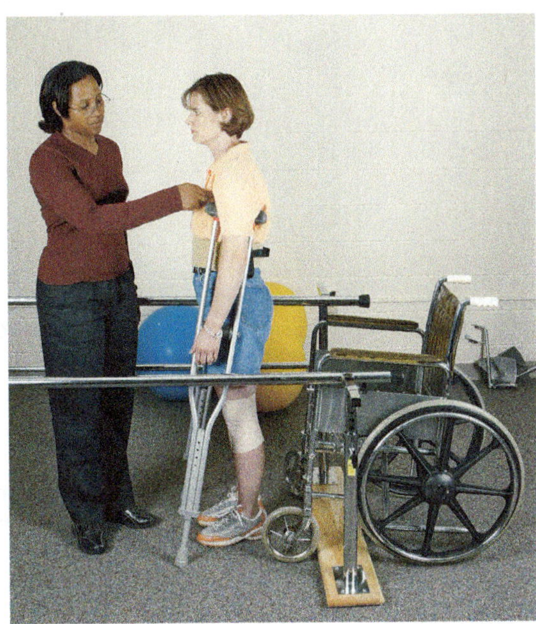

FIGURE 10–39 ■ Fitting axillary crutches at the parallel bars.

SITTING TO STANDING AND STANDING TO SITTING Initial instruction will most likely be related to using chairs with armrests. Patients must be taught to sit in a controlled manner, rather than collapsing into a sitting position. Varying seat height, availability of armrests, and type of cushioning is necessary to promote problem-solving abilities of a patient and generalizability of a patient's skills.

AMBULATING ON LEVEL OR UNEVEN SURFACES Initial training in the performance of gait training is on level surfaces. When patients can perform safely on a level surface, instruction in the use of ramps and uneven surfaces is provided. Instruction on how to fall safely is also provided.

Uneven surfaces may present specific problems for patients. Gravel, grass, broken sidewalks and paving, and floor thresholds may require additional instruction and practice. Patients should be cautioned to avoid small throw rugs that may slip or become entangled with their feet or ambulatory assistive devices. Wet or highly polished floors can be slippery and should also be avoided whenever possible. When ambulating on icy, wet, or highly polished surfaces, smaller movements and shorter step lengths should be used. Taking shorter steps applies forces placed on ambulatory assistive devices more directly downward, which is more stable and avoids horizontal forces that may cause ambulatory assistive devices to slip.

■ **Take Note**

Caution—Crutch and cane tips wear from use on rough and uneven surfaces. Teach patients to check them regularly.

AMBULATING THROUGH DOORWAYS Instruction in moving through doorways of different types and configurations is necessary. Doors may or may not have automatic door openers and automatic closing devices. The arc of door opening, force necessary to open a door, speed of door closing, right- versus left-hinged doors, the direction of door opening (toward, or away from the patient), and the type of doorknob are variables to be considered.

ASCENDING AND DESCENDING STAIRS Patients should be taught to ascend and descend stairs on the appropriate side when possible. In the United States this is the patient's right side when facing the stairs. Handrails may not exist, be placed only on one side, be of different shapes and sizes, and be placed at different heights. Stairs may have different riser heights or tread depths. Traversing curbs is similar to stairs, but curbs usually do not have handrails. In addition, curb cuts may not exist, and curb heights vary.

PROCEDURE 10–1 Assumption of Standing and Sitting

Preparing the Wheelchair

When the patient is assuming standing from a wheelchair or assuming sitting in a wheelchair, the physical therapist/assistant places the wheelchair against a stable surface, such as a wall or heavy table if possible, and engages the wheel locks. The physical therapist/assistant raises the footplates and removes the footrests and places them out of the way of the physical therapist/assistant or patient.

Positioning the Patient

To ease the assumption of a standing position, the patient moves to sitting at the front edge of the seat, as shown in Chapter 9. The patient places both feet flat on the floor below the front edge of the seat. In this position the patient's knees are flexed to approximately 110 degrees, and ankles are in slight dorsiflexion. The patient's center of gravity can be brought over the base of support quickly from this position as the patient assumes standing. The patient may place her feet side by side or in a short stride position. Using a stride position increases the patient's anterior/posterior base of support. When moving to standing with the feet in stride, the patient places the foot of the uninvolved lower extremity slightly behind the involved lower extremity. This allows the patient to use the uninvolved lower extremity efficiently for rising to standing. Having the patient place the hands on the armrests also increases the base of support and provides initial assistance to push to a standing position.

Assumption of Standing

1. To assume a standing position, the patient must lean forward to shift the center of gravity over the feet and extend the knees and hips to rise from the seat.

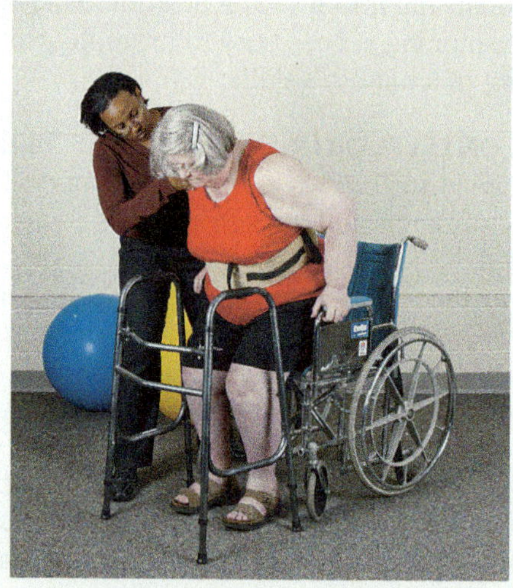

2. Initially, the patient pushes directly downward on the armrests. Pushing at an angle creates a horizontal component of the pushing force vector that does not assist the patient in rising and may also propel the patient horizontally and, thus, off balance.

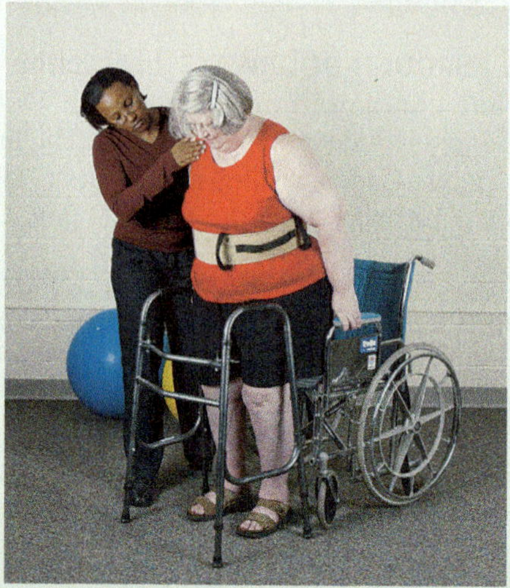

Ambulatory assistive devices must be accessible to patients when they are sitting in a chair and after the assumption of standing. Initially, ambulatory assistive devices may not be used during the assumption of standing. During initial learning, the patient places both hands on the armrests of the chair to assist with pushing to standing. In such cases, the ambulatory assistive device must be accessible to the physical therapist/assistant, who hands it to the patient once standing has been achieved. When using ambulatory assistive devices to assume standing, the patient may place one hand on the ambulatory assistive device and the other hand on the armrest. Whichever hand position is used, the movement to assume standing should be a controlled continuous motion.

Assumption of Sitting

1. To assume a sitting position after walking, the patient must approach the front edge of a chair and then turn away from the chair. When performing this maneuver, the patient may initially feel more confident turning toward the uninvolved side. This occurs because the patient is turning into his or her strength. However, the patient must be able to turn in both directions, toward the involved and uninvolved sides. As the patient approaches a chair, he or she must ensure that the chair is secure and, if the chair is a wheelchair, that the footrests are out of the way.
2. With the patient standing close to the front edge of the seat and facing away from the chair, the patient's center of gravity can be maintained over the base of support during the assumption of sitting. The patient may place the feet side by side or in a short stride position. Using a stride position increases a patient's base of support. When moving to sitting with the feet in stride, the foot of the uninvolved lower extremity is slightly farther back than the foot of the involved lower extremity. Having patients reach for and use armrests while lowering to the seat also increases a patient's base of support and provides assistance to control the latter stages of lowering.

■ Take Note

When assuming a sitting position, the patient's feet are in stride, with the uninvolved lower extremity closest to wheelchair.

Initially, ambulatory assistive devices may not be used for the assumption of sitting. In such cases, the patient may hand the ambulatory assistive device, such as crutches and canes, but not walkers, to the physical therapist/assistant before beginning to lower to sitting. Then the patient uses both hands to grasp the armrests of the chair to assist with the controlled lowering to sitting. When using ambulatory assistive devices during assumption of sitting, the patient places one hand, usually the hand on the side of the involved lower extremity, on the assistive device and the other hand on the armrest. The patient then assumes sitting in a controlled manner.

PROCEDURE 10–2 Ascending and Descending Stairs

Generally, patients ascend and descend stairs toward the right side when facing the stairs (refer to Figures 10–35 and 10–36). When ascending or descending stairs, the patient places the tips of the ambulatory assistive device one-half to two-thirds of the way forward onto the stair tread, in the direction the patient is facing. When two ambulatory assistive devices are used, the patient places them far enough apart to allow room for the patient to move between them. When a stair rail is available, the patient should use it for greater stability. When the patient is using two ambulatory assistive devices, he can place both in one hand to free the other hand for use on the stair rail. When only the right upper extremity can be used, the patient can hold the ambulatory

■ Take Note

The involved lower extremity is never left without support, either from the uninvolved lower extremity or the ambulatory assistive device.

(continued)

PROCEDURE 10–2 Ascending and Descending Stairs (*continued*)

assistive device in the hand on the stair rail. When the right upper extremity is unable to be used, patients may use the assistive device only or ascend and descend toward the left side when facing the stairs.

When first learning to ascend and descend stairs, patients usually use a step-to gait pattern. As a patient's condition permits, the patient may progress to a step-over-step gait pattern to ascend and descend stairs.

Ascending Stairs

1. When ascending stairs, the patient moves the uninvolved lower extremity to the next higher stair first because it must lift the body. To do so, the patient shifts weight to the handrail and as permitted to the involved lower extremity, freeing the uninvolved lower extremity to move.

■ Take Note

When ascending stairs, lead with the uninvolved lower extremity—up with the good.

2. Once the patient has appropriately placed the uninvolved lower extremity on the next stair, he shifts weight to the uninvolved lower extremity. He extends the uninvolved lower extremity to lift the body.
3. The patient advances the involved lower extremity and the ambulatory assistive device(s) to the same stair while he lifts the body.
4. An alternative is to have the patient move the involved lower extremity to the same stair as the uninvolved lower extremity, followed by the ambulatory assistive device.

Descending Stairs

1. When descending stairs, the patient moves the ambulatory assistive devices to the next lower stair first to provide support for the involved lower extremity.
2. The patient shifts weight to the handrail and uninvolved lower extremity, permitting the ambulatory assistive device(s) and involved lower extremity to be moved.

■ Take Note

When descending stairs, lead with the assistive device and then the involved lower extremity—down with the bad.

3. The patient uses the uninvolved lower extremity to lower the body until the ambulatory assistive device(s) and the involved lower extremity are on the next lower stair.

   An alternative is to lower the ambulatory assistive device(s) first, followed by the involved lower extremity once the ambulatory assistive device is in place.
4. The patient shifts weight to the ambulatory assistive device(s) and involved lower extremity. Then the patient moves the uninvolved lower extremity down to the same stair.

Curbs

The sequence for ascending and descending curbs is the same as the sequence for ascending and descending stairs. Only ambulatory assistive devices are available for support when ascending and descending curbs because of the absence of handrails.

Moving Through Doorways

There are many combinations of extremity involvement and doorway configurations. A patient may have one or two functional upper extremities, and the impairment of the patient's lower extremities may involve one or both. Doors may open toward or away from the patient, they may be hinged on the left or right, the space around the door available for maneuvering may be ample or limited, and doors may or may not have automatic openers or closers. Each combination of factors will require modifications to the general method of ambulating through doorways. Patient safety must not be compromised regardless of patient level of function and physical configuration of the environment.

■ **Take Note**

Caution—Doorways require movement into spaces where there is no initial visibility because of the door. Proceed carefully when opening and progressing through doorways.

Often balance is a major concern. Patients may be required to lean in all directions, moving their center of gravity with respect to their base of support while pushing or pulling on doors. Another concern is the danger of a door with an automatic closer striking a patient as it closes. Should a door strike a patient with sufficient force, the patient may lose balance control, resulting in more weight bearing on the involved lower extremity than is permitted or the patient falling to the ground. To avoid an automatic closing door from forcefully striking a patient, such doors should be opened wider than the minimal width for a patient to progress through the doorway. This allows the patient time to progress through the doorway before the automatic closing door impedes progress. An alternative technique is to use the tips of ambulatory assistive devices as temporary doorstops while progressing through these doorways. Patients should avoid rushing through doorways because rushing may cause loss of control of the ambulatory assistive device or balance.

The physical therapist's/assistant's position for guarding the patient during movement through doorways is the same position as for guarding during other gait training activities. Recognizing that shorter steps and abrupt turns may be required, the physical therapist/assistant must be prepared to move with the patient, avoiding interference with the patient's freedom of movement or the arc of movement of a door. During initial gait training through doorways, the physical therapist/assistant may need to control opening and closing of the door to protect the patient.

When a door does not have an automatic closer, the door does not have to be opened greater than the width of the patient because the door closes forcefully or quickly on a patient before he progresses through the doorway. Doors that do not have automatic closers require that the patient turn and close the door after moving through the doorway.

Tilt Table

A tilt table may be used when patients have restrictions on sitting or the amount of hip flexion allowed. When individuals move from sitting to standing, the hips ordinarily flex more than 90 degrees. Following total hip replacement, patients are restricted to no more than 90 degrees of hip flexion. For patients unable to assume standing from sitting while maintaining hip precautions, a tilt table can be used to rise to a standing position.

Some patients must be reacclimated to upright posture in a safe manner before standing or gait training can be initiated. This is usually necessitated by the existence of orthostatic hypotension in patients who have been in bed for extended periods. Accommodation by the cardiovascular system may be necessary to avoid dizziness or fainting as these patients assume an upright posture. Tilt tables are a safe method to provide maximum support for such patients. Support is provided while the patient is raised slowly to an upright position by the tilt table, leaving the physical therapist/assistant free to control the tilt table and monitor the patient. Abdominal binders and elastic wraps or elastic hose on the lower extremities may be used to assist venous return. Use of lower extremity muscles, such as isometric contractions, often called *muscle setting* exercises, or active range of motion exercises also assists venous return.

■ **Take Note**

Use a tilt table to assist patients to achieve and maintain an upright posture. These patients may be non–weight bearing or partial weight bearing.

PROCEDURE 10–3 Tilt Table

Measure vital signs, as presented in Chapter 5, before, during, and after the process of raising patients to an upright posture. Lower patients when they report feeling faint. Monitor a patient who is lowered after feeling faint until vital signs return to normal and the patient no longer reports feeling faint. Obtain medical assistance when necessary.

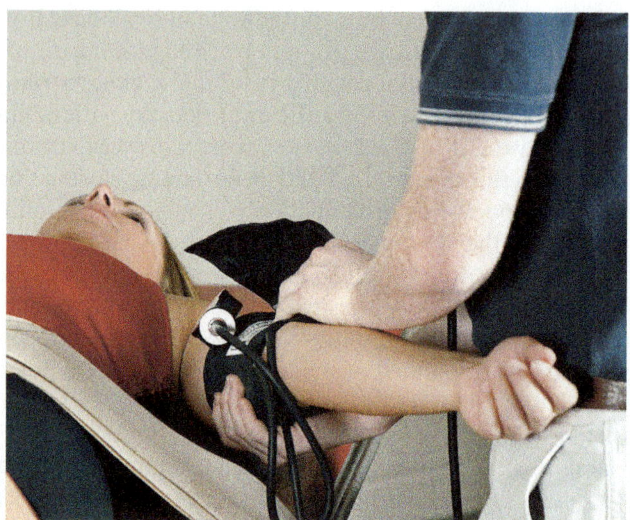

Use straps to secure patients on a tilt table. A variety of styles of straps are available. A bar extends along each side of the tilt table surface. Straps used to secure the patient on the tilt table are attached to the bar on one side of the table.

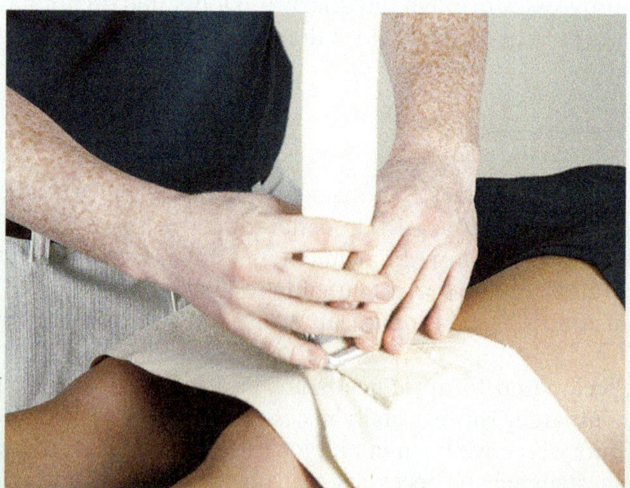

Straps are passed over the patient and secured around the bar on the other side. The location of the straps across the patient depends on the patient's condition. When upper trunk stability is required, use a chest strap leaving the upper extremities free. A strap over the pelvis stabilizes the lower trunk. Use a strap at knee level when the patient cannot maintain knee extension.

Adjust the angle of tilt to a position the patient can tolerate safely. Perform changes in the position of the table slowly and steadily. Greater degrees of tilt may be assumed as the patient's cardiovascular system adjusts to the demands of an upright posture. For many patients a full upright position provides a sensation of falling forward; therefore, this position is usually avoided.

Patients with non–weight-bearing status on one lower extremity can be placed on a tilt table. Place a lift under the foot of the uninvolved lower extremity, preventing the involved lower extremity from reaching the supporting surface. Thus, the involved lower extremity is non–weight bearing.

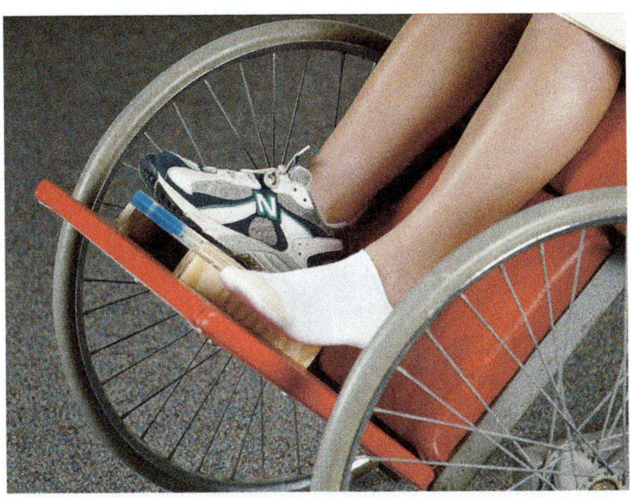

When an exercise program for one lower extremity is to be implemented, loosen the strap across the knees or place it only around the opposite lower extremity. This permits the physical therapist/assistant to implement the patient's lower extremity exercise program. Upper extremity and trunk exercises can also be performed on the tilt table.

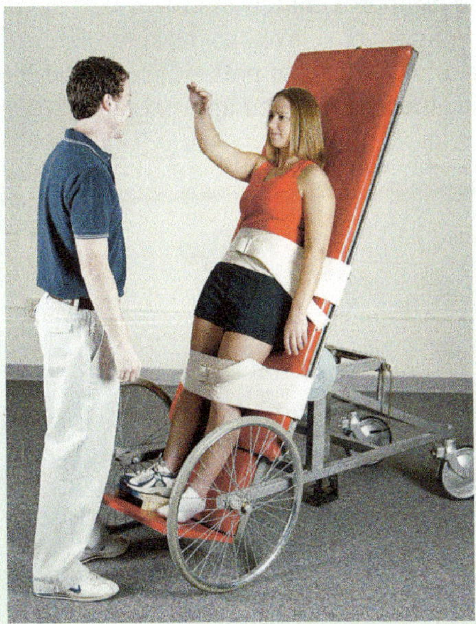

(continued)

PROCEDURE 10–3 Tilt Table (*continued*)

Patients can be fitted with ambulatory assistive devices while on a tilt table and "walk," with guarding, off the tilt table for gait training.

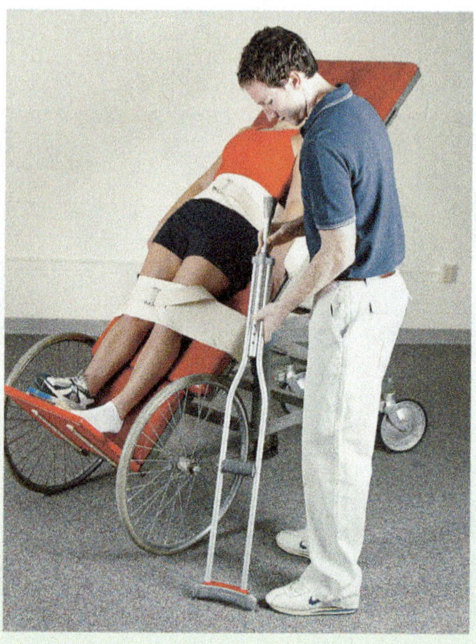

Walkers

Fitting

To measure a walker for proper height adjustment, the patient stands upright with the shoulder girdle relaxed within the walker with the crossbar in front. The top of the handgrips should be approximately at the level of the patient's ulnar styloid processes when the upper extremities are relaxed at the side (Figure 10–40 ■). This fitting can be done within the parallel bars. When the patient grasps the handgrips with shoulder girdles level and relaxed, the elbows are flexed approximately 20 to 30 degrees (Figure 10–41 ■).

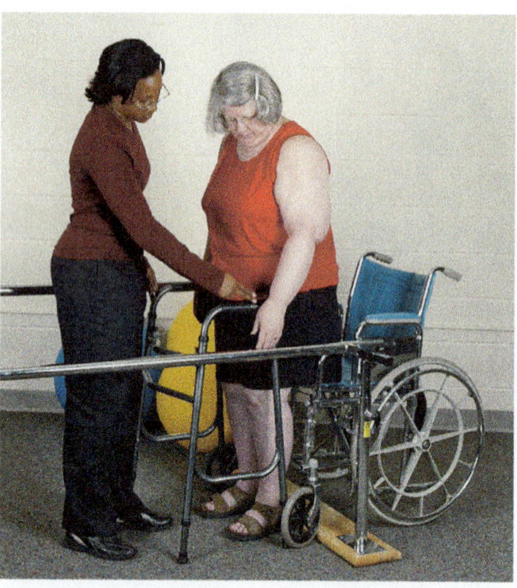

FIGURE 10–40 ■ Checking handgrip height when fitting a walker.

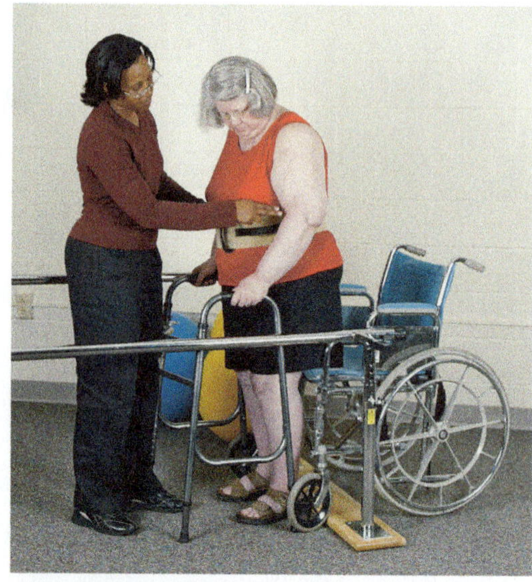

FIGURE 10–41 ■ Checking elbow flexion angle when fitting a walker.

PROCEDURE 10–4 In and Out of a Wheelchair with a Walker

Two methods of getting in and out of a wheelchair will be described. In both methods, the physical therapist/assistant prepares a wheelchair and positions the patient in the manner presented earlier in this chapter under *Assumption of Standing and Sitting*. Reversing wheelchair desk armrests so the higher portion is at the front of the wheelchair will assist patients in pushing to standing and lowering to sitting. A physical therapist/assistant is positioned in the manner described earlier in this chapter under *Guarding*.

Assuming Standing Using a Walker

The physical therapist/assistant engages wheelchair wheel locks and moves footrests out of the way. The patient is positioned at the front edge of the seat, with her feet in stride or side by side. A physical therapist/assistant is positioned in stride, behind and to one side of the patient. The physical therapist/assistant grasps the patient's gait belt with one hand. The other hand may be on the patient's shoulder girdle if necessary. If a hand is placed on the patient's shoulder girdle, it should not interfere with a patient's ability to move smoothly using the upper extremity.

The physical therapist/assistant performs the same actions when guarding on the patient's involved or uninvolved side.

1. The patient uses the hand on the uninvolved side to grasp and push down on the crossbar of the walker. The patient places the hand on the involved side on the armrest of the wheelchair. This ensures that the patient is moving into her strength.

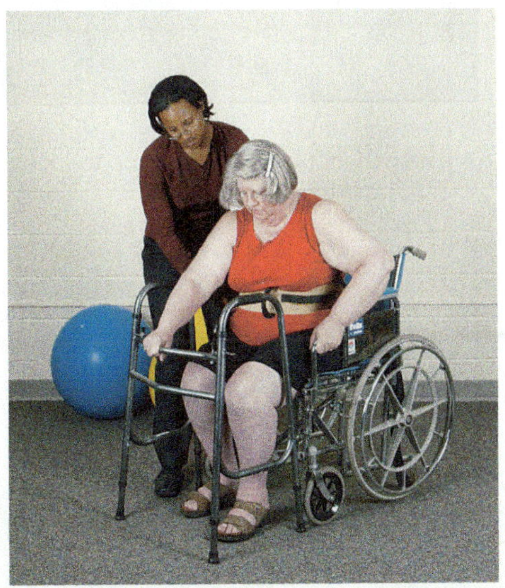

2. The patient pushes to standing.

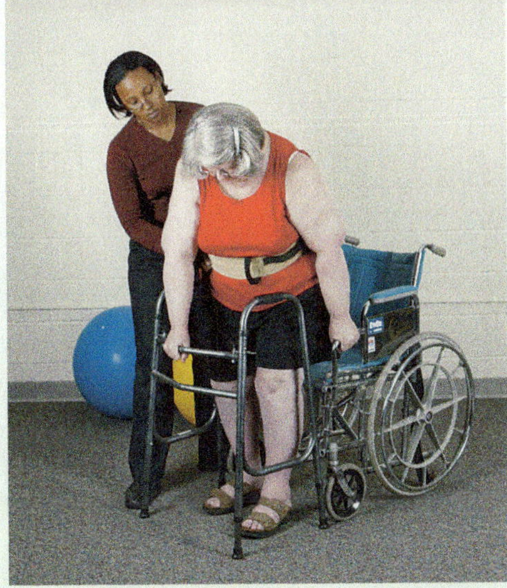

(continued)

PROCEDURE 10–4 In and Out of a Wheelchair with a Walker (*continued*)

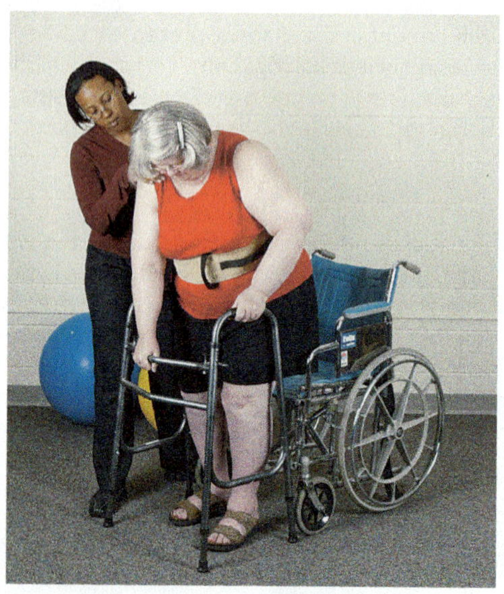

3. The patient moves the hand on the involved side from the armrest of the wheelchair and grasps the handgrip of the walker.

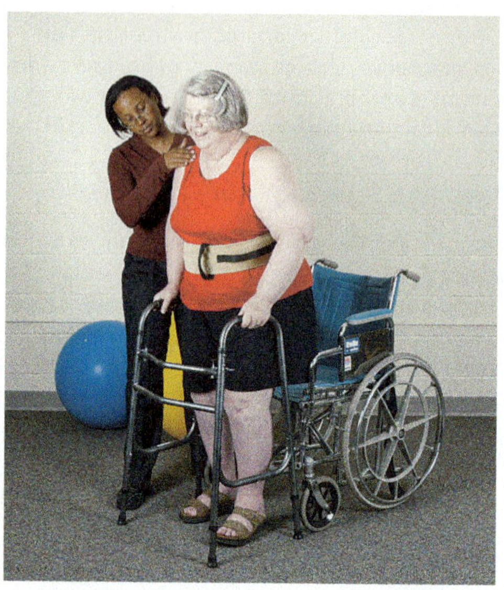

4. The patient moves the hand on the uninvolved side from the crossbar to grasp the other handgrip. The patient is now correctly positioned in the walker to begin ambulation.

Force exerted on the crossbar of a walker must be exerted directly downward to avoid tipping the walker.

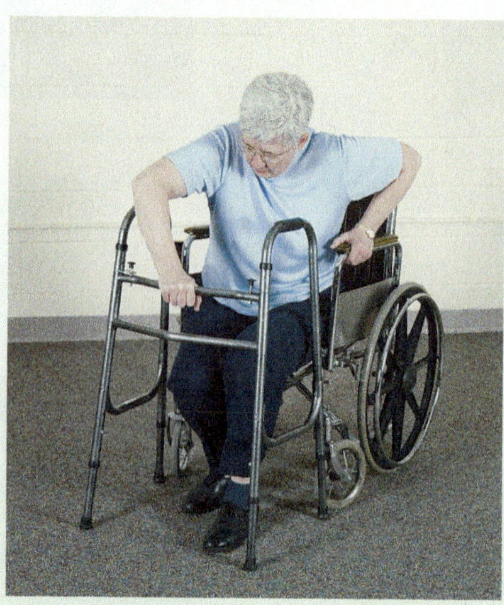

If force is not exerted directly downward when a patient's hand is placed on the crossbar of a walker, the walker tips forward.

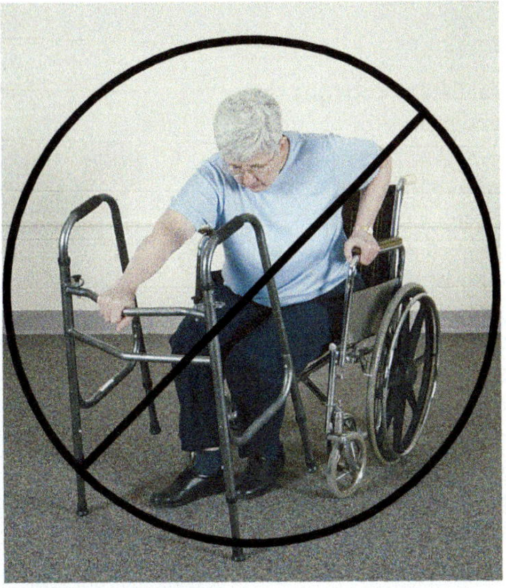

■ Take Note

When a patient uses the crossbar of the walker to assume standing, the force on the crossbar must be directly downward to prevent tipping of the walker.

The patient may place the hand on the uninvolved side on the walker's handgrip instead of crossbar. There are two disadvantages to this method. First, a walker's handgrip is higher than the crossbar. The height of the handgrip may make pushing directly downward more difficult for a patient. Second, the handgrip is at the very outside of the walker's base of support. Slight deviation from pushing directly downward will cause the walker to tip sideways.

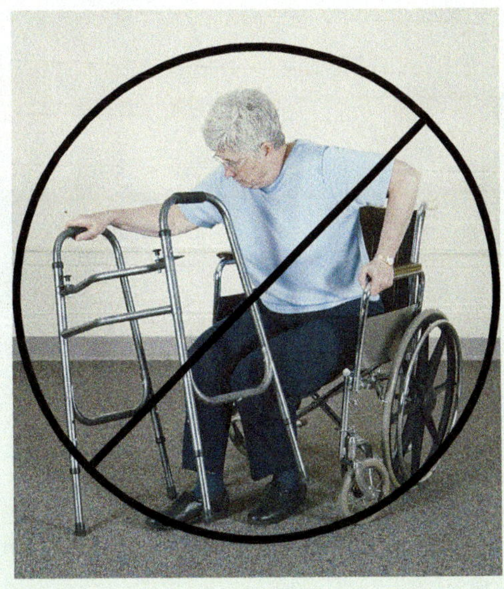

(continued)

PROCEDURE 10–4 In and Out of a Wheelchair with a Walker (*continued*)

Assuming Sitting Using a Walker

1. The physical therapist/assistant engages the wheelchair wheel locks and moves the footrests out of the way. To sit, the patient is positioned facing away from the wheelchair at the front edge of the wheelchair seat, close enough so she can feel the front edge of wheelchair seat against the backs of the lower extremities. The patient can position her feet either in stride or side by side. Positioned in stride behind and to one side of the patient, the physical therapist/assistant grasps the patient's gait belt and shoulder girdle.

   The physical therapist/assistant performs the same actions when guarding on the patient's involved or uninvolved side.

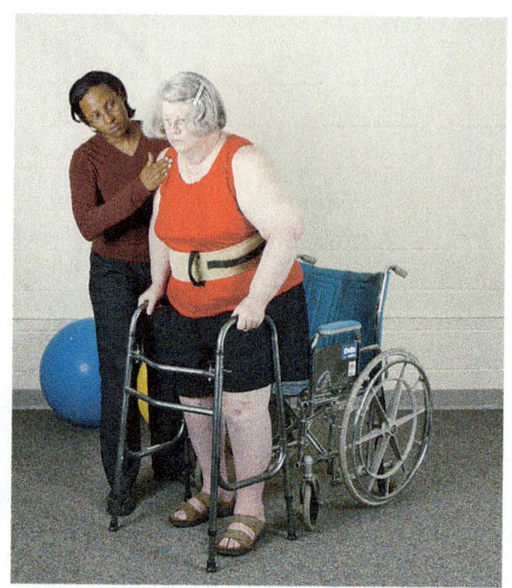

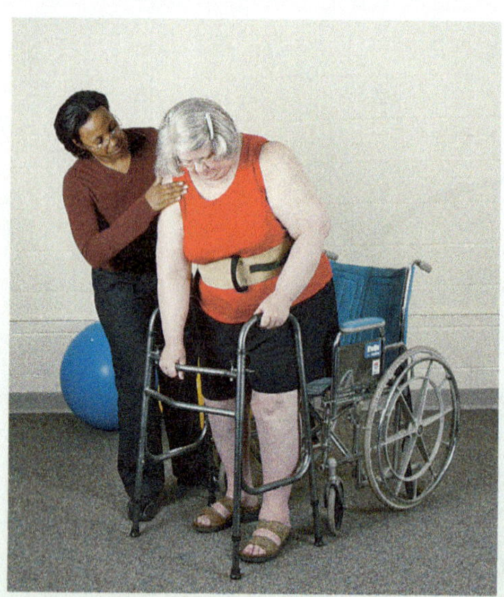

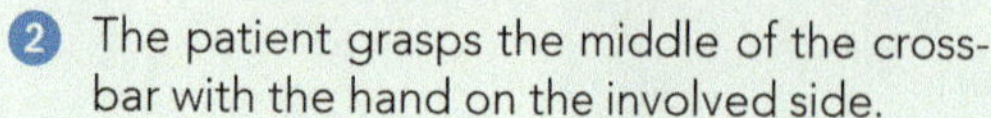

2. The patient grasps the middle of the crossbar with the hand on the involved side.

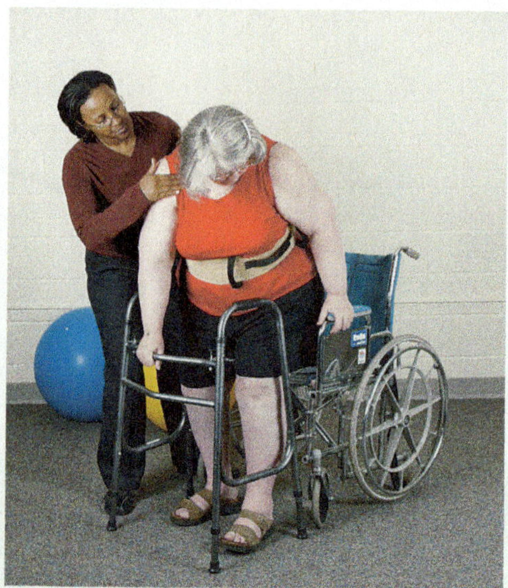

3. The patient reaches backward and grasps the armrest with the hand on the uninvolved side.

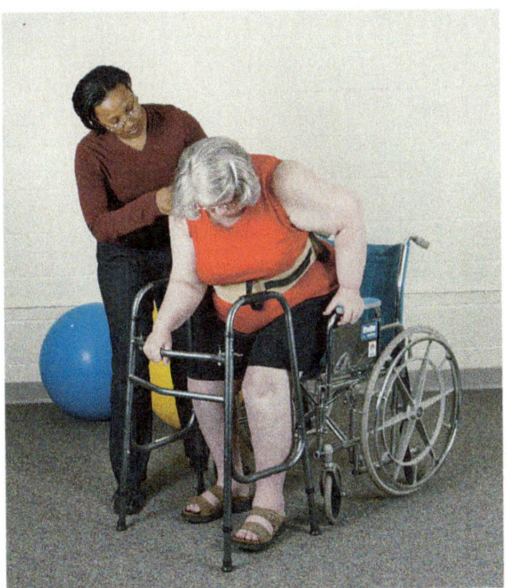

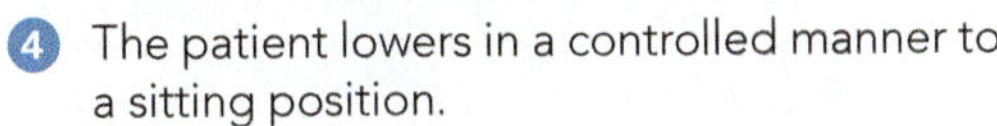

4 The patient lowers in a controlled manner to a sitting position.

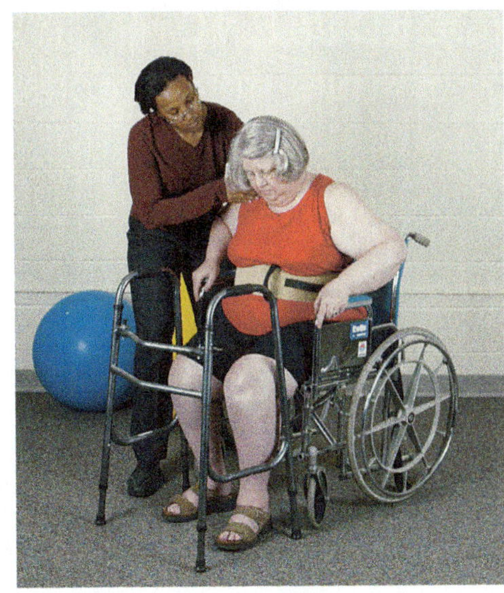

5 The patient moves the hand from the crossbar to the armrest and adjusts the sitting position in the wheelchair.

Assuming Standing Using Both Armrests

1 The physical therapist/assistant engages the wheelchair wheel locks and moves the footrests out of the way. The patient is positioned at the front edge of the seat with the feet in stride or side by side. Positioned in stride behind and to one side of the patient, the physical therapist/assistant grasps the patient's gait belt and shoulder girdle. Sitting on the front edge of the seat, the patient places both hands on the armrests.

The physical therapist/assistant performs the same actions when guarding on the patient's involved or uninvolved side.

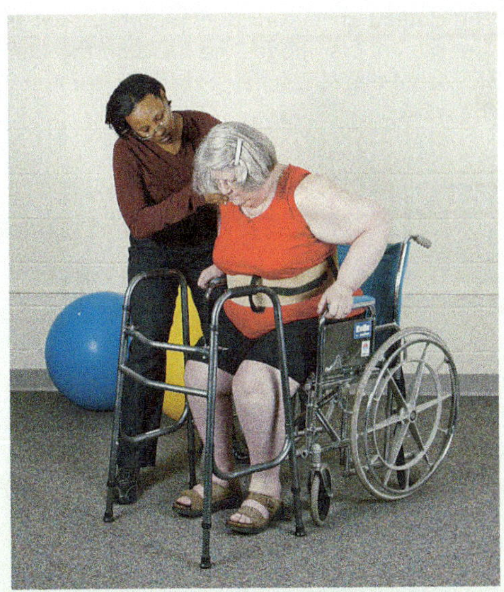

(continued)

PROCEDURE 10–4 In and Out of a Wheelchair with a Walker (*continued*)

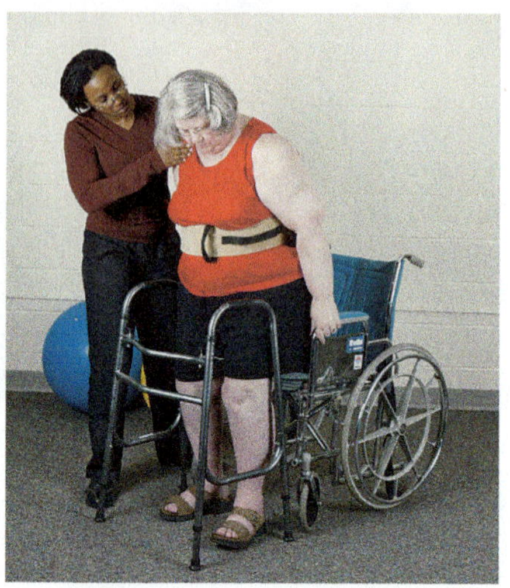

2 Using the armrests, the patient pushes to standing.

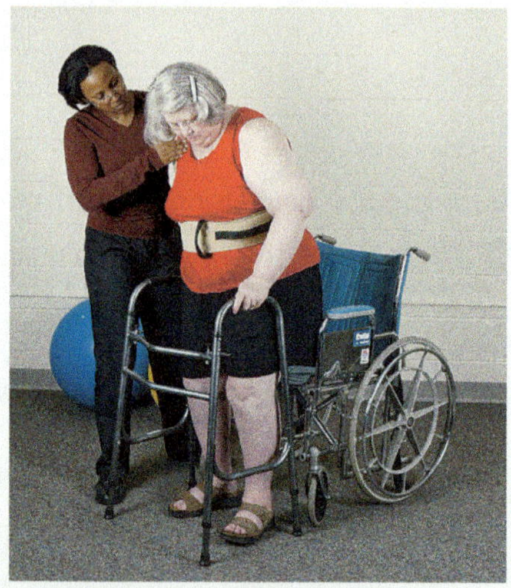

3 The patient shifts weight completely over the feet. The patient first moves the hand on the uninvolved side from the wheelchair armrest to the handgrip of the walker.

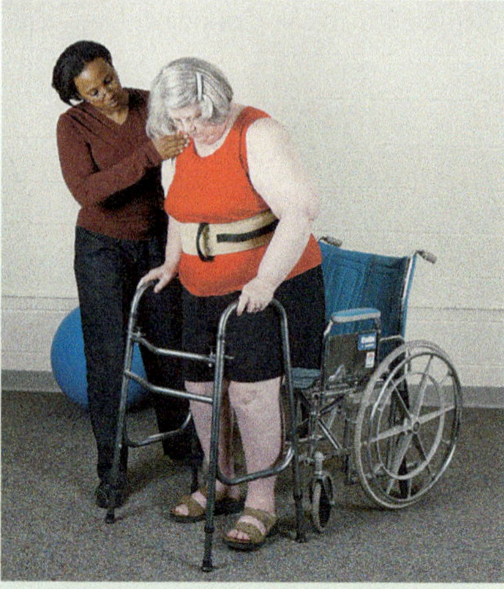

4 Once the patient has the hand on the uninvolved side properly positioned, the patient moves the hand on the involved side from the wheelchair armrest to the handgrip of the walker.

Assuming Sitting Using Both Armrests

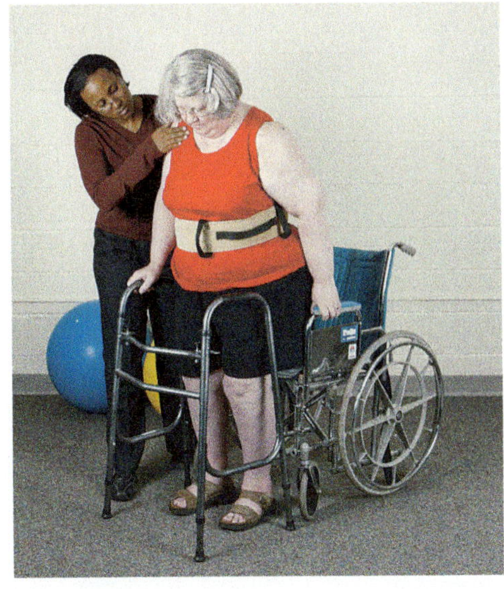

1. The physical therapist/assistant engages the wheelchair wheel locks and moves the footrests out of the way. To sit, the patient is positioned facing away from the wheelchair at the front edge of the wheelchair seat, close enough so she can feel the front edge of the wheelchair seat against the backs of the lower extremities. The patient positions her feet in stride or side by side. Positioned in stride behind and to one side of the patient, the physical therapist/assistant grasps the patient's gait belt and shoulder girdle.

   The physical therapist/assistant performs the same actions when guarding on the patient's involved or uninvolved side.

   The patient retains a grasp on the handgrip of the walker with the hand on the involved side while reaching back with the hand on the uninvolved side to grasp the wheelchair armrest.

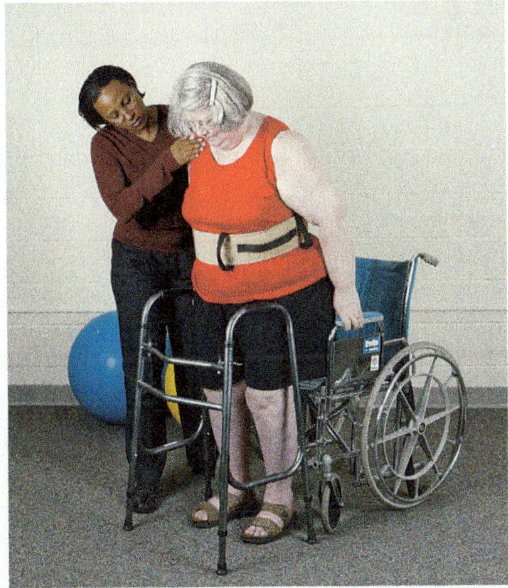

2. After grasping the armrest with the hand on the uninvolved side, the patient moves the hand on the involved side from the handgrip of the walker and grasps the other wheelchair armrest.

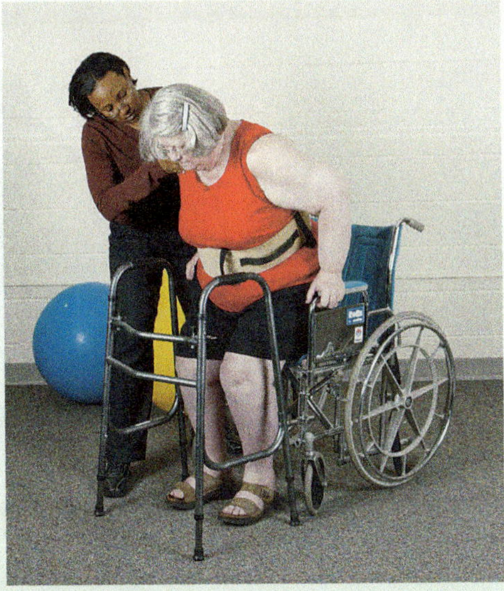

3. The patient then lowers to a sitting position in a controlled manner.

(continued)

PROCEDURE 10–4 In and Out of a Wheelchair with a Walker (*continued*)

4. Once seated, the patient adjusts the sitting position.

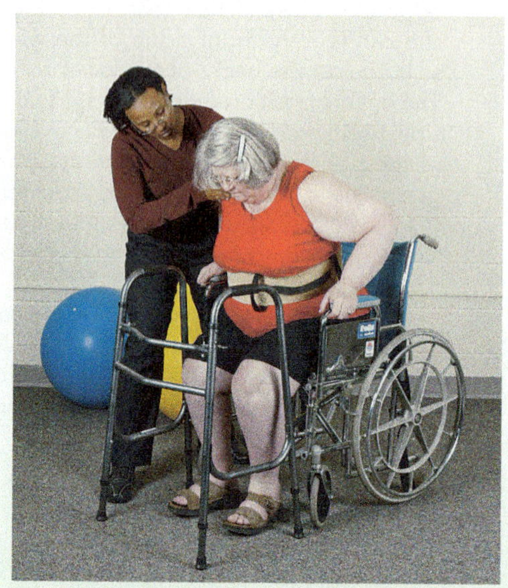

PROCEDURE 10–5 Ambulating with a Walker

When ambulating with a walker, the patient can lift her body to decrease weight bearing by shoulder depression and elbow extension. The patient moves a walker by picking it up, moving it a step-length forward, and placing it on the floor. Walkers should be lifted and set down so that all four legs clear or contact the floor simultaneously.

Some patients will "rock" the walker, lifting and setting down two legs and rocking onto the other two legs. Rocking the walker reduces the base of support and stability a walker provides when used properly. *Rocking the walker should be discouraged.*

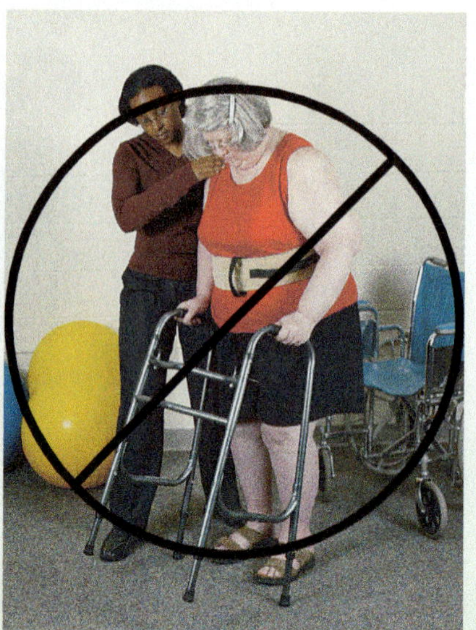

■ Take Note

Caution—Place the walker so that all four legs of the walker clear or contact the floor simultaneously.

The patient should not place her leading lower extremity beyond the crossbar. Doing so prevents appropriate weight shifting over this lower extremity. When stepping beyond the crossbar occurs, the base of support and stability provided by a walker are compromised.

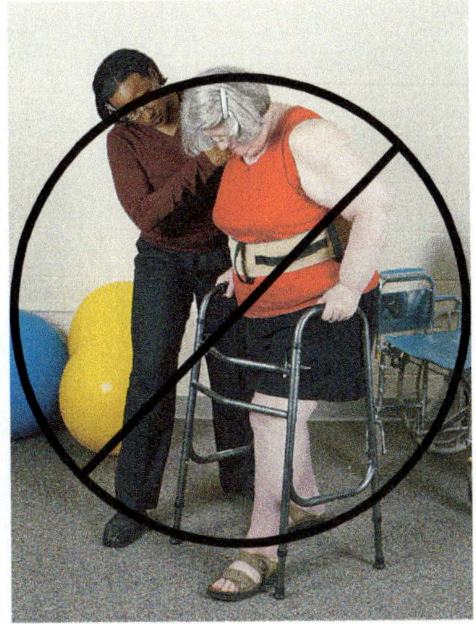

■ **Take Note**

Caution—The patient should not step beyond the crossbar of the walker.

Three-Point Step-To Gait Pattern

Partial to Full Weight Bearing

1. For contact guarding, the physical therapist/assistant is positioned in stride behind and to one side of the patient, grasping the patient's gait belt and shoulder girdle. To ambulate using the three-point gait pattern, the patient stands centered within the walker. The patient lifts and advances the walker. All four legs of the walker are lifted from or lowered to the floor simultaneously. As the patient moves the walker, the physical therapist/assistant advances the outside foot.

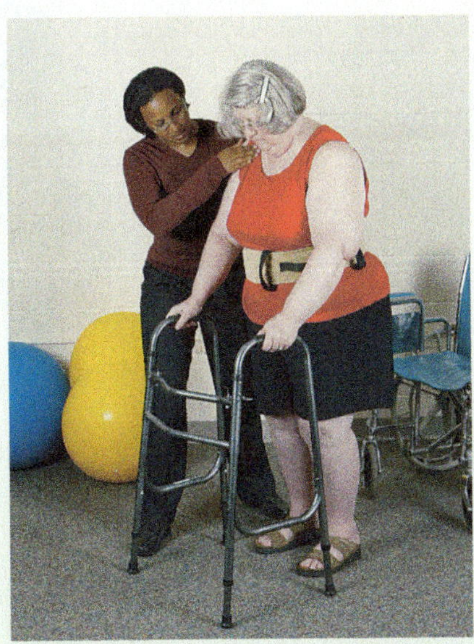

(continued)

PROCEDURE 10–5 Ambulating with a Walker (*continued*)

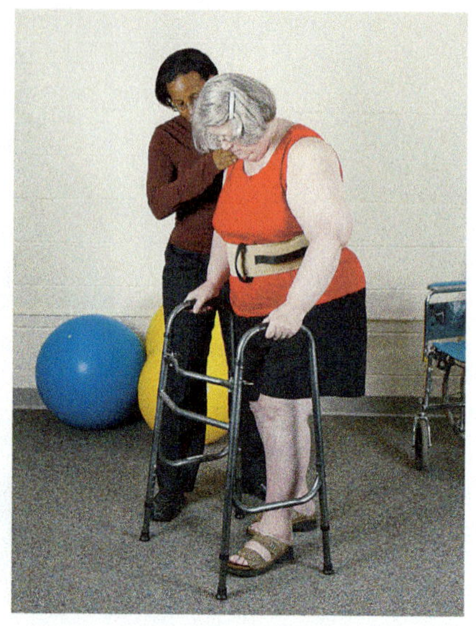

2 The patient advances the involved lower extremity, moving it into the base of support and stability of the walker.

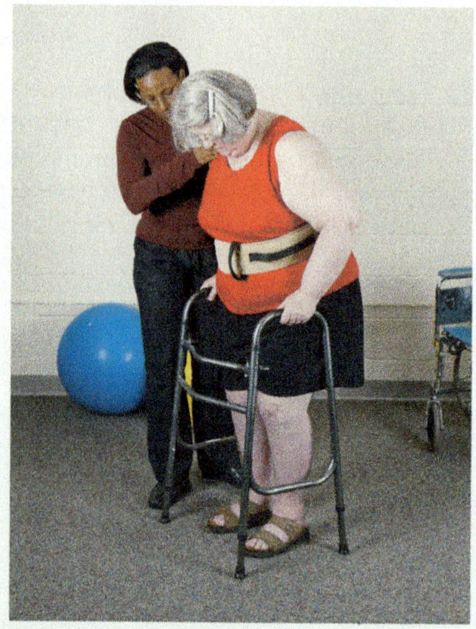

3 Supporting weight as necessary to achieve the desired weight-bearing status, the patient bears weight through the upper extremities as she advances the uninvolved lower extremity. The patient may step to or slightly beyond the involved foot, but not beyond the crossbar. The physical therapist/assistant should encourage equal step lengths. The physical therapist/assistant advances the inside foot to move with the patient. The total sequence is repeated for continued progression.

Non–Weight Bearing

For contact guarding, the physical therapist/assistant is positioned in stride behind and to one side of the patient, grasping the patient's gait belt and shoulder girdle. To ambulate using the three-point gait pattern non–weight bearing on the involved lower extremity, the patient stands centered within the walker. The patient does not rest the involved lower extremity on the floor. The patient may hold the involved lower extremity with the knee extended and the foot in front or with the knee flexed and the foot behind the patient. The uninvolved lower extremity and both upper extremities provide support.

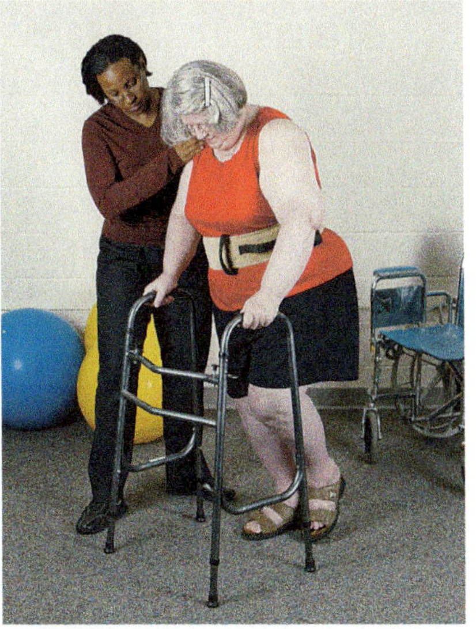

1 The patient lifts and advances the walker. All four legs of a walker are lifted from or lowered to the floor simultaneously. As the patient moves the walker, the physical therapist/assistant advances the outside foot.

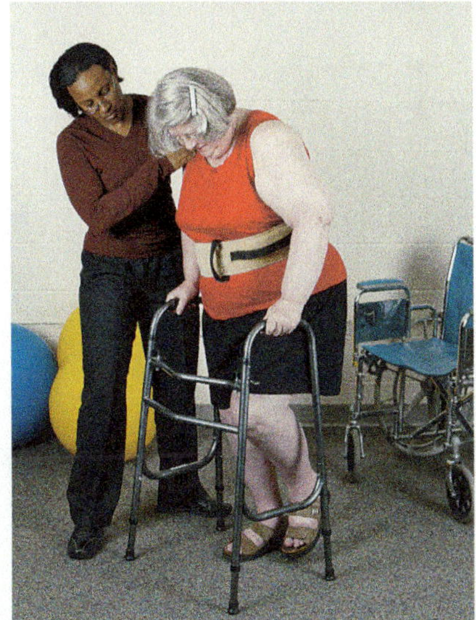

2 Supporting weight as necessary through the upper extremities to achieve non–weight-bearing status, the patient steps into the walker with the uninvolved lower extremity. The physical therapist/assistant advances the inside foot to move with the patient. The total sequence is repeated for continued progression.

Swing-To Gait Pattern

1 For contact guarding, the physical therapist/assistant is positioned in stride behind and to one side of a patient, grasping the patient's gait belt and shoulder girdle. To ambulate using a swing-to gait pattern, the patient stands centered within the walker. The patient lifts and advances the walker. All four legs of a walker are lifted from or lowered to the floor simultaneously. As the patient moves the walker, the physical therapist/assistant advances the outside foot.

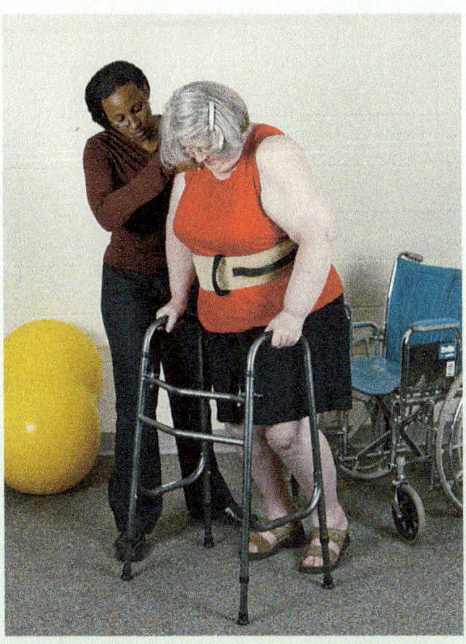

(continued)

PROCEDURE 10–5 Ambulating with a Walker *(continued)*

2 Bearing weight through the upper extremities, the patient lifts the body. The patient then lets the body swing forward ("swing-to") into the walker. The physical therapist/assistant moves the inside foot as the patient swings forward.

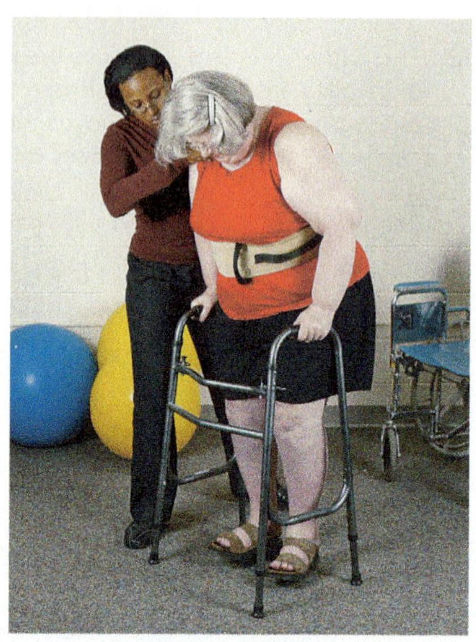

3 The patient lowers at the end of the swing and bears weight on the lower extremities. The sequence is repeated for continued progression.

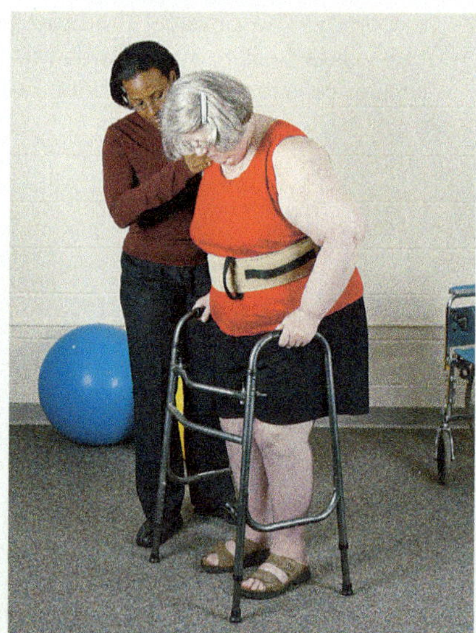

PROCEDURE 10–6 Ambulating on Stairs with a Walker

Ambulation on the stairs using a walker can be accomplished with a standard walker or with a stair-climbing walker. When the patient must negotiate stairs frequently, a stair-climbing walker should be considered.

Stair-Climbing Walker

A standard walker can be used when ambulating on stairs, although it is not a stable device in this case.

Ascending Stairs

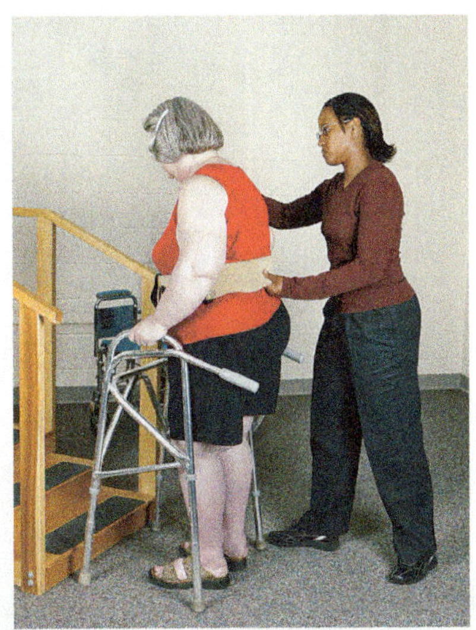

1. For contact guarding, the physical therapist/assistant is positioned in stride behind and to one side of the patient, grasping the patient's gait belt and shoulder girdle. The patient stands facing up the stairs with the walker in the usual position for ambulation.

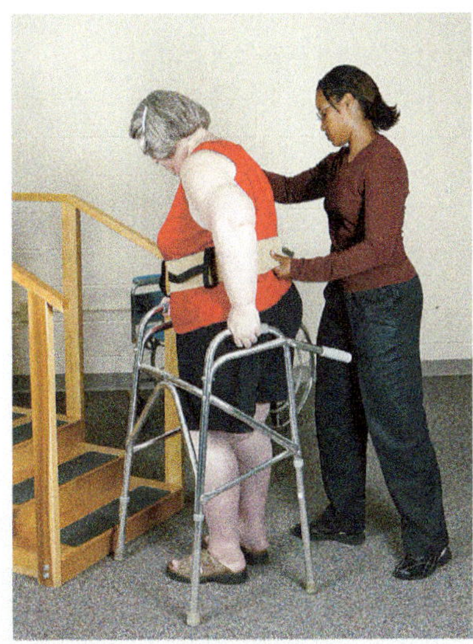

2. The patient turns the stair-climbing walker so the crossbar is to the side of the patient.

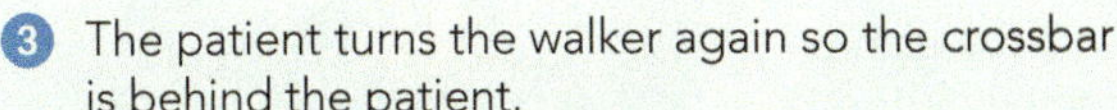

3. The patient turns the walker again so the crossbar is behind the patient.

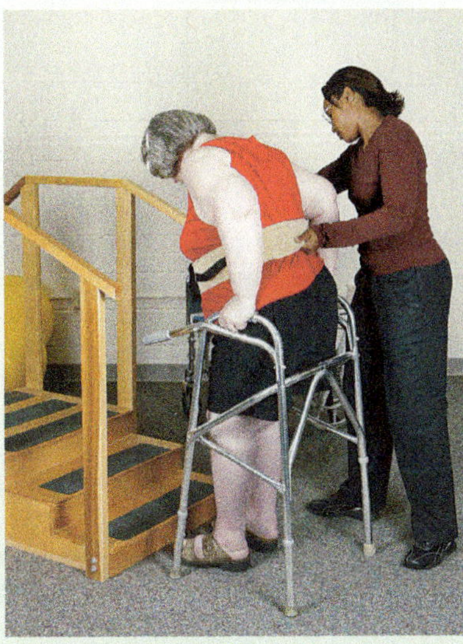

(continued)

PROCEDURE 10–6 Ambulating on Stairs with a Walker (*continued*)

4. The patient places the two legs of the stair-climbing walker closest to the stairs on the first stair.

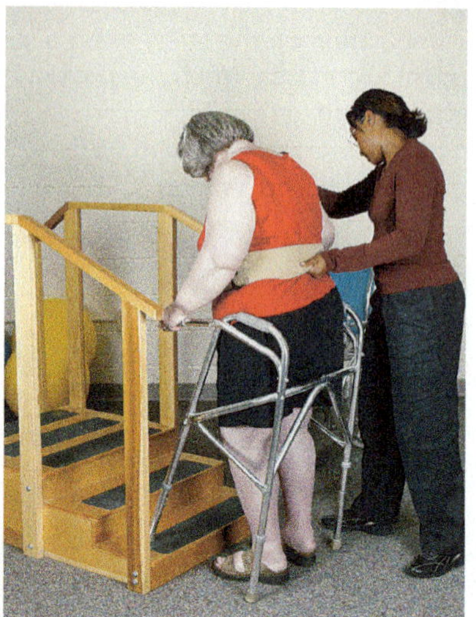

5. Grasping the handgrips, the patient can support weight on the upper extremities. The physical therapist/assistant places one hand on the stair rail and the other on the patient's gait belt. Supporting weight on the upper extremities and the involved lower extremity as permitted, the patient advances the uninvolved lower extremity up onto the same stair as the forwardmost legs of the walker.

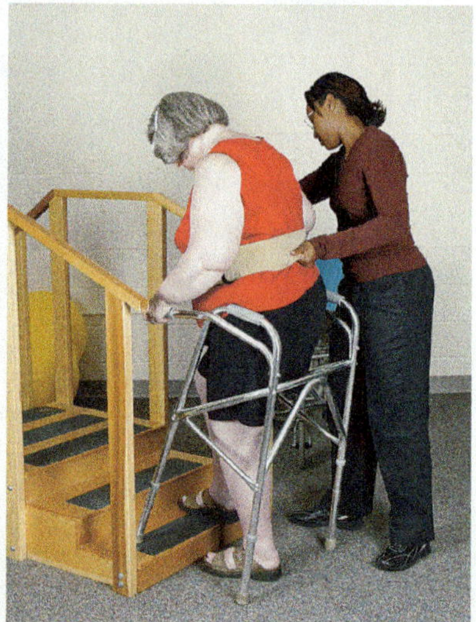

6. Shifting weight and extending the uninvolved lower extremity, the patient lifts the body and places the involved lower extremity on the same stair as the uninvolved lower extremity. The patient can advance the walker and involved lower extremity simultaneously.

   Guarding becomes more difficult for the physical therapist/assistant because placement of the walker may prevent the physical therapist/assistant from maintaining a position close behind the patient.

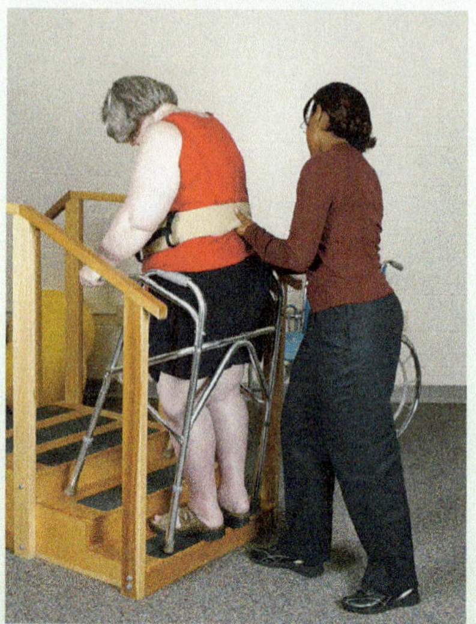

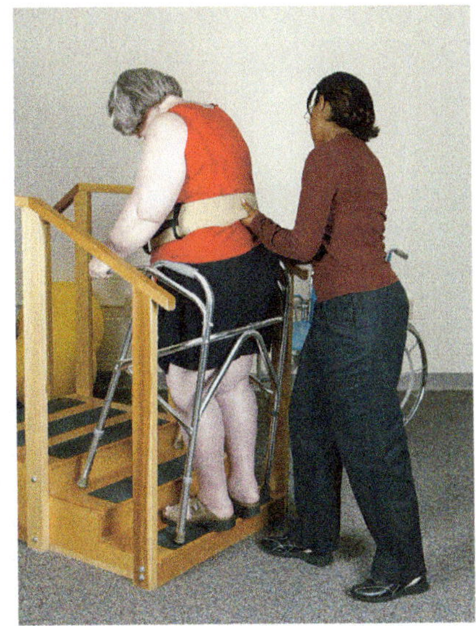

7 The patient lifts the walker and advances it to the next stair. At this time the physical therapist/assistant can again move to a closer position behind the patient. The sequence is repeated to ascend the remaining stairs.

Descending Stairs

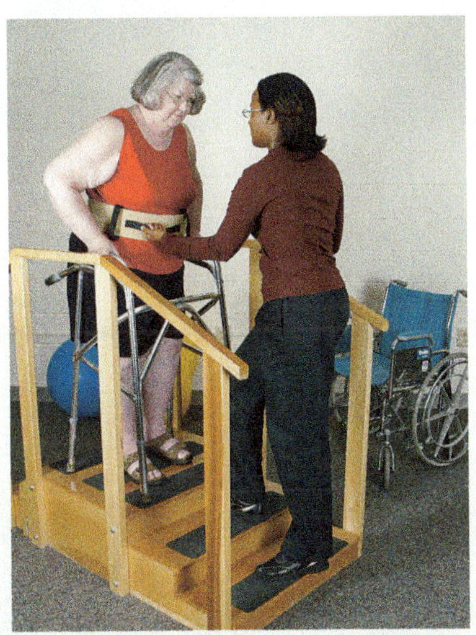

1 To descend stairs using a stair-climbing walker, the patient stands facing down the stairs. The patient positions the walker with the crossbar in front of her. The patient grasps the handgrips and positions the walker so the forwardmost legs are on the lower stair. Positioned in stride in front of the patient, the physical therapist/assistant grasps the patient's gait belt and handrail.

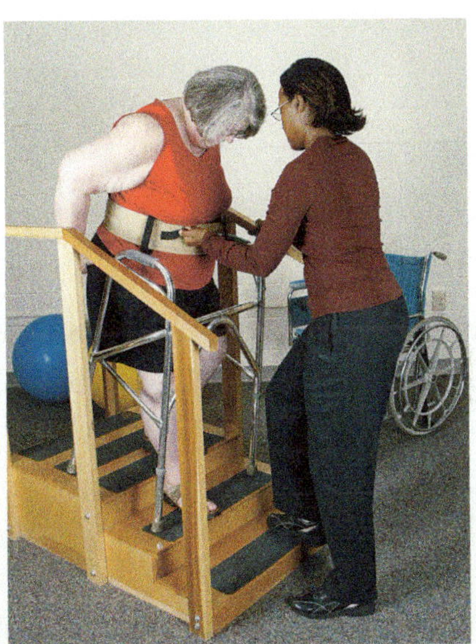

2 Supporting weight on the upper extremities and uninvolved lower extremity, the patient lowers the involved lower extremity down to the same stair as the front legs of the walker by flexing the uninvolved lower extremity.

(continued)

PROCEDURE 10–6 Ambulating on Stairs with a Walker (*continued*)

3 Continuing to support weight with the upper extremities on the walker and the involved lower extremity as permitted, the patient lowers the uninvolved lower extremity down to the same stair as the walker's front legs.

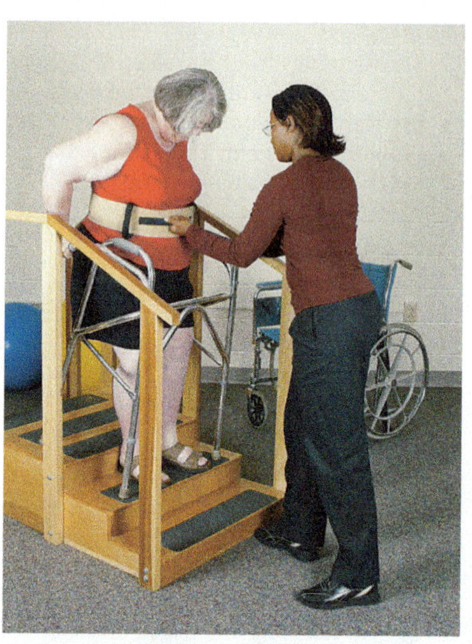

4 The sequence is repeated until the patient finishes descending the stairs. When the patient has completed descending the stairs and reaches the landing or floor level, she grasps the handgrips of the walker and positions the walker for ambulation.

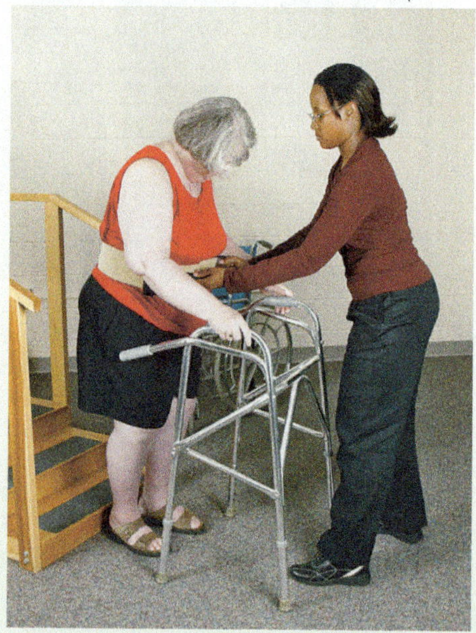

PROCEDURE 10–7 Ambulating Through Doorways with a Walker

Door Opens Toward Patient

Note: In this section, text and photographs depict independent ambulation. This method was used so a physical therapist/assistant does not obscure the desired photographic views of the patient.

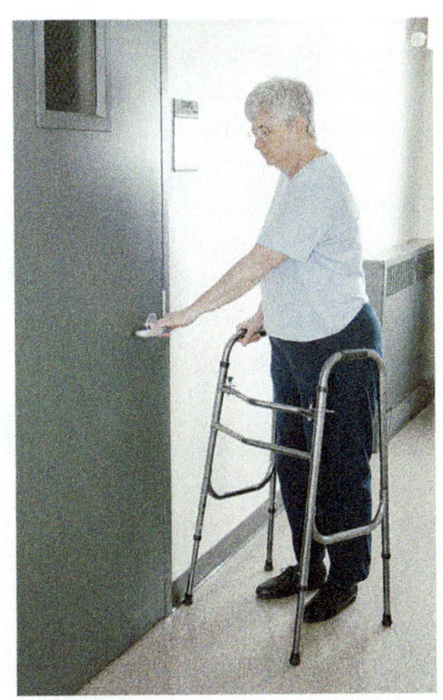

1. The patient approaches the latch edge of the door, standing outside the arc through which the opening door will move. The patient shifts the weight to the side of the walker away from the hand that will be placed on the door handle. The patient then places the unweighted hand on the door handle.

■ Take Note

When a door opens toward the patient, the patient should stand at the latch side of the door.

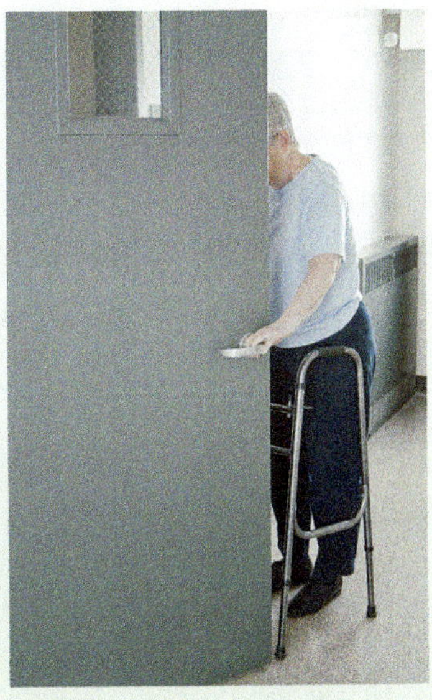

2. Using a pulling motion, the patient opens the door wider than the width of the patient and walker. This is necessary because the door will start to close automatically before the patient can progress through the doorway. The patient must block the door from closing with the walker to allow time to progress through the doorway.

(continued)

PROCEDURE 10–7 Ambulating Through Doorways with a Walker (*continued*)

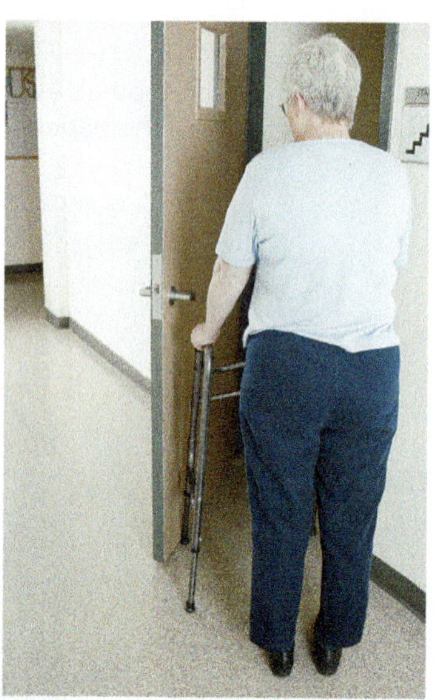

3 The patient quickly returns the hand used to open the door to the walker. The patient lifts the walker and moves it forward into the doorway. The patient places all four legs of the walker on the floor, with the legs closest to the door serving as doorstops. Using this method, the closing door hits the walker's legs, not the patient.

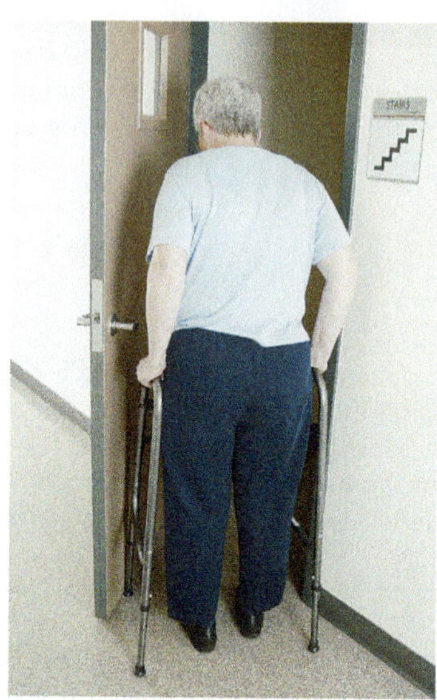

4 Once the walker has absorbed the contact of a closing door, the patient can step into the walker to advance through the doorway.

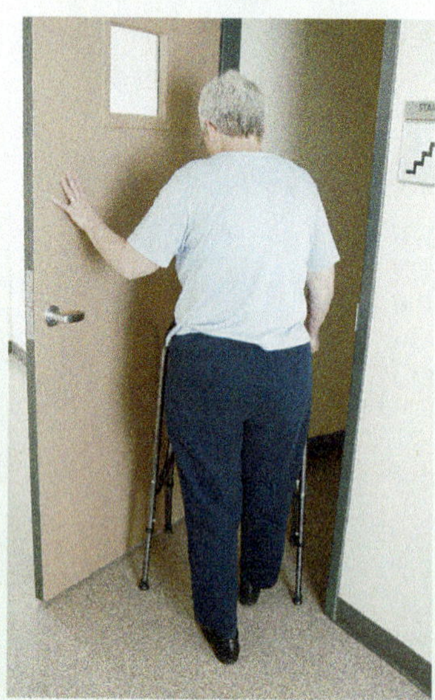

5 The patient may have to push the door farther open during transit through the doorway to allow a walker to be moved.

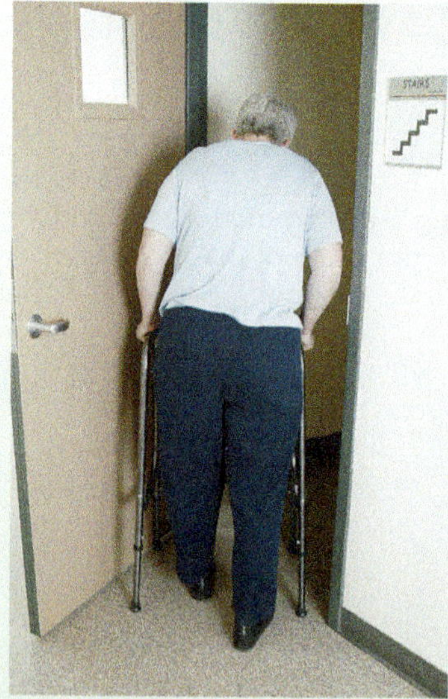

6 The patient should wait until the walker's legs have absorbed the contact of the closing door before moving forward. Once the patient has moved completely through the doorway, the door closes behind the patient.

Door Opens Away from Patient

1. When a door with an automatic door closer opens away from a patient, the patient should approach the door and shift the weight to the side of the walker away from the hand that is closest to the door handle. The patient then places the unweighted hand on the door handle.

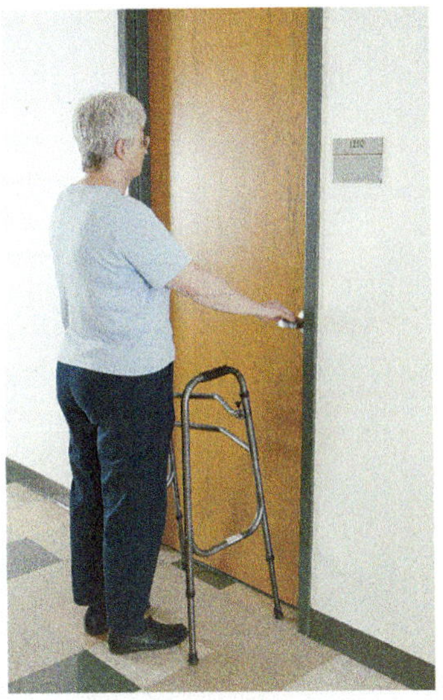

2. Using a pushing motion, the patient opens the door wider than the width of the patient. The patient quickly returns the hand used to open the door to the walker. The patient lifts the walker and moves it forward into the doorway. The patient places all four legs of the walker on the floor, with the legs closest to the door serving as doorstops. Using this method, the closing door hits the walker's legs, not the patient. Once a walker has absorbed the contact of a closing door, the patient can step into the walker to advance through the doorway.

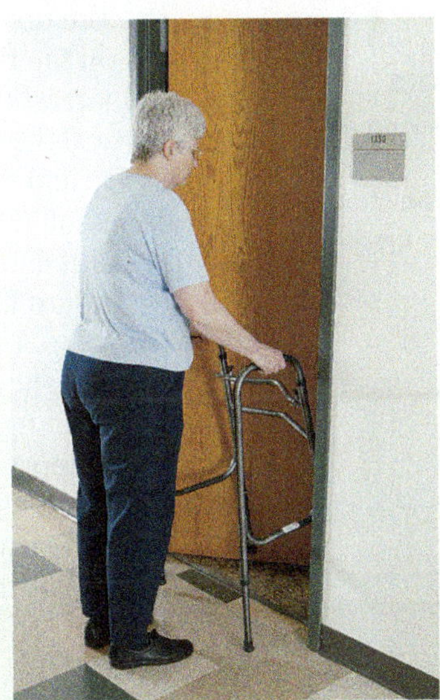

3. Using a walker's legs as doorstops, the patient progresses through the doorway. The patient may have to push a door farther open during transit through the doorway to allow a walker to be moved. Whenever this is done, the patient should wait until the walker's legs have absorbed the contact of the closing door before moving forward. Once the patient has moved completely through the doorway, the door closes behind the patient.

Axillary Crutches

Fitting

Axillary crutches are fitted with the patient standing and with shoulder girdles relaxed. Proper adjustment requires appropriate posture because of the potential for injury. When crutches are too long or when a patient rests on the tops of the crutches, injury to nerves and blockage of blood vessels in the axillae can occur. Patients may report pain or tingling in the upper extremities, and muscle weakness or paralysis may occur.

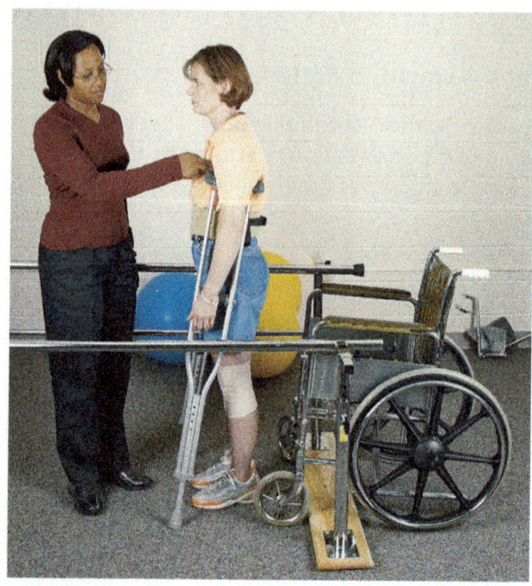

FIGURE 10–42 ■ Checking overall height of axillary crutches.

■ **Take Note**

When checking for the correct length of axillary crutches, the shoulder girdle must be relaxed.

The first adjustment is the overall length of the crutch (Figure 10–42 ■). Position crutch tips on the floor, approximately 6 inches away from the toes at a 45-degree angle anterior and lateral to the small toe. With the patient's shoulder girdles in a relaxed position, the physical therapist/assistant should be able to put two or three fingers between the patient's axillae and the top of the crutch on each side. When axillary pads are to be used on crutches, they should be in place during fitting. In some styles of crutches, nuts and bolts should not be tightened completely until all adjustments are completed.

Adjust handgrip height after overall length of the crutch is determined (Figure 10–43 ■). The top of the handgrip should be approximately at the level of the patient's ulnar styloid process when the upper extremities are in a relaxed position at the patient's side. When the patient grasps the handgrips with shoulder girdles level and relaxed, elbows should be flexed approximately 20 to 30 degrees.

When all length and handgrip adjustments are made, check all nuts, bolts, and button locks to ensure that they are tightened or fully positioned to maintain crutch integrity during gait training.

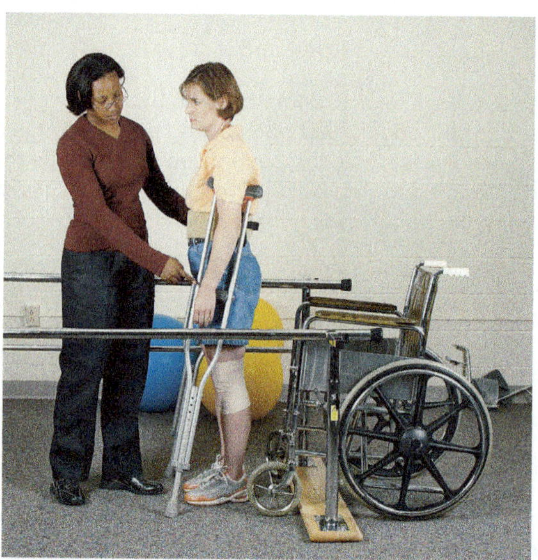

FIGURE 10–43 ■ Checking handgrip height of axillary crutches.

PROCEDURE 10–8 In and Out of a Wheelchair with Axillary Crutches

The procedure for a patient assuming standing or assuming sitting is the same whether you are guarding from the side of involved lower extremity or from the side of the uninvolved lower extremity.

Assuming Standing—Guarding from the Side of the Patient's Involved Lower Extremity

1. The physical therapist/assistant engages the wheelchair wheel locks and moves the footrests out of the way. The physical therapist/assistant places crutches within reach before the patient starts to stand.

   As the patient moves to the front edge of the seat, the physical therapist/assistant may need to support the involved lower extremity the first few times a patient assumes standing.

2. To provide assistance, the physical therapist/assistant squats on the involved side of the patient while supporting the involved lower extremity.

   When the patient is unable to flex the knee of the involved lower extremity, an elevating legrest is used for support during sitting. The legrest must be removed or lowered and pivoted to the side before the involved extremity is lowered to the floor.

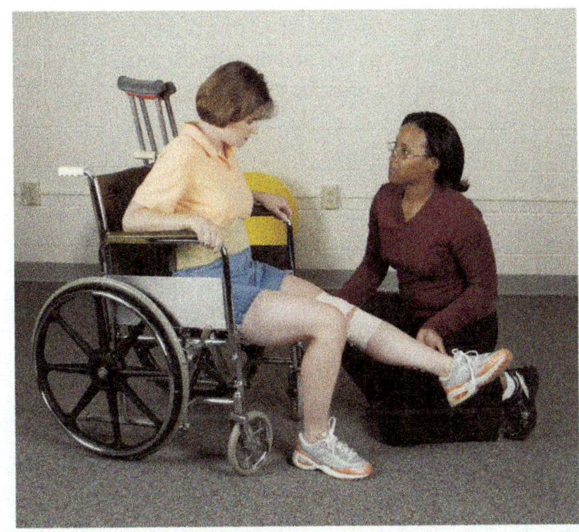

3. The physical therapist/assistant supports the involved lower extremity with one hand and arm while removing the legrest with the other hand. The involved lower extremity is lowered carefully to the floor before the patient attempts to stand.

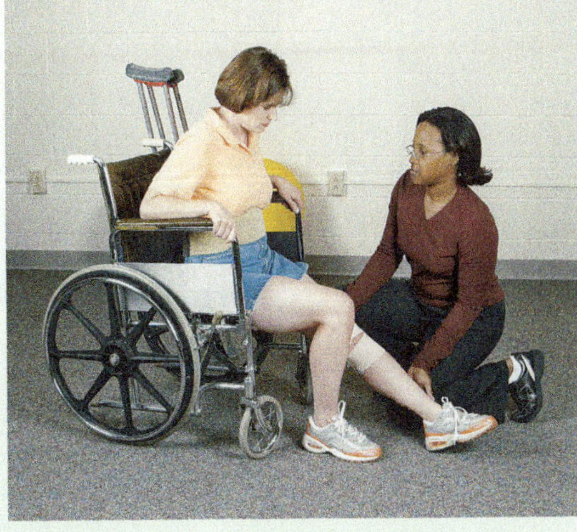

(continued)

PROCEDURE 10–8 In and Out of a Wheelchair with Axillary Crutches (*continued*)

4 Both crutches are placed together in front of and slightly lateral to the patient's foot on the uninvolved side. The patient grasps both crutch handgrips with the hand on the uninvolved side while grasping the wheelchair armrest on the involved side. Positioned in stride to one side of the patient, the physical therapist/ assistant grasps the patient's gait belt and maintains contact with the patient's shoulder girdle.

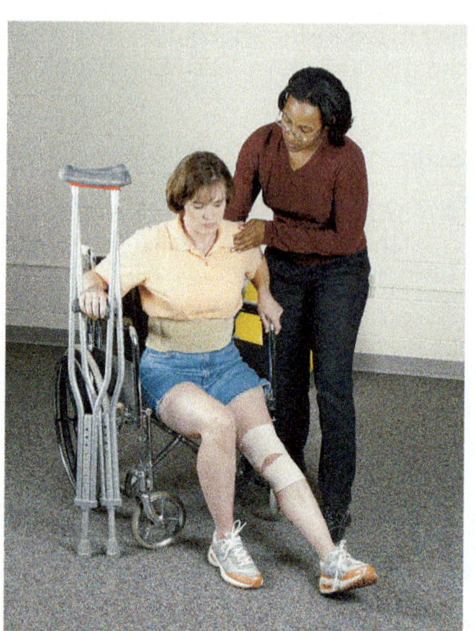

■ Take Note

Caution—The hand on the patient's shoulder girdle should guide, not impede, movement.

5 The patient assumes standing using the upper extremities and extending the uninvolved lower extremity. The involved lower extremity must be maintained within the desired weight-bearing status.

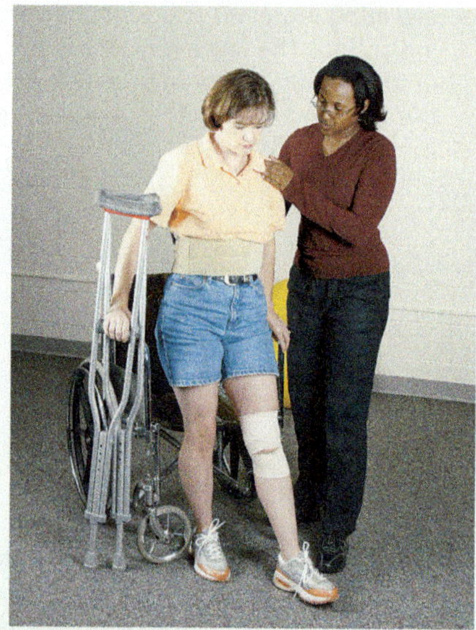

6 Once the patient has assumed a standing position, the physical therapist/assistant ensures the patient is stable and able to maintain an upright posture. One at a time, crutches are positioned properly under the axillae. The patient reaches across the body with the hand on the involved side for a crutch.

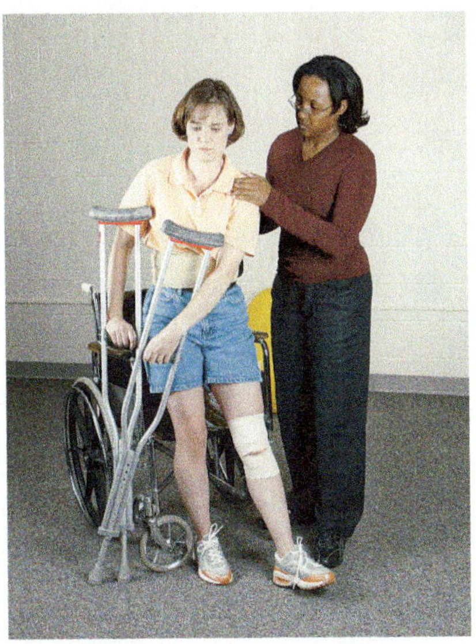

7 The patient first positions the crutch that was retrieved by the hand on the involved side under the axillae.

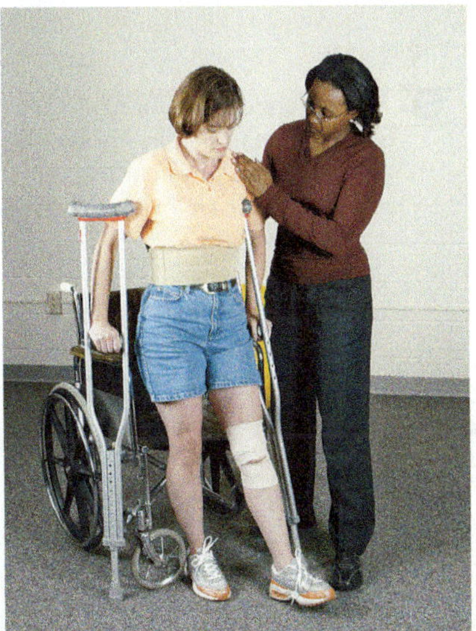

8 The patient positions the crutch that remains in the hand on the uninvolved side. The patient is ready to ambulate.

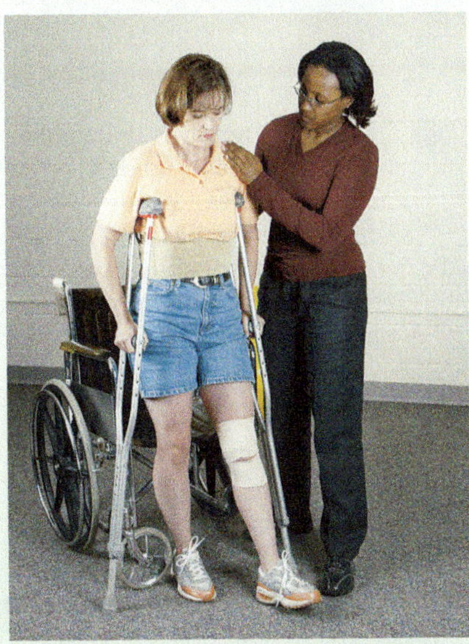

(continued)

PROCEDURE 10–8 In and Out of a Wheelchair with Axillary Crutches (*continued*)

Assuming Sitting—Physical Therapist/Assistant on Involved Side

1. The physical therapist/assistant engages the wheelchair wheel locks and moves the footrests out of the way. To sit, the patient is positioned facing away from the wheelchair at the front edge of a wheelchair seat, close enough so that she can feel the front edge of wheelchair seat against the backs of the lower extremities.

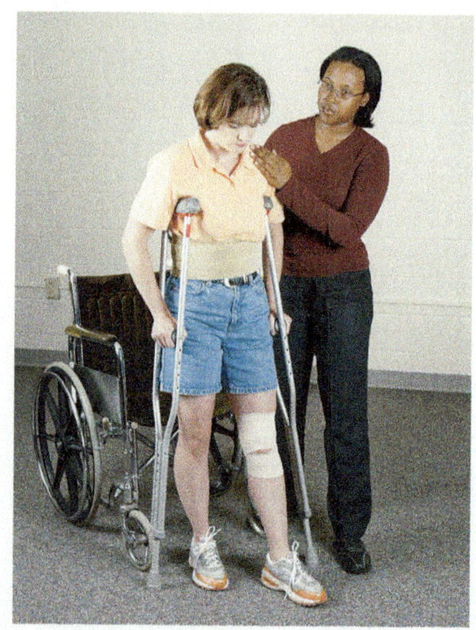

2. The patient can position her feet either in stride or side by side. Positioned in stride behind and to one side of a patient, the physical therapist/assistant grasps the patient's gait belt and shoulder girdle.

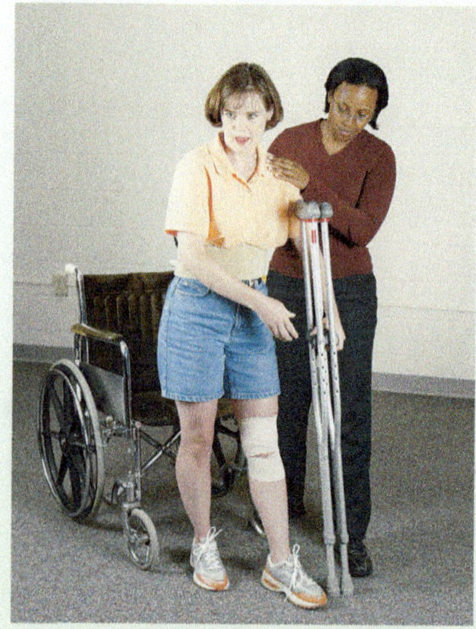

3. The patient removes the crutch from the axilla on the involved side and holds it by the handgrip only. The patient removes the crutch from the axilla on the uninvolved side and passes it to the hand on the involved side. The patient holds both crutches by the handgrips and places them in front of and slightly lateral to the patient's foot on the involved side.

4 Reaching back with the hand on the uninvolved side, the patient grasps the wheelchair armrest.

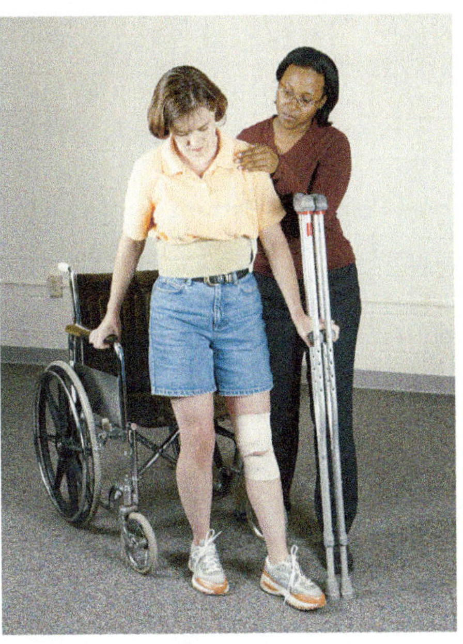

5 Using support from the handgrip and armrest, the patient lowers to sitting.

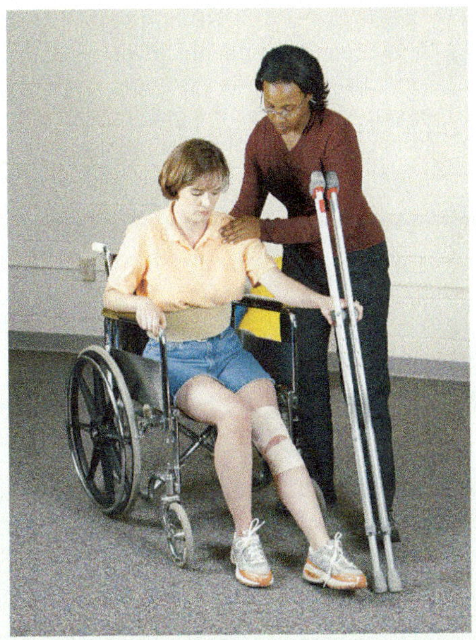

6 Setting crutches aside, the patient grasps both armrests and moves completely into the seat. A physical therapist/assistant may or may not need to assist with an involved lower extremity. When necessary, a patient's involved lower extremity is placed on the elevating legrest.

PROCEDURE 10–9 Ambulating on Level Surfaces with Axillary Crutches

Three-Point Gait Pattern

Partial to Full Weight Bearing

When ambulating with crutches, the patent can lift the body to decrease weight bearing by shoulder depression and elbow extension. The patient must also adduct the upper extremities to keep crutches in place under the axillae.

1. The physical therapist/assistant is positioned in stride behind and to one side of the patient. When contact guarding is required, the physical therapist/assistant maintains contact with the patient's gait belt and shoulder when necessary. In the starting position, the patient stands with crutches approximately 6 inches away from the toes at a 45-degree angle anterior and lateral to the small toe. The patient's feet are side by side.

2. To ambulate, the patient advances both crutches simultaneously the same distance. The physical therapist/assistant advances the outside foot either at the same time or immediately after the crutches are advanced.

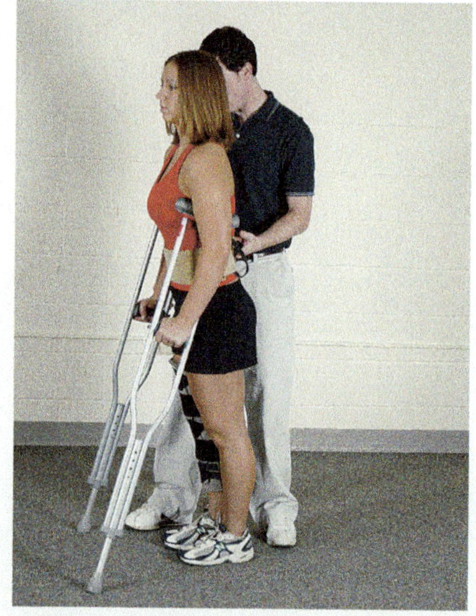

3. The patient advances the involved lower extremity so the ball of the foot is approximately even with the crutch tips. As the patient improves, she may move the crutches and involved lower extremity at the same time, permitting a faster gait.

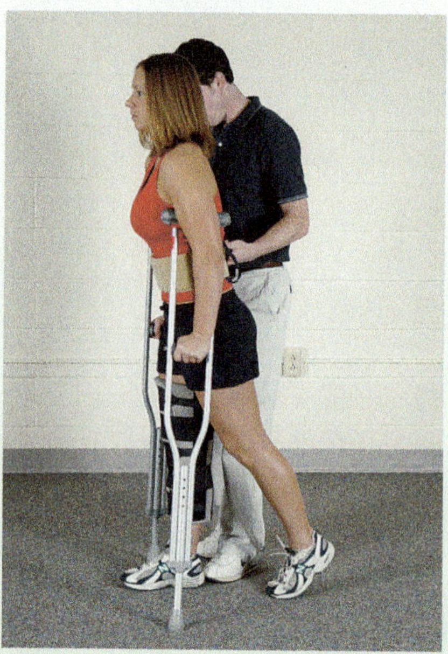

4 Using the upper extremities and involved lower extremity weight bearing as permitted to support body weight, the patient advances the uninvolved lower extremity beyond the crutches. Initially, the patient may "step to" the involved lower extremity. Stepping through is a normal gait pattern and should be encouraged. The physical therapist/assistant advances the inside foot as the patient moves the uninvolved lower extremity. The sequence is repeated for continued progression.

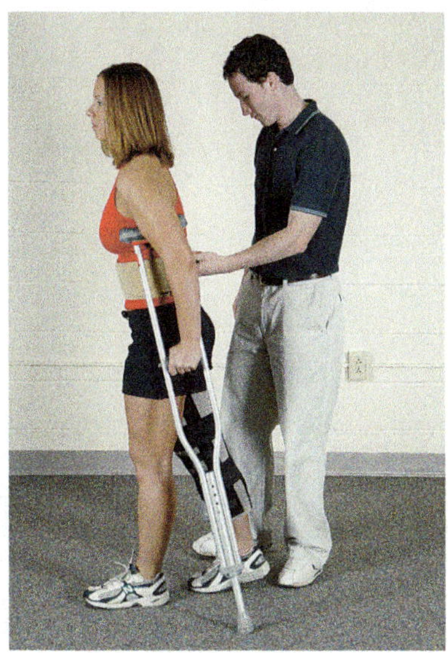

Non–Weight Bearing

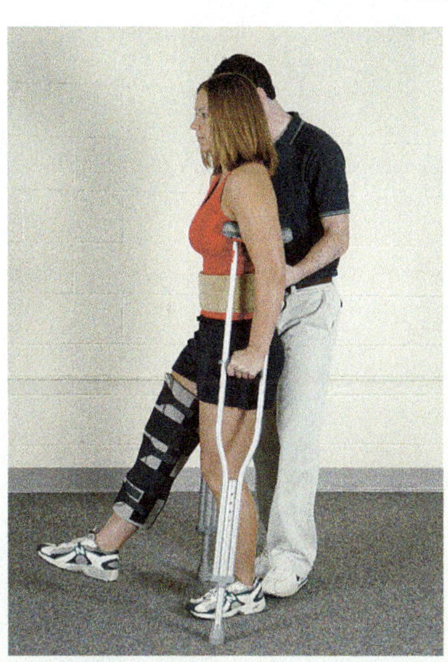

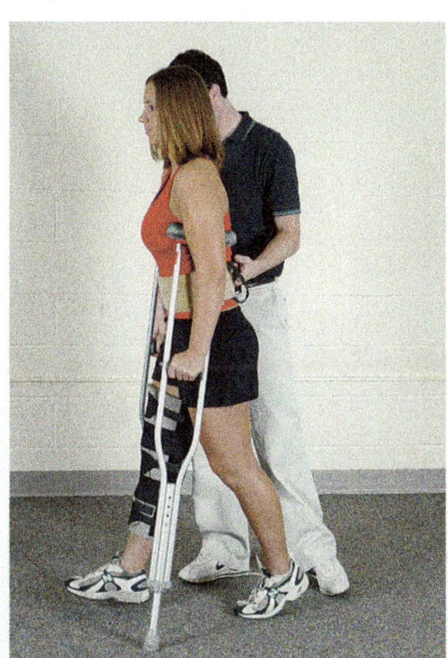

1 The physical therapist/assistant is positioned in stride behind and to one side of the patient, grasping the patient's gait belt. When contact guarding is required, the physical therapist/assistant maintains contact with the patient's gait belt and shoulder when necessary. In the starting position, the patient stands with crutches approximately 6 inches away from the toes at a 45-degree angle anterior and lateral to the small toe. The patient's involved lower extremity is not on the floor. Generally, patients hold the involved lower extremity in front when the knee cannot be flexed and behind when the knee can be flexed.

2 To ambulate, the patient advances both crutches and the involved lower extremity simultaneously the same distance. The physical therapist/assistant advances the outside foot at the same time or immediately after the crutches are advanced.

(continued)

PROCEDURE 10–9 Ambulating on Level Surfaces with Axillary Crutches (*continued*)

3. Using the upper extremities to support all body weight, the patient advances the uninvolved lower extremity beyond the crutches. Initially, the patient may "step to" the crutches. Stepping through is a normal gait pattern and should be encouraged. The physical therapist/assistant advances the inside foot as the patient moves the uninvolved lower extremity. The sequence is repeated for continued progression.

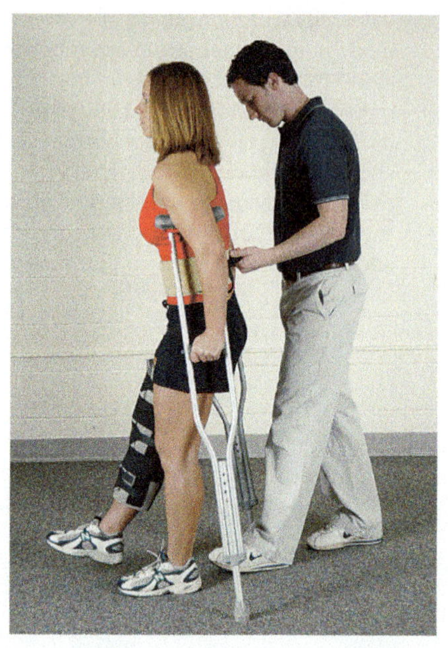

Four-Point Gait Pattern

1. The physical therapist/assistant is positioned in stride behind and to one side of a patient, grasping the patient's gait belt. In the starting position, the patient stands with crutches approximately 6 inches away from the toes at a 45-degree angle anterior and lateral to the small toe. The patient's feet are side by side. To ambulate, the patient advances one crutch. The physical therapist/assistant advances the outside foot when the crutch closest to the physical therapist/assistant is advanced.

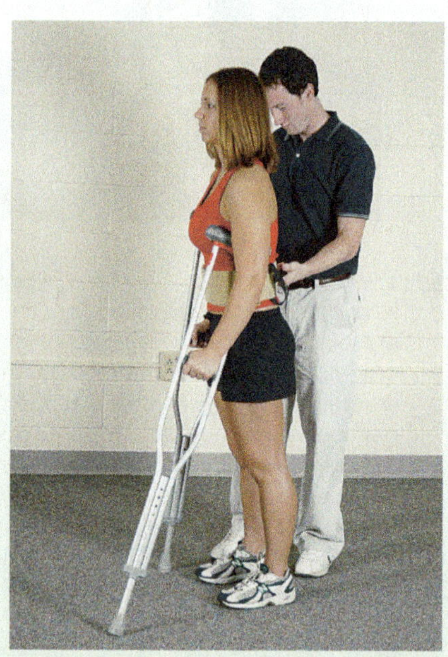

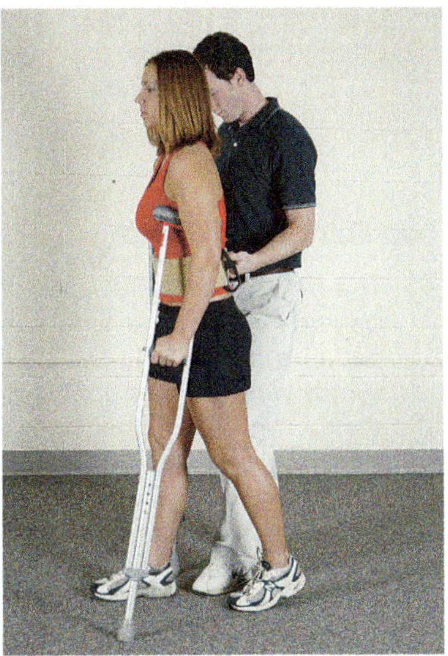

2 The patient then advances the opposite lower extremity so the ball of the foot is approximately even with the tip of the crutch. The physical therapist/assistant advances his inside foot when the patient advances the lower extremity closest to the physical therapist/assistant.

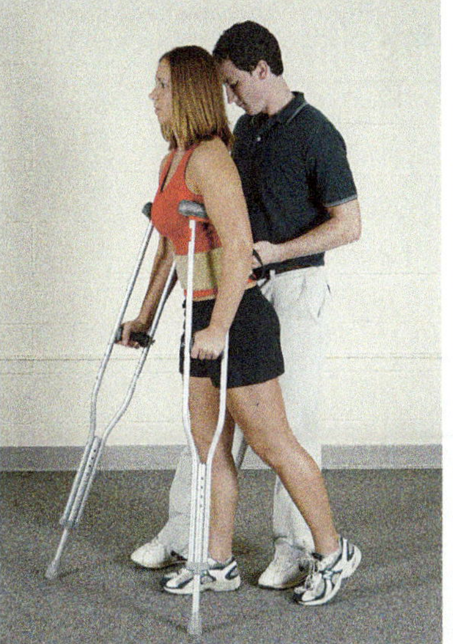

3 The patient shifts weight to the crutch and lower extremity just advanced and then advances the remaining crutch beyond the other crutch.

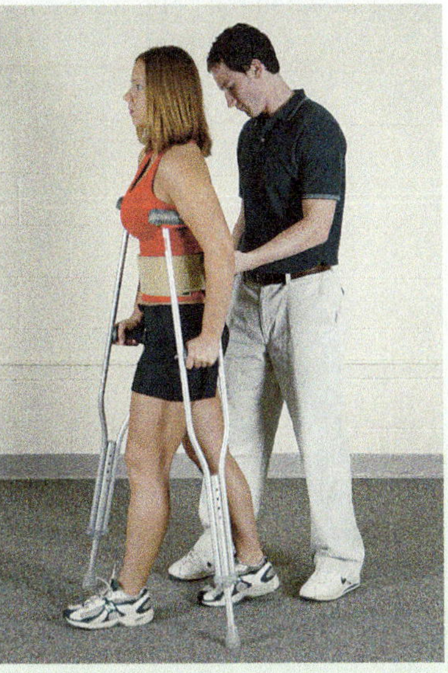

4 The patient advances the remaining lower extremity so the ball of the foot is approximately even with the tip of the crutch just advanced. The patient shifts weight to the crutch and lower extremity just advanced. The sequence is repeated for continued progression.

(continued)

PROCEDURE 10–9 Ambulating on Level Surfaces with Axillary Crutches (*continued*)

Two-Point Gait Pattern

1. The physical therapist/assistant is positioned in stride behind and to one side of a patient, grasping the patient's gait belt. In the starting position, the patient stands with crutches approximately 6 inches away from the toes at a 45-degree angle anterior and lateral to the small toe. The patient's feet are side by side. To ambulate, the patient advances one crutch and the opposite lower extremity simultaneously, placing the ball of the foot approximately even with the tip of the crutch. The patient shifts weight onto this crutch and lower extremity. The physical therapist/assistant advances the inside foot when the patient advances the crutch closest to the physical therapist/assistant.

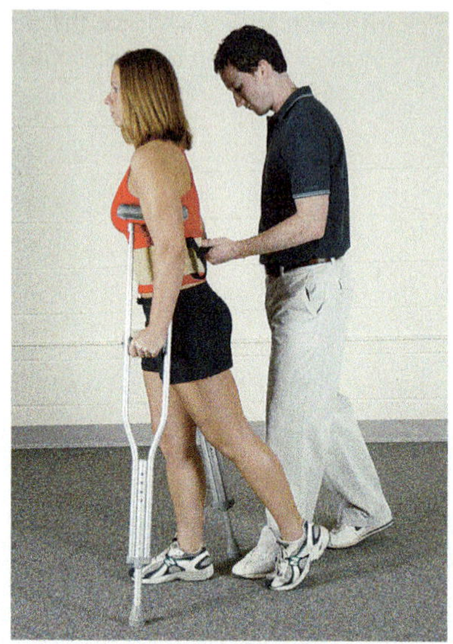

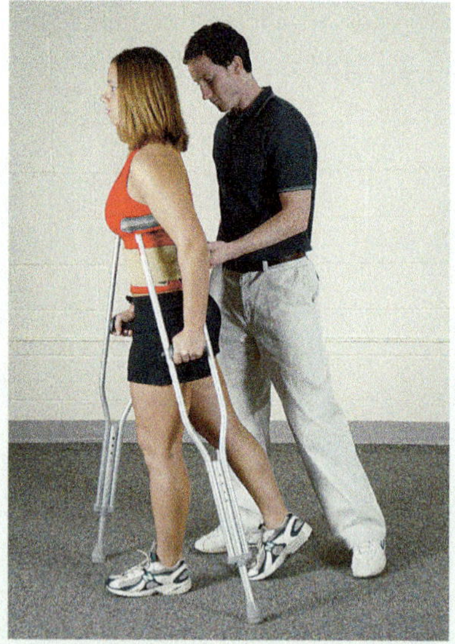

2. The patient advances the remaining crutch and lower extremity together beyond the first crutch and lower extremity in a normal step length. The patient shifts weight onto the just-advanced crutch and lower extremity. The physical therapist/assistant advances the outside foot when the patient advances the crutch closest to the physical therapist/assistant. The sequence is repeated for continued progression.

Falling

Patients must be taught how to control a fall, as falls may occur during gait training or after discharge. When the patient starts to fall, the physical therapist/assistant must decide whether to prevent the fall or to permit a controlled fall in a manner that will prevent injury to the patient or physical therapist/assistant. The physical therapist/assistant must be alert to the patient's movements at all times and react quickly to prevent or control a fall. Proper guarding and attention focused on the patient are required at all times.

▪ Take Note

Patients should practice falling so they will know what to do if a fall should occur.

1. The physical therapist/assistant prevents a fall by using the biomechanical advantages of standing in stride behind and slightly to the side of a patient. By standing in stride, the physical therapist/assistant is able to shift weight onto the back foot and pull the patient into the physical therapist's/assistant's base of support.

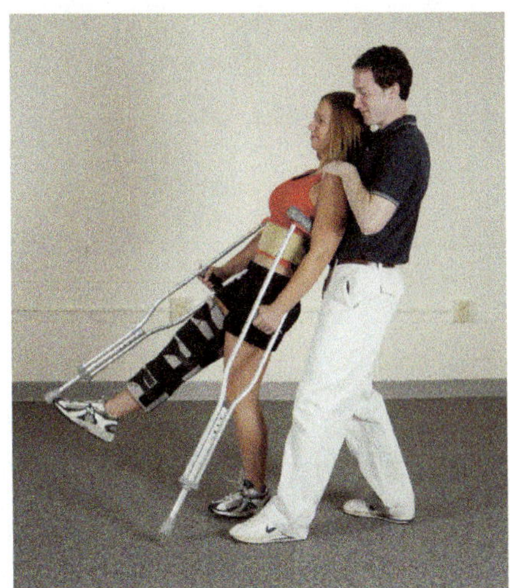

2. When the physical therapist/assistant cannot prevent a fall, the fall must be controlled. The physical therapist/assistant instructs the patient to let the crutches fall to the sides, away from the area in which the patient will land, avoiding injury from landing on the crutches. The physical therapist/assistant steps forward in a stride position to widen the base of support while slowing the rate at which the patient falls.

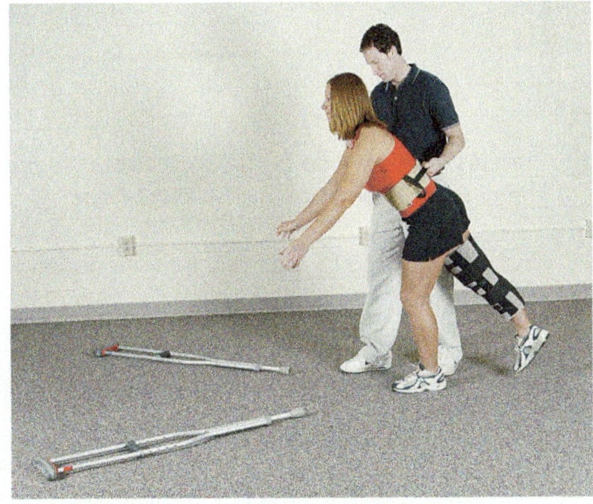

3. Patients can catch themselves on outstretched upper extremities, making sure that the elbows flex slightly to absorb impact. If the elbow does not flex, the patient's upper extremities may be injured.

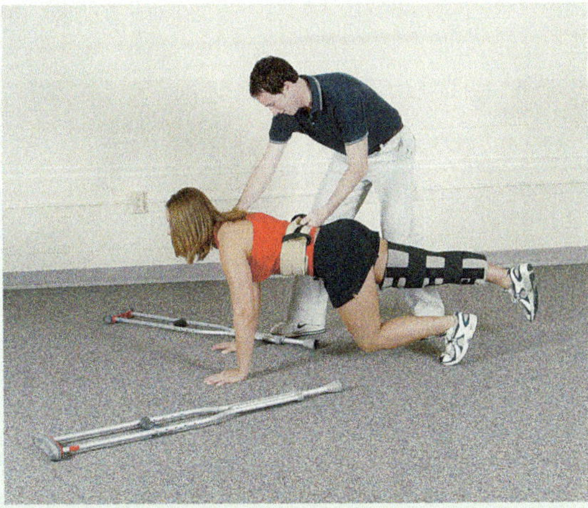

(continued)

PROCEDURE 10–9 Ambulating on Level Surfaces with Axillary Crutches (*continued*)

4. The physical therapist/assistant continues lowering the patient to the floor slowly, and the patient turns onto the side of the uninvolved lower extremity to avoid additional injury to the involved lower extremity.

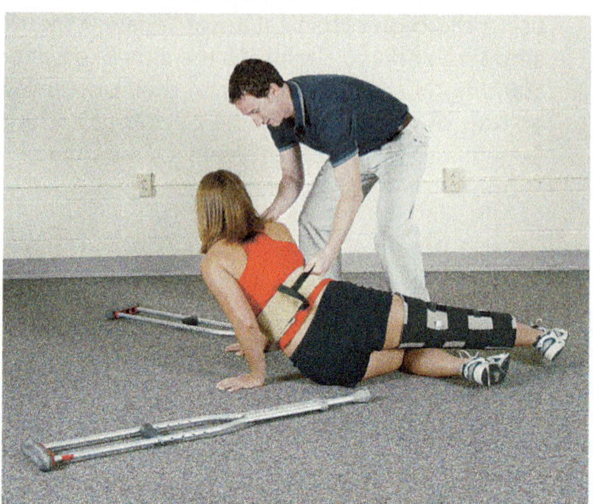

5. Turning from the side of the uninvolved lower extremity into a long sitting position, the patient is then in a position to get up from the floor.

The method used to rise from the floor depends on the patient's initial problem and any additional injury the fall may have caused. When the patient is unsure of the ability to arise after having fallen, she should call for assistance. Usually the patient can move on the floor to a sitting position near a chair or couch. Using furniture for stability and assistance, the patient can usually assume standing again. Methods of moving from the floor to a sitting position in a chair are described in Chapter 9, *Independent Transfer from Wheelchair to Floor and Return.*

PROCEDURE 10–10 Ambulating on Stairs with Axillary Crutches

Holding the Crutches

Patients can perform ambulation on stairs using two crutches without the use of a handrail. Use of a handrail, however, provides stability and, thus, is an added safety feature. When using a handrail, it takes the place of the crutch on one side. There are several methods of holding crutches when using a handrail. Whichever method of holding crutches is used, the sequence of movements for the lower extremities and ambulatory assistive devices is the same.

There are three common methods of holding crutches while ambulating on stairs.

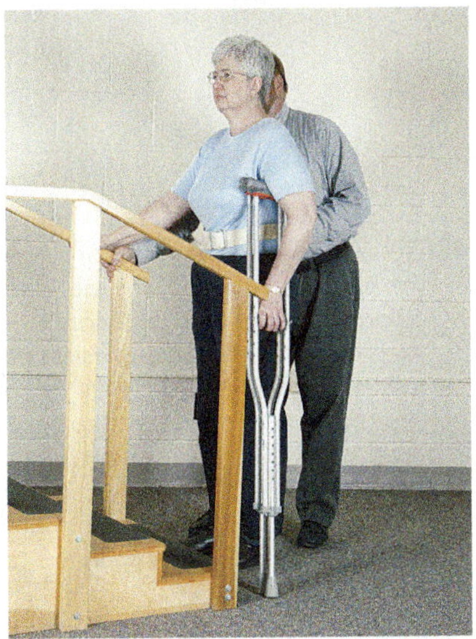

1. One method of holding two crutches while using a handrail is to place both crutches together under the upper extremity on the side opposite the handrail. This is the preferred method.

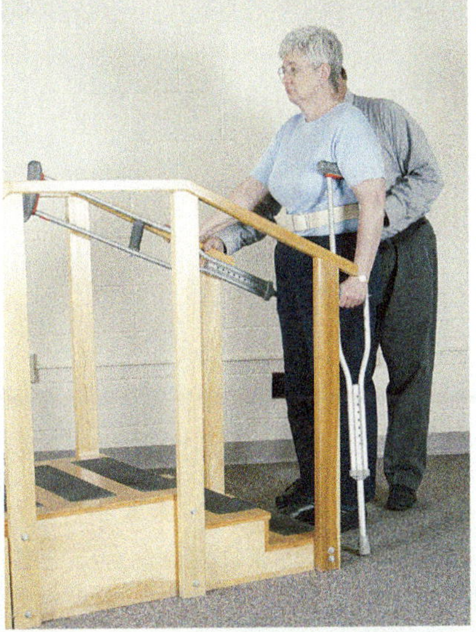

2. A second method of holding two crutches while using a handrail is to hold the crutch on the side of the handrail in the hand that grasps the handrail. The patient holds this crutch by one of its uprights, parallel to the handrail. The patient uses the crutch on the side opposite the handrail in the usual manner.

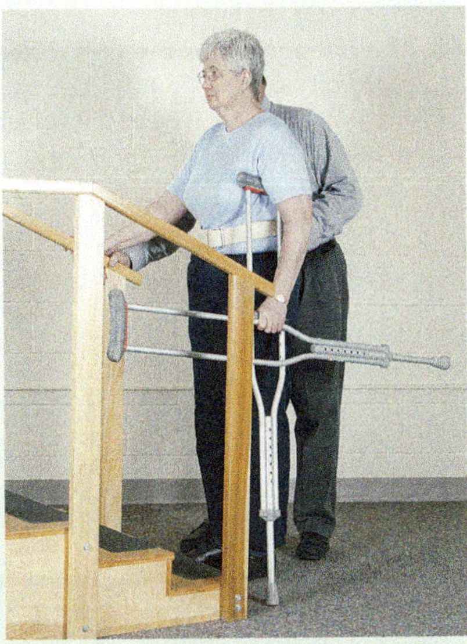

3. A third method of holding two crutches while using a handrail is to hold the handrail with one hand. The patient holds both crutches in the hand on the side opposite the handrail, one in the usual manner and the other by one of its uprights perpendicular to the first crutch.

(continued)

PROCEDURE 10–10 Ambulating on Stairs with Axillary Crutches (*continued*)

Ascending Using a Handrail

1. To ascend stairs using any of the methods of holding crutches, the patient stands facing up the stairs. Positioned in stride behind the patient, the physical therapist/assistant grasps the patient's gait belt and the handrail. For the method illustrated in this section, the patient places both crutches under the upper extremity on the side opposite the handrail and grasps the handrail with the other hand.

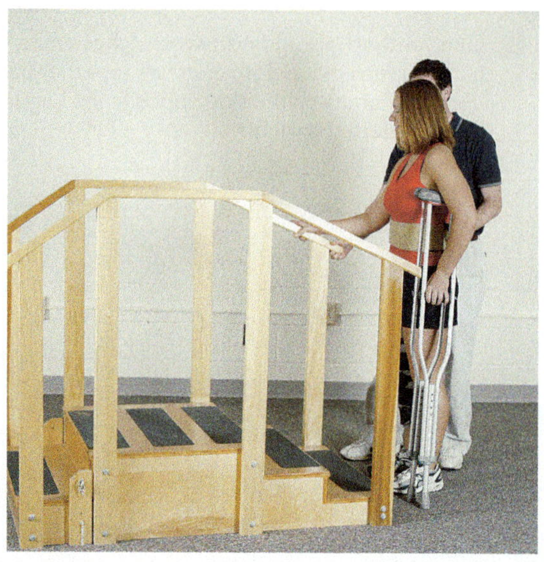

2. The patient places the uninvolved lower extremity on the next higher stair while the upper extremities and involved lower extremity support the body weight.

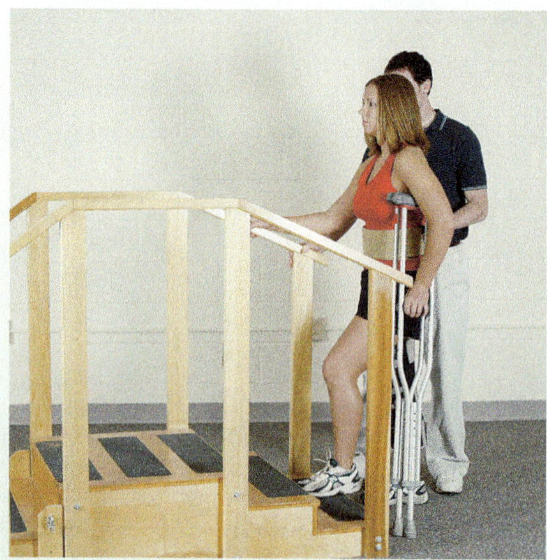

3 The patient shifts weight to the uninvolved lower extremity on the next higher stair. Extending the uninvolved lower extremity, the patient lifts up to the next higher stair. The patient advances the crutches and involved lower extremity to the same stair at the same time.

Patients must place the crutches on the step, midway from front to back. Proper crutch placement on stairs provides stability and space for patients to maneuver.

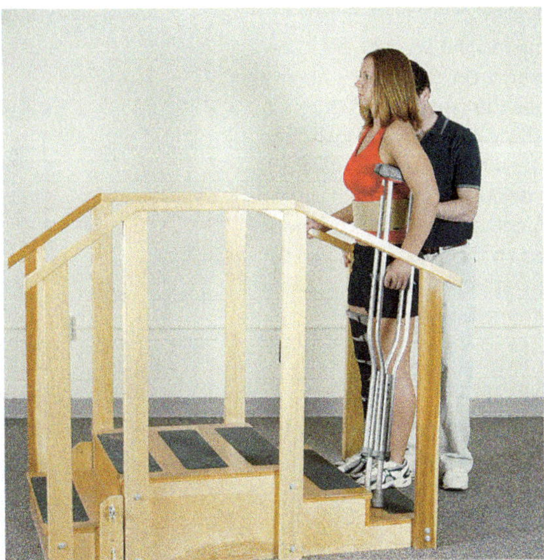

■ Take Note

Caution—Physical therapists/assistants must check that the placement of crutches on each stair tread is appropriate for safety purposes.

4 The physical therapist/assistant ascends with the patient. This sequence is repeated to ascend an entire flight of stairs.

Descending Using a Handrail

1 To descend stairs using any of the methods of holding crutches, the patient stands facing down the stairs. Positioned in stride in front of the patient, the physical therapist/assistant grasps the patient's gait belt and the handrail. For the method illustrated in this section, the patient places both crutches under the upper extremity on the side opposite the handrails and grasps the handrail with the other hand.

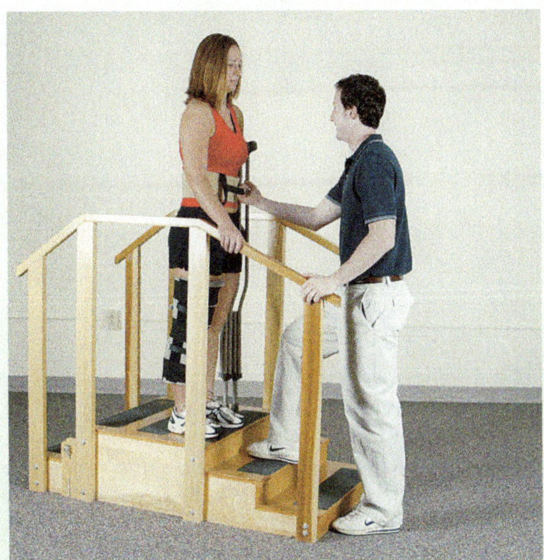

(continued)

PROCEDURE 10–10 Ambulating on Stairs with Axillary Crutches (*continued*)

2. Maintaining support using the uninvolved lower extremity and the hand on the handrail, the patient securely places the crutches on the next lower stair. The patient must place crutches midway on the stair tread and far enough from the handrail or far enough from each other when no handrail is used, to permit movement through the crutches to the next stair. Proper crutch placement on stairs provides stability and space for the patient to maneuver.

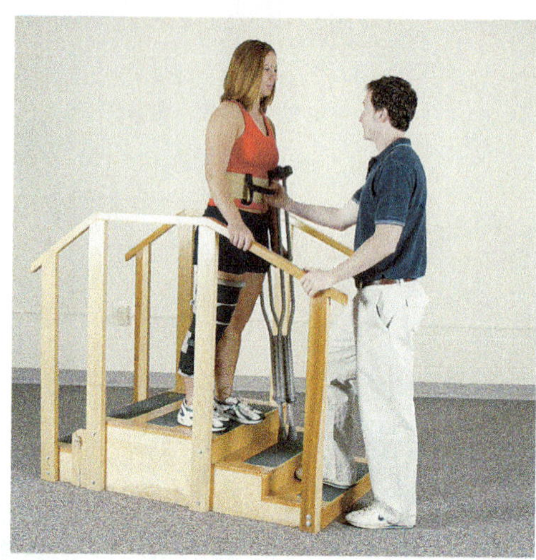

3. With the body supported by the upper extremities and the uninvolved lower extremity, the patient moves the involved lower extremity to the same stair as the crutches. As the patient improves, the involved lower extremity and crutches advance simultaneously.

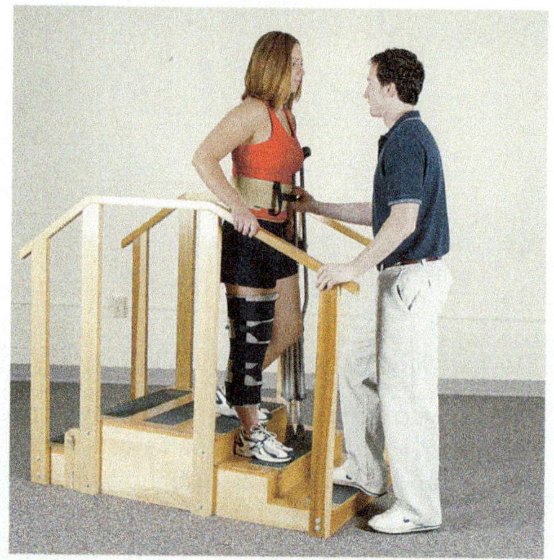

4. Bearing weight on the upper extremities and on the involved lower extremity if weight bearing is permitted, the patient moves the uninvolved lower extremity to the same stair as the crutches and involved lower extremity.

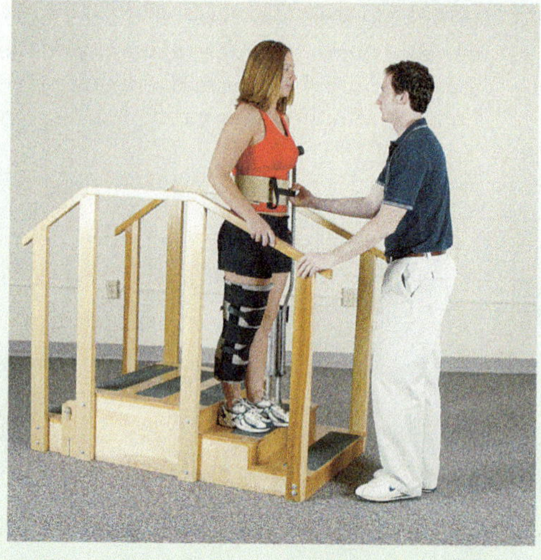

5. The physical therapist/assistant descends with the patient. This sequence is repeated to descend an entire flight of stairs.

Ascending and Descending Stairs Without Using a Handrail

To ascend or descend stairs without using a handrail, the patient retains the crutches in the same position used for ambulating on level surfaces. Rather than using a handrail for support on one side, patients use one crutch on each side for support. The physical therapist's/assistant's position, and the sequence of moving the crutches and lower extremities, remains the same as for ascending stairs using a handrail and descending stairs using a handrail. The physical therapist/assistant holds the handrail, when available, for stability, whether or not a patient is using a handrail. The patient must place the crutches widely enough from side to side to permit patient movement through the crutches without hitting and disrupting stability of the crutches.

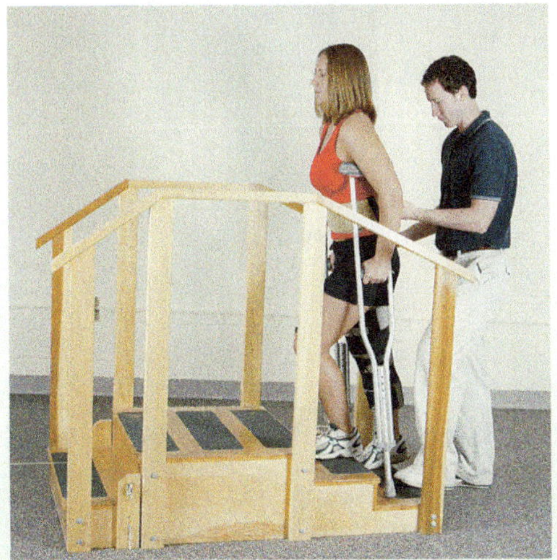

Ascending stairs without using a handrail.

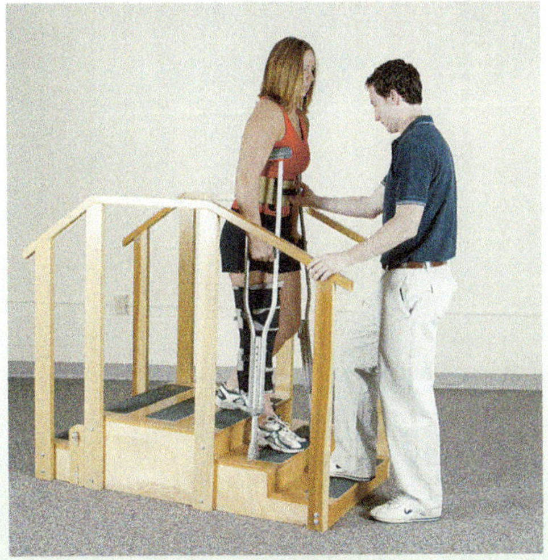

Descending stairs without using a handrail.

PROCEDURE 10–11 Ambulating Through Doorways with Axillary Crutches

Door with Automatic Door Closer

Door Opens Toward Patient

1. The patient approaches the latch edge of the door, standing outside the arc through which the opening door will move. The patient shifts weight onto the crutch on the side away from the hand that will be placed on the door handle. The patient places the unweighted hand on the door handle. Preferably, the patient shifts weight to the side closer to the door handle and uses the hand farthest from the door handle to pull open the door. Using the hand farther from the door permits a patient to open a door wider than using the hand closer to the door.

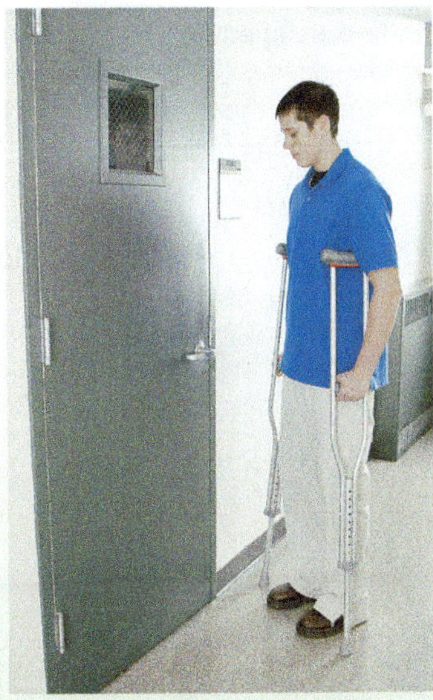

(continued)

PROCEDURE 10–11 Ambulating Through Doorways with Axillary Crutches (*continued*)

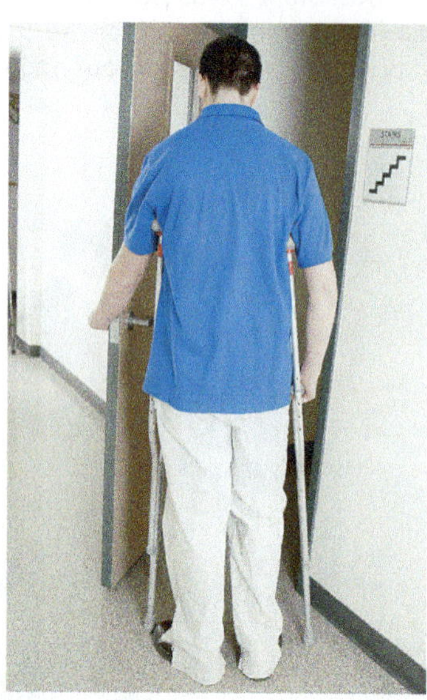

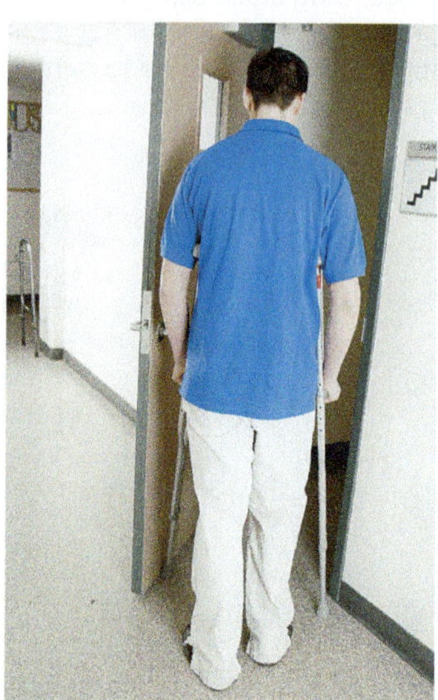

2. Using a pulling motion, the patient opens the door wider than the width of the patient and crutches. This is necessary because a door will start to close automatically before patients can progress through the doorway.

3. The patient quickly returns the hand used to open the door to the crutch. To block automatic closing of the door, the patient turns into the doorway and places the tip of the crutch closer to the door on the floor in the path of the door. This crutch tip acts as a doorstop, permitting the patient to progress through the doorway without being struck by the closing door.

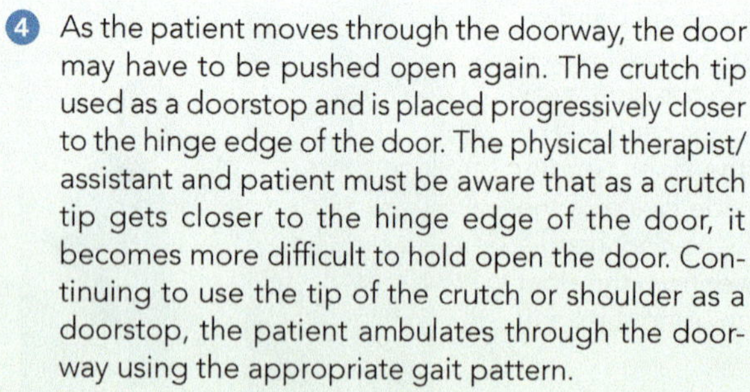

4. As the patient moves through the doorway, the door may have to be pushed open again. The crutch tip used as a doorstop and is placed progressively closer to the hinge edge of the door. The physical therapist/assistant and patient must be aware that as a crutch tip gets closer to the hinge edge of the door, it becomes more difficult to hold open the door. Continuing to use the tip of the crutch or shoulder as a doorstop, the patient ambulates through the doorway using the appropriate gait pattern.

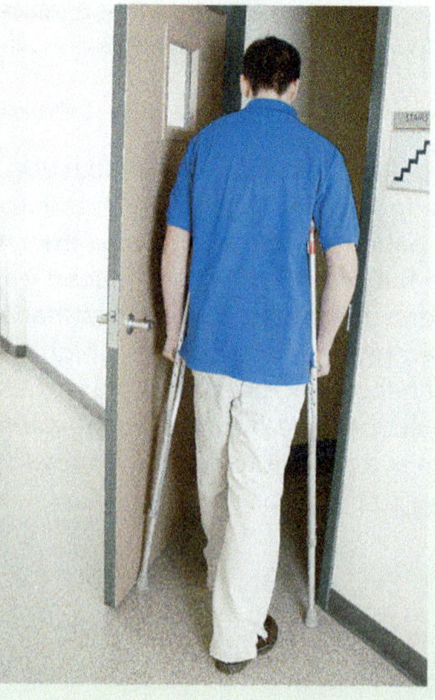

5. Once the patient has moved completely through the doorway, the door closes behind the patient.

Door Opens Away from Patient

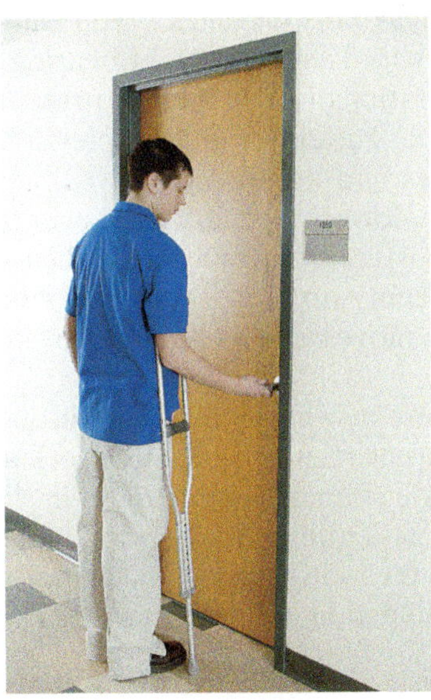

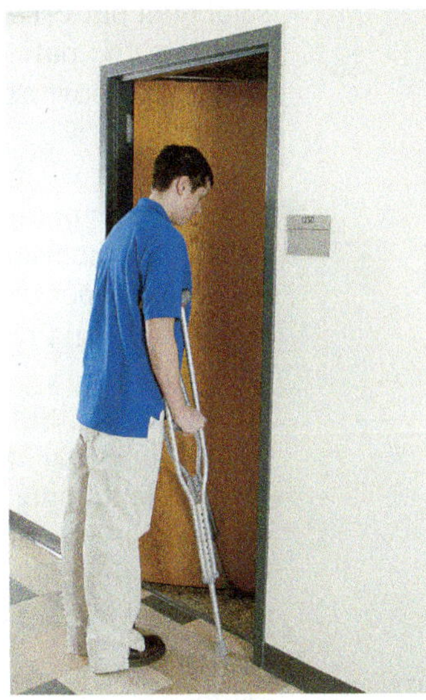

1. The patient faces the door and shifts weight onto the crutch away from the hand that is closer to the door handle. Using the hand closer to the door handle permits a patient to open a door wider than using the hand farther from the door. The patient places the unweighted hand on the door handle.
2. Using a pushing motion, the door is opened wider than the width of the patient and crutches because the door will start to close automatically before a patient can move through the doorway. The patient quickly returns the hand used to open the door to the crutch. Automatic closing of the door must be blocked by the tip of the crutch closer to the door, permitting the patient time to progress through the doorway. The patient advances the crutch closer to the door into the doorway to act as a doorstop.
3. As the patient moves through the doorway, the door may have to be pushed open again. Continuing to use the tip of the crutch or shoulder as a doorstop, the patient ambulates through the doorway using the appropriate gait pattern.
4. Once a patient has moved completely through the doorway, the door closes behind the patient.

Door Without Automatic Door Closer

When a door does not have an automatic closer, the patient's initial rapid movement to place a crutch tip on the ground as a doorstop is not necessary. Extra wide opening of a door is also not necessary. The patient can perform crutch movement more slowly, and the patient is not required to place a crutch tip as a doorstop between a door and a patient. Patients must turn to close the door because the door will not close automatically.

Forearm (Lofstrand) Crutches

Forearm crutches can be used by patients with the same impairments and with the same gait patterns as patients who use axillary crutches. When ambulating with forearm crutches, the patient can lift the body to decrease weight bearing by shoulder depression and elbow extension. The illustrations in this section present the use of forearm crutches for a patient with paraplegia. Patients with paraplegia have paralysis of the musculature of the lower extremities and usually some weakness of trunk muscles. Patients with paraplegia lack sufficient lower extremity and lower trunk muscle strength to support themselves in an upright posture. To overcome this lack of strength, a greater degree of upper trunk and upper extremity strength is required. Ambulation for patients with paraplegia requires upper body movement to control paretic or paralyzed lower extremities.

Patients with paraplegia usually use a swing-to or swing-through gait pattern. They will use bilateral knee-ankle-foot orthoses (KAFOs). KAFOs lock at the knee and ankle joints, maintaining the patient's knees in extension and ankles in slight dorsiflexion during ambulation training. Initially, the patient may use a swing-to gait pattern. As ability improves, the patient may progress to the swing-through pattern. The swing-through gait pattern is more efficient, permitting the patient to move more quickly.

Fitting

Setting the length of forearm crutches determines handgrip height. Position forearm crutches with the crutch tip on the floor, approximately 6 inches away from the toes at a 45-degree angle anterior and lateral to the small toe. Handgrips are level with the ulnar styloid processes when the upper extremities are relaxed at the side (**Figure 10–44** ■).

When handgrips are held with the shoulders relaxed, the elbows should be in 20 to 30 degrees of flexion. Adjust forearm cuff height after crutch length has been adjusted. Adjust cuff height to a point as high as possible on the forearm without interfering with elbow flexion. Cuff width should be tight enough to stay on the upper extremity when a handgrip is released but loose enough not to bind. Adjust cuff width by squeezing the cuff together or spreading it apart (**Figure 10–45** ■).

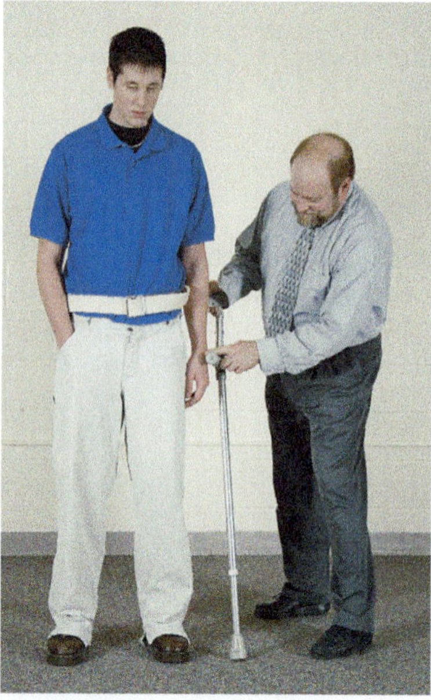

FIGURE 10–44 ■ Measuring forearm crutch length.

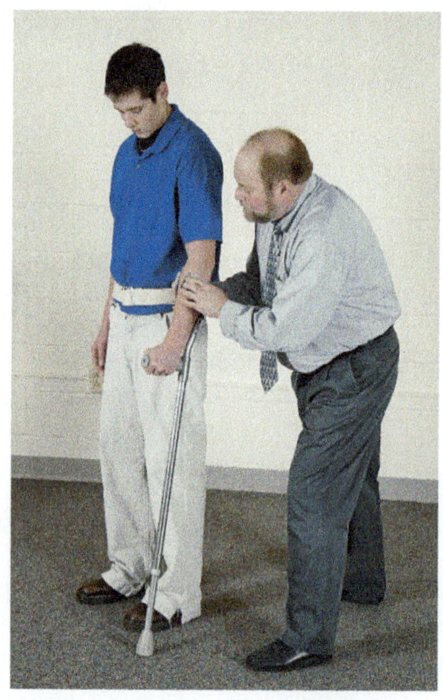

FIGURE 10–45 ■ Ensuring proper elbow flexion and cuff tightness.

PROCEDURE 10–12 In and Out of a Wheelchair with Forearm Crutches

Two methods, the turn-around method and the power method, may be used to assume standing using forearm crutches and KAFOs. The turn-around method requires less strength than the power method.

1. The physical therapist/assistant locks the wheelchair wheels and moves the footrests out of the way. The patient is positioned at the front edge of the seat. Positioned in stride behind and to one side of the patient, the physical therapist/assistant grasps the patient's gait belt and shoulder.
2. The patient positions one forearm crutch on either side of the wheelchair. Crutches must be supported securely enough so they will not fall as the patient moves, yet be accessible to the patient.
3. The patient moves forward on the seat of the wheelchair and secures the knee locks of the KAFOs in knee extension.

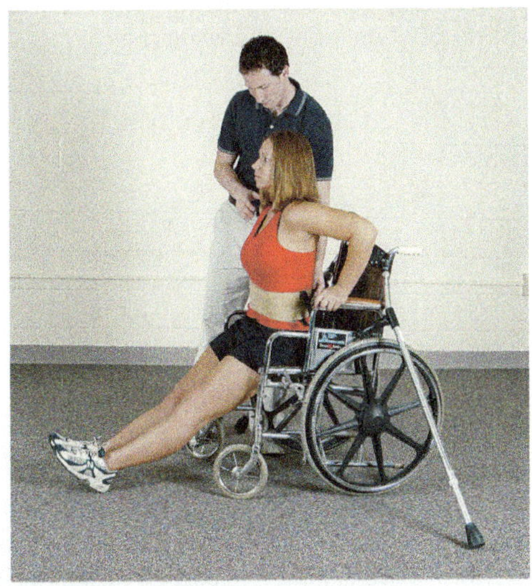

Assuming Standing Using the Turn-Around Method

For this method, the physical therapist/assistant initially assumes the proper position on the side from which the patient will turn. In the illustrations for this section, this is on the patient's right side. The physical therapist/assistant must be prepared to move with the patient so as not to inhibit the patient's fluid motion. Initially, the physical therapist/assistant may assist by lifting or guiding the patient.

1. When the patient turns to the left, she begins by hooking the medial upright of the right orthosis over the medial upright of the left orthosis. This aids in placement of the lower extremities as the patient stands. The patient then turns onto the left side. As the patient turns, she reaches behind with the left hand to grasp the right armrest and in front with the right hand to grasp the left armrest.

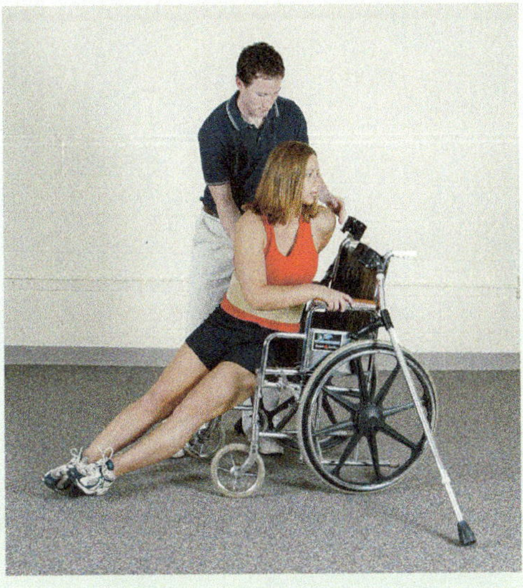

(continued)

PROCEDURE 10–12 In and Out of a Wheelchair with Forearm Crutches (*continued*)

2 Using the upper extremities, the patient pushes to standing, completing the turn to assume a standing position facing the wheelchair.

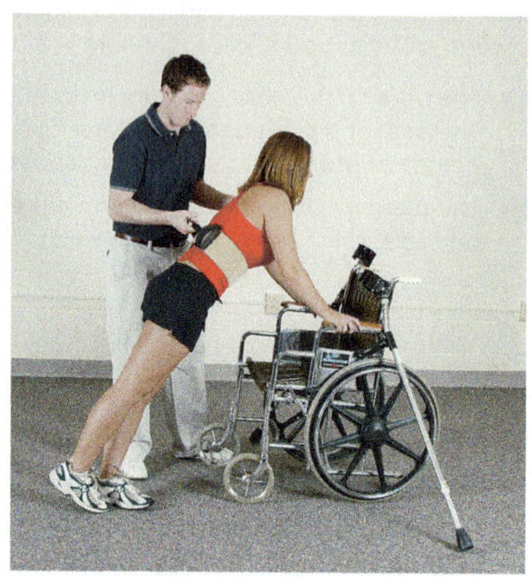

3 Using the armrests for support, the patient performs a push-up, lifting the body to position the lower extremities. Feet must be positioned so the patient is centered in front of the wheelchair at a distance that will permit support with one upper extremity as the crutches are retrieved.

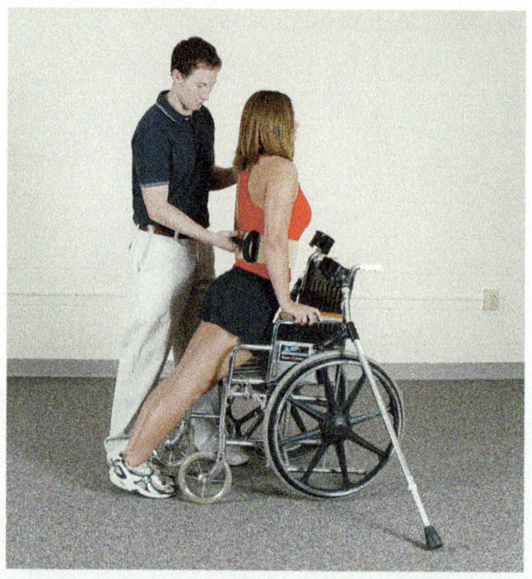

4 The patient shifts weight to one side and grasps and positions the forearm crutch on the side that has been unweighted.

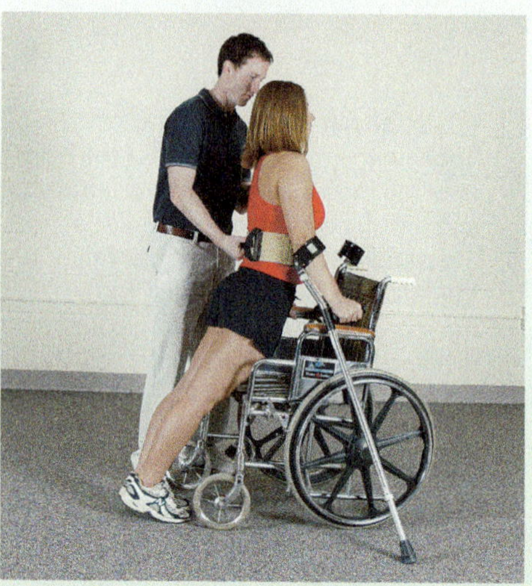

5 Shifting weight onto one forearm crutch, the patient grasps the second forearm crutch and places it properly.

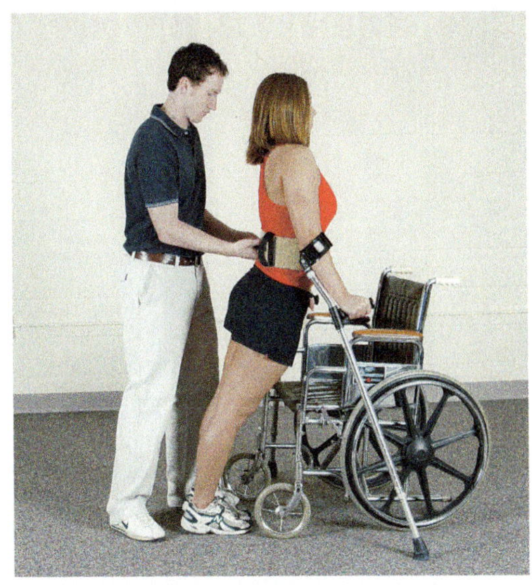

6 Using both crutches for support, the patient pushes to a fully upright position, shoulders behind hips to maintain hip extension. This posture is called a "C" curve.

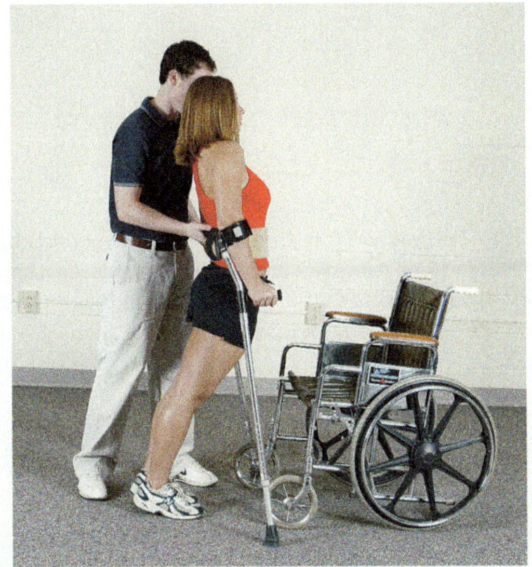

Assuming Sitting Using the Turn-Around Method

1 The physical therapist/assistant engages the wheelchair wheel locks and moves the footrests out of the way. Positioned in stride slightly behind and to the side to which the patient will turn, the physical therapist/assistant grasps the patient's gait belt. The physical therapist/assistant must be prepared to move as the patient moves to avoid interfering with the patient's fluid motion. Initially, the physical therapist/assistant may guide or control the rate at which the patient turns and lowers into the seat.

(continued)

PROCEDURE 10–12 In and Out of a Wheelchair with Forearm Crutches (*continued*)

2. To assume sitting using the turn-around method, the patient approaches and faces the wheelchair.

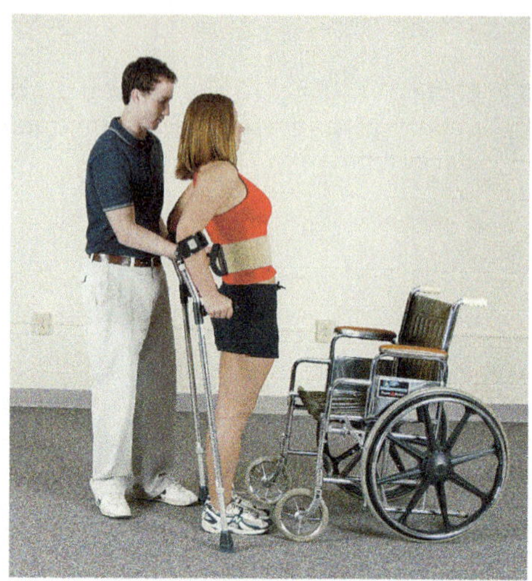

3. Shifting weight onto one forearm crutch, the patient removes the other forearm crutch. The patient places the crutch that has been removed against the wheelchair.

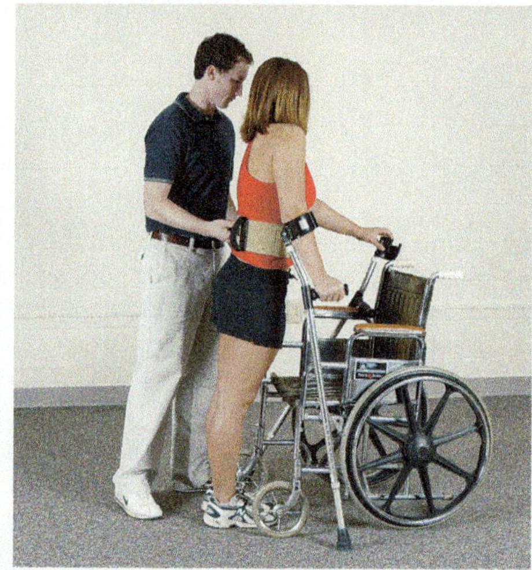

4. The patient then grasps the armrest with the free hand and shifts weight onto the upper extremity that is grasping the armrest. The patient removes the remaining crutch and places it against the wheelchair.

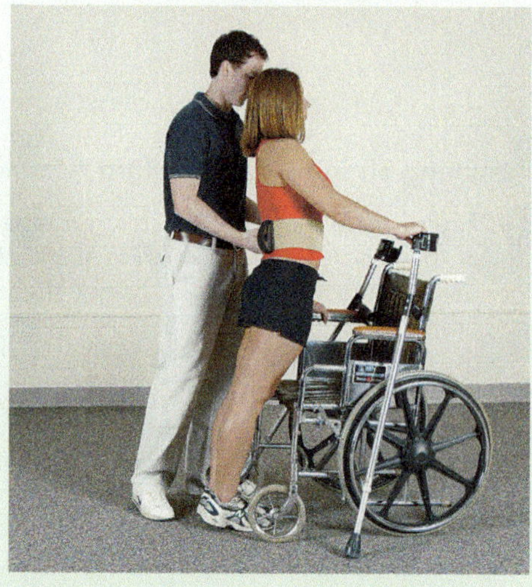

5 The patient is then able to grasp the remaining armrest.

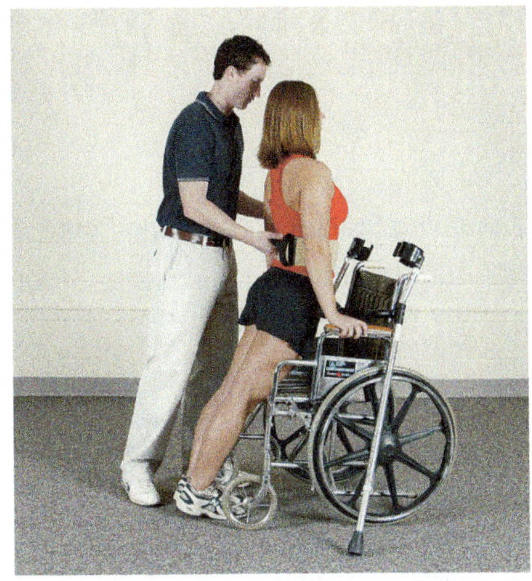

6 Turning, the patient then lowers into the wheelchair.

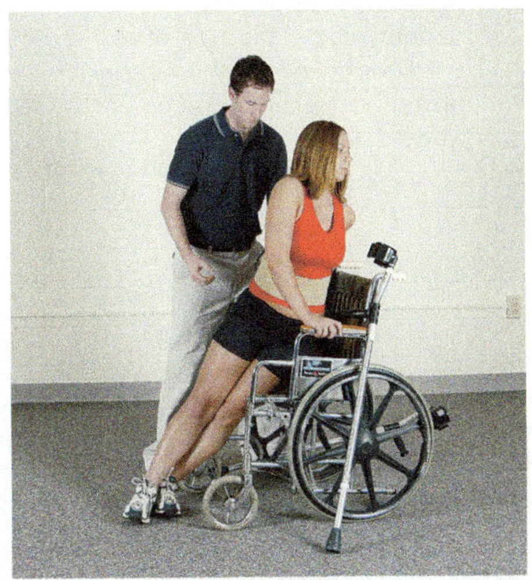

7 Repositioning the upper extremities, the patient adjusts her position in the wheelchair. Knee locks on the KAFOs are released. Once KAFO knee locks are released, the patient replaces the wheelchair footrests and assumes a proper sitting position.

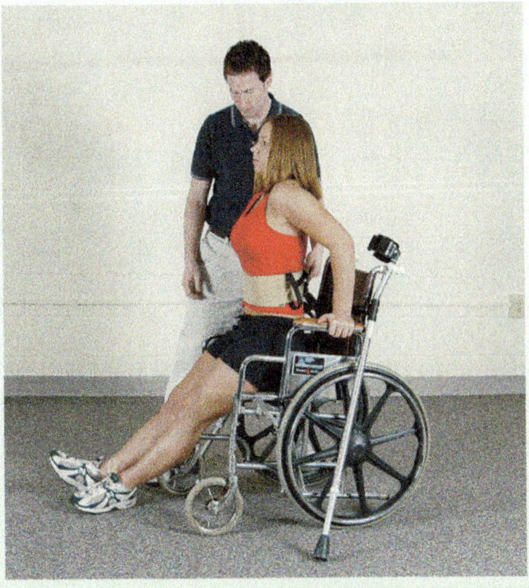

(continued)

PROCEDURE 10–12 In and Out of a Wheelchair with Forearm Crutches (*continued*)

Assuming Standing Using the Power Method

1. The physical therapist/assistant engages the wheelchair wheel locks and moves the footrests out of the way. The patient is positioned toward the front edge of the seat. Positioned in stride behind and to one side of the patient, the physical therapist/assistant grasps the patient's gait belt and shoulder. The physical therapist/assistant must be prepared to move as the patient moves to avoid interfering with the patient's fluid motion.

2. With knee locks of the KAFOs secured, the patient grasps one crutch in each hand. The patient places the tips of the crutches on the floor even with the hips in the anterior/posterior direction, one on each side of the wheelchair.

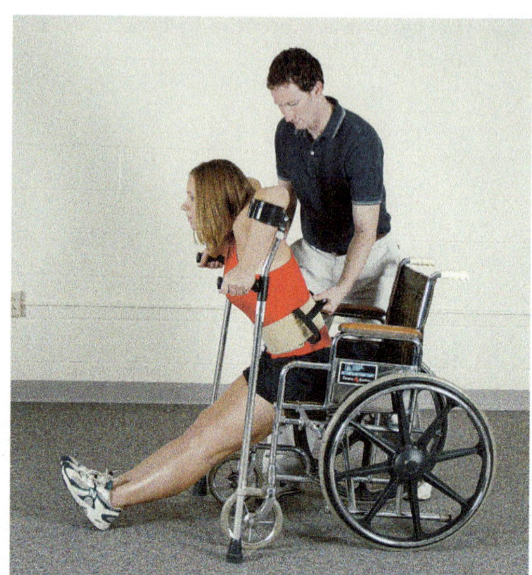

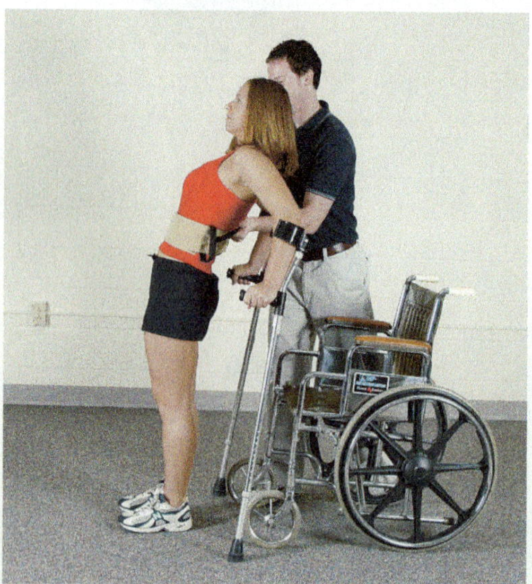

3. Pushing on the crutches, the patient extends the upper extremities and depresses the shoulders, producing a quick thrusting movement to propel the body upward and forward into a standing position.

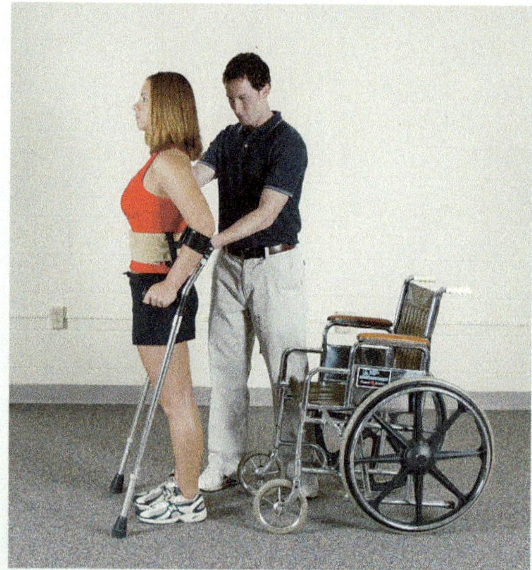

4. The patient must move the crutches forward quickly to halt the forward momentum. Placing the crutches slightly ahead and to the side of the toes, the patient assumes a "C" curve. The physical therapist/assistant can assist the patient into a "C" curve position by pushing forward on the gait belt and pulling backward on the patient's shoulder.

Assuming Sitting Using the Power Method

1. The physical therapist/assistant engages the wheelchair wheel locks and moves the footrests out of the way. Positioned in stride slightly behind and to the side, the physical therapist/assistant grasps the patient's gait belt and shoulder. The physical therapist/assistant must be prepared to move as the patient moves to avoid interfering with the patient's fluid motion.

■ Take Note

Caution—When using the power method to assume sitting, the wheelchair should be placed against a wall so the wheelchair does not slide backward or tip during the maneuver.

2. To sit, the patient stands facing away from the wheelchair with the feet approximately 12 to 18 inches in front of the front edge of the seat. The position of the feet must permit the patient to end up sitting securely in the seat as she lowers.

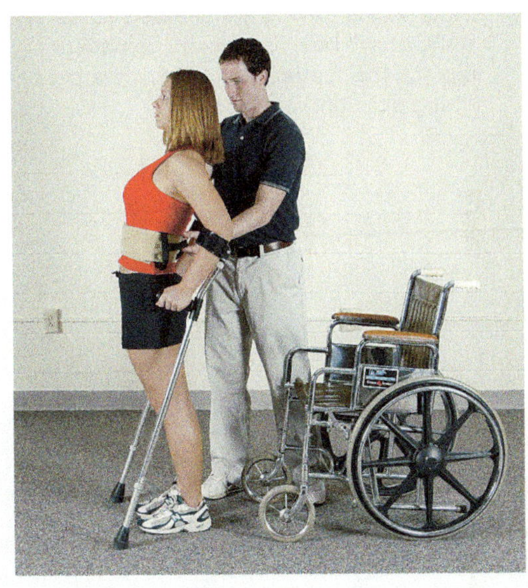

3. Moving the shoulders anterior to the hips, the patient flexes at the hips into a "jackknife" position. The patient starts falling backward, initiating lowering into the wheelchair.

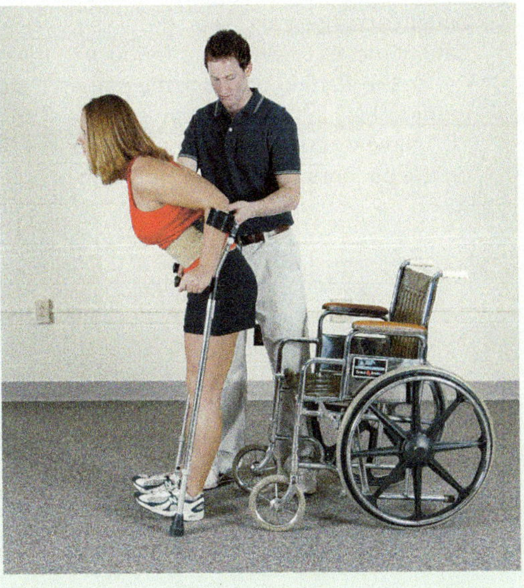

(continued)

PROCEDURE 10–12 In and Out of a Wheelchair with Forearm Crutches (*continued*)

4. As the patient sits, she lifts the crutches. After the patient is seated, the crutches are removed and placed to one side. Then knee locks on the KAFOs are released. Once the KAFOs have been unlocked, the patient can replace the footrests and assume a proper sitting position.

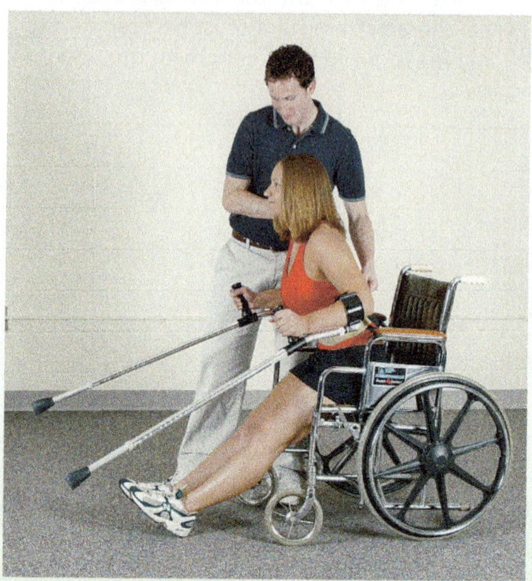

PROCEDURE 10–13 Ambulating on Level Ground with Forearm Crutches

Swing-To Gait Pattern

1. Positioned in stride slightly behind and to the side, the physical therapist/assistant grasps the patient's gait belt and shoulder. The physical therapist/assistant must be prepared to move as the patient moves to avoid interfering with the patient's fluid motion.

   In the starting position, the patient maintains her hips in extension by keeping shoulders posterior to hips in the "C" curve posture. The physical therapist/assistant can assist in maintaining a "C" curve by pushing forward with the hand on the gait belt while pulling backward with the hand on the patient's shoulder.

2. To initiate the swing-to gait pattern, the patient advances the crutches one step length beyond the patient's toes. The physical therapist/assistant advances the outside foot.

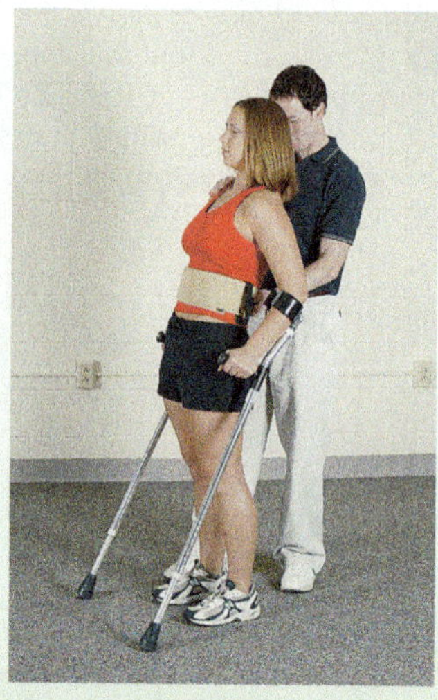

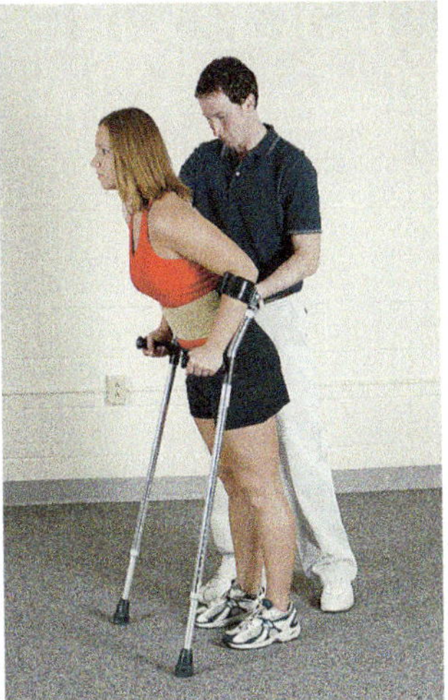

3 Pushing down on the crutches, the patient extends the upper extremities and depresses the shoulders. At the same time, she flexes the trunk to lift the feet off the ground. The physical therapist/assistant may assist by lifting with the hand on the gait belt.

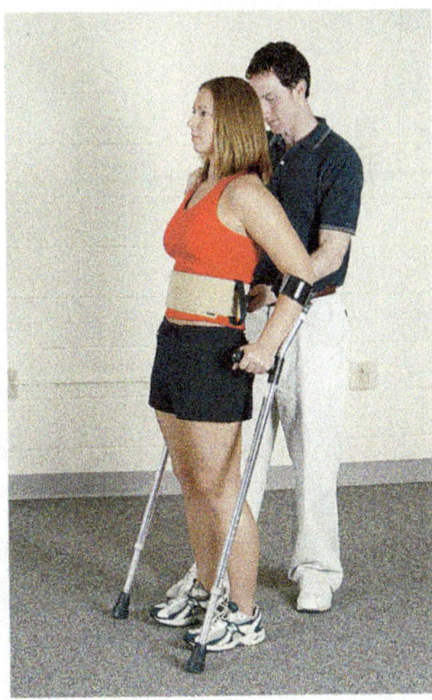

4 With the feet off the ground and trunk flexed, the patient's lower extremities will be swung forward by gravity. As the lower extremities swing forward, the patient begins to extend the neck and trunk to regain a "C" curve. With the feet placed on the floor between the crutches, momentum continues to move the patient's hips anterior to the shoulders. As the patient swings forward, the physical therapist/assistant steps forward with the inside foot. The physical therapist/assistant may assist a patient to regain a "C" curve by pushing forward with the hand on the gait belt and pulling backward with the hand on the patient's shoulder. Once a "C" curve is regained, the patient advances the crutches. The sequence is repeated for continued progression.

Swing-Through Gait Pattern

A swing-through gait pattern is essentially the same as a swing-to gait pattern. The difference is that during the swing phase of the swing-through gait pattern, the patient swings beyond the crutches and lands anterior to the crutch tips.

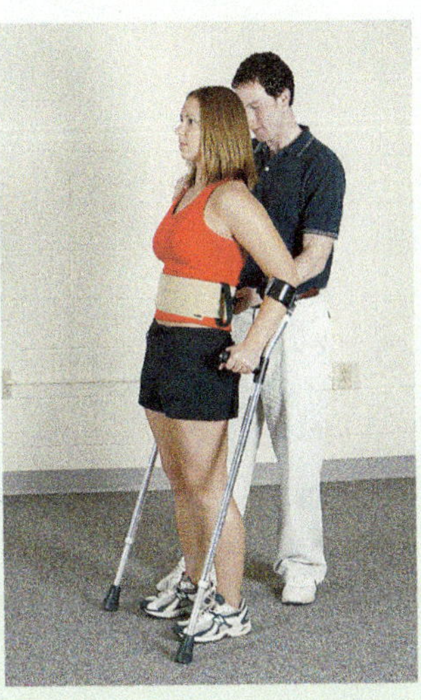

1 In the starting position for a swing-through gait pattern, the patient is in a "C" curve, with crutch tips beyond the toes. The role and position of the physical therapist/assistant is the same as for a swing-to gait pattern.

(continued)

PROCEDURE 10–13 Ambulating on Level Ground with Forearm Crutches (*continued*)

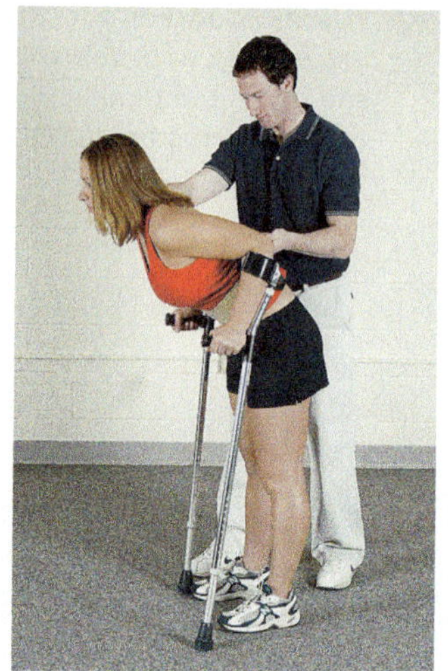

2. Pushing down on the crutches, the patient extends the upper extremities and depresses the shoulders. At the same time, she flexes the trunk to lift the feet off the ground. The physical therapist/assistant may assist by lifting with the hand on the gait belt.

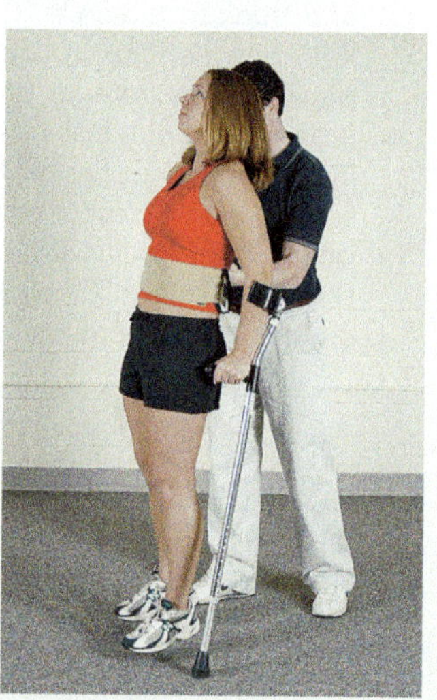

3. With the feet off the ground and trunk flexed, the patient's lower extremities will be swung forward by gravity. As the lower extremities swing forward, the patient extends the neck and trunk to regain a "C" curve.

■ Take Note

Caution—The physical therapist/assistant must be prepared to move quickly because patients cover a greater distance in less time when using a swing-through gait pattern.

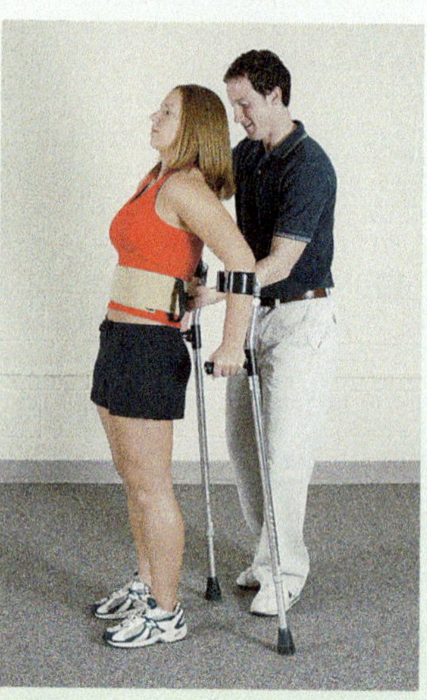

4. The patient lands with the feet anterior to the crutches. As the patient swings forward, the physical therapist/assistant steps forward with the inside foot.

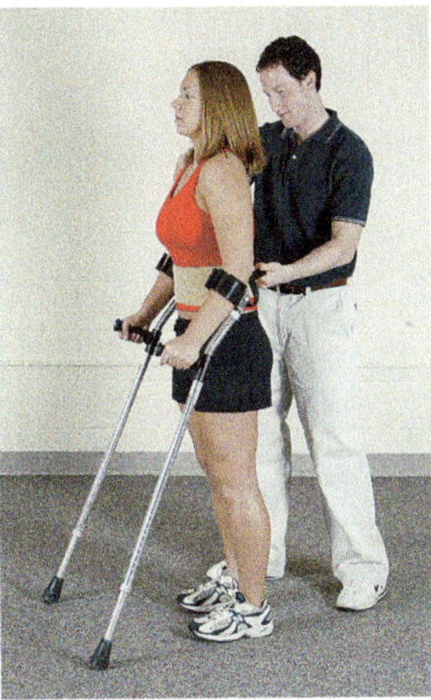

5 Because of momentum generated by a larger swing, the patient must advance the crutches quickly to prevent falling. As the patient advances the crutches, the physical therapist/assistant steps forward with the outside foot.

Falling

The patient must be taught how to control a fall, as falls may occur during gait training or after discharge. When the patient starts to fall, the physical therapist/assistant must decide whether to prevent the fall or to permit a controlled fall in a manner that will prevent injury to the patient or physical therapist/assistant. The physical therapist/assistant must be alert to the patient's movements at all times and react quickly to prevent or control a fall. Proper guarding and attention focused on the patient are required at all times.

Patients with paraplegia tend to fall when they lose their "C" curve or when momentum into the "C" curve is interrupted, causing them to "jackknife." The most effective method of preventing falls in these situations is for a physical therapist/assistant to assist the patient in regaining the "C" curve. This is achieved by pulling the patient's shoulders backward while pushing forward with the hand on the gait belt.

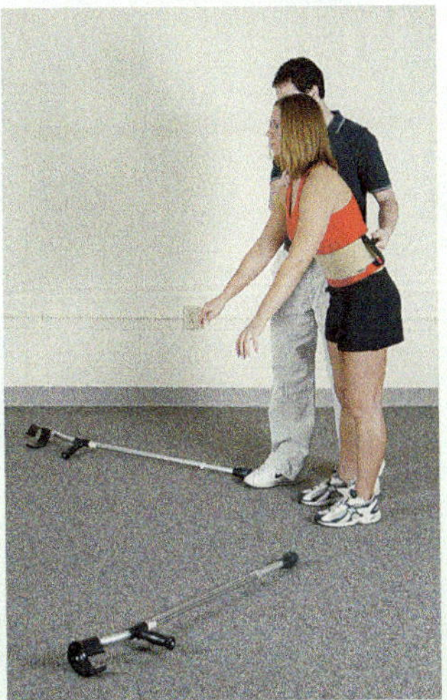

1 When the physical therapist/assistant cannot prevent a fall, he must control the fall. The physical therapist/assistant instructs the patient to let the crutches fall to the sides, away from the area in which the patient will land, to avoid injury from landing on the crutches. The physical therapist/assistant steps forward in a stride position to widen the base of support while slowing the rate at which the patient falls.

(continued)

PROCEDURE 10–13 Ambulating on Level Ground with Forearm Crutches (*continued*)

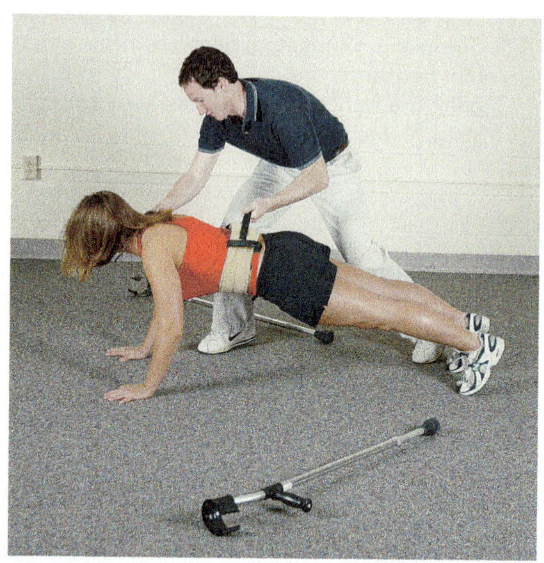

2 The patient catches herself on outstretched hands, flexing the elbows to absorb the impact. If elbows are not flexed, the patient's upper extremities may be injured.

■ Take Note

Caution—When falling, patients catch themselves with their arms, flexing at the elbows to absorb the force of falling.

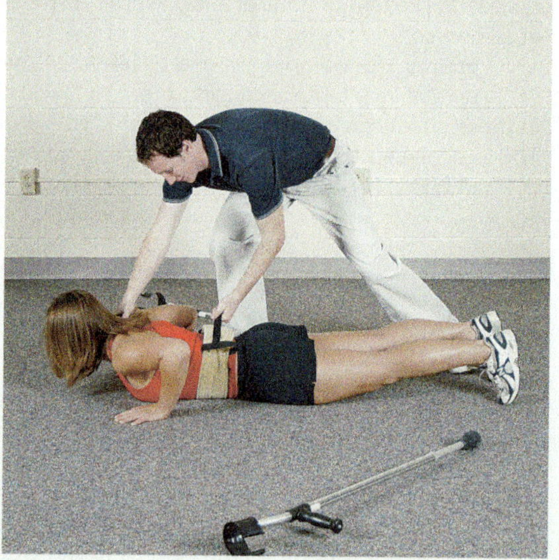

3 The physical therapist/assistant continues to control the lowering of the patient to the floor.

Assuming Standing from the Floor

To assume standing from the floor independently is a difficult maneuver for patients using KAFOs and forearm crutches. The most practical method is to move along the floor to a chair or other sturdy object and then use the object as support to rise from the floor. Methods of moving from the floor to a sitting position in a chair are described in the Chapter 9 section, *Independent Transfer from Wheelchair to Floor and Return.*

1. To assume standing directly from a prone position on the floor, the patient must first retrieve and position the crutches.

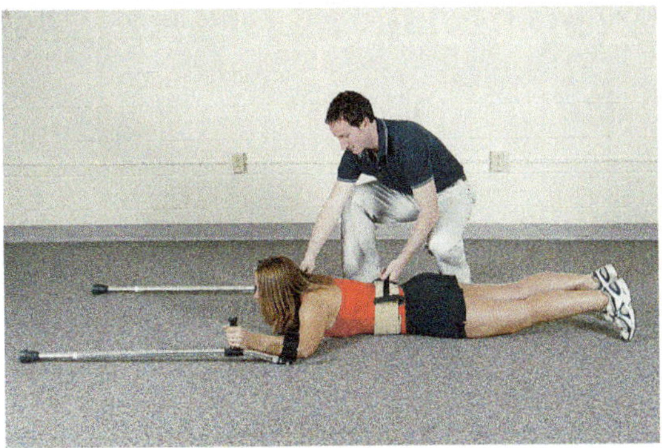

2. Grasping one crutch, the patient places it upright with the tip of the crutch on the floor. The patient places the other hand on the other crutch or on the floor at the level of the shoulder.

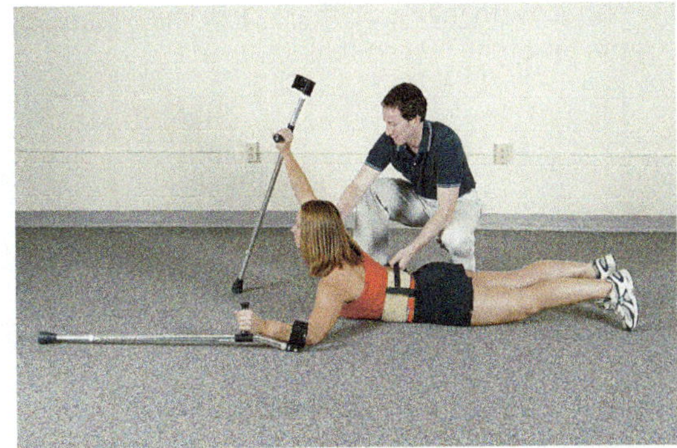

The following sequence of movements must be performed quickly, without pauses.

3. Pushing with the hand on the floor and pulling with the hand on the crutch, the patient raises the trunk. Positioned in stride slightly behind and to the side, the physical therapist/assistant grasps the patient's gait belt and shoulder. The physical therapist/assistant may assist by lifting with the hand on the gait belt.

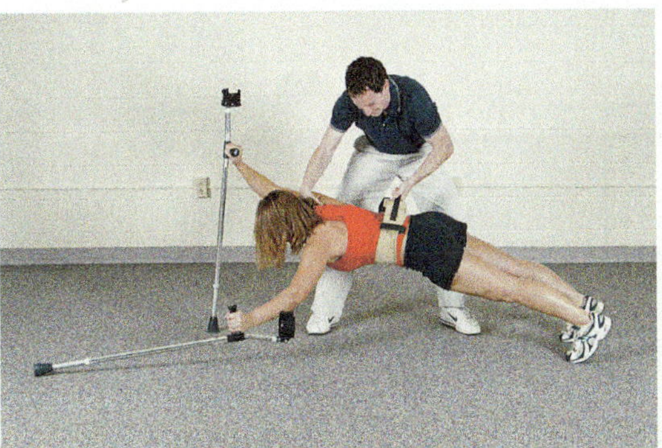

4. With weight shifted onto the upper extremity that is on the floor, the patient pushes down on the handgrip and floor to assume a "jackknife" position. During initial training, the physical therapist/assistant assists by lifting on the gait belt. The physical therapist/assistant may also need to block the patient's feet to prevent them from sliding posteriorly. After shifting weight onto the upright crutch, the patient grasps the handgrip of the remaining crutch.

(continued)

PROCEDURE 10–13 Ambulating on Level Ground with Forearm Crutches (*continued*)

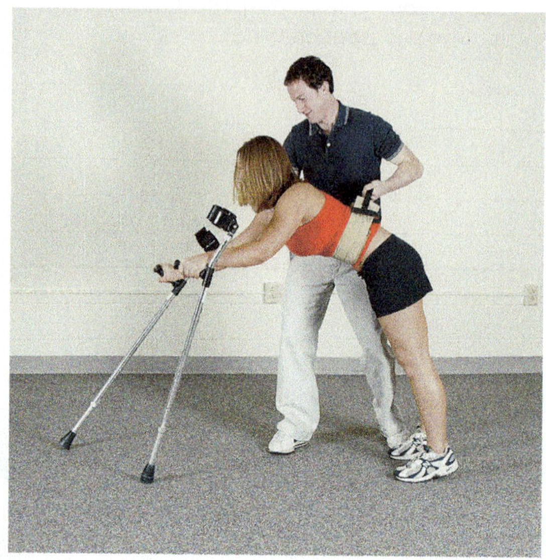

5 The patient positions the second crutch upright with the tip on the floor in line with the tip of the first crutch.

6 The patient then uses both crutches to push through an upright position, into a "C" curve.

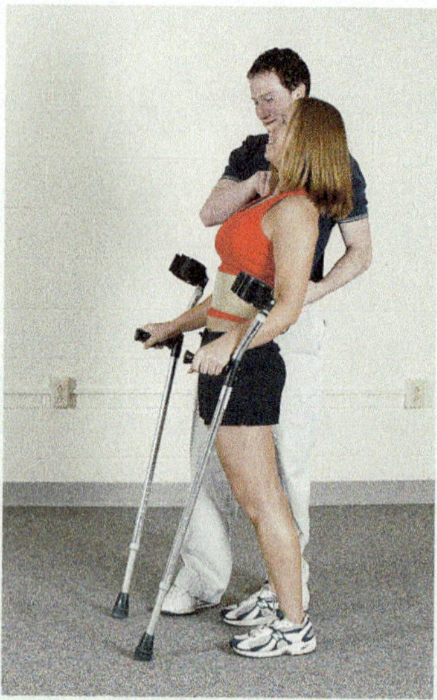

7 The patient properly positions the first crutch.

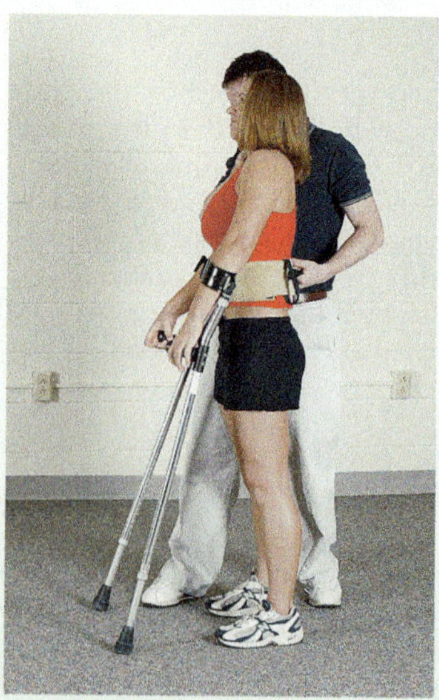

8 The patient properly positions the second crutch.

9 The patient is then ready to ambulate.

Doorways

Patients using forearm crutches maneuver through doorways in the same manner as do patients using axillary crutches.

PROCEDURE 10–14 Ambulating on Stairs with Forearm Crutches

There are two basic methods for patients using KAFOs and forearm crutches to ambulate on stairs: the forward method and the backward method. In both methods, the patient may use a handrail and one crutch or no handrail and two crutches. In both methods, the physical therapist/assistant is positioned in stride on the stairs below the patient and grasps the patient's gait belt and the handrail. Initially, gait training on stairs may require assistance by two people to ensure patient safety.

Ascending—Forward Method

1 To ascend stairs using the forward method, the patient starts in a "C" curve position facing up the stairs. The patient's feet and crutch tips are parallel with the base of the stair.

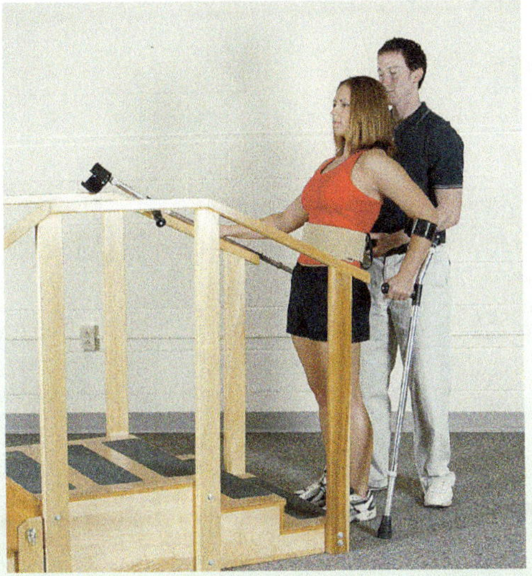

(continued)

PROCEDURE 10–14 Ambulating on Stairs with Forearm Crutches (*continued*)

2. The same motion used to initiate ambulation on level surfaces is used to initiate ambulation on stairs. Flexing the neck and upper trunk, the patient extends the upper extremities and depresses the shoulders to lift the body. As the patient's feet are lifted from the ground, gravity swings the lower extremities forward onto the next higher stair. The physical therapist/assistant may assist by lifting on the gait belt as the patient raises the body.

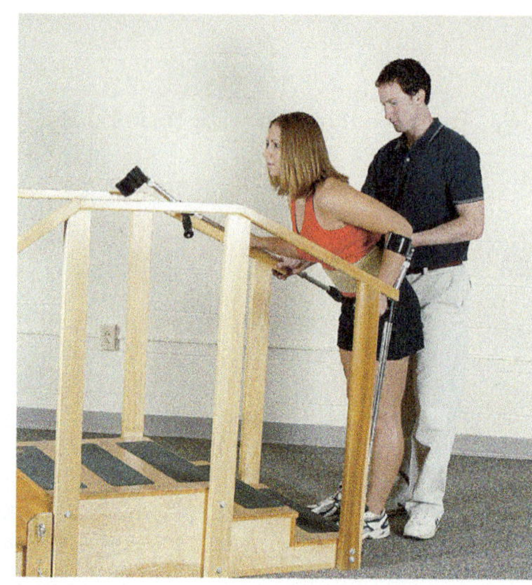

3. The patient extends the neck and trunk to regain a "C" curve while placing the lower extremities onto the next higher stair. The physical therapist/assistant may assist the patient in regaining a "C" curve by pushing forward on the gait belt.

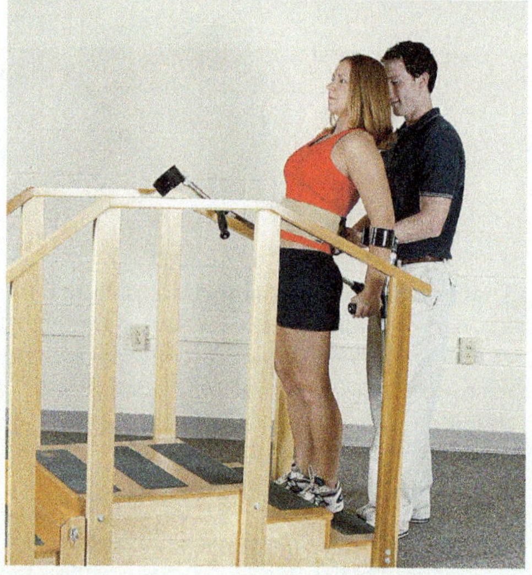

4. The patient advances the crutch(es) to the same stair as the lower extremities. The sequence is repeated to ascend an entire flight of stairs.

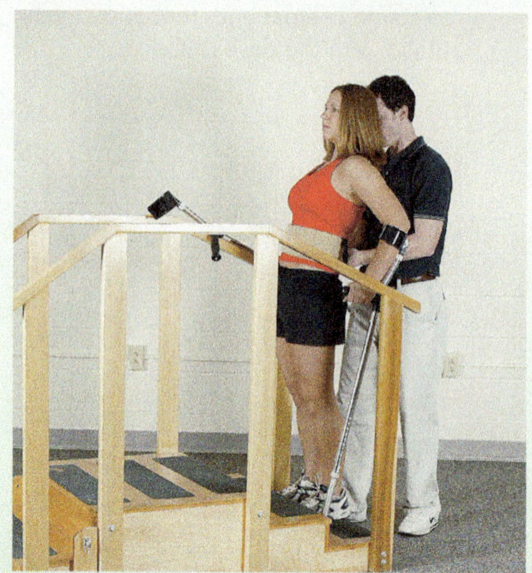

Descending—Forward Method

1. To descend stairs using the forward method, the patient starts in a "C" curve position facing down the stairs. The feet and crutch tip(s) are parallel with the top of the stairs.

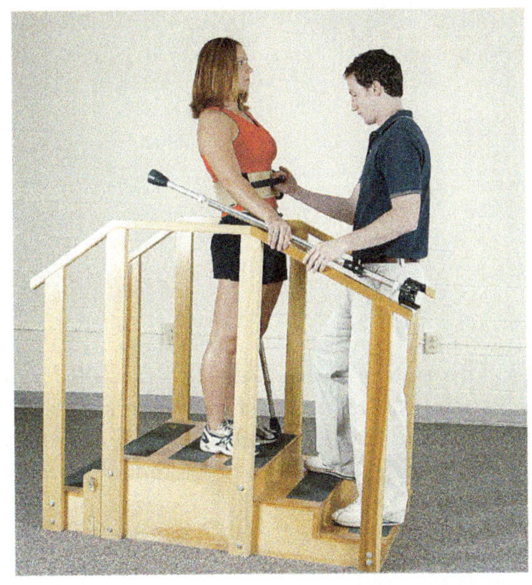

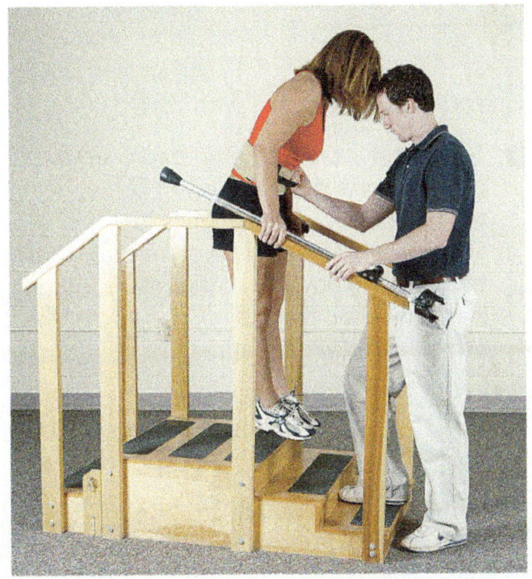

2. The same motion used to initiate ambulation on level surfaces is used to initiate ambulation on stairs. Flexing the neck and upper trunk, the patient extends the upper extremities and depresses the shoulders to lift the body. The physical therapist/assistant may assist by lifting on the gait belt as the patient raises the body. As the patient's feet are lifted from the ground, gravity swings the lower extremities forward over the next lower stair.

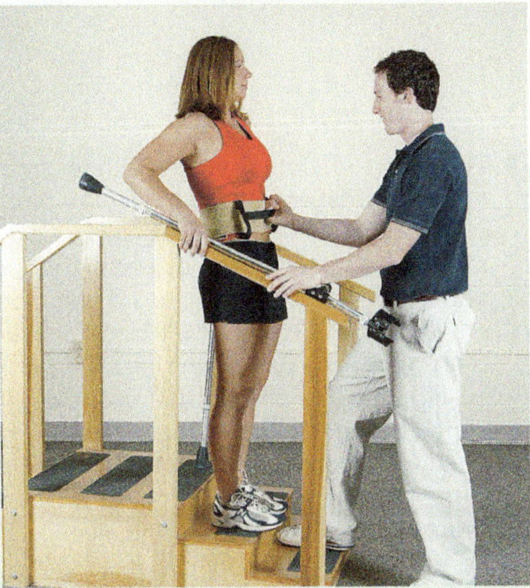

3. As the lower extremities swing over the stair, the patient uses the upper extremities to lower in a controlled manner onto the next lower stair.

   Extending the neck and trunk, the patient regains a "C" curve while placing the lower extremities on the next lower stair. The physical therapist/assistant may assist the patient in regaining a "C" curve by pulling forward on the gait belt.

(continued)

PROCEDURE 10–14 Ambulating on Stairs with Forearm Crutches (*continued*)

4. The patient advances the crutch(es) onto the same stair as the lower extremities. Patients often descend two steps at a time. The sequence is repeated to descend an entire flight of stairs.

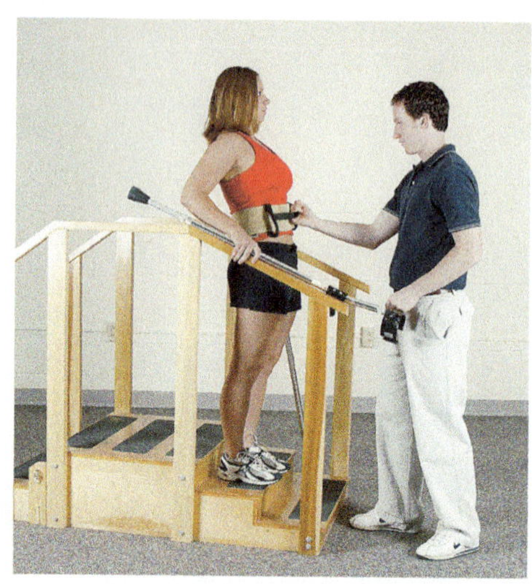

Ascending—Backward Method

1. To ascend stairs using the backward method, the patient starts in a "C" curve position facing away from the stairs. The patient's feet and crutch tips are parallel with the base of the stair. During initial training, two physical therapists/assistants may be positioned on the stairs, one above the patient and one below the patient.

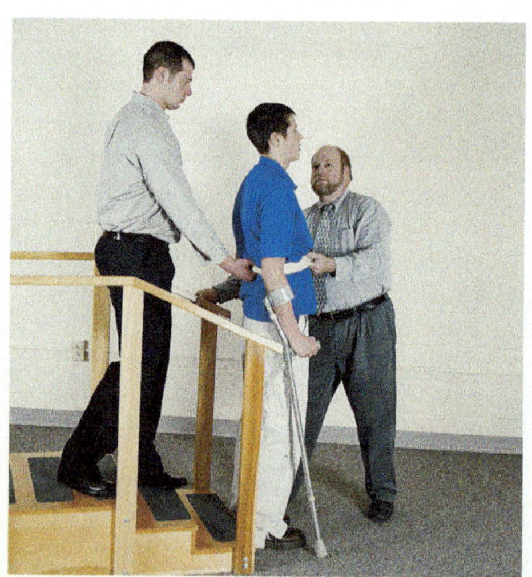

2. The same motion used to initiate ambulation on level surfaces is used to initiate ambulation on stairs. Flexing the neck and upper trunk, the patient extends the upper extremities and depresses the shoulders to lift the body. The physical therapist/assistant positioned on the stairs above the patient may assist by lifting and pulling back. The physical therapist/assistant positioned below the patient pushes on the gait belt as the patient raises the body. When the physical therapist/assistant exerts force into the abdominal area to assist patient positioning, he must be careful not to injure the patient.

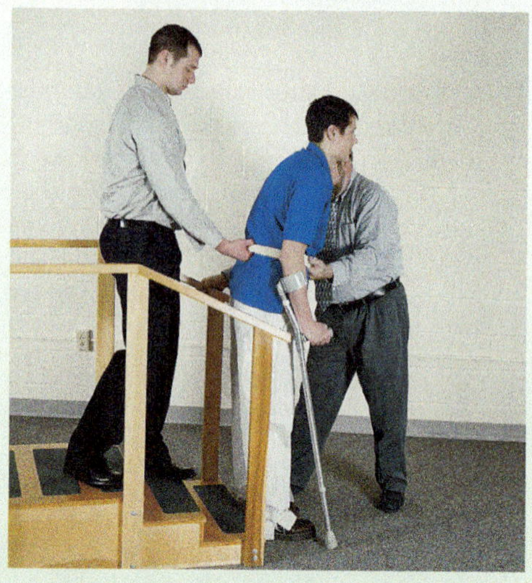

3 As the patient lifts into a "jackknife" position, backward momentum of the lower extremities moves the patient up and over the higher stair. The patient uses the upper extremities to lower onto the next higher stair.

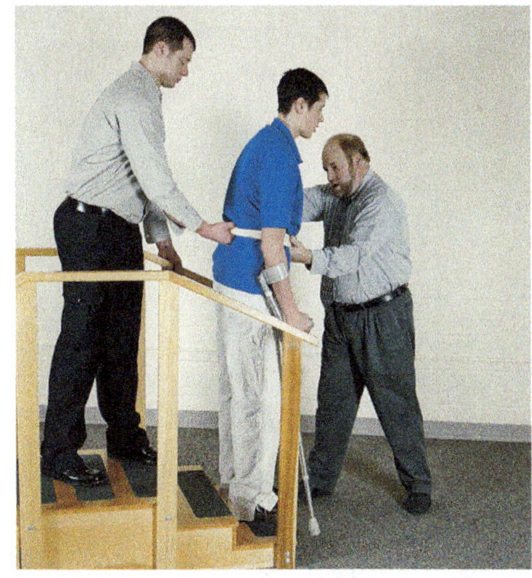

4 Once the patient's lower extremities are on the next higher stair, the patient permits the pelvis to move forward. As this movement occurs, the patient extends the neck and trunk to regain a "C" curve, while moving the crutches onto the same stair as the lower extremities. The physical therapist/assistant positioned below the patient may assist the patient in regaining a "C" curve by pulling forward on the gait belt. The sequence is repeated to ascend an entire flight of stairs.

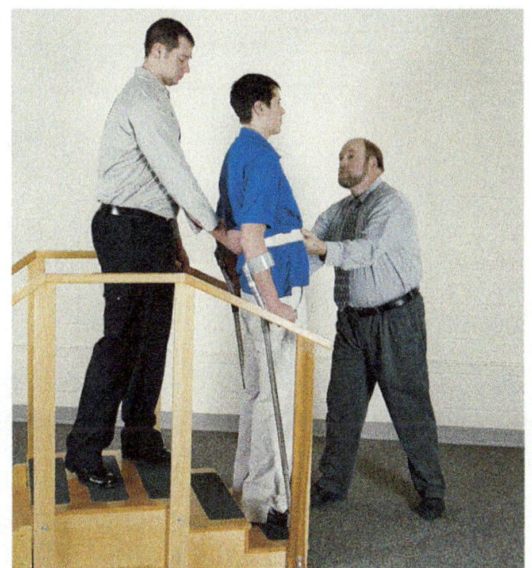

Descending—Backward Method

1 To descend stairs using the backward method, the patient starts in a "C" curve position facing away from the stairs. The patient's feet and crutch tips are parallel at the top of the stairs. During initial training, two physical therapists/assistants may be positioned on the stairs, one above the patient and one below the patient.

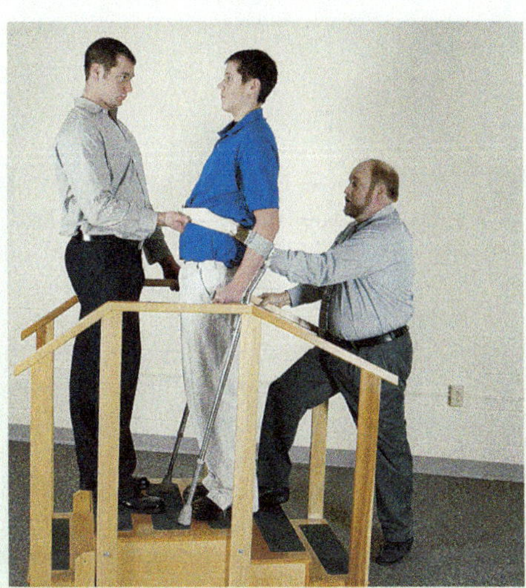

(continued)

PROCEDURE 10–14 Ambulating on Stairs with Forearm Crutches (*continued*)

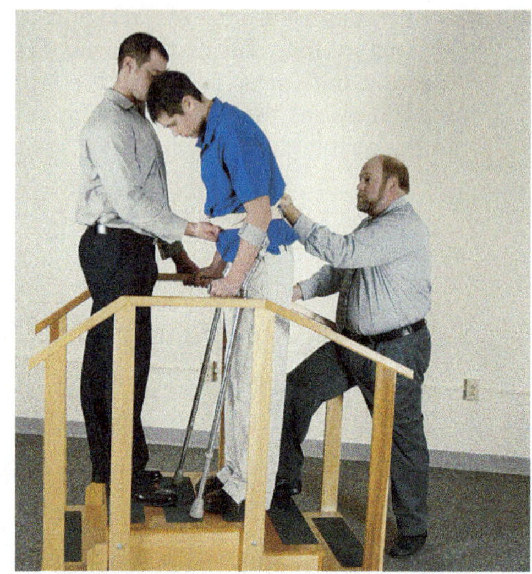

2. The same motion used to initiate ambulation on level surfaces is used to initiate ambulation on stairs. Flexing the neck and upper trunk, the patient extends the upper extremities and depresses the shoulders to lift the body. The physical therapist/assistant positioned on the stairs above the patient may assist by pushing on the gait belt. The physical therapist/assistant positioned on the stairs below the patient may assist by lifting on the gait belt as the patient raises the body.

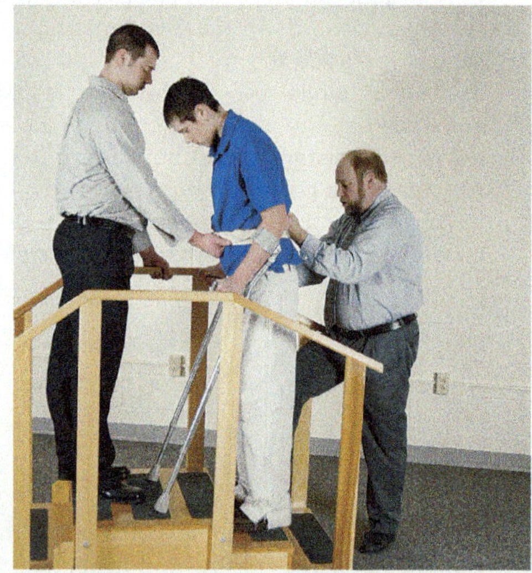

3. As the patient lifts into a "jackknife" position, the backward momentum of the lower extremities moves the patient over the next lower stair. Once the lower extremities are over the stair, the patient uses the upper extremities to lower in a controlled manner onto the next lower stair.

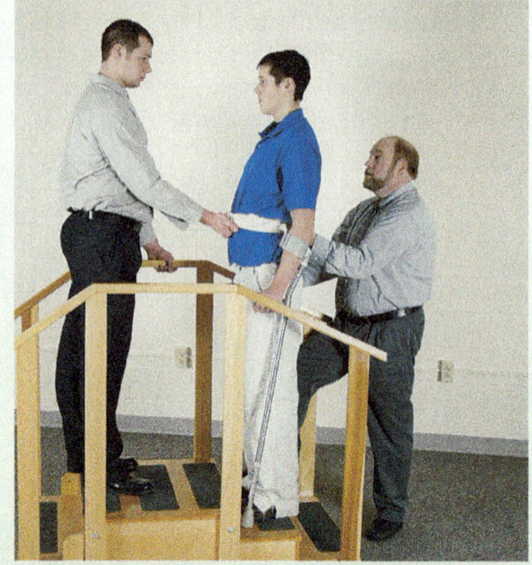

4. After the lower extremities are on the next lower stair, the patient extends the neck and trunk to regain a "C" curve. This movement allows the hips to remain in extension. Then the patient moves the crutches onto the same stair as the lower extremities. The physical therapist/assistant positioned on the stairs above the patient may assist by pulling on the gait belt to assist the patient in assuming a "C" curve. The physical therapist/assistant positioned on the stairs below the patient may assist by pushing on the gait belt.
5. The sequence is repeated to descend an entire flight of stairs.

Canes

Fitting

When using one cane to limit weight bearing on one lower extremity, the cane is initially used in the hand on the side opposite the involved lower extremity. Use of a cane on the uninvolved side reduces the amount of force required by muscles to stabilize the pelvis during stance on the involved lower extremity. This placement also provides an additional point of support, which increases the base of support on the uninvolved side. Increasing the base of support on the uninvolved side permits a patient to shift weight to the uninvolved side during stance on the involved lower extremity. When weight bearing on the involved lower extremity is permitted, the cane may be used on the involved side, which increases the base of support on that side. Increasing the base of support on the involved side encourages weight shifting onto the involved lower extremity. Depending on the severity of a patient's problem, either one or two canes may be required. Two canes are used primarily for bilateral involvement or for assistance with balance.

Canes are fitted with the patient standing with shoulders relaxed. The cane is positioned upright, with the tip on the floor alongside the small toe. With the cane in this position, adjust the top of the cane to be at the level of the patient's ulnar styloid process (Figure 10–46 ■). This permits 20 to 30 degrees of elbow flexion when the cane is held in the patient's hand (Figure 10–47 ■). When used properly, forces on a cane should be exerted directly downward.

When using a quad cane, the longer legs of the cane are positioned facing away from the patient's lower extremity (Figure 10–48 ■). This reduces the risk of the patient's foot becoming entangled in the legs of the quad cane. Quad canes are measured and used in the same manner as standard canes.

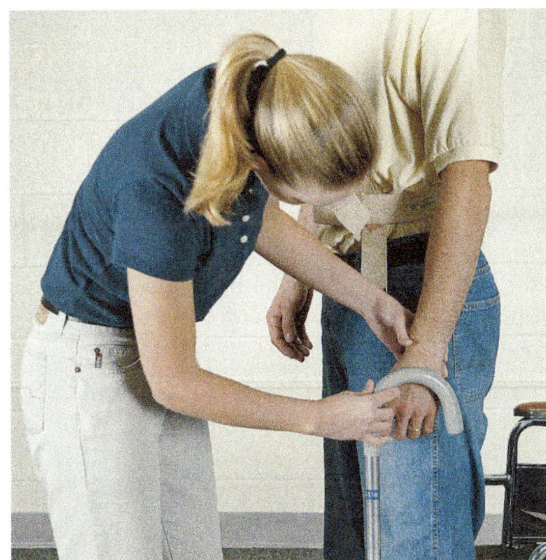

FIGURE 10–46 ■ Measuring cane height.

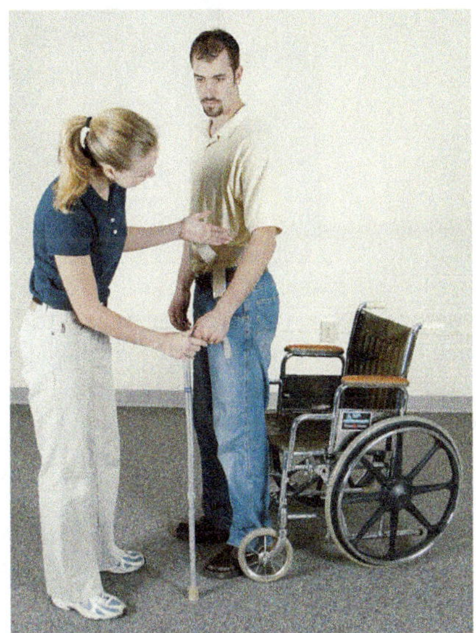

FIGURE 10–47 ■ Ensuring proper elbow flexion.

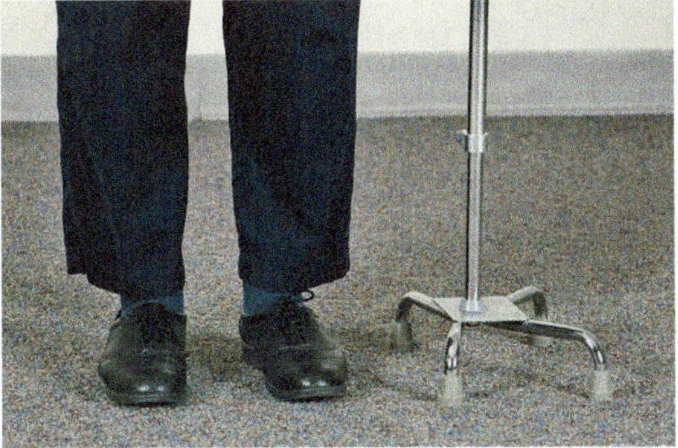

FIGURE 10–48 ■ Proper positioning of a quad cane for ambulation.

PROCEDURE 10–15 In and Out of a Wheelchair with One Cane

Assuming Standing—Quad Cane and Armrest

1. The physical therapist/assistant engages the wheelchair wheel locks and moves the footrests out of the way. The patient is positioned at the front edge of the seat, with the feet in stride or side by side. Positioned in stride behind and to one side of a patient, the physical therapist/assistant grasps the patient's gait belt and shoulder.

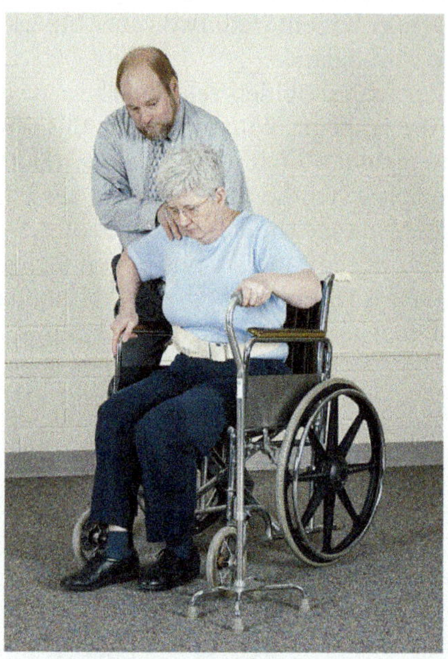

2. The patient positions the quad cane alongside the foot on the side on which it will be held. The patient may place both hands on the respective armrests or place one hand on the cane and one on the armrest to push to standing. When the patient has only one functional upper extremity, that upper extremity is used on the armrest to push to standing. Once the patient is standing, she grasps the cane.

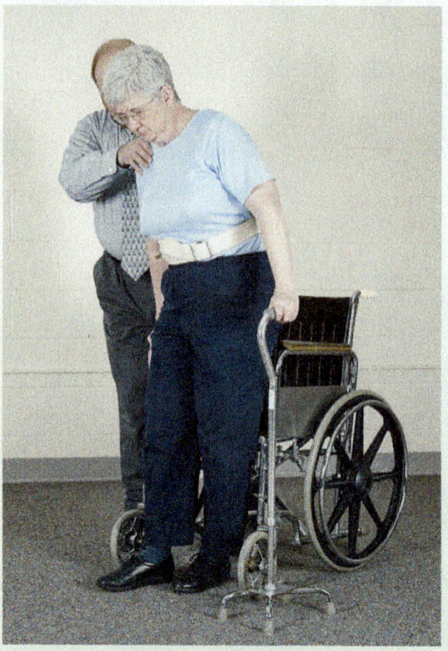

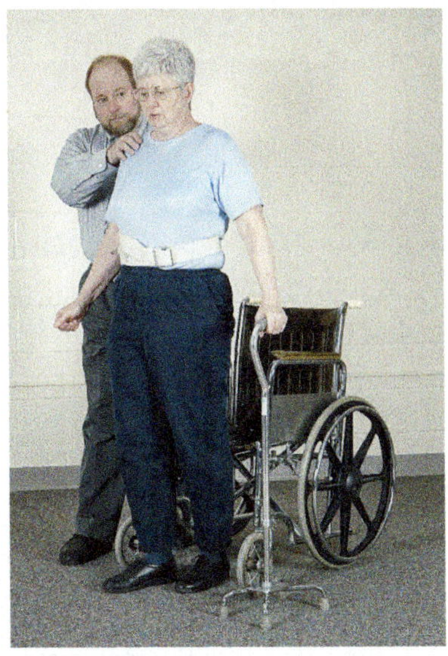

3 The patient pushes to standing and straightens, making sure to be erect and balanced. The patient is then ready to ambulate.

Assuming Sitting—Quad Cane and Armrest

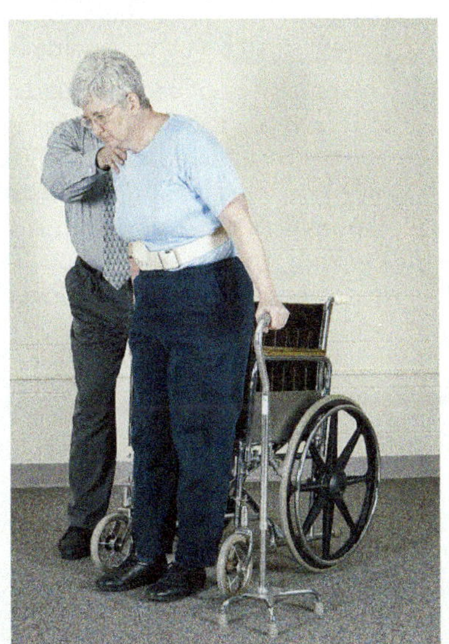

1 The physical therapist/assistant engages the wheelchair wheel locks and moves the footrests out of the way. To sit, the patient is positioned at the front edge of the wheelchair seat, facing away from the wheelchair, so she can feel the front edge of the wheelchair seat against the backs of the lower extremities. The patient positions her feet in stride or side by side. Positioned in stride behind and to one side of a patient, the physical therapist/assistant grasps the patient's gait belt and shoulder. The patient reaches for the armrest with one hand while maintaining a grasp on the cane with the other hand.

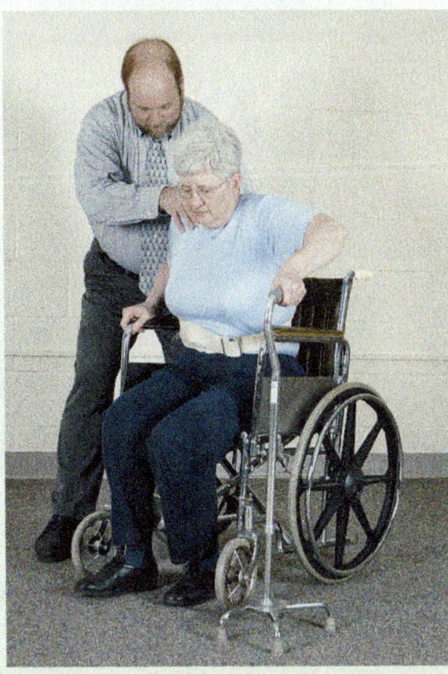

2 While grasping the armrest and the cane, the patient lowers in a controlled manner onto the seat. The patient moves completely onto the seat and positions appropriately.

(continued)

PROCEDURE 10–15 In and Out of a Wheelchair with One Cane (*continued*)

Assuming Standing—Quad Cane Only

The patient with sufficient strength and balance may assume standing using a quad cane instead of the armrest for support.

1. The physical therapist/assistant engages the wheelchair wheel locks and moves the footrests out of the way. The patient is positioned at the front edge of the seat, with the feet in stride or side by side. Positioned in stride behind and to one side of a patient, the physical therapist/assistant grasps the patient's gait belt and shoulder.
2. The patient positions the quad cane alongside the foot on the side on which it will be held. She places one hand on the quad cane. When the patient has only one functional upper extremity, that upper extremity is used on the quad cane to push to standing. The patient must push directly downward to prevent the cane from tipping.

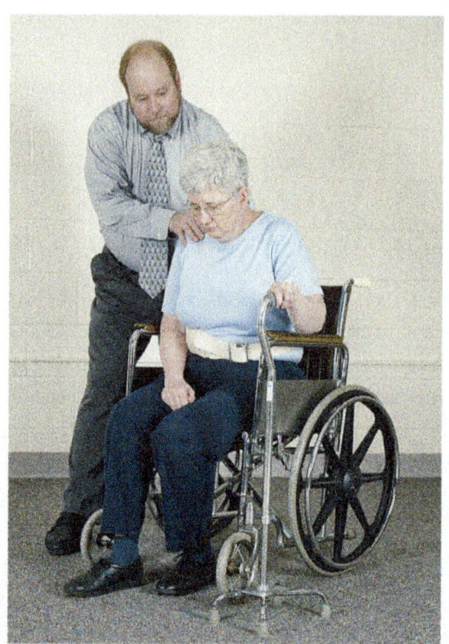

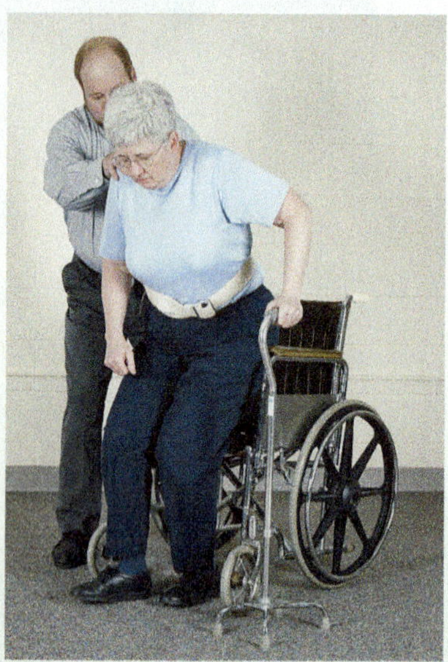

3. The patient leans forward, pushes downward on the quad cane, and extends the lower extremities to assume standing.

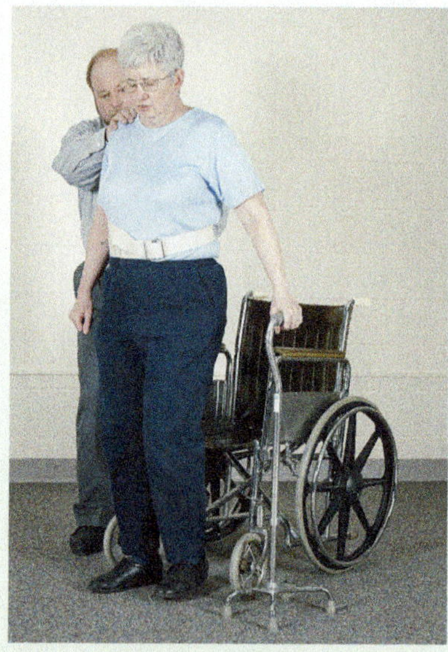

4. The patient must be erect and balanced before initiating ambulation.

Assuming Sitting—Quad Cane Only

1. The physical therapist/assistant engages the wheelchair wheel locks and moves the footrests out of the way. To sit, the patient is positioned at the front edge of the wheelchair seat, facing away from the wheelchair, so she can feel the front edge of the wheelchair seat against the backs of the lower extremities. The patient positions her feet in stride or side by side. Positioned in stride behind and to one side of a patient, the physical therapist/assistant grasps the patient's gait belt and shoulder.

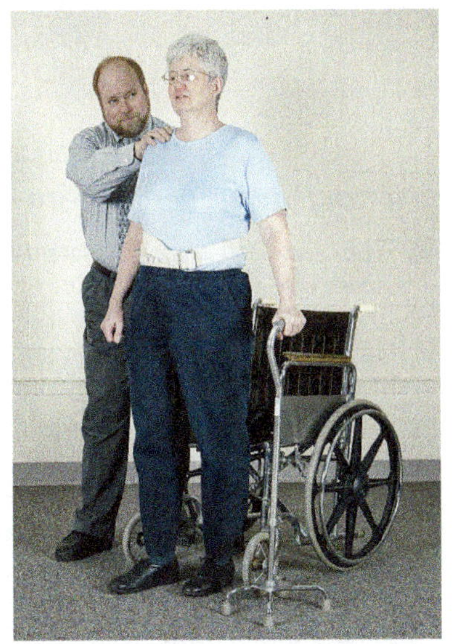

2. While grasping the quad cane, the patient lowers in a controlled manner onto the seat.

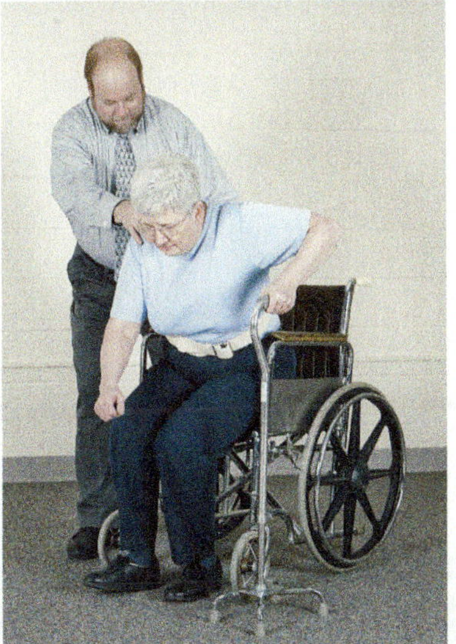

3. The physical therapist/assistant continues to guard the patient until safely seated and appropriately positioned.

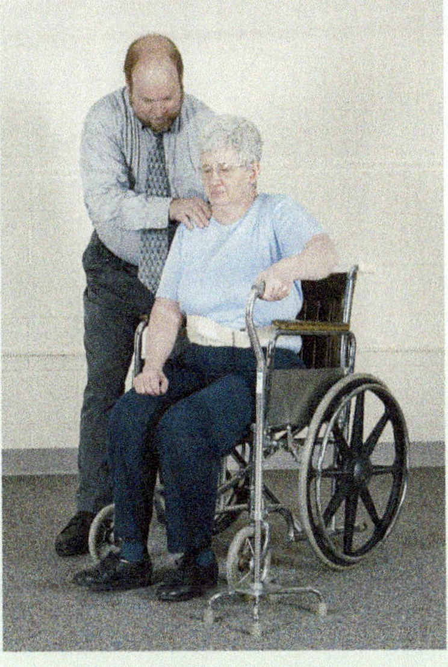

(continued)

PROCEDURE 10–15 In and Out of a Wheelchair with One Cane (*continued*)

Assuming Standing—Standard Cane and Two Armrests

1. The physical therapist/assistant engages the wheelchair wheel locks and moves the footrests out of the way. The patient is positioned at the front edge of the seat with the feet in stride or side by side. Positioned in stride behind and to one side of a patient, the physical therapist/assistant grasps the patient's gait belt and shoulder.
2. The patient places both hands on their respective armrests. while grasping the cane in the same hand as will be used for ambulation. Thus, the patient must grasp both the cane and armrest at the same time with this hand.

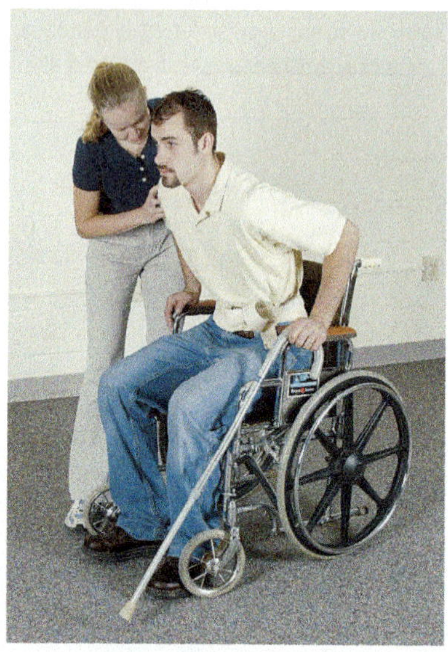

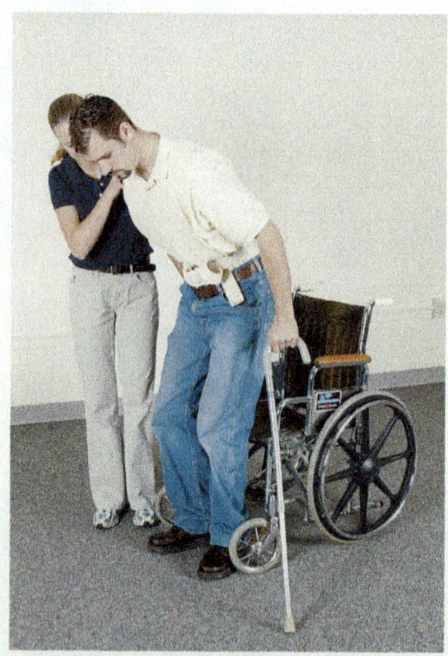

3. Pushing downward on both armrests, the patient pushes to standing.

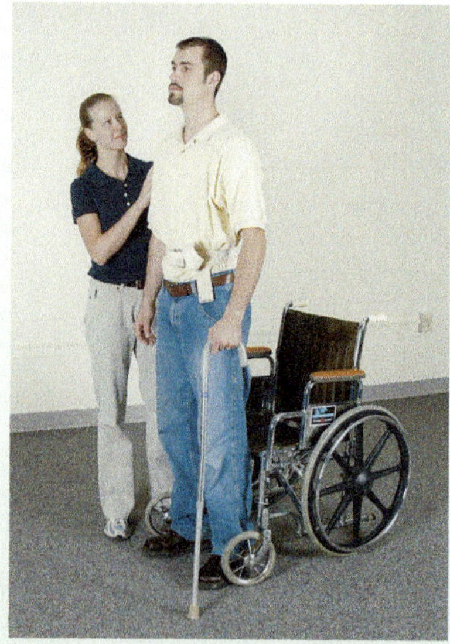

4. Once standing, the patient releases the grasp on the armrests, stands erect, and positions the cane. The patient is then ready to ambulate.

Assuming Sitting—Standard Cane and Two Armrests

1. The physical therapist/assistant engages the wheelchair wheel locks and moves the footrests out of the way. To sit, the patient is positioned at the front edge of the wheelchair seat, facing away from the wheelchair, so he can feel the front edge of the wheelchair seat against the backs of the lower extremities. The patient positions his feet in stride or side by side. Positioned in stride behind and to one side of the patient, the physical therapist/assistant grasps the patient's gait belt and shoulder.

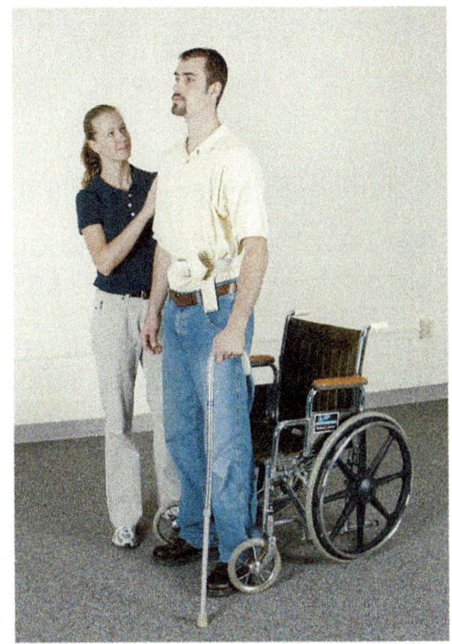

2. The patient grasps both armrests. This may be performed with both hands simultaneously or the patient may move the hands one at a time. The patient keeps the cane grasped in the same hand in which it was used for ambulation. The patient holds both the cane and armrest by the hand that grasps the cane.

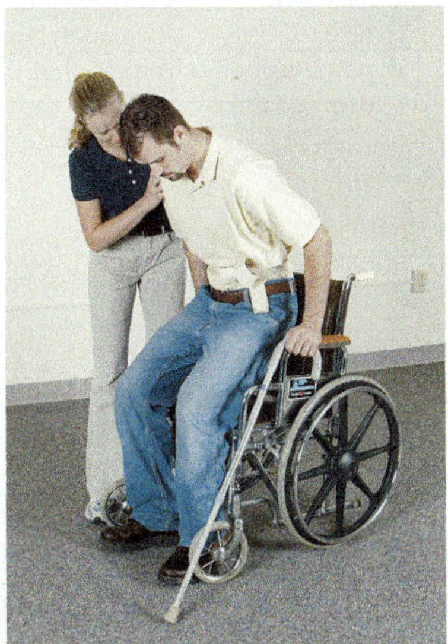

3. The patient lowers in a controlled manner onto the seat. Setting the cane aside, the patient moves completely onto the seat and positions himself appropriately.

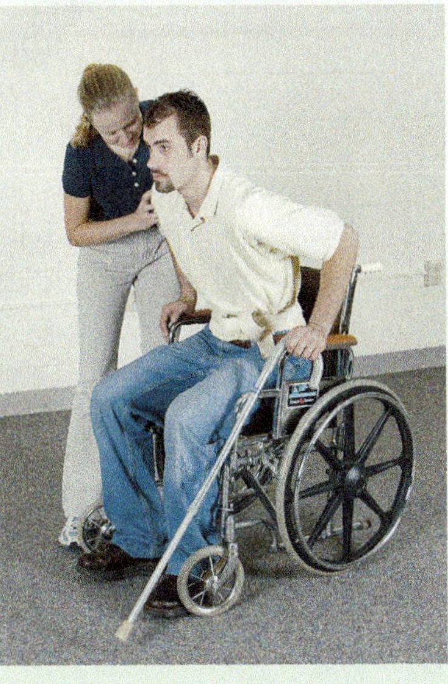

(continued)

PROCEDURE 10–15 In and Out of a Wheelchair with One Cane (*continued*)

Assuming Standing—Standard Cane and One Armrest

1. The physical therapist/assistant engages the wheelchair wheel locks and moves the footrests out of the way. The patient is positioned at the front edge of the seat, with the feet in stride or side by side. Positioned in stride behind and to one side of the patient, the physical therapist/assistant grasps the patient's gait belt and shoulder.

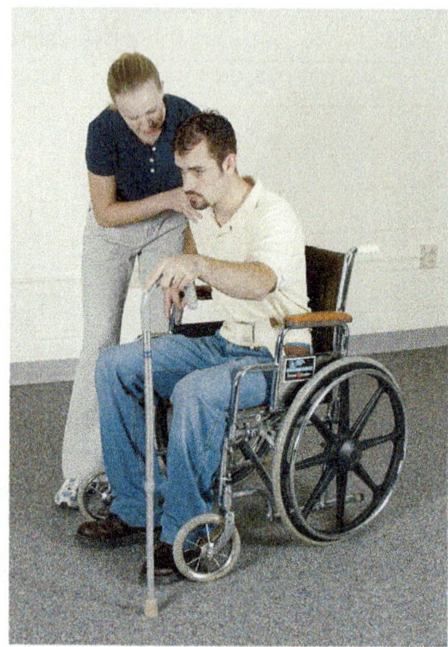

2. The patient positions the cane alongside the foot on the side on which it will be held. The patient places one hand on the armrest and the other hand on the cane. The patient must push directly downward on the cane to prevent the cane from tipping. When the patient has only one functional upper extremity, that upper extremity is used on the cane to push to standing.

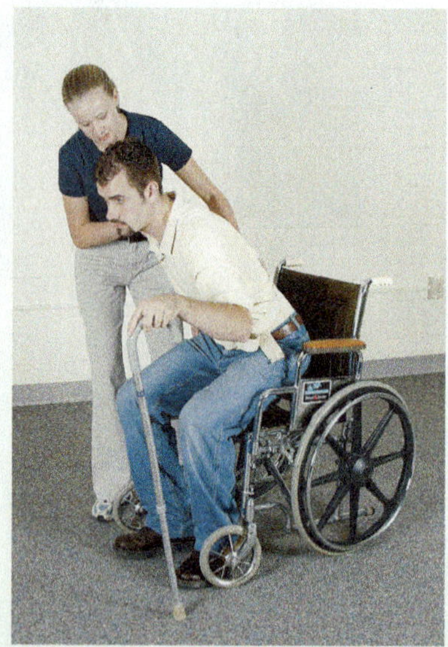

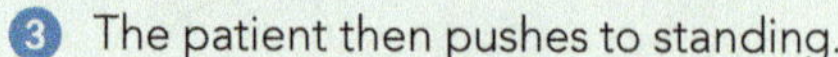

3. The patient then pushes to standing.

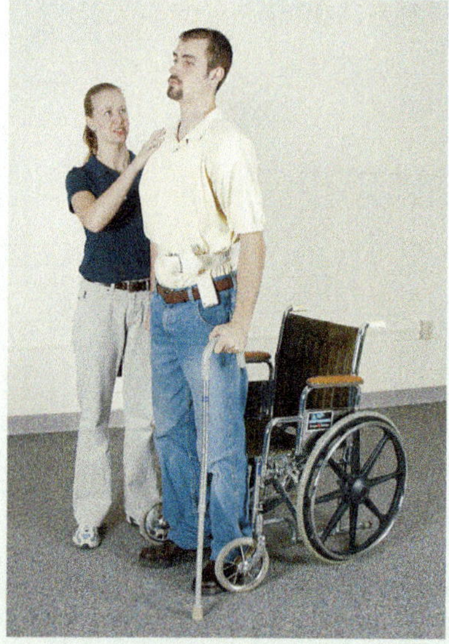

4. The patient releases the grasp on the armrest and stands erect. The patient is then ready to ambulate.

Assuming Sitting—Standard Cane and One Armrest

1. The physical therapist/assistant engages the wheelchair wheel locks and moves the footrests out of the way. To sit, the patient is positioned at the front edge of the wheelchair seat, facing away from the wheelchair, so he can feel the front edge of the wheelchair seat against the backs of the lower extremities. The patient positions his feet in stride or side by side. Positioned in stride behind and to one side of the patient, the physical therapist/assistant grasps the patient's gait belt and shoulder.

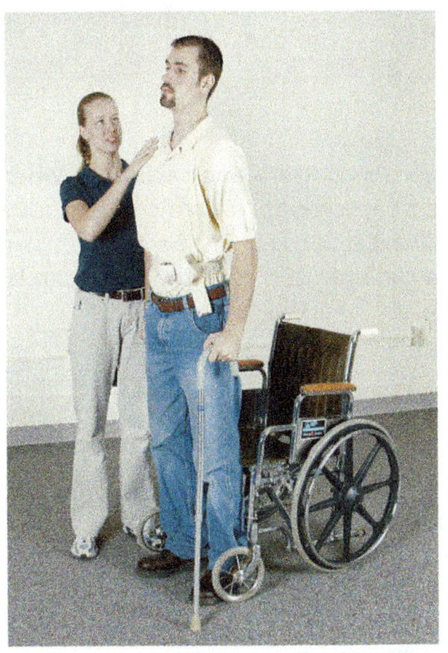

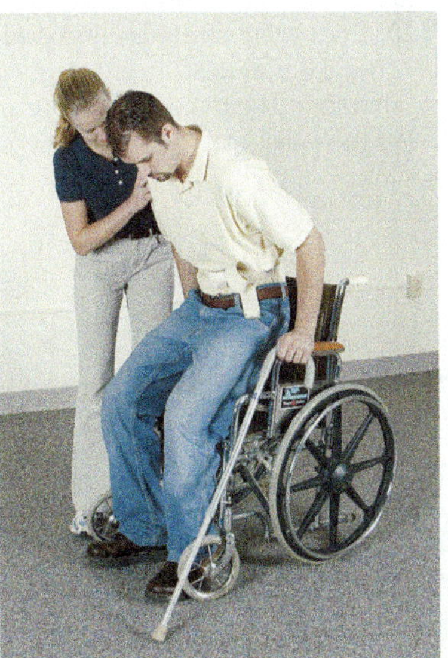

2. While continuing to use the cane, the patient reaches back and grasps the armrest with the opposite hand.

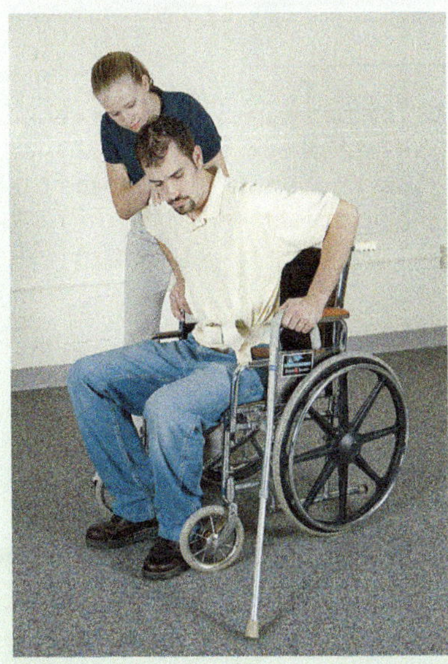

3. The patient then lowers in a controlled manner onto the seat. Setting the cane aside, the patient moves completely into the seat and positions himself appropriately.

PROCEDURE 10–16 Ambulating on Level Surfaces with One Cane

The gait pattern and sequence when using one standard cane or one quad cane are the same. To decrease weight bearing on an involved lower extremity, the patient uses the cane on the uninvolved side. This allows a minimal reduction of weight bearing on the involved lower extremity. As patients improve, the cane can be used on the side of the involved lower extremity to increase weight bearing.

1 Positioned in stride behind and to one side of a patient, the physical therapist/assistant grasps the patient's gait belt and shoulder. The patient's feet are side by side, with the cane next to the small toe.

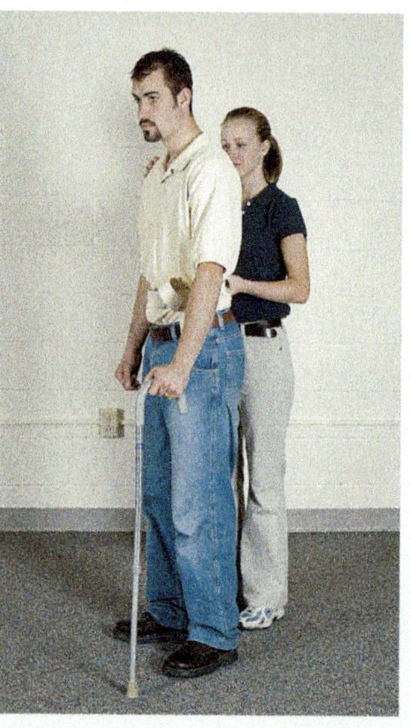

2 The patient advances the cane first, approximately one step length ahead. When the physical therapist/assistant is guarding on the side opposite the cane, she steps forward with the outside foot.

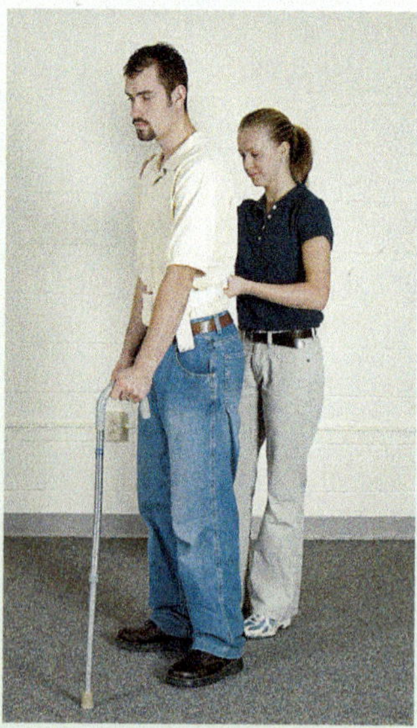

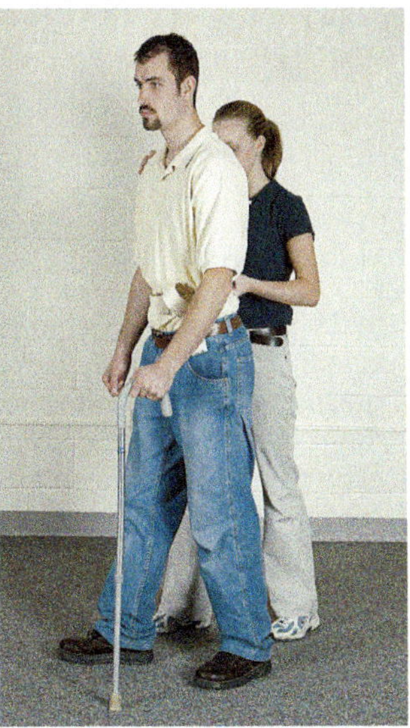

3. The patient advances the lower extremity on the side opposite the cane so the ball of the foot is approximately even with the cane. When the physical therapist/assistant is guarding on the side opposite the cane, she steps forward with the inside foot.

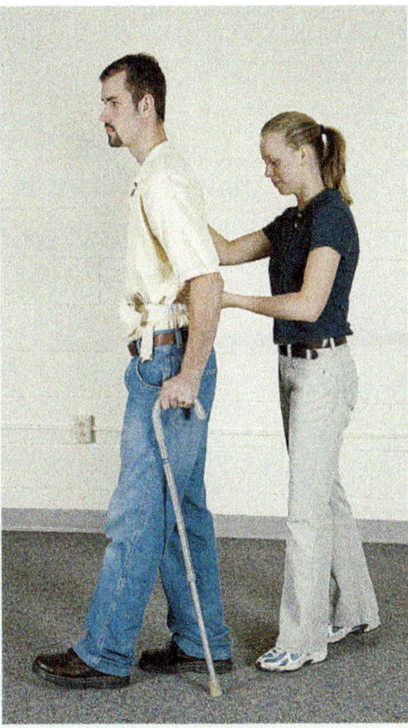

4. The patient advances the lower extremity on the same side as the cane. Initially, the patient may only step to the other lower extremity and cane. However, the patient should be encouraged to step beyond the other lower extremity and cane, to develop a normal gait pattern.

5. The sequence is repeated for continued progression. The patient should remain erect during this progression and avoid leaning on the cane.

6. As patients improve, they may move the cane and involved lower extremity at the same time, permitting a faster pace of gait. As patients are able, they may use the cane on the involved side, moving the cane and involved lower extremity simultaneously. Using a cane on the involved side encourages weight bearing on the involved lower extremity.

PROCEDURE 10–17 Ambulating on Stairs with One Cane

Holding the Cane

Initially, the physical therapist/assistant should teach the patient to use a handrail for increased stability. Patients who use a cane on the left side continue to grasp the cane with the left hand and grasp the handrail with the right hand. Patients who use a cane in the right hand must do one of three things: (1) continue to use the cane in the right hand and not use the handrail, (2) switch the cane to the left hand and grasp the handrail with the right hand, or (3) grasp both the handrail and cane with the right hand. Patients with a functional right upper extremity only must either (1) continue to use the cane without using the handrail or (2) grasp both the handrail and cane with the right hand.

There are two methods for grasping both the cane and handrail in one hand. Note that the method is the same whether the patient uses one cane or two.

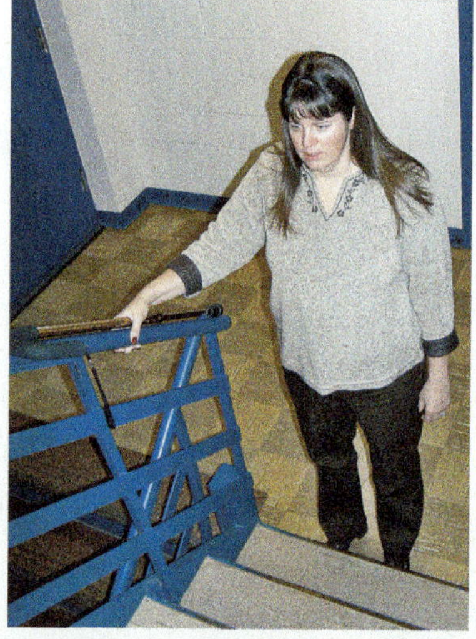

1 The patient holds the cane at midshaft, parallel to the handrail.

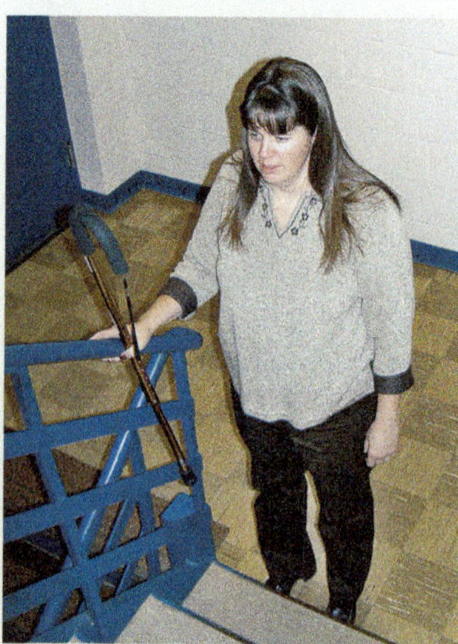

2 The patient holds the cane at midshaft, perpendicular to the handrail.

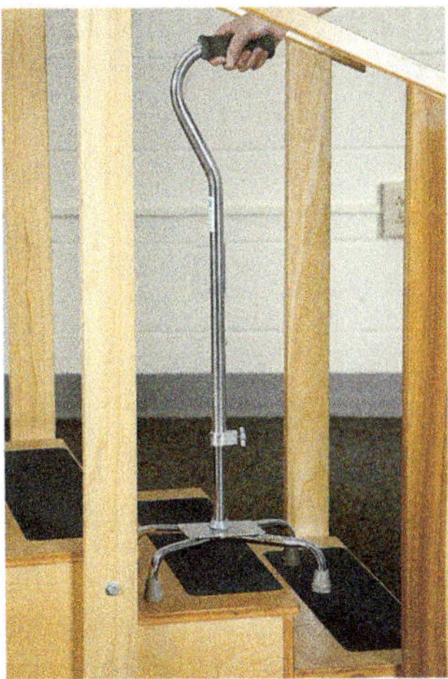

3 The base of a quad cane may be longer than the depth of a stair tread.

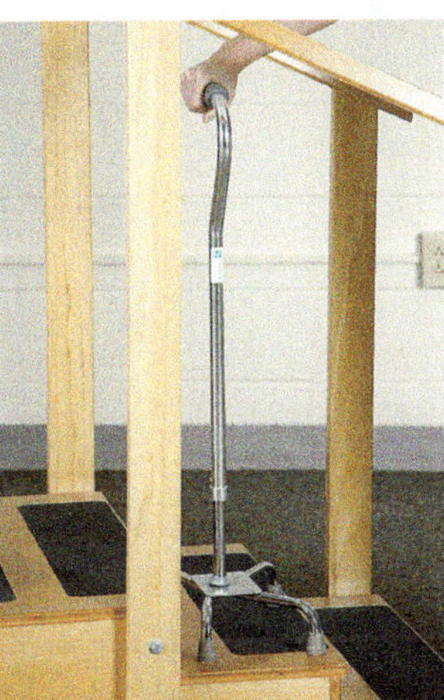

4 Turning a quad cane sideways permits all four legs of the cane to be supported on the stair tread.

Ascending Using a Cane and Handrail

1 Positioned in stride behind the patient, the physical therapist/assistant grasps the patient's gait belt and the handrail. To ascend stairs, the patient stands facing up the stairs with the feet and cane parallel to the base of the first stair.

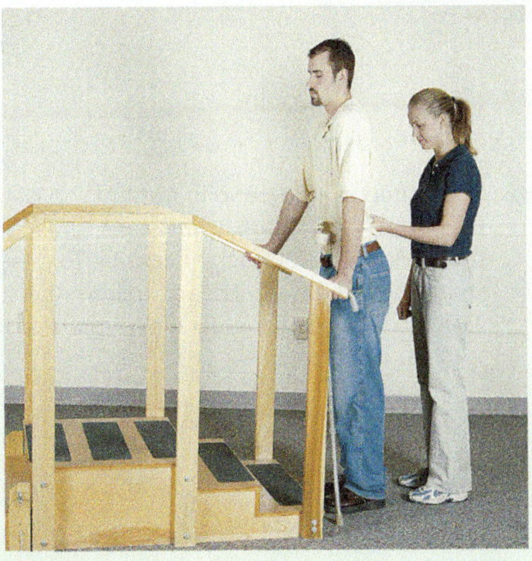

(continued)

PROCEDURE 10–17 Ambulating on Stairs with One Cane (*continued*)

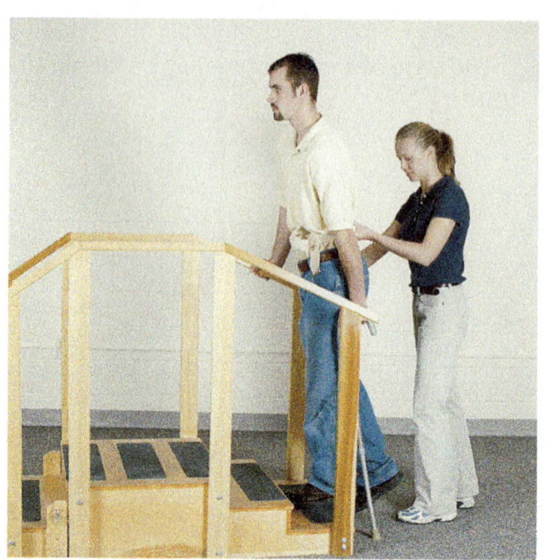

2. The patient moves the uninvolved lower extremity to the next higher stair and shifts weight onto this extremity.

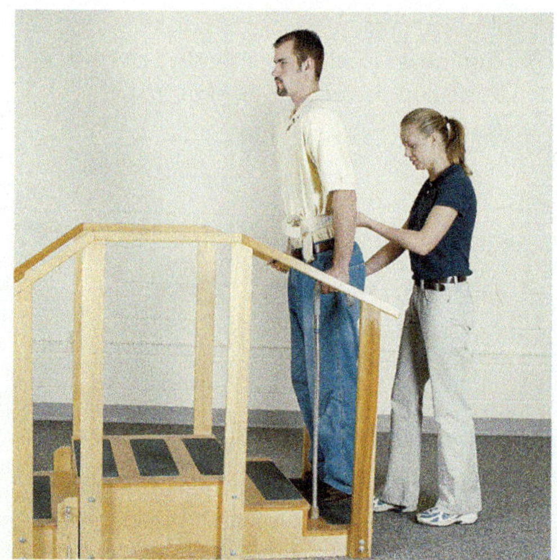

3. The patient extends the uninvolved lower extremity, lifting the body. The patient places the involved lower extremity and cane on the same stair as the uninvolved lower extremity.
4. The sequence is repeated to ascend the remaining stairs.

Descending Using a Cane and Handrail

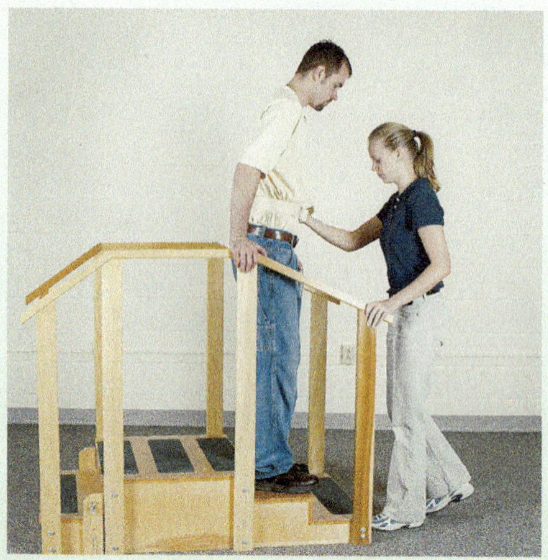

1. Positioned in stride and in front of the patient, the physical therapist/assistant grasps the patient's gait belt and the handrail. To descend stairs, the patient stands facing down the stairs, with the feet and cane parallel to the stair.

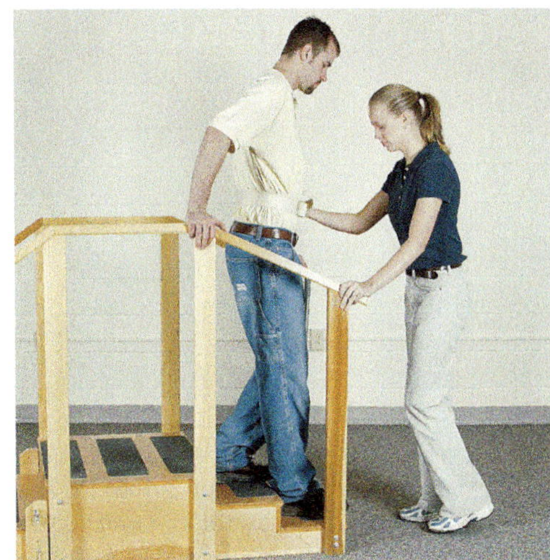

2 The patient lowers the cane to the next lower stair and places it securely on the stair tread. The patient lowers the involved lower extremity to the next lower stair by flexing the uninvolved lower extremity. As the patient's balance and strength improve, the patient may move the cane and involved lower extremity simultaneously.

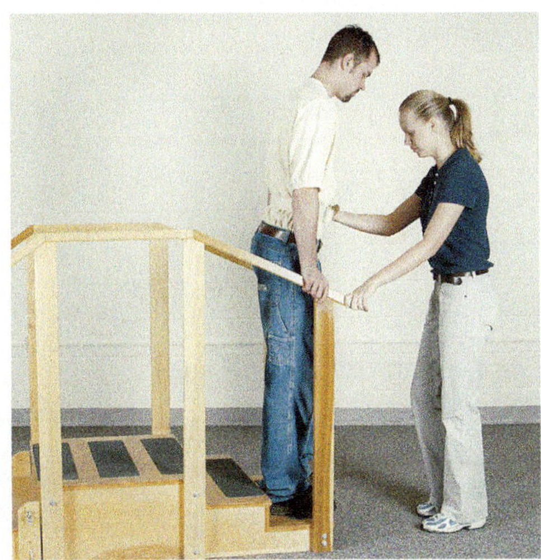

3 The patient shifts weight to the involved lower extremity, cane, and handrail and lowers the uninvolved lower extremity to the same stair as the cane and involved lower extremity.

4 The sequence is repeated to descend the remaining stairs.

Ascending Using One Cane

When not using a handrail, the gait pattern for ascending stairs with one cane is similar to that used when both a cane and handrail are used. As the patient improves, he should practice using only a cane and no handrail, which prepares the patient for situations in which no handrail is available.

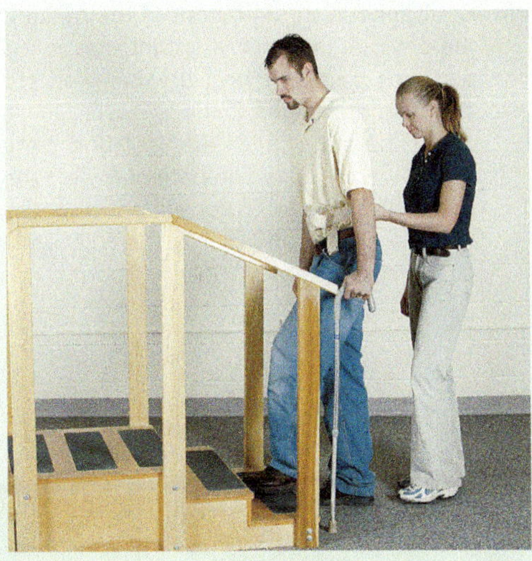

1 Positioned in stride behind the patient, the physical therapist/assistant grasps the patient's gait belt and the handrail. To ascend stairs, the patient stands facing up the stairs with the feet and cane parallel to the base of the first stair. The patient moves the uninvolved lower extremity to the next higher stair and shifts weight onto this extremity.

(continued)

PROCEDURE 10–17 Ambulating on Stairs with One Cane (*continued*)

2. The patient extends the uninvolved lower extremity, lifting the body. The patient places the involved lower extremity and cane on the same stair as the uninvolved lower extremity.
3. The sequence is repeated to ascend the remaining stairs.

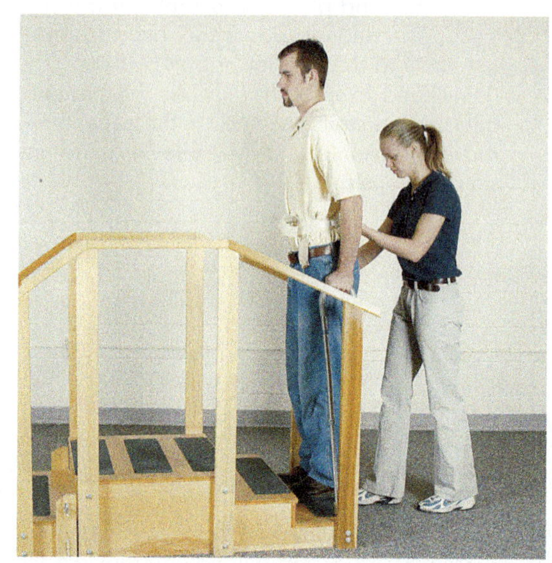

Descending Using One Cane

When not using a handrail, the gait pattern for descending stairs with one cane is similar to that used when both a cane and handrail are used. As the patient improves, he should practice using only a cane and no handrail, which prepares the patient for situations in which no handrail is available.

1. Positioned in stride in front of the patient, the physical therapist/assistant grasps the patient's gait belt and the handrail. To descend stairs, the patient starts facing down the stairs, with the feet and cane parallel to the stair. The patient lowers the cane and involved lower extremity to the next lower stair and places them securely on the stair tread.

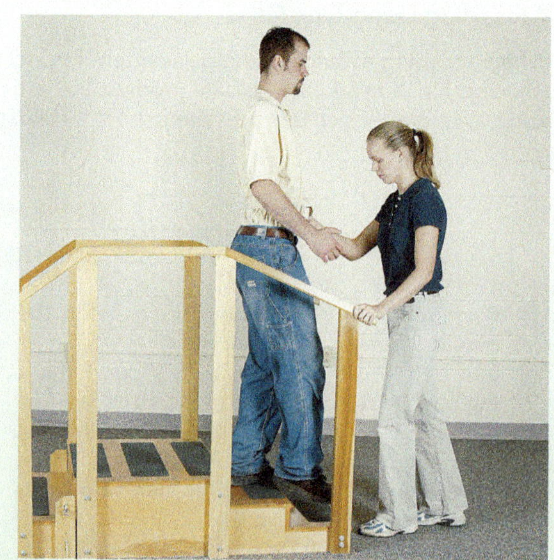

2. The patient shifts weight to the involved lower extremity and cane and lowers the uninvolved lower extremity to the same stair as the cane and involved lower extremity.
3. The sequence is repeated to descend the remaining stairs.

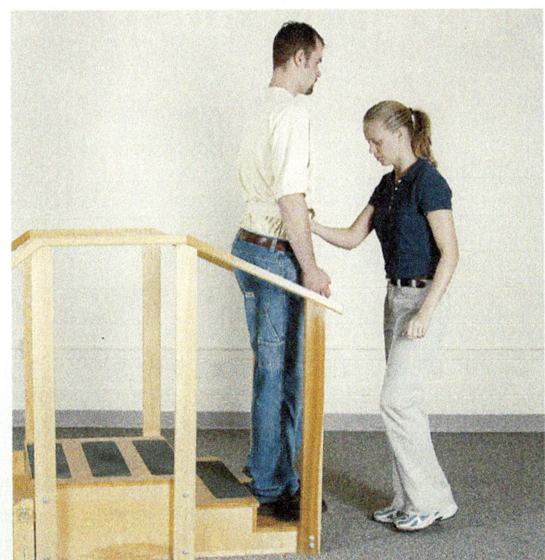

PROCEDURE 10–18 Ambulating Through Doorways with One Cane

Door with Automatic Door Closers

Door Opens Toward Patient—Cane at Hinge Edge

Note: In the illustrations for this section, a cane is used in the patient's left hand, the hand closer to the hinge edge of the door when facing the door.

1. The patient approaches the door and stands at the latch edge of the door, out of the arc of the opening door. The patient places his right hand on the door handle.

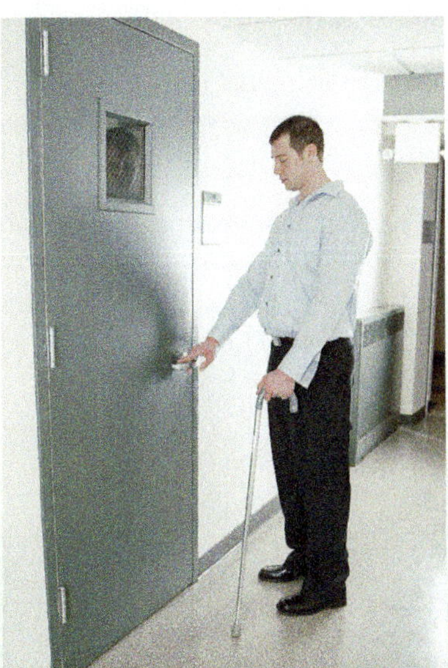

(continued)

PROCEDURE 10–18 Ambulating Through Doorways with One Cane (*continued*)

2. The patient opens the door wide enough to permit movement into the doorway before the door closes. Unlike the sequences for a walker or crutches, the patient does not open a door completely in a single motion. Opening a door in a single motion when using one cane is often not possible when patients must move the upper extremity across the body. Attempting to do so can compromise a patient's safety.

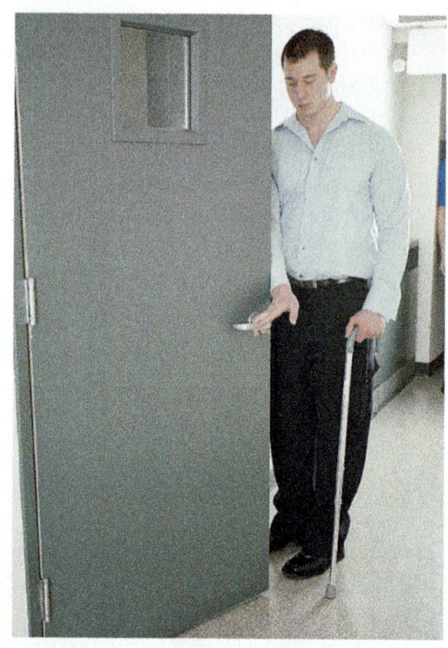

3. The patient opens the door farther and places the tip of the cane on the floor to serve as a doorstop.

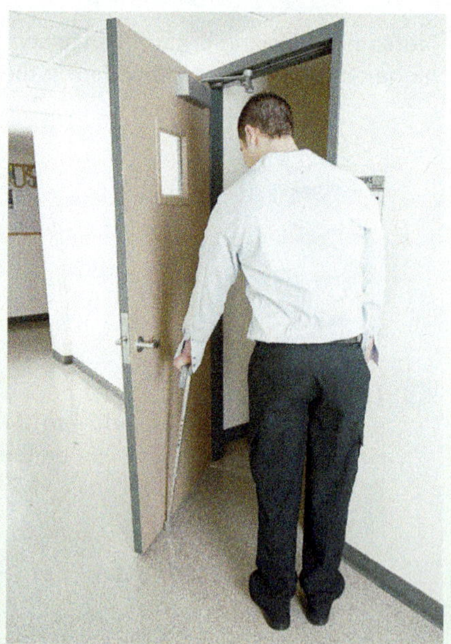

4 As the patient moves through a doorway, he places the tip of the cane progressively closer to the hinge edge of the door to serve as a doorstop. The patient may need to use a hand or hip to maintain an open door. The physical therapist/assistant and patient must be aware that as the tip of a cane is placed closer to the hinge edge of the door, the door becomes more difficult to block. Once a patient has moved completely through the doorway, the door closes behind the patient.

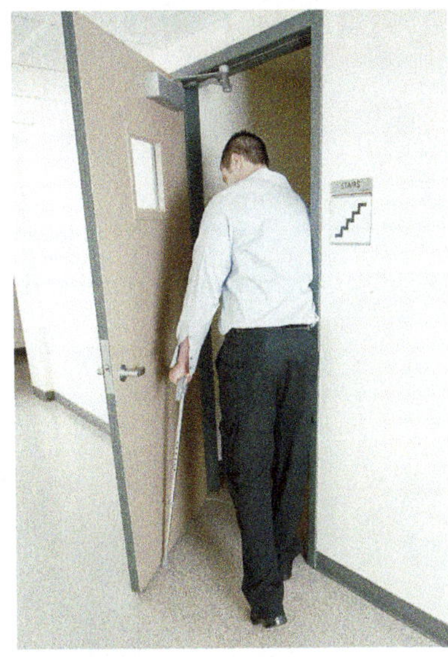

Door Opens Away from Patient—Cane at Hinge Edge

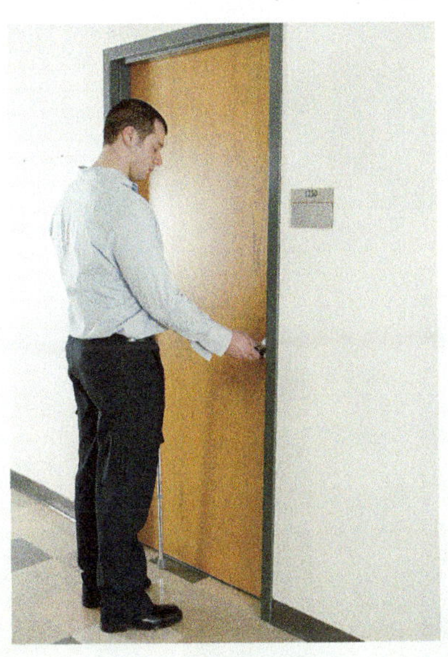

1 The patient approaches the door and places his right hand on the door handle.

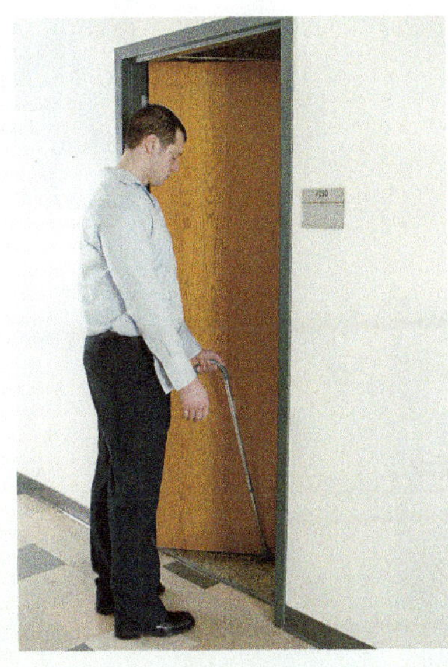

2 The patient opens the door wide enough to permit a patient to enter the doorway. The patient places the tip of the cane on the floor to serve as a doorstop. A door is not opened completely in a single motion. As the patient moves through a doorway, he places the tip of the cane progressively closer to the latch edge of the door to serve as a doorstop. The patient may need to use a hand or hip to maintain an open door. Once the patient has moved completely through a doorway, the door closes behind him.

(continued)

PROCEDURE 10–18 Ambulating Through Doorways with One Cane (*continued*)

Door Opens Away from Patient—Cane at Latch Edge

1. The patient approaches the door and places the right hand on the door handle.

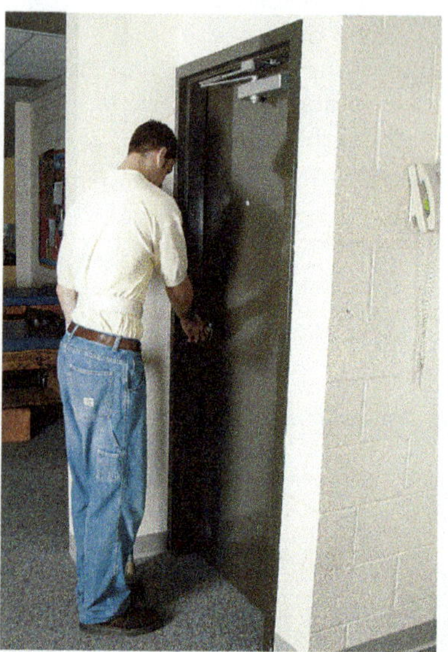

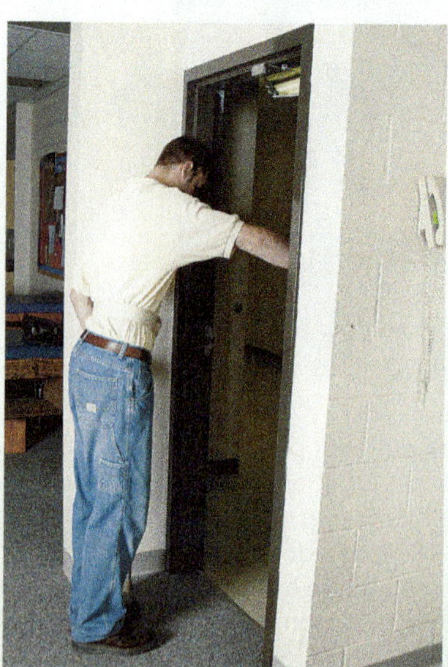

2. The patient pushes the door open wide enough to permit movement into the doorway. The patient moves the right hand from the door handle to the door and uses this hand to hold open the door.

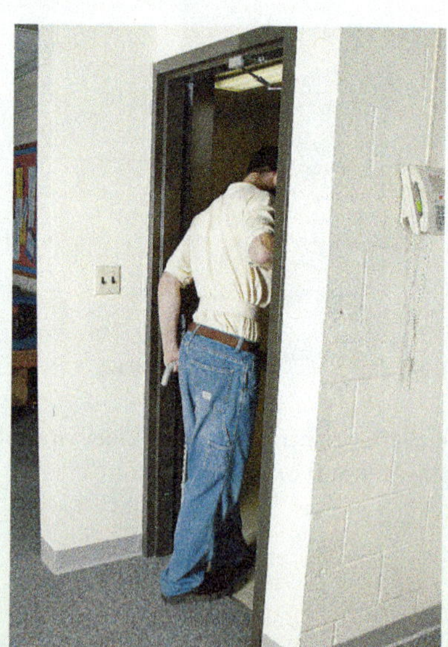

3. The patient continues to move through the doorway, using the hand to hold open the door. Once the patient has moved completely through the doorway, the door closes behind him.

PROCEDURE 10–19 Ambulating on Level Surfaces with Two Canes

Assuming standing and sitting when preparing for and finishing ambulation using two canes is performed in a manner similar to those maneuvers when using one cane.

Three-Point Gait Pattern

1. Positioned in stride behind and to one side of a patient, the physical therapist/assistant grasps the patient's gait belt and shoulder. In the starting position, the patient stands with one cane in each hand in the same position used for measuring cane fit. The patient's feet are side by side.

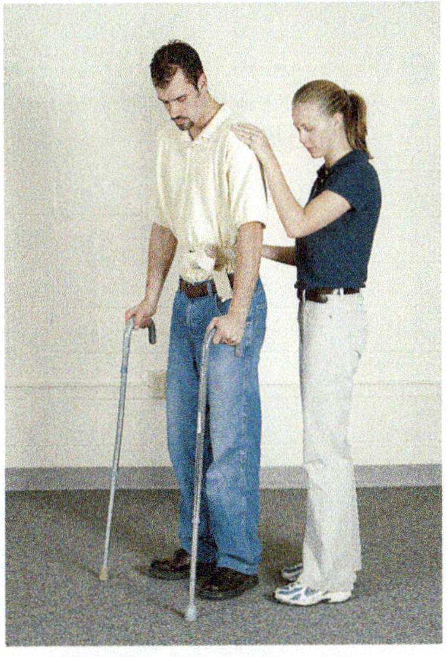

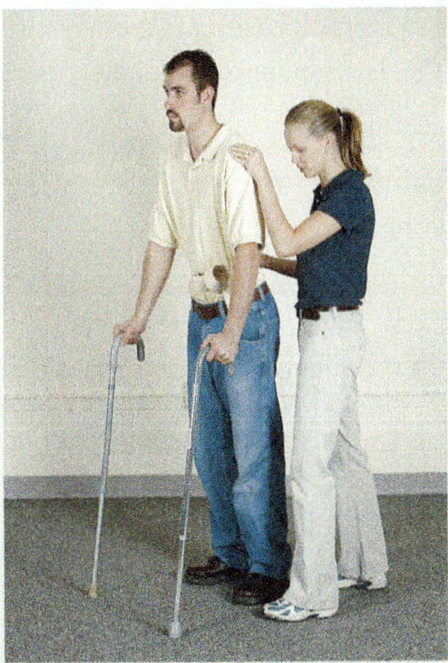

2. To ambulate, the patient advances both canes and then advances the involved lower extremity to the canes. As the patient improves, he can advance the canes and the involved lower extremity simultaneously the same amount.

(continued)

PROCEDURE 10–19 Ambulating on Level Surfaces with Two Canes (*continued*)

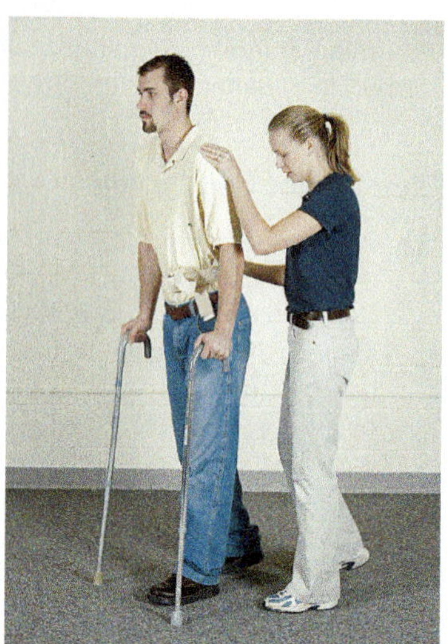

3. The physical therapist/assistant advances the outside foot either at the same time or immediately after the canes are advanced.

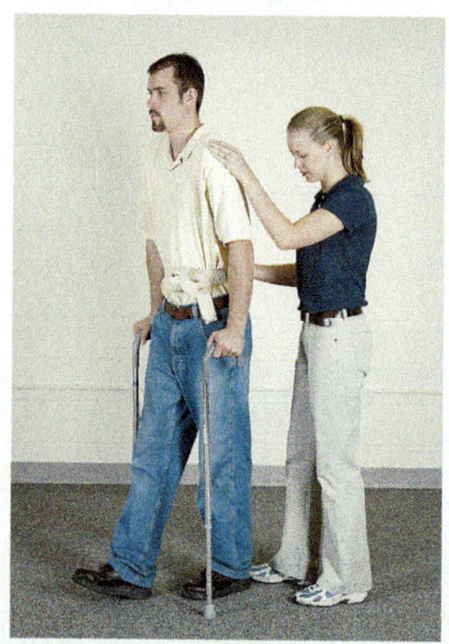

4. The patient then advances the uninvolved lower extremity beyond the canes. Initially, the patient may "step to" the involved lower extremity. Stepping through is the normal gait pattern and should be encouraged. The physical therapist/assistant advances the inside foot as the patient moves the uninvolved lower extremity.
5. The sequence is repeated for continued progression.

Four-Point Gait Pattern

1. Positioned in stride behind and to one side of the patient, the physical therapist/assistant grasps the patient's gait belt. In the starting position, the patient stands with one cane in each hand in the same position used for measuring cane fit. The patient's feet are side by side.

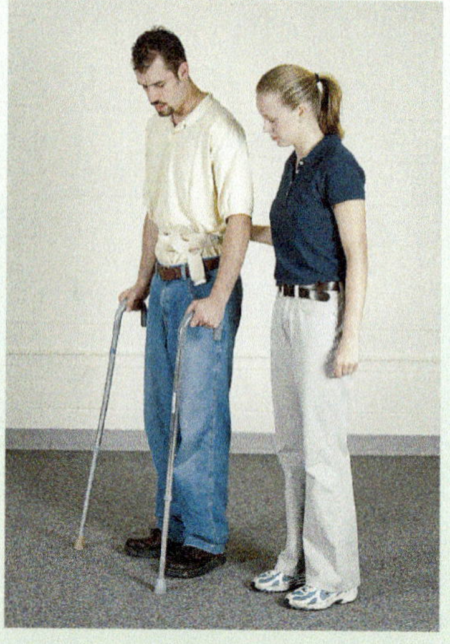

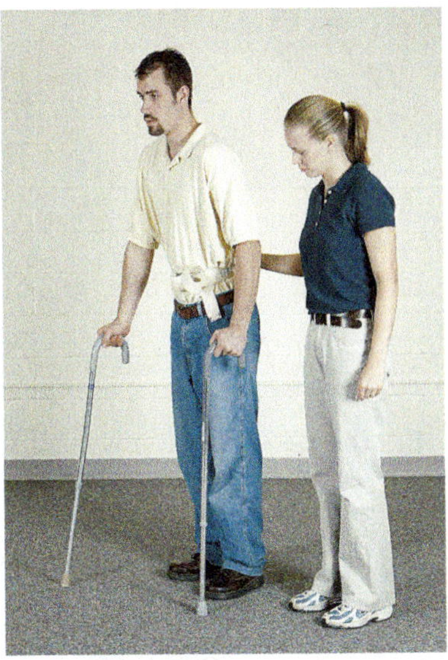

2 To ambulate, the patient advances one cane. In this example, the right cane is advanced first.

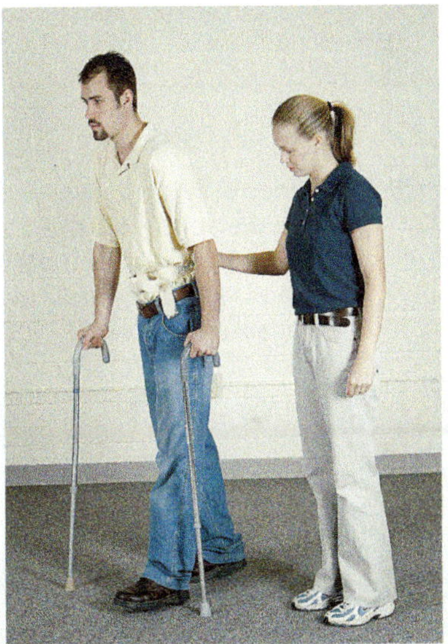

3 The patient then advances the opposite (left) lower extremity to a point even with the tip of the right cane. The physical therapist/assistant advances the inside foot.

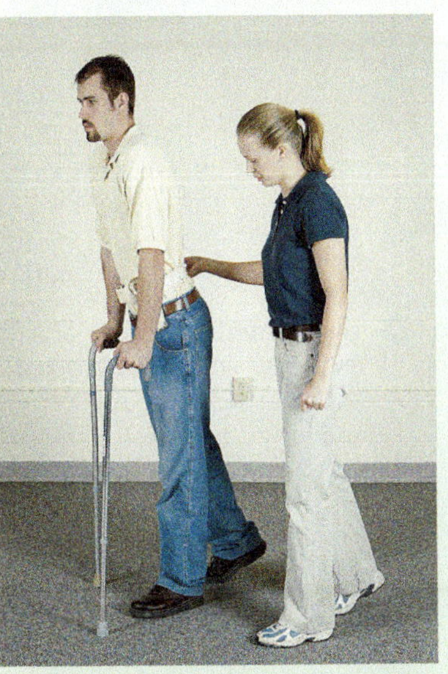

4 The patient shifts weight to the right cane and left lower extremity and advances the left cane beyond the right cane.

(continued)

PROCEDURE 10–19 Ambulating on Level Surfaces with Two Canes (*continued*)

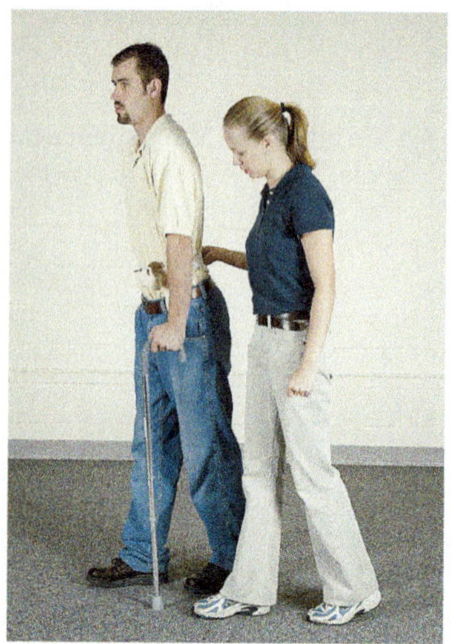

5. The patient then advances the right lower extremity to a point even with the tip of the left cane. The physical therapist/assistant advances the outside foot.
6. The sequence is repeated for continued progression.

Two-Point Gait Pattern

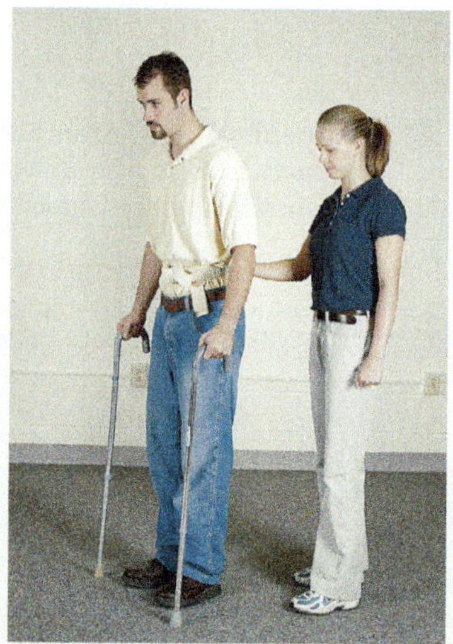

1. Positioned in stride behind and to one side of a patient, the physical therapist/assistant grasps the patient's gait belt. In the starting position, the patient stands with one cane in each hand in the same position used for measuring cane fit. The patient's feet are side by side.

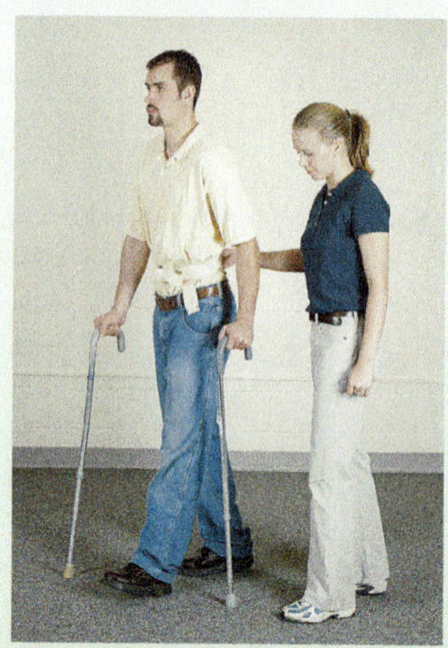

2. The patient advances one cane and the opposite lower extremity simultaneously, placing the toes even with the tip of the cane. The patient then shifts weight onto this cane and lower extremity. In this example, the right cane and left foot have been advanced together. The physical therapist/assistant moves the inside foot at this time.

3. The patient then advances the left cane and right lower extremity together. This cane and lower extremity are advanced beyond the other cane and lower extremity in a normal step length. The physical therapist/assistant moves the outside foot at this time.
4. The sequence is repeated for continued progression.

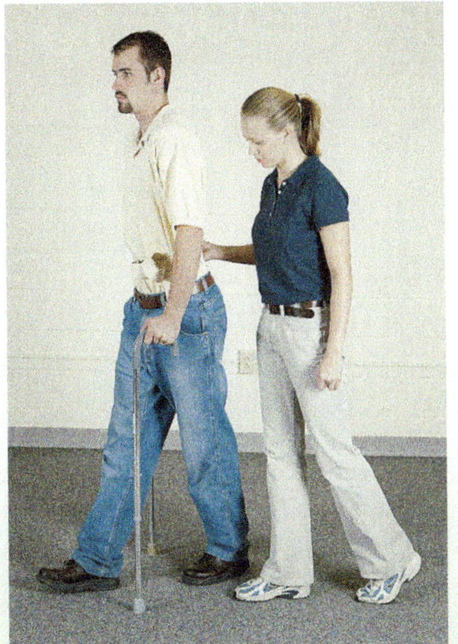

PROCEDURE 10–20 Ambulating on Stairs with Two Canes

Holding the Canes

A patient can perform ambulation on stairs using two canes, with or without the use of a handrail. Use of a handrail provides stability and is an added safety feature. When using a handrail, the handrail takes the place of the cane on one side. There are several methods of holding canes when using a handrail. Whatever method of holding canes is used, the sequence of movements for the lower extremities and ambulatory assistive devices is the same.

A practical method of holding two canes while using a handrail is for the patient to place both canes in one hand. There are two methods of holding a cane in the hand that is grasping a handrail and cane simultaneously.

1. One method of grasping a cane and handrail in the same hand is for the patient to hold the cane at mid-shaft parallel to the handrail.

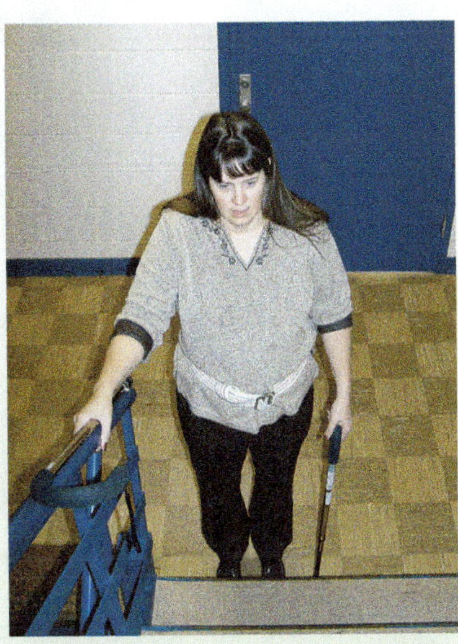

(continued)

PROCEDURE 10–20 Ambulating on Stairs with Two Canes (*continued*)

2 A second method of grasping a cane and handrail in the same hand is for the patient to hold the cane at midshaft in a vertical orientation.

The patient uses the cane on the side opposite the handrail in the usual manner.

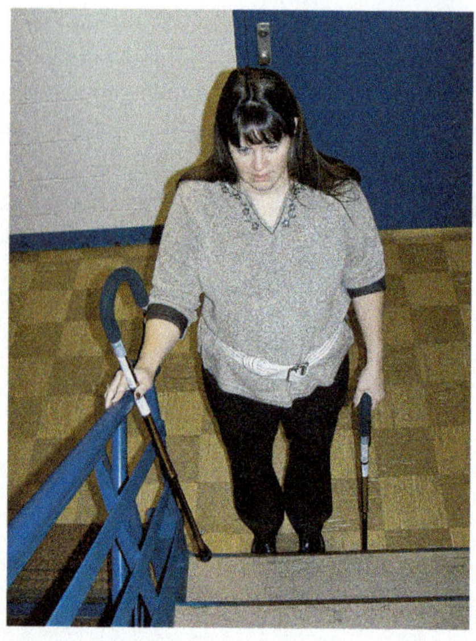

Three-Point Gait Pattern

Ascending Stairs

1 To ascend stairs, the patient stands facing up the stairs with feet and canes parallel to the base of the first stair. Positioned in stride behind a patient, the physical therapist/assistant grasps the patient's gait belt and the handrail.

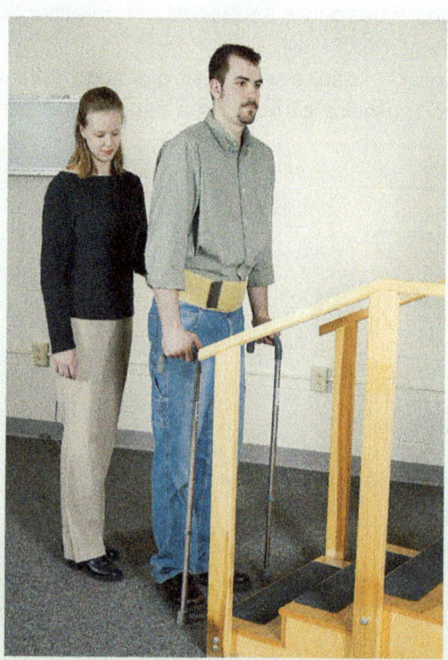

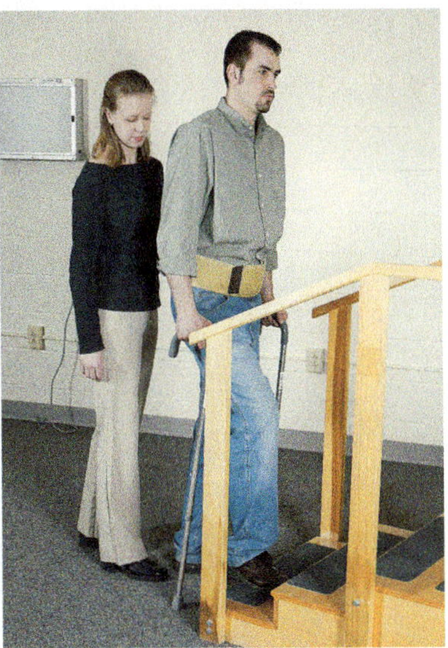

2 The patient places the uninvolved lower extremity on the next higher stair and shifts weight onto this extremity.

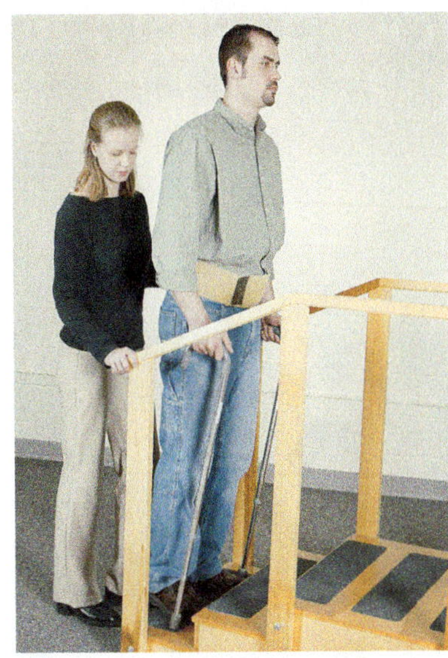

3 The patient extends the uninvolved lower extremity to raise the body. The patient advances the canes and involved lower extremity to the same stair simultaneously. The canes must be properly placed on the stair for stability and to provide room for the patient to maneuver.

4 The sequence is repeated to ascend the remaining stairs.

Descending Stairs

1 To descend stairs, the patient stands facing down the stairs. Positioned in stride in front of the patient, the physical therapist/assistant grasps the patient's gait belt and the handrail.

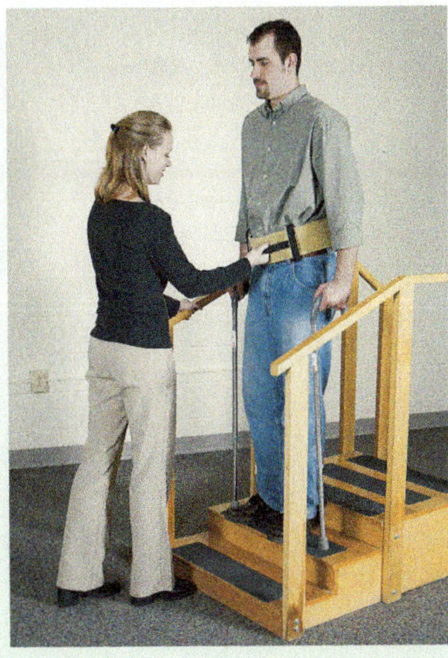

(continued)

PROCEDURE 10–20 Ambulating on Stairs with Two Canes (*continued*)

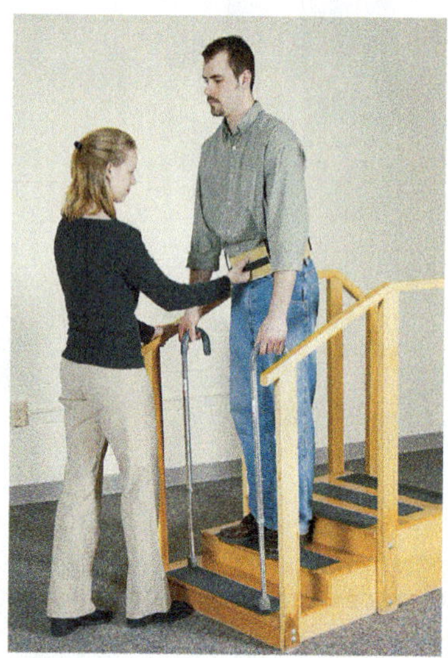

2 The patient lowers the two canes to the next lower stair.

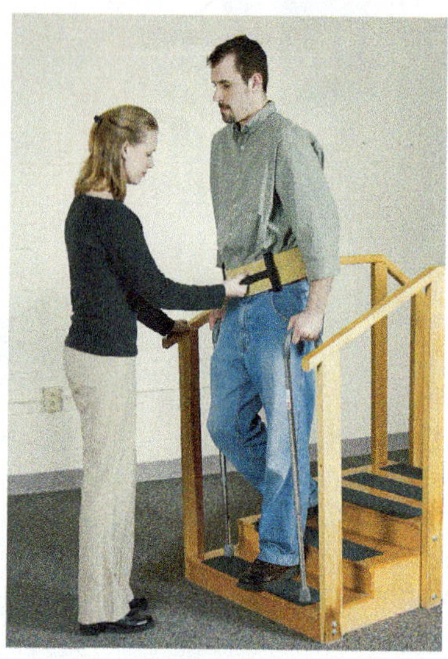

3 The patient lowers the involved lower extremity to the same stair as the two canes. The canes and involved lower extremity may be moved simultaneously.

4 The patient shifts weight to the involved lower extremity and canes and moves the uninvolved lower extremity to the same stair.

5 The sequence is repeated to descend the remaining stairs.

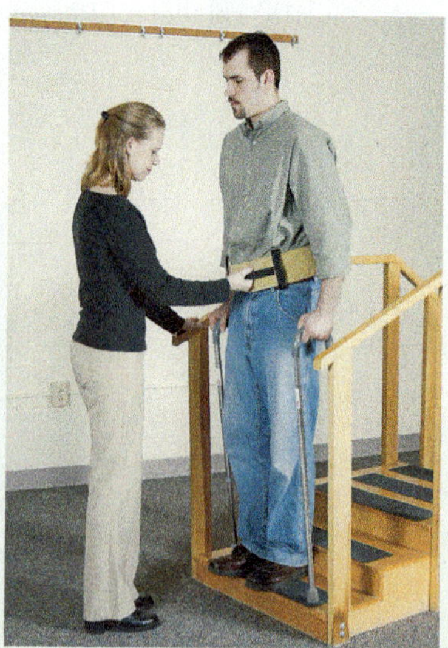

Four-Point Gait Pattern

Ascending Stairs

1. To ascend stairs, the patient stands facing up the stairs with feet and canes parallel to the base of the stair. Positioned in stride behind the patient, the physical therapist/assistant grasps the patient's gait belt.

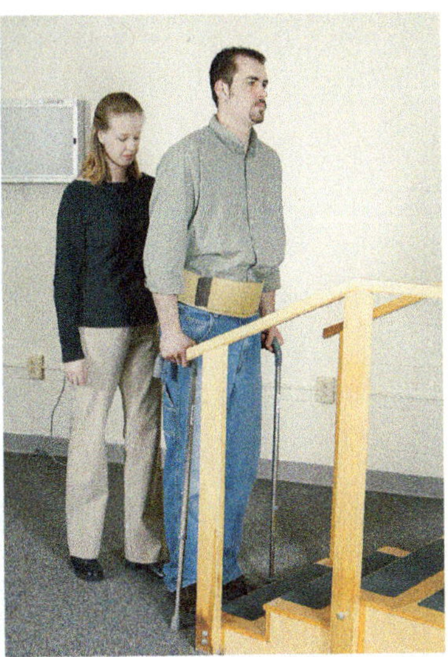

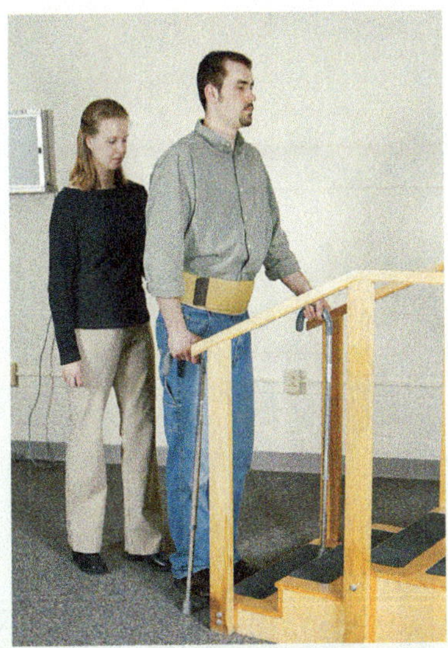

2. The patient advances one cane to the next higher stair.

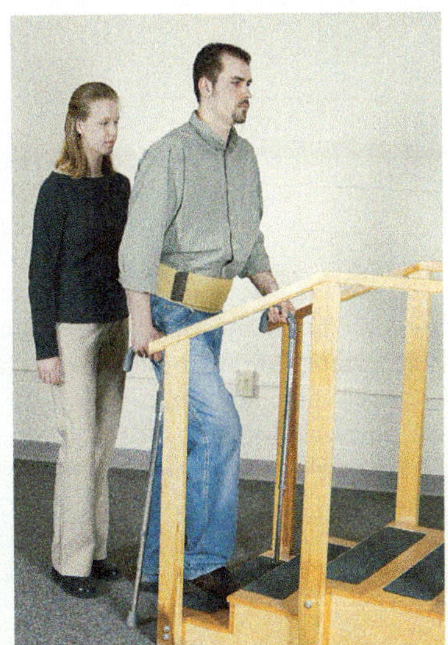

3. The patient then advances the opposite lower extremity to the same stair and shifts weight onto the cane and lower extremity that have been placed on the next higher stair.

(continued)

PROCEDURE 10–20 Ambulating on Stairs with Two Canes (*continued*)

4. The patient advances the second cane to the same stair.

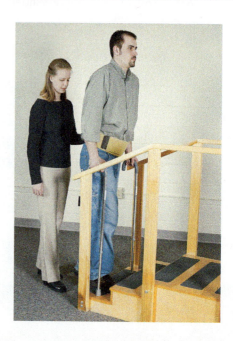

5. The patient then extends the lower extremity on the higher stair to lift the body. The patient places the second lower extremity on the same stair. Thus, both lower extremities and both canes are on the same stair. As the physical therapist/assistant gets close enough to the stairs, she grabs the handrail for stability.
6. The sequence is repeated to ascend the remaining stairs.

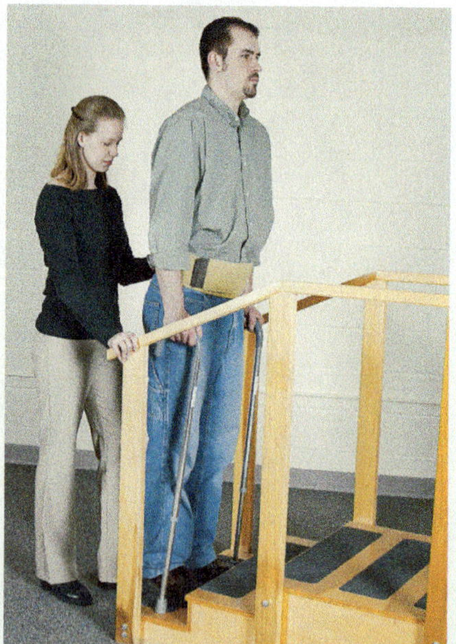

Descending Stairs

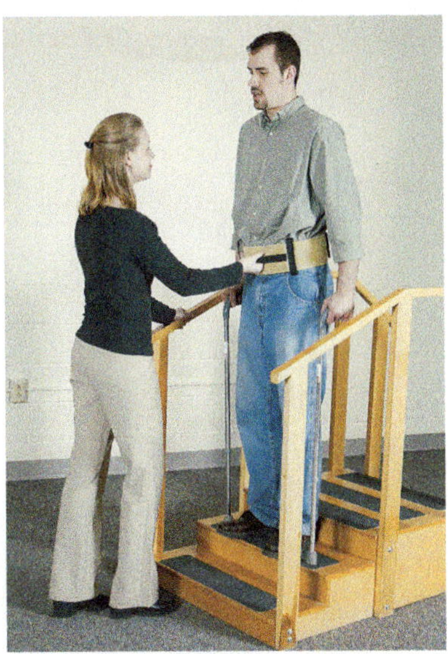

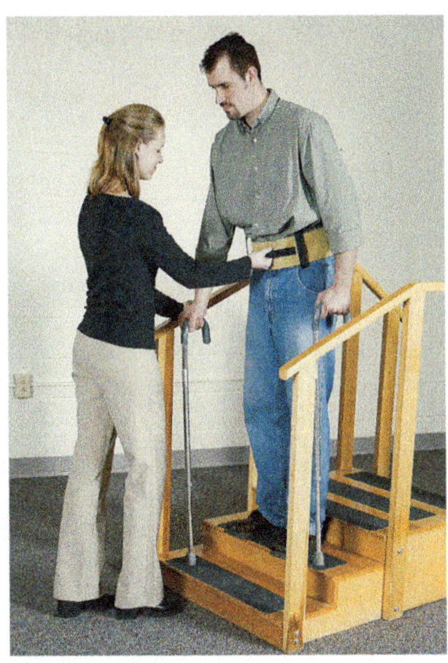

1. To descend stairs, the patient stands facing down the stairs. Positioned in stride in front of the patient, the physical therapist/assistant grasps the patient's gait belt and the handrail.

2. The patient moves one cane to the next lower stair.

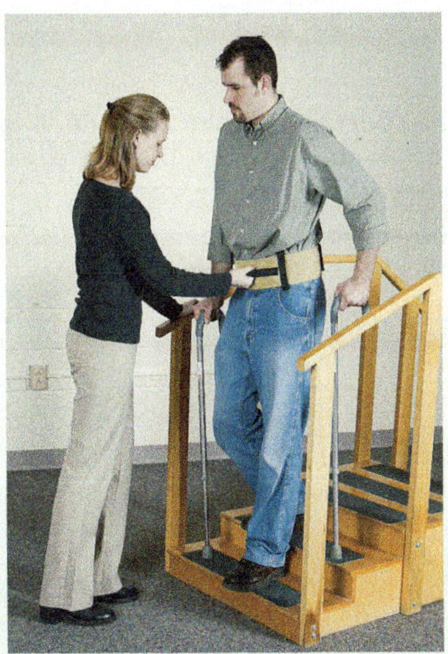

3. The patient flexes the lower extremity on the same side to lower the body, placing the opposite lower extremity on the same stair as the lowered cane.

(*continued*)

PROCEDURE 10–20 Ambulating on Stairs with Two Canes (*continued*)

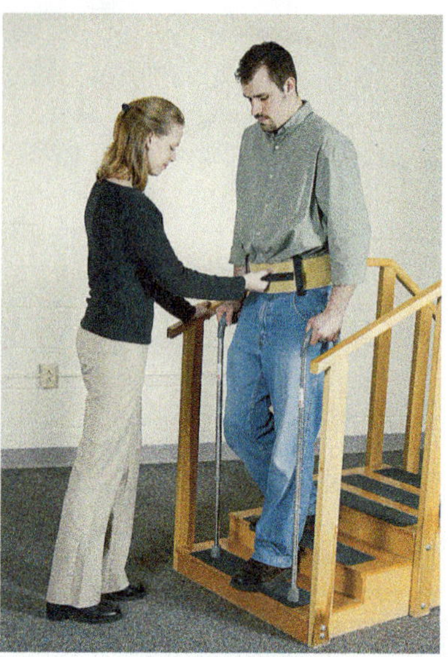

4. Shifting weight onto the cane and lower extremity on the lower stair, the patient moves the second cane to the same lower stair.

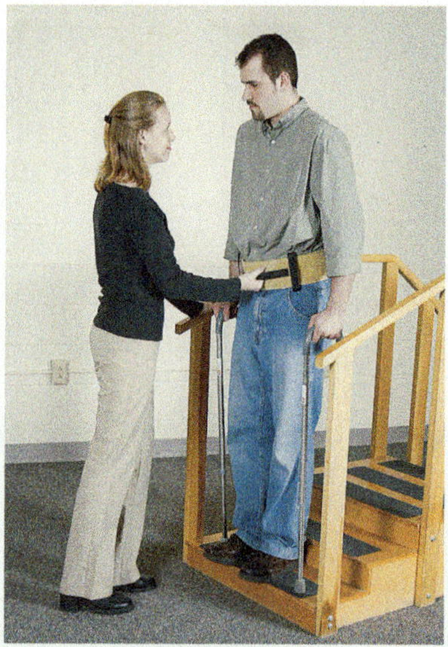

5. The patient moves the opposite lower extremity to the same lower stair. Thus, both lower extremities and both canes are on the same stair.
6. The sequence is repeated to descend the remaining stairs.

Two-Point Gait Pattern

Ascending Stairs

Ascending stairs using two canes and a two-point gait pattern is very similar to using a four-point gait pattern. The difference is that in a two-point gait pattern, the patient moves one cane and the opposite lower extremity simultaneously.

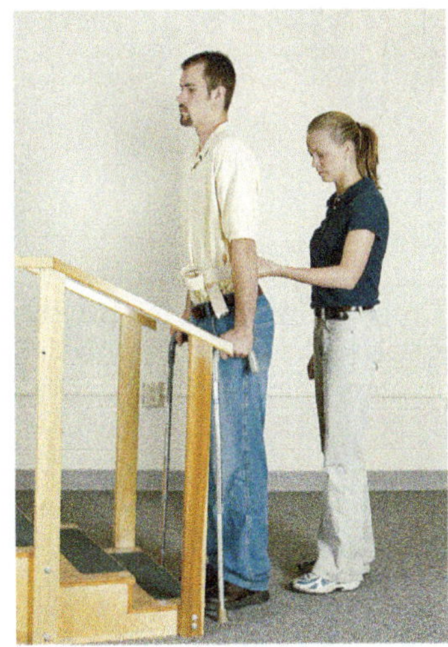

1. To ascend stairs, the patient stands facing up the stairs with feet and canes parallel to the base of the stair. Positioned in stride behind the patient, the physical therapist/assistant grasps the patient's gait belt.

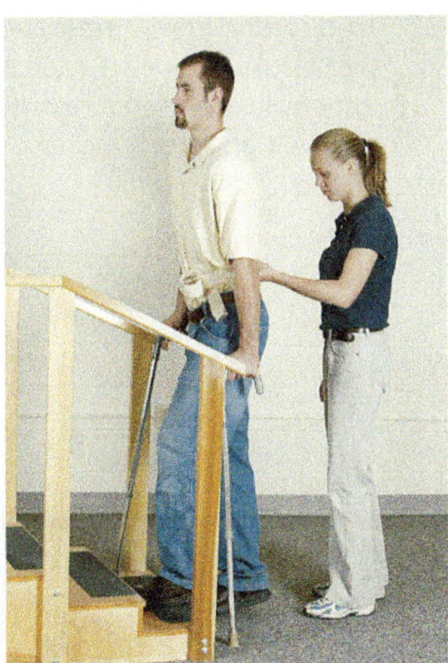

2. The patient moves one cane and the opposite lower extremity to the next higher stair.

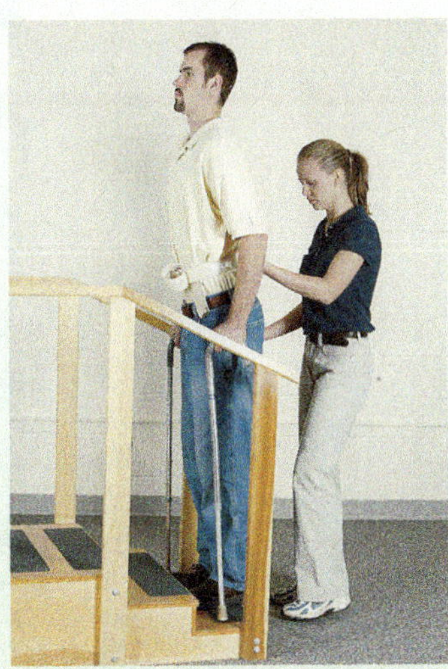

3. Then the patient moves the second cane and opposite lower extremity to the same stair. As the physical therapist/assistant gets close enough to the stairs, she grabs the handrail for stability.
4. The sequence is repeated to ascend the remaining stairs.

(continued)

PROCEDURE 10–20 Ambulating on Stairs with Two Canes (*continued*)

Descending Stairs

Descending stairs using two canes and a two-point gait pattern is very similar to using a four-point gait pattern. The difference is that in a two-point gait pattern, the patient moves one cane and the opposite lower extremity simultaneously.

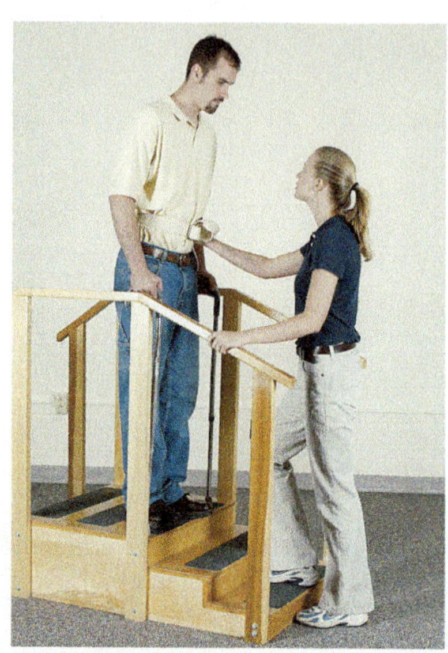

1. To descend stairs, the patient stands facing down the stairs. Positioned in stride in front of the patient, the physical therapist/assistant grasps the patient's gait belt and the handrail.

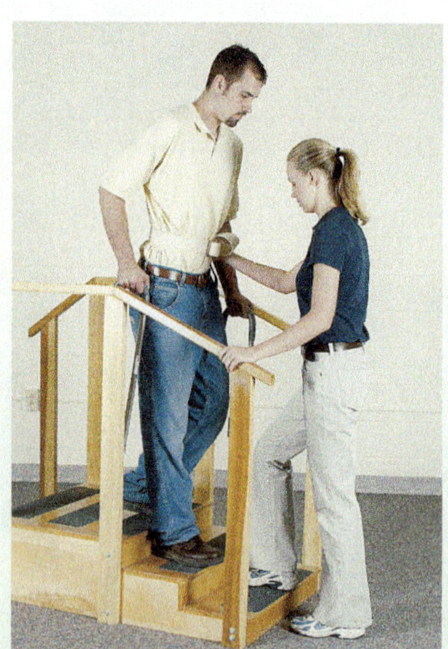

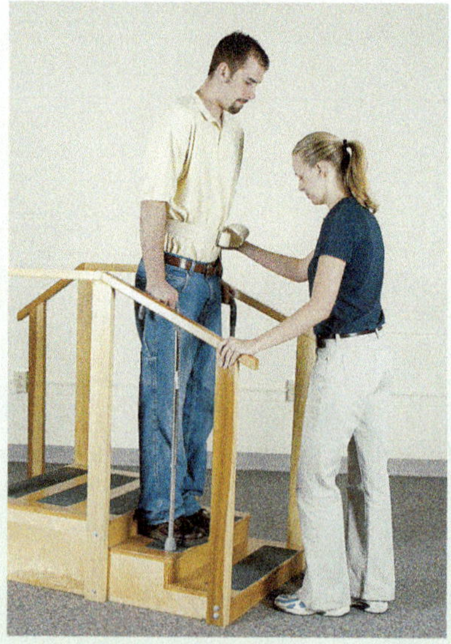

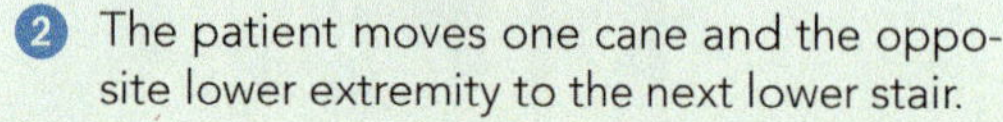

2. The patient moves one cane and the opposite lower extremity to the next lower stair.
3. The patient lowers the second cane and opposite lower extremity to the same stair.
4. The sequence is repeated to descend the remaining stairs.

PROCEDURE 10–21 Ambulating Through Doorways with Two Canes

When moving through a doorway, patients can use one cane in each hand or may place both canes in one hand. The method of moving through doorways with both canes in one hand is the same as when using one cane.

Door with Automatic Door Closer

Door Opens Away from Patient

1. The patient faces the door and shifts the weight onto the cane away from the hand that is closer to the door handle. Holding the cane, the patient uses the unweighted hand to grasp the door handle.

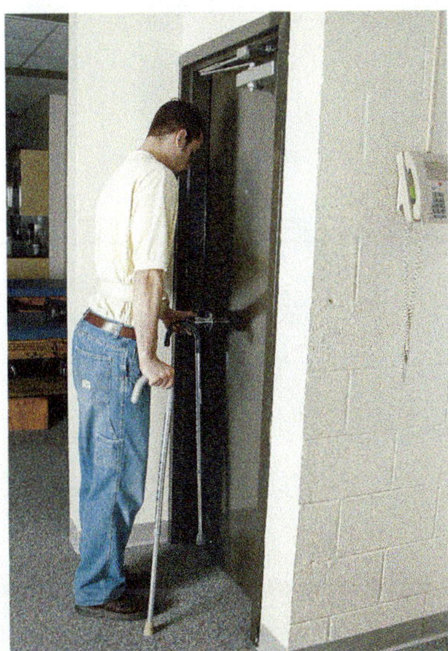

2. Using a pushing motion, the patient opens the door part way and blocks the door the tip of the cane closer to the door.

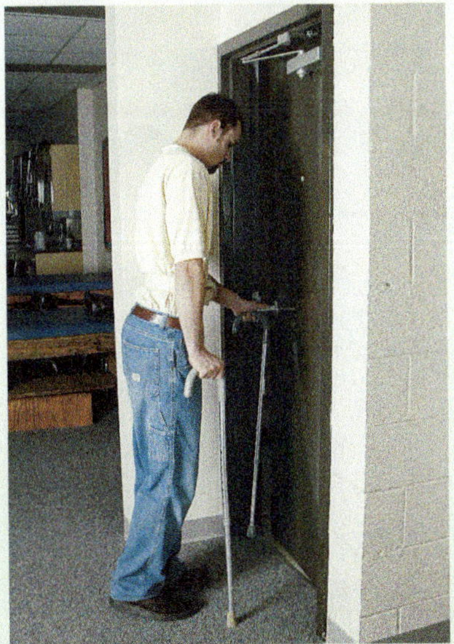

(continued)

PROCEDURE 10–21 Ambulating Through Doorways with Two Canes (*continued*)

3 As the patient moves through the doorway, he pushes the door open in increments. Continuing to use the tip of the cane as a doorstop, the patient progresses through the doorway. The door closes behind the patient.

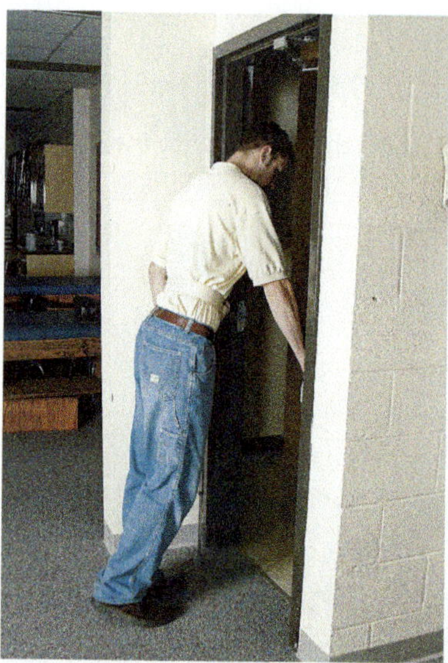

Door Opens Toward Patient

1 The patient approaches the latch edge of the door, standing outside the arc through which the opening door will move. The patient shifts weight onto the cane on the side away from the hand that will be placed on the door handle. Holding the cane, the patient uses the unweighted hand to grasp the door handle. Preferably, the patient shifts weight to the side closer to the door handle and uses the hand toward the hinge edge to pull open the door.

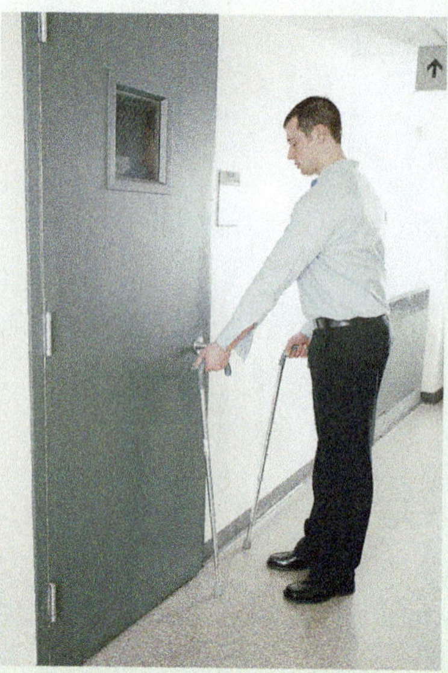

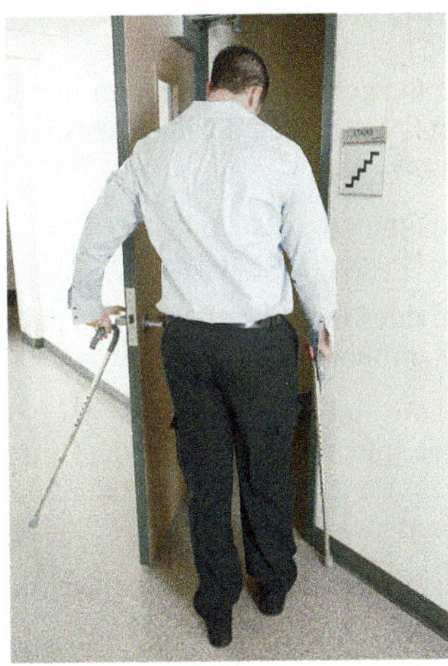

2 Using a pulling motion, the patient opens the door wider than the width of the patient because the door will start to close automatically before the patient can progress through the doorway. To block the automatic closing of the door, the patient moves into the doorway and places the tip of the cane closer to the door on the floor in the path of the door. This serves as a doorstop, permitting the patient to move into the doorway without being struck by the closing door.

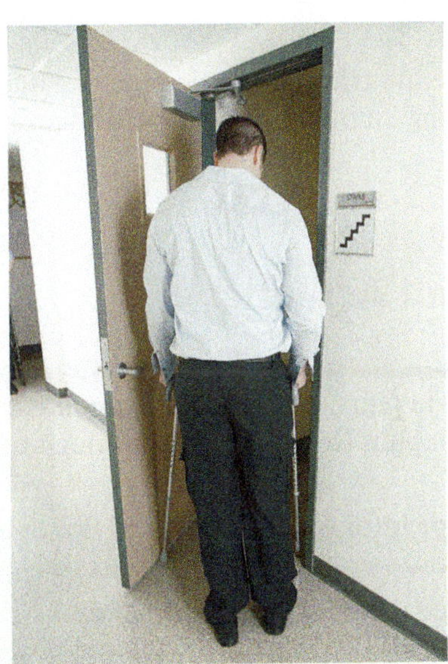

3 Continuing to use the tip of the cane as a doorstop, the patient progresses through the doorway using an appropriate gait pattern. As the patient moves through the doorway, he uses the tip of the cane as a doorstop by placing it progressively closer to the hinge edge of the door. The physical therapist/assistant and patient must be aware that as the tip of a cane gets closer to the hinge edge of the door, it becomes more difficult to hold open the door.

4 Once the patient has moved completely through the doorway, the door closes behind the patient.

Doors Without Automatic Closers

Patients using two canes can negotiate doorways without automatic door closers using the same sequences presented earlier in this chapter in the section *Axillary Crutches*.

Review Questions

1. What are the general guidelines for instructing a patient in the use of ambulatory assistive devices and gait patterns?
2. Which components of ambulatory assistive devices should be checked for safety?
3. What activities should be taught to a patient learning to use an ambulatory assistive device?
4. What are the ambulatory assistive devices that (1) provide the most stability to the least stability; and (2) require the most patient coordination to the least patient coordination?
5. What are the indications for the selection of specific ambulatory assistive devices?
6. What are the five major gait patterns used with ambulatory assistive devices?
7. Which gait patterns can be used with each assistive device?
8. What are the criteria for selection of gait patterns when using ambulatory assistive devices?
9. What is the purpose of using the tilt table in gait training?
10. What is the proper method of fitting each ambulatory assistive device?
11. What are the proper methods for a physical therapist/assistant to guard a patient ambulating using an assistive device on level surfaces, stairs, and through doorways?
12. How is the wheelchair prepared properly for a patient to move into or out of the wheelchair when using ambulatory assistive devices?
13. What are the indications for the use of ambulatory assistive devices?
14. What are causes of patient fatigue during gait training?
15. What is the proper lower extremity to be moved first when descending stairs?

Suggested Activities

1. Working in pairs, practice the procedures presented in this chapter. Rotate partners during the practice session.
   a. Practice fitting each assistive device to at least three different people.
   b. Practice demonstrating gait patterns with each assistive device.
   c. Practice guarding partners using each assistive device with each appropriate gait pattern on level surfaces, stairs, and curbs; the assumption of sitting from standing and standing from sitting; moving through doorways; falling without injury; and resumption of ambulation after falling.
2. Practice teaching partners how to use ambulatory assistive devices on level surfaces, stairs, and curbs; the assumption of sitting from standing and standing from sitting; moving through doorways; falling without injury; and resumption of ambulation after falling, as partners role-play various diagnoses. Students role-playing a patient can add "character" to the role play by being cooperative, uncooperative, in pain, hard of hearing, or faint, to enhance the activity. The patient must role-play the diagnosis and character consistently (see *Case Studies* for suggested patient roles).
3. Monitor vital signs and check for signs of circulatory problems of the lower extremities as appropriate.
4. Document interventions.

Case Studies

Use these case studies to complete Suggested Activities 2 above.

1. The patient is a 16-year-old male high school soccer player who sustained a left knee injury in a game the previous night. He is to ambulate using axillary crutches with a non–weight-bearing gait pattern until a diagnosis is determined following an MRI in 2 days.
2. The patient is a 63-year-old female with a left CVA presenting with right hemiplegia. She has sufficient motor control and balance to ambulate with a small-base quad cane.
3. The patient is a 78-year-old male who had a left total hip replacement 1 day ago. He is to ambulate using a walker with weight bearing as tolerated.
4. The patient is a 49-year-old female with severe rheumatoid arthritis who received a right total knee joint replacement 2 days ago. She is to ambulate using a platform walker, with weight bearing as tolerated.
5. The patient is a 21-year-old male with a complete L3–4 spinal cord injury. He is ready to begin gait training using Lofstrand (forearm) crutches and knee-ankle-foot orthoses (KAFOs). His upper extremity strength is adequate for ambulating with these ambulatory assistive devices.

References

1. Uniform Data System for Medical Rehabilitation, A Division of UB Foundation Activities, Inc. ($UDS_{MR}{}^{SM}$). (1997). *Guide for the Universal Data Set for Medical Rehabilitation, version 5.1.* Buffalo: State University of New York at Buffalo.
2. Guccione, A. A., & Scalzitti, D. A. (2007). Examination of functional status and activity level. In S. B. O'Sullivan & T. J. Schmitz (Eds.), *Physical rehabilitation* (5th ed.). Philadelphia: F. A. Davis.

Glossary

A

Abduction movement in the frontal plane that is the result of the limb segment surfaces moving away from the midline of the body; does not include the thumb

Accessible route public path from public transportation, accessible parking spaces, and public streets to a building that meets accessibility requirements

Active assisted range of motion (AAROM) exercises performed by a physical therapist/assistant assisting a patient in performing movement

Active listening techniques used to promote effective communication

Active pathology part of Nagi model; interruption of normal body function at the cellular level

Active range of motion (AROM) exercises performed independently by a patient, although they may be supervised by a physical therapist/assistant to ensure correct performance

Adduction movement in the frontal plane that is the result of the limb segment surfaces moving toward the midline of the body; does not include the thumb

Afebrile when a patient's oral temperature remains below 100°F (37.8°C)

Airborne precautions prevent transmission of infectious agents that remain infectious over long distances when suspended in the air

Airborne transmission occurs by two modes: (1) airborne droplet nuclei (particle residue 5 μm or smaller in size) that are evaporated droplets containing microorganisms that remain suspended in the air for long periods of time; and (2) in dust particles containing the infectious agent that are dispersed widely by air currents and inhaled by a susceptible host

Alcohol-based hand rub alcohol-containing preparation designed for application to the hands for reducing the number of viable microorganisms on the hands. In the United States, such preparations usually contain 60% to 95% ethanol or isopropanol

Ambulation a mobility activity

Ambulatory assistive devices provide external support for the musculoskeletal system to permit upright ambulation

Americans with Disabilities Act (1990; ADA) Public Law 101–336, that contains five titles and provides "a clear and comprehensive national mandate for the elimination of discrimination against individuals with disabilities"

Analysis (SOAP note) list of patient problems and professional opinions concerning a patient's problems and reasoning used as the basis for the plan of care; also includes diagnosis and prognosis related to physical therapy care

Anatomical planes of movement three cardinal planes—sagittal, frontal, and transverse—used to move body segments to perform ROM exercises

Anatomical position position in which a person is standing upright, eyes looking straight ahead, arms at the sides with palms facing forward, and the feet approximately 4 inches apart at the heels with the toes pointing forward

Anthropometric measures measurements of physical characteristics such as height and weight

Antimicrobial soap soap (i.e., detergent) containing an antiseptic agent

Antiseptic agent antimicrobial substances that are applied to the skin to reduce the number of microbial flora. Examples include alcohols, chlorhexidine, chlorine, hexachlorophene, iodine, chloroxylenol (PCMX), quaternary ammonium compounds, and triclosan

Antiseptic hand rub applied to all surfaces of the hands to reduce the number of microorganisms present

Antiseptic hand wash washing hands with water and soap or other detergents containing an antiseptic agent

Anti-tipping devices small extensions, with or without wheels, attached to the lower horizontal support bar to prevent accidental backward tipping of a wheelchair

Architectural Barriers Act (1968; ABA) federal law that requires access to facilities designed, built, altered, or leased with federal funds

Armrests arm supports on a wheelchair

Aseptic technique the methods and procedures used to create and maintain a sterile field

Assessment analysis of data about a patient (Part 3 of a SOAP note)

Assisted transfers transfers in which a patient participates actively and requires assistance by additional (one or more) personnel; examples include two-person lift, sliding board transfer, squat pivot, and assisted standing pivot transfer

Audit systematic reviews of documentation that examine the efficacy and efficiency of patient-care outcomes with respect to interventions used

Auscultation monitoring of the heart and lungs using a stethoscope; also used to obtain heart rate

B

Bacterial barrier a barrier that keeps microorganisms from coming in contact with sterile items

Basal heart rate pulse rate measured after an extended period of rest; one indication of cardiovascular function in the absence of physical stress

Base of support part of the body in contact with the supporting surface

Biarticular muscles that cross more than one joint

Blanching a noted loss of color of the skin resulting from decreased circulation

Blood pressure a measure of vascular resistance to blood flow

Body mass index (BMI) used to classify a person's weight and height relationship with respect to being underweight, normal, overweight, or obese

Body mechanics requires strength, range of motion (ROM), and motor control to maintain proper skeletal alignment during standing and proper skeletal movement during activity by maintaining the center of gravity within the base of support

Bradycardia a very slow resting heart rate; less than 60 bpm

C

Caster wheels the small front wheels of a wheelchair

Center of gravity the point at which the three cardinal planes intersect

Centers for Disease Control and Prevention (CDC) federal agency responsible for safety and health issues

Chart review review of a patient's chart prior to interacting with the patient

Cleaning the physical removal of organic material or soil from objects. The process of cleaning is usually performed with water, with or without detergents. Cleaning is the least rigorous of the three levels and is designed to remove microorganisms rather than kill them. Cleaning usually precedes either of the next two levels, disinfection or sterilization

Cleanliness degree of lack of contamination; three levels of cleanliness—cleaning, disinfection, and sterilization—have been established for equipment use in patient care

Clear-space areas include the floor dimensions of an accessible route and clearances for use of certain facilities, such as toilet stalls and drinking fountains

Close guarding physical therapist/assistant is close to the patient without contact, and the likelihood of physical assistance being required is fair

Closed-ended question used to obtain or confirm specific information and often answered with a single word or a brief phrase

Combining components occurs when more than one plane of joint motion is performed simultaneously

Common vehicle transmission applies to microorganisms transmitted by contaminated items such as food, water, medications, devices, and equipment

Compression wrap bandage applied to control edema in a limb segment or to provide some support for a joint

Contact guarding physical therapist/assistant is close to the patient with hands on patient/gait belt, and the likelihood of physical assistance being required is high

Contact precautions intended to prevent transmission of infectious agents, including epidemiologically important microorganisms, that are spread by direct or indirect contact with the patient or the patient's environment

Contact transmission the most important and frequent mode of nosocomial infection transmission

Contaminated an item, surface, or field whenever it comes in contact with anything that is not sterile

Control mechanisms switches, dial, handles, and the like that are used to manipulate or turn a device on/off

Critical items introduced directly into the circulatory system or other normally sterile areas of the body. Surgical instruments, implants, and the blood compartment of a hemodialyzer are examples of critical items

Cues spoken directions provided during performance of an activity

Curb cut a ramp to permit smooth transition from sidewalk to street level

D

Daily note part of POMR method; brief presentation or description documenting treatment and patient responses for each day

Damp-to-damp dressing application of a moistened gauze pad to a wound, and re-moistened just before removal

Database part of POMR method; contains subjective and objective information, including medical, family, and social history, and medical examination and test results

Decontaminate hands to reduce bacterial counts on hands by performing antiseptic hand rub or antiseptic hand wash

Department of Health and Human Services (DHHS) federal agency that administers Medicare and Medicaid, among other programs

Department of Justice (DOJ) primary federal criminal investigation and enforcement agency

Dependent transfers transfers in which a patient does not participate actively, or participates only minimally, and additional personnel perform all aspects of the transfer; examples include sliding transfer from cart to treatment table, three-person carry, dependent standing pivot transfer, and hydraulic lift transfer

Detergent compounds that possess a cleaning action. Detergents (i.e., surfactants) are composed of both hydrophilic and lipophilic parts and can be divided into four groups: anionic, cationic, amphoteric, and nonionic detergents. Although products used for hand-washing or antiseptic hand wash in healthcare settings represent various types of detergents, the term "soap" is used to refer to such detergents in this guideline

Diagnosis assignment of a label that states the categorization or classification of a patient's problems; physical therapists diagnose based on the practice pattern or diagnostic category that most closely describes a patient's impairments and functional limitations as presented in the *Guide to Physical Therapist Practice*

Diagonal patterns of movement combining components of motion at one joint as well as all the joints of an extremity

Diastolic pressure a measure of the pressure exerted by arterial walls against blood when the heart is not contracting

Direct-contact transmission involves direct body-surface-to-body-surface contact and physical transfer of microorganisms between a susceptible host and an infected or colonized person, such as when turning or transferring a patient or when performing other patient-care activities that require direct personal contact

Disability part of Nagi model; functional limitations that prevent an individual from fulfilling his/her life roles

Discharge note part of POMR method; present documentation of the status of patient problems, and the current course of treatment, at the time of patient discharge

Discharge plan plan indicating duration of care, referrals and follow-ups, and equipment requirements; a plan to obtain necessary equipment for a patient to achieve goals

Disinfection an intermediate level between cleaning and sterilization. Three levels of disinfection—high, intermediate, and low—have been defined. Disinfection is usually performed using pasteurization or chemical germicides

Documentation medico-legal record of patient care provided by all practitioners for a given patient

Doppler measurements used to examine patency using frequency changes during blood flow

Draping covering a patient appropriately in a manner that maintains patient modesty and comfort

Drive wheels the large rear wheels of a wheelchair; used for propulsion

Droplet precautions intended to prevent transmission of pathogens spread through close respiratory or mucous-membrane contact with respiratory secretions

Droplet transmission theoretically a form of contact transmission but quite distinct from either direct- or indirect-contact transmission, so considered a separate route of transmission; droplets generated from a source person (during coughing, sneezing, talking, performance of certain procedures such as suctioning or wound care) are propelled a short distance through the air and deposited on a host's conjunctivae, nasal mucosa, or mouth

Dry-to-dry dressing application of a dry dressing to cover a wound

E

ECHOWS a physical therapist's patient-interview assessment tool

Education for All Handicapped Children Act of 1975 (PL 94–142) (EHA) focuses on ensuring all children, including those with disabilities, have access to free and appropriate public education (FAPE)

Effective communication characterized by being timely, accurate, appropriate, clear, precise, concise, and organized

End feel quality of restriction felt by a physical therapist/assistant when a limit of motion is reached

Episode of physical therapy all physical therapist services provided without a break in care for a given condition or problem

Equal Employment Opportunity Commission (EEOC) the agency of the U.S. government that enforces the federal employment discrimination laws

Evaluation process whereby physical therapists use examination data, professional knowledge, and clinical judgment, to identify impairments and functional limitations and generate diagnoses, prognoses, and a plan of care

Eversion movement of the foot that occurs in the frontal plane about the long axis of the foot such that the plantar surface of the foot faces away from the midline of the body

Examination process of generating a patient/client history, reviewing all physiologic systems, and applying tests and measures

Explanatory model an approach to develop an understanding of a patient's perspective or explanation of their condition

Extension movement in the sagittal plane; does not include the thumb

F

Febrile when a patient's oral temperature exceeds 100°F

Feedback information provided after performing an activity

Fixed frame the wheelchair frame is solid and cannot be folded

Flexion movement in a sagittal plane; does not include the thumb

Folding-frame wheelchair can be folded or collapsed for storage or transport by raising footplates and pulling up on the handles located on either side of the seat

Footrest front rigging with only a footplate

Front rigging consists of a footplate attached to either a footrest or an elevating legrest on a wheelchair; purpose is to provide support for the lower extremities

Frontal (coronal) plane divides the body into front and back portions

Full weight bearing (FWB) the patient is permitted full weight bearing on the involved lower extremity

Functional limitations part of Nagi model; loss of a system is sufficient to prevent the performance of routine tasks by an individual, such as performing activities of daily living (ADLs), independently and in a timely manner

G

Gait pattern a selected sequence of movements for the ambulatory assistive device(s) and lower extremities to permit ambulation

Gait training process of training a patient to ambulate

Gait or transfer belts belts secured around a patient's waist, providing a secure point of contact and control for a physical therapist/assistant

Gauze wrap application of gauze from a roll of gauze to secure a dressing

Generalizability ability to use skills learned for one activity when performing other similar activities

Grab bar bar to hold onto for support during standing or transitions

Guidelines interpretations for the implementation of laws; recommendations to follow when implementing a procedure or process

H

Hand antisepsis either antiseptic hand wash or antiseptic hand rub

Hand hygiene a general term that applies to hand washing, antiseptic hand wash, antiseptic hand rub, or surgical hand antisepsis

Hand washing washing hands with plain (i.e., nonantimicrobial) soap and water

Health Insurance Portability and Accountability Act (HIPAA) of 1996 (PL 104-191) protects confidentiality of patient medical information and records when stored, when discussed by healthcare providers, and as they are conveyed between healthcare providers or between healthcare providers and insurers

Heel loops constructed of clothstrapping or webbing; attach to footplates and prevent the feet from sliding off the footplates and under the wheelchair

Horizontal abduction movement of the upper extremity posteriorly when the shoulder has already been abducted to 90 degrees in the frontal plane

Horizontal adduction movement of the upper extremity anteriorly when the shoulder has already been abducted to 90 degrees in the frontal plane

Hospital Infection Control Practices Advisory Committee (HICPAC) a federal advisory committee made up of 14 external infection control experts who provide advice and guidance to the Centers for Disease Control and Prevention (CDC) and the Secretary of the Department of Health and Human Services (HHS) regarding the practice of healthcare infection control, strategies for surveillance and prevention and control of healthcare-associated infections in U.S. healthcare facilities

Hyperthermia a rectal temperature greater than 106°F (41.1°C)

Hypothermia a rectal temperature less than 94°F (34.4°C)

I

Identifiers could allow identification of an individual and the individual's medical information and thus are to be protected under HIPPA to prevent inappropriate use of this information

Impairment part of Nagi model; the body cannot compensate or heal itself, so the individual sustains loss of normal function of a body system

Independent transfers transfers in which a patient consistently performs all aspects of the transfer, including setup, in a safe manner and without assistance by additional personnel; an example is a push up transfer

Indirect-contact transmission involves contact of a susceptible host with a contaminated intermediate object, usually inanimate, such as whirlpool water that is not changed between patient treatments, reuse of self-adhesive electrodes on more than one patient, contaminated hands that are not washed, and gloves that are not changed between patients

Individually identifiable health information eighteen specific identifiers that are protected information for purposes of confidentiality

Individuals with Disabilities Education Act of 1990 (PL 101–476)13/2004 (PL 108–446)(IDEA) replaces the EHA, and extends services to infants and toddlers

Initial note part of POMR method; documentation of initial findings, from patient interview and evaluation, and plan of care

Instructions inform patients of what is to be done and provide information as part of the teaching process; may include oral description, visual demonstration, and written description

Intake form form completed by patient prior to patient interview

International Classification of Function (ICF) model a model of health and function generated by the World Health Organization (WHO) that considers a person's health influences, and is influenced by, any disease or disorder that affects body functions and structures

Intervention services provided based on plan of care; may include treatment, communication, education, and planning

Interview the process of soliciting information by talking with another person(s)

Inversion movement of the foot that occurs in the frontal plane about the long axis of the foot such that the plantar surface of the foot faces toward the midline of the body

Isolation the separation and placement of patients in environments that reduce the potential for transmission of infectious microorganisms

Isometric muscle contractions contractions of muscles that result in development of muscle tension without joint movement

J

Joint range of motion moving a joint in all planes of motion appropriate for the specific joint

K

Knee walker ambulatory assistive device permitting upright ambulation while removing the requirement for weight bearing through the foot, ankle, and lower leg

L

Lateral (external) rotation movement in the transverse plane that results in anterior limb segment surfaces turning outward, away from the midline of the body

Legrest wheelchair front rigging with a footplate and calf pad support

Levels of assistance stated as supervision, close guarding, contact guarding, minimal, moderate, and maximum assistance

Long sitting position in which a person sits with hips flexed to 90° and knees fully extended on a supporting surface

Long-term goals (LTGs) statements describing functional capabilities a patient will have on discharge

M

Mask a nonactive device that filters environmental air

Maximal heart rate the highest heart rate a person should achieve on exertion with respect to age and medical condition

Maximum assistance indicated for patients who can perform 25% or less of an activity

Medial (internal) rotation movement in the transverse plane that results in anterior limb segment surfaces turning inward, toward the midline of the body

Midsagittal plane divides the body into equal right and left halves

Minimal assistance indicated for patients who can perform 75% or more of an activity

Moderate assistance indicated for patients who can perform approximately 50% of an activity

Multiarticular muscles crossing more than one joint

Muscle range of motion lengthening a muscle through its available length for all appropriate joint motions

N

Nagi model a model of health and function with four sequential phases

Narrative note documentation method for entering patient information in the medical record that may include headings and subheadings to organize information

National Center for Medical Rehabilitation and Research (NCMRR) model a disablement model derived from both the Nagi and World Health Organization models

Noncritical items do not touch the patient or touch the patient in areas that are normally not sterile, such as intact areas of skin; examples are blood pressure cuffs and crutches

Non–weight bearing (NWB) the involved lower extremity is not to be weight bearing and is usually not permitted to touch the ground

Nosing front edge of a stair tread

Nosocomial infection infection acquired while hospitalized for treatment of other conditions

O

Objective (SOAP note) documentation that includes the verifiable data such as: examination results, observations by healthcare providers, interventions, and patient response to interventions (Part 2 of a SOAP note)

Occlusive dressing bandage applied to provide a semipermeable barrier to air and moisture penetration

One-arm drive wheelchair has two hand rims on one drive wheel with a linking mechanism between the drive wheels, providing control for both drive wheels using one upper extremity

Open-ended question allows a patient to tell his or her story in his or her own words

Opposition multiplanar movement of the carpometacarpal joint of the thumb that results in approximation of the tip of the thumb and the tip of a finger of the same hand

Orthostatic hypotension the inability of the cardiovascular system to adapt to upright postures after prolonged horizontal positioning

Outcome functional capacity of a patient/client at discharge

P

Pain subjective perception described by patients; difficult to measure

Partial weight bearing (PWB) a limited amount of weight bearing, such as five pounds, is permitted for the involved lower extremity

Passive range of motion (PROM) exercise performed with the patient relaxed and a physical therapist/assistant moving the body segment without patient assistance

Patency openness of the arteries; can be determined by measurements of pulse

Patient's Bill of Rights a list of guarantees for those receiving medical care

Patient-care equipment categories three categories of patient care equipment—critical, semi-critical, and noncritical—provide a basis for the level of cleanliness deemed necessary

Patient/client management note documentation method based on the Physical Therapy Patient/Client Management process; has components of both the narrative and SOAP note formats

Patient Protection and Affordable Care Act of 2010 (PL 111–148) commonly called the Affordable Care Act, or ACA, provides major health care reform and access, which among other elements requires that hospitals provide patients with a copy of the Patient's Bill of Rights

Pelvic positioners devices that stabilize a patient's pelvis in the proper position while seated in a wheelchair

Plain soap detergents that do not contain antimicrobial agents or that contain low concentrations of antimicrobial agents that are effective solely as preservatives

Plan (SOAP note) documentation of the plan of care developed by the physical therapist for providing patient treatment (Part 4 of a SOAP note)

Plan of care statement that specifies outcomes, interventions to be provided to achieve the stated outcomes, and a timeline for reaching the stated outcomes

Platform lifts used for building entrances, in building interiors, and with transportation vehicles

Preferred practice pattern element of evidence-based patient management for specific diagnoses that guides management of patients but does not prescribe specifics of patient/client management

Problem list part of POMR method; list of the patient's problems identified from information contained in the database; problems may be identified by any professional in a discipline providing patient care and may be listed as an abnormal test result, chief complaint, diagnosis, physical finding, physiological finding, or symptom

Problem-oriented medical record (POMR) method organizes each medical record in a format based on identified patient problems rather than by professional discipline

Prognosis determination of an optimal level of improvement and the time necessary to achieve projected outcomes

Progress (weekly) notes documentation of the POMR method; progression of treatment, patient responses to treatment, and changes in the plan of care over specific intervals

Pronation defined differently for the upper and lower extremities; for the upper extremity, pronation of the forearm occurs when the arm is stabilized and the forearm is rotated so that the palm of the hand faces posteriorly; for the lower extremity, pronation of the foot occurs when the leg is stabilized and the foot is rotated about the oblique axis of the subtalar and other midfoot joints in direction of dorsiflexion, forefoot adduction, and eversion

Prone position in which a person lies on his or her stomach on a supporting surface

Proper posture appropriate alignment of the musculoskeletal system such that the stresses and strains placed on bones, muscles, ligaments, and cartilage are as low as possible

Proprioceptive Neuromuscular Facilitation (PNF) an approach to therapeutic exercise

Protraction multiplanar movement of the scapula around the lateral aspect of the ribs toward the anterior aspect of the thorax; often termed scapular abduction

Pulse a measurement of heart rate in beats per minute

R

Radial deviation when the wrist is moved such that the hand moves away from the midline of the body

Ramp slanted portion of a route

Range of motion (ROM) movement of each joint and muscle through its available arc of motion

Reach range unobstructed space a person is able to reach such as distance to some type of controls

Reclining-back wheelchairs type of wheelchair that has a back that can be adjusted from vertical to horizontal and points between

Recommendations ranking scheme CDC's Center for Infectious Diseases has established four categories to indicate the scientific support for their recommendations

Red flag a sign or symptom noted that does not fit with a known medical diagnosis for the specific patient

Regularity evenness of heart rate or respiratory rate

Regulations rules for the implementation of laws

Rehabilitation Act of 1973 (PL93–112) addresses civil rights of individuals with disabilities (often called the 504 Act)

Respirator a mechanical device that provides a source of air not associated with the immediate environment

Respiratory rate rate of breathing

Resting heart rate pulse rate measured during rest; a measurement of heart rate without imposed stresses

Retraction multiplanar movement of the scapula around the lateral aspect of the ribs as the scapula moves toward the spine; often termed scapular adduction

Rigid dressing bandage that prevents motion to provide physical protection to a wound and the adjacent area and joint

Rigidity resistance to passive movement that is not affected by movement velocity

Riser vertical dimension that separates one stair tread from the next stair tread

Rules regulations for the implementation of laws

S

Sacral sitting occurs when an individual slouches, sliding the buttocks forward and tilting the pelvis posteriorly

Sagittal plane divides the body into two sides, left and right, but not equally

Semicritical items devices introduced into body cavities not usually considered sterile, and include, but are not limited to, endotracheal tubes and fiberoptic endoscopes. There is a lower degree of risk of infection associated with semicritical items

Shelf life the length of time an unopened sterilized package is considered to remain sterile

Short-term goals (STGs) more discrete activities a patient will achieve to perform functional activities stated as long-term goals

Sidelying position in which a patient is lying on one side

Signs objective evidence of disease perceptible by a healthcare provider and reported in the objective data

SOAP note documentation method that originated with POMR system and now is used more widely for medical chart notes

Source-oriented method charts are divided into sections for each health profession providing service for a patient, thereby segregating patient information by discipline (source)

Spasticity increased resistance to movement, especially as the velocity of movement is increased

Spiral wrap application of a wrap in a continuous manner around a limb segment

Standard precautions precautions designed for the care of all patients, particularly hospitalized patients, regardless of their diagnosis or presumed infection status. This is new terminology to replace the term universal precautions

Sterile an item or environment free from living microorganisms

Sterile field an area considered free from living microorganisms

Sterilization the highest level of cleanliness. Sterilization is the destruction of all forms of microbial life by steam under pressure, liquid or gaseous chemicals, or dry heat

Subjective (SOAP note) documentation of relevant data concerning the patient's history that are not verifiable in medical records; includes the patient's description of functional problems, pain, and the date of onset; could also include patient's name, gender, age and date of birth, primary and secondary diagnoses, and physicians (Part 1 of a SOAP note)

Supervision physical therapist/assistant is near the patient and able to provide physical or verbal assistance as appropriate, and the likelihood of assistance being required is minimal

Supination defined differently for the upper and lower extremities; for the upper extremity, supination of the forearm occurs when the arm is stabilized and the forearm is rotated so that the palm of the hand faces anteriorly; for the lower extremity, supination of the foot occurs when the leg is stabilized and the foot is rotated about the oblique axis of the subtalar and other midfoot joints in the direction of plantarflexion, forefoot abduction, and inversion

Supine position in which a person lies on his or her back on a supporting surface

Surgical hand antisepsis antiseptic hand wash or antiseptic hand rub performed preoperatively by surgical personnel to eliminate transient, and reduce resident, hand flora. Antiseptic detergent preparations often have persistent antimicrobial activity

Symptoms subjective perceptions of patients that may be indicative of disease

Systems review brief or limited examination of (1) the anatomical and physiological status of the cardiovascular/pulmonary, integumentary, musculoskeletal, and neuromuscular systems and (2) the communication ability, affect, cognition, language, and learning style of the patient

Systolic pressure measurement of pressure exerted by blood against arterial walls when the heart is contracting

T

Tachycardia a very fast heart rate; greater than 100 bpm

Target heart rate heart rate that an individual should achieve during exercise for cardiovascular conditioning with respect to age and medical condition

Temperature provides information concerning basal metabolic state, potential presence of infection, and metabolic response to exercise

Tenodesis functional use of shortened muscles

Tests and measures examination methods to obtain objective data pertaining to a patient

Tilt-in-space wheelchair reclining wheelchair that has a fixed seat-to-back angle, even when reclined

Toe touch weight bearing (TTWB) the patient can rest the foot of the involved lower extremity on the ground for balance but not for weight bearing

Transitions the act of moving from one position or activity to another

Transmission-based precautions based on the concept of avoiding infection by limiting the potential for transmission of microorganisms, these are designed for the care of only specified patients: patients known, or suspected, to be infected by epidemiologically important pathogens, highly transmissible pathogens for which additional precautions, beyond standard precautions, are needed to interrupt transmission in healthcare settings

Transverse (horizontal) plane divides body into upper and lower portions

Tread horizontal dimension of a stair

Trophic physiological sequels to decreased circulation, such as loss of hair, dry or flaky skin, and muscle atrophy

U

Ulnar deviation when the wrist is moved such that the hand moves toward the midline of the body

Uniarticular muscles that cross only a single joint

United States Access Board (USAB) independent federal agency whose primary mission is accessibility for people with disabilities

Unsterile (nonsterile) any item or environment that has not been sterilized, has come into contact with an item that is no longer considered sterile, has entered a field that is not sterile, or has exceeded its shelf life

V

Valsalva maneuver closing of the glottis during heavy exertion resulting in increased intra-thoracic and intra-abdominal pressure, which can cause a rapid increase in blood pressure

Vectorborne transmission occurs when vectors such as mosquitoes, flies, rats, and other vermin transmit microorganisms

Verbal cues auditory cues to patients that are provided during activity performance

Visual analog scale a straight horizontal line with 0 at the left side (representing a complete absence of pain) and 10 at the right side (representing the worst pain a patient can imagine)

W

Waterless antiseptic agent does not require use of exogenous water; after application, the hands are rubbed together until the agent has dried

Weight bearing the amount of weight that can be borne on a lower extremity during standing or ambulation

Weight bearing as tolerated (WBAT) the patient determines the amount of weight bearing that will occur on the involved lower extremity

Wheel locks devices that stabilize the wheels of a wheelchair after the wheelchair has been stopped

Y

Yellow flag risk factors indicating to proceed with caution because of the potential for adverse effects

Glossary of Abbreviations

A

A Assessment
AAROM Active-assisted range of motion
AFO Ankle foot orthosis
ALS Amyotrophic lateral sclerosis
AROM Active range of motion
ATNR Asymmetric tonic neck reflex

B

B or bil Bilateral
B/C Because
B/S Bedside
BE Below elbow
BID or bid Twice a day
BK Below knee
BM Bowel movement
BOS Base of support
BP Blood pressure
bpm Beats per minute
BR Bedrest

C

c̄ With
C&S Culture and sensitivity
c/o Complains of
CA Cancer
CABG Coronary artery bypass graft
CAD Coronary artery disease
CAT Computerized axial tomography
CBC Complete blood cell count
CC or C/C Chief complaint
CG Contact guard
CHF Congestive heart failure
CNS Central nervous system
Cont. or cont'd Continue; continued
COLD Chronic obstructive lung disease
COPD Chronic obstructive pulmonary disease
COTA Certified occupational therapy assistant
CPM or cpm Continuous passive motion
CPR Cardiopulmonary resuscitation
CPT Chest physical therapy
CS Close supervision

D

D/C Discontinue or discharge
DJD Degenerative joint disease
DM Diabetes mellitus
DME Durable medical equipment
DNR Do not resuscitate
DO Doctor of osteopathy
DOB Date of birth
DOE Dyspnea on exertion
DPT Doctor of Physical Therapy
DTR Deep tendon reflex
DVT Deep vein thrombosis
Dx or dx Diagnosis

E

ECF Extended care facility
ECG or EKG Electrocardiogram
EEG Electroencephalogram
EENT Ear, eyes, nose, throat
EMG Electromyogram
eval Evaluation
ex Exercise
ext. Extension; external
ext rot or ER External (lateral) rotation
e-stim Electrical stimulation

F

F Fair (as a muscle grade)
FBS Fasting blood sugar
FES Functional electrical stimulation
FEV Forced expiratory volume
FH Family history
fl or flex Flexion
FRC Functional residual capacity
FUO Fever, unknown origin

FVC Forced vital capacity
F/U Follow-up
FWB Full weight bearing
Fx Fracture; function

G

G Good (as a muscle grade)
GCS Glasgow Coma Scale
GI Gastrointestinal
G-tube Gastrointestinal tube
GSW Gunshot wound
GYN Gynecology

H

H or hr. Hour
H&P History and physical
H/O or h/o History of
HA or H/A Headache
HEENT Head, ear, eye, nose, throat
HEP Home exercise program
HHA Home health aide
HNP Herniated nucleus pulposus
HOB Head of bed
HR Heart rate
HTN Hypertension
hs At bedtime
ht. Height
Hx or hx History

I

I or indep Independent
I&O or IO Intake and output
ICU Intensive care unit
Imp. Impression
inf Inferior
int rot or IR Internal (medial) rotation
IP Interphalangeal joint
IV Intravenous

J

J-tube Jejunsotomy tube

K

KAFO Knee-ankle-foot orthosis

L

L or [L] Left
Lat Lateral
LBBB Left bundle branch block
LBP Low back pain
LBQC Large-base quad cane
LE Lower extremity
Lig Ligament
LLL Left lower lobe
LLQ Left lower quadrant
LMN Lower motor neuron
LOB Loss of balance
LOC Loss of consciousness; level of consciousness
LOS Length of stay
LPN Licensed practical nurse
lat rot or LR Lateral (external) rotation
LTG Long-term goal
LTC Long-term care
LUL Left upper lobe
LUQ Left upper quadrant
LVH Left ventricular hypertrophy

M

Max Maximum; maximal
MCA Middle cerebral artery
MCP Metacarpal phalangeal joint
MD Medical doctor
MED Minimal erythemal dose
med rot or MR Medial (internal) rotation
Meds. Medications
min Minimum; minimal
MMT Manual muscle test
mod Moderate
MRI Magnetic resonance imaging
MS Multiple sclerosis
MVA Motor vehicle accident
mvt Movement

N

N Normal (as a muscle grade)
N/A Not applicable
NBCQ Narrow-base quad cane
NDT Neurodevelopmental treatment
neg. Negative

NG Nasogastric

NICU Neonatal intensive care unit

nn Nerve

NO or n/o Not observed

noc Night; at night

NPO or npo Nothing by mouth

NSR Normal sinus rhythm

N/T Not tested

NWB Non–weight bearing

O

O Objective

OA Osteoarthritis

OB Obstetrics

OBS Organic brain syndrome

od Once daily

OOB Out of bed

O.P. Out patient

O.R. or OR Operating room

ORIF Open reduction internal fixation

OT or OTR Occupational therapy; occupational therapist

P

p̄ After

P Poor (as a muscle grade)

P Plan

P.A. Physician's assistant

PA Posterior/anterior

pc After meals

PCA Posterior cerebral artery

PE Pulmonary embolus

per By/through

PERRLA Pupils equal, round, reactive to light, and accommodation

PET Positron emission tomography

PF Plantar flexion

PH Past history

PIP Proximal interphalangeal joint

PMH Past medical history

PNF Proprioceptive Neuromuscular Facilitation

PNI Peripheral nerve injury

PO Per oral (by mouth)

POMR Problem-oriented medical record

pos. Positive

post Posterior

post op Postoperative

PRE Progressive resistive exercise

pre op Before surgery

prn As often as necessary

PROM Passive range of motion

prox Proximal

Pt Patient

PT Physical therapy; physical therapist

PTA Physical therapist assistant; prior to admission

PVD Peripheral vascular disease

PWB Partial weight bearing

Q

q Every

qd Every day

qh Every hour

qid Four times a day

qn Every night

quads Quadriceps

R

R or [R] Right

RA Rheumatoid arthritis

RBBB Right bundle branch block

re Concerning; about

RBC Red blood cell

R.D. Registered dietician

Rehab Rehabilitation

reps Repetitions

resp Respiratory; respiration

RLL Right lower lobe

RLQ Right lower quadrant

RML Right middle lobe

RN Registered nurse

R/O or r/o Rule out

ROM Range of motion

ROS Review of systems

RR Respiratory rate

RROM Resistive range of motion

R.T. Respiratory therapy; respiratory therapist

R/T Related to

RUQ Right upper quadrant

Rx Prescription; treatment; orders; intervention; therapy

S

S Supervision

s̄ Without

S Subjective

SAQ Short arc quads

SBA Stand by assist

SBQC Small-base quad cane

SCI Spinal cord injury

SED Suberythemal dose

SLE Systemic lupus erythematosus

SLP Speech language pathologist

sig Significant

SLR Straight leg raise

SNF Skilled nursing facility

SOAP Subjective, objective, assessment, plan

S/O Standing order

SOB Short of breath

SOS Step over step

s/p Status post

stat Immediately; at once

STG Short-term goal

STNR Symmetrical tonic neck reflex

sup Superior

surg Surgical; surgery

sx Symptoms

T

T Trace (as a muscle grade)

TBA To be assessed

TBI Traumatic brain injury

TDWB Touch down weight bearing

temp Temperature

TENS Transcutaneous electrical nerve stimulator

ther. ex Therapeutic exercise

THR Total hip replacement

TIA Transient ischemic attack

tid Three times a day

TKA Total knee arthroplasty

TKR Total knee replacement

TMJ Temporomandibular joint

TNR Tonic neck reflex

t.o. Telephone order

T/O Throughout

TPR Temperature, pulse, and respiration

TTWB Toe touch weight bearing

Tx Treatment; traction

U

UA Urine analysis

UE Upper extremity

U/L Unilateral

UMN Upper motor neuron

URI Upper respiratory infection

US Ultrasound

UTI Urinary tract infection

UV Ultraviolet

V

VAS Visual analog scale

VC Vital capacity; verbal cues

v.o., VO or V/O Verbal orders

vol. Volume

v.s. or VS Vital signs

Vtach Ventricular tachycardia

W

WB Weight bearing

WBAT Weight bearing as tolerated

WBQC Wide-base quad cane

w/c Wheelchair

WBC White blood cell

wk. Week

WFL Within functional limits

WNL Within normal limits

wt. Weight

X

x Times

Y

y/o or y.o. Years old

yr. Year

Z

Z Zero (as a muscle grade)

Index

I

J

K

L

M

N

O

P

U

V

W

Y